Nunn's
Applied Respiratory Physiology

SEVENTH EDITION

Andrew B Lumb MB BS FRCA
Consultant Anaesthetist, St James's University Hospital; Senior Clinical Lecturer in Anaesthesia,
University of Leeds, Leeds, UK

Foreword by
Ronald G Pearl MD PhD
Dr Richard K and Erika N Richards Professor and Chairman, Department of Anesthesia, Stanford University School of
Medicine, Stanford, CA, USA

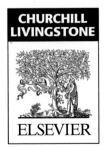

CHURCHILL LIVINGSTONE

ELSEVIER

EDINBURGH   LONDON   NEW YORK   OXFORD   PHILADELPHIA   ST LOUIS   SYDNEY   TORONTO 2010

CHURCHILL LIVINGSTONE
ELSEVIER

© 2010 Elsevier Ltd. All rights reserved

First edition 1969
Second edition 1977
Third edition 1987
Fourth edition 1993
Fifth edition 1999
Sixth edition 2005
Seventh edition 2010
  Reprinted 2011 (twice)

ISBN 978 0 7020 2996 7

British Library Cataloguing-in-Publication Data
A catalogue record for this book is available from the British Library

Library of Congress Cataloging-in-Publication Data
A catalog record for this book is available from the Library of Congress

ELSEVIER your source for books, journals and multimedia in the health sciences

www.elsevierhealth.com

Working together to grow libraries in developing countries

www.elsevier.com | www.bookaid.org | www.sabre.org

 ELSEVIER   BOOK AID International   Sabre Foundation

The Publisher's policy is to use **paper manufactured from sustainable forests**

Printed in China

Contents

Foreword

It is a great honor to write the foreword for the seventh edition of *Nunn's Applied Respiratory Physiology*. Since publication of the first edition in 1969, *Nunn's Applied Respiratory Physiology* has been the classic textbook on this critical subject. The challenge for any textbook on respiratory physiology has been to present the information in a manner which provides for the changing needs of the reader throughout his or her career. The beginning student often learns respiratory physiology from the mathematical analysis of gas exchange; the more advanced student may be interested in the underlying cellular and molecular mechanisms; and the clinician needs to understand the impact of altered respiratory physiology on specific disease states. The ideal textbook therefore has the daunting challenge of providing a comprehensive but easily understood approach for all three readers. Despite the rapid evolution of knowledge in this field, Nunn's *Applied Respiratory Physiology* has accomplished this task throughout the past four decades. In this age of multi-authored contributions, it is a tribute to Andrew Lumb that he has been the sole author for the past three editions (with the exception of the first chapter on the atmosphere which continues to be written by Dr. Nunn). The cohesion inherent in a single-authored textbook allows for internal consistency so that interrelated concepts can be readily appreciated by the reader. In addition, a single-authored textbook avoids duplication of material, so that a vast topic is comprehensively covered in just over 500 pages.

This seventh edition maintains the tradition of presenting respiratory physiology in a manner which can be readily understood by students, clinicians and investigators. The book continues the three part approach which was first adopted in the fifth edition. The first section on basic principles covers anatomy, mechanics, control of breathing, ventilation, circulation, ventilation-perfusion matching, diffusion, carbon dioxide, oxygen, and non-respiratory functions of the lung. Although the basic concepts have not changed, the content has been updated with recent advances such as alternative models to explain lung recoil and expanded sections on tissue oxygen and on airway lining fluid and cilial activity. The second section on applied physiology discusses the effects of pregnancy, exercise, sleep, altitude, pressure, drowning, smoking, anesthesia, hypocapnia, hypercarbia, hypoxia, hyperoxia, and anemia. The third part on physiology of pulmonary disease discusses specific clinical disorders (ventilatory failure, airways disease, pulmonary vascular disease, parenchymal lung disease, acute lung injury), ventilatory support, and pulmonary surgery. These chapters have been extensively updated as new information has entered the literature in areas such as pulmonary hypertension and management of patients with acute respiratory failure. Valuable changes which were made in the last edition have been continued, including double column pages, color figures, and the key points section of each chapter.

For more than four decades, *Nunn's Applied Respiratory Physiology* has been the standard text for understanding this challenging but critical subject. I congratulate Dr. Lumb on continuing this tradition with a superb seventh edition which deserves its place on the bookshelves of students, researchers, and clinicians interested in understanding normal respiratory physiology and in treating patients with respiratory disorders.

Ronald G Pearl
Stanford
2010

Preface to the seventh edition

Over the past 41 years *Nunn's Applied Respiratory Physiology* has developed into a renowned textbook on respiration, providing both physiologists and clinicians with a unique fusion of underlying principles and their applications. With Dr John Nunn's retirement in 1991 a new author was required, and, as Dr Nunn's final research fellow in the Clinical Research Centre in Harrow, I was honoured to be chosen as his successor. As a practising clinician with a fascination for physiology and an interest in medical education, the seventh edition has again focussed on combining a clear, logical and comprehensive account of basic respiratory physiology with a wide range of applications, both physiological and clinical. This approach acknowledges the popularity of the book among doctors from many medical specialties and will hopefully provide readers with a scientific background with an even greater insight into the applications of respiratory physiology. Clinical chapters in Part 3 of the book are not intended to be comprehensive reviews of the pulmonary diseases considered, but in each case they provide a detailed description of the physiological changes that occur, accompanied by a brief account of the clinical features and treatment of the disease.

Key references are identified by an asterisk in the reference list following each chapter. These references are highlighted because they either provide outstanding recent reviews of their subject or describe research that has had a major impact on the topic under consideration.

Advances in respiratory physiology since the last edition are too numerous to mention individually. Clarification of some fundamental concepts has been provided, e.g. the definitions of oxygen saturation and haemoglobin oxygen carrying capacity (Hufners constant). Other new topics include the contribution of airway lining fluid to lung defence mechanisms, the biphasic nature of hypoxic pulmonary vasoconstriction, and a new look at tissue oxygen diffusion patterns based on work done by Krogh more than 100 years ago that identifies tissue regions where hypoxia is most likely to occur, referred to as the 'lethal corner'.

New topics for Part 3 of the seventh edition include pleural diseases and lung cancer. Pneumothorax and pleural effusions occur in many different clinical specialties, and the physiology and pathophysiology of the pleural space is now included in Chapter 30. Whilst many, sometimes rare, lung diseases have been covered in Part 3 for years, lung cancer has been a significant omission. Lung cancer remains common, is mostly preventable by avoiding tobacco smoke and environmental radon, and, relative to many other cancers, remains difficult to treat due to its usually late presentation. A detailed description of how lung cancer develops from a molecular level to its clinical presentation is now included in Chapter 30, along with a brief account of its treatment.

Pulmonary surgery (Chapter 33) is new for the seventh edition. Although surgery of the lungs and pleura is only performed in specialised hospitals, the prevalence of smoking worldwide means that these operations, a majority of which are for cancer treatment, will remain common for some decades yet. Thoracic surgery procedures are also evolving, with less invasive techniques for accessing the lungs and pleura slowly replacing the trauma of a thoracotomy. Safe and successful use of these techniques relies on all staff involved having a thorough understanding of the physiological changes that occur.

I wish to personally thank the many people who have helped with the preparation of the book, including the numerous colleagues who have encouraged and assisted my acquisition of knowledge in subjects not so close to my own areas of expertise. I am indebted to Professor Pearl for his kind words in the Foreword, and would like to thank Professor Hedenstierna for providing the excellent CT scans in Figure 33.3. I remain especially indebted to Dr Nunn for his continued support of the book and its author, and would like to thank him for once again providing an excellent Chapter 1 on the origins of Earth's atmosphere. His statement that 'Fossil fuels were buried over the course of 350 million years, and probably all that is recoverable will be burned in 300' is thought provoking. Last, but by no means least, I would like to thank Lorraine, Emma and Jenny for again tolerating a preoccupied and reclusive husband/father for so long. Jenny, when aged 5, often enquired about my activities in the study, until one evening she nicely summarised my years of work by confidently informing me that 'if you don't breathe, you die'. So what were the other 527 pages about?

Andrew Lumb
Leeds 2010

PART 1

Basic principles

PART 1

Basic principles

Chapter 1

The atmosphere

John F Nunn

KEY POINTS

- The mass of the Earth and its distance from the sun provide optimal conditions of gravity and temperature for long-term liquid surface water and the retention in its atmosphere of oxygen, nitrogen and carbon dioxide.
- Primitive life-forms generated energy by photosynthetic reactions, producing oxygen, and so facilitating the development of an oxygen-containing atmosphere and aerobic organisms.
- Carbon dioxide was initially the main component of the Earth's atmosphere, but by 300 million years ago rock weathering and photosynthesis had reduced its concentration to current low levels.
- There is now an acceptance that human activity is causing an increase in atmospheric carbon dioxide, unprecedented in the last 40 million years.

The atmosphere of Earth is radically different from that of any other planet in the solar system (Table 1.1) and may well be rare on planets of other stars in the universe as a whole. The unique character of our atmosphere is because of two main reasons. First, temperature has permitted the existence of liquid surface water for at least 3800 million years (Ma), and this has resulted in weathering of silicate rocks, reducing the concentration of carbon dioxide far below the levels still pertaining in the rocky planets Venus and Mars. Secondly, the existence of liquid surface water enabled living organisms to appear at a very early stage: life forms then evolved to undertake oxygenic photosynthesis. When oxygen sinks were saturated, oxygen appeared in the atmosphere and some organisms began to utilise highly efficient oxidative metabolic pathways. An atmosphere containing oxygen is in inorganic chemical disequilibrium, and is an indication of the existence of life.

EVOLUTION OF THE ATMOSPHERE

FORMATION OF THE EARTH AND THE PRE–BIOTIC ATMOSPHERE

The earth was formed by a relatively short lived, but intense, gravitational accretion of rather large planetesimals, orbiting the newly formed sun some 4560 Ma ago. The kinetic energy of the impacting bodies was sufficient to raise the temperature to a few thousand degrees Celsius. This would have melted the entire Earth, resulting in loss of the primary atmosphere.

Earth cooled rapidly by radiation when the initial bombardment abated, and the very high temperature (Hadean) phase is not thought to have lasted longer than a few hundred Ma. The crust solidified, but massive outgassing continued, resulting in an atmosphere mainly comprising carbon dioxide and steam (Table 1.2) as probably occurred on Venus and Mars.[1,2] In the case of Earth, the water vapour condensed to surface water, and there is good evidence that oceans existed about 3800 Ma ago and perhaps even earlier.[3] Once Earth's crust was cool, and surface water was in existence, it was possible for comets and meteorites to leave a secondary veneer of their contents, including water and a wide range of organic compounds.[4]

Important physico-chemical changes occurred in the early secondary atmosphere. Helium and

DOI: 10.1016/B978-0-7020-2996-7.00001-5

Table 1.1 Composition of the atmosphere of Earth and the nearer planets

PLANET	ATMOSPHERE			
Mercury	Extremely tenuous			
Venus	Carbon dioxide	96.5%	+ Traces: Argon, Helium, Neon,	
	Nitrogen	3.5%	Krypton (all < 20 ppmv)	
Earth	Nitrogen	78.08%	Water vapour – variable	
	Oxygen	20.95%	Neon	18.2 ppmv
	Argon	0.93%	Helium	5.2 ppmv
	Carbon dioxide	0.039%	Methane	1.8 ppmv
Mars	Carbon dioxide	95.3%	Oxygen	0.13 %
	Nitrogen	2.7%	Carbon monoxide	0.27 %
	Argon	1.6%	+ traces: Neon, Krypton, Xenon	
Jupiter	Hydrogen	89%	Methane	1750 ppmv
	Helium	11%	+ Traces: Ammonia, Water vapour etc.	
Saturn	Hydrogen	94%	Methane	4500 ppmv
	Helium	6%	+ Traces: Ethylene, Phosphine	

ppmv, parts per million volume.
Earth's data for carbon dioxide has been updated (see text).
(Planetary data are from Taylor,[1] reproduced from Nunn[2] by permission of the Geologists' Association.)

Table 1.2 Average composition of gas evolved from Hawaiian volcanoes

CONSTITUENT	PERCENT
Water vapour	70.75
Carbon dioxide	14.07
Sulphur dioxide	6.40
Nitrogen	5.45
Sulphur trioxide	1.92
Carbon monoxide	0.40
Hydrogen	0.33
Argon	0.18
Sulphur	0.10
Chlorine	0.05

(Data are from reference 5, reproduced from reference 2 by permission of the Geologists' Association.)

hydrogen tended to be lost from the Earth's gravitational field. Ammonia dissociated to nitrogen and hydrogen, the former retained and the latter lost from the atmosphere. Some carbon dioxide might have been reduced by hydrogen to form traces of methane, but very large quantities slowly reacted with surface silicates to become trapped as carbonates, while forming silica (weathering). Traces of water vapour underwent photodissociation to hydrogen and oxygen. However, oxygen from this source was present in only minimal quantities, and the early atmosphere is no longer thought to have been as strongly reducing as was formerly believed.[6]

The initial very high partial pressure of carbon dioxide, and probably some methane, would have provided a powerful greenhouse effect to offset the early minimal weak solar radiation, which was some 30% less than today (Figure 1.1). However, the Sun commenced its main sequence of thermonuclear fusion of hydrogen to helium about 3000 Ma ago. Since then solar radiation has been increasing steadily as the Sun proceeds remorselessly towards becoming a red giant, which will ultimately envelop the inner planets. It is fortunate that increasing solar radiation has been approximately offset by a diminishing greenhouse effect, due mainly to decreasing levels of carbon dioxide (see below). As a result, Earth's temperature has remained relatively stable, permitting the existence of surface water for the last 3800 Ma.

SIGNIFICANCE OF MASS OF EARTH AND DISTANCE FROM SUN

Small bodies, such as Mercury and most of the planets' satellites, have a gravitational field which is too weak for the retention of any significant

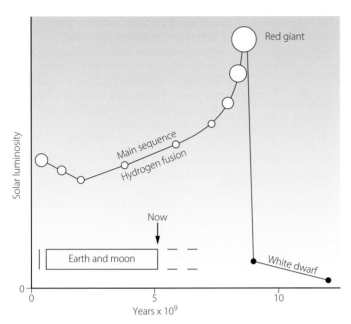

Fig. 1.1 Solar luminosity plotted against the age of the Sun, with the open circles giving a qualitative impression of the diameter of the Sun. Superimposed is an indication of the life of the Earth and Moon, which is now about half way through the main sequence of the Sun deriving its energy from hydrogen fusion to helium. The times can only be very approximate. (After reference 7 with kind permission of Springer Link and Business Media.)

atmosphere (Figure 1.2). The gas-giants (Jupiter, Saturn, Uranus and Neptune) have a gravitational field which is sufficiently strong to retain all gases, including helium and hydrogen, thereby ensuring the retention of a reducing atmosphere. The gravitational field of the Earth is intermediate, resulting in a differential retention of the heavier gases (oxygen, carbon dioxide and nitrogen), while permitting the escape of hydrogen and helium. This is essential for the development of an oxidising atmosphere and life as we know it. Water vapour (molecular weight only 18) would be lost from the atmosphere were it not for the cold trap at the tropopause.

Surface temperature of a planetary body is crucial for the existence of liquid water, which is essential for life and therefore the composition of our atmosphere. To a first approximation, temperature is dependent on the distance of a planet from the Sun, and the intensity of solar radiation (Figure 1.2). The major secondary factor is the greenhouse effect of any atmosphere which the planet may possess. Mercury and Venus have surface temperatures far above the boiling point of water. All planets (and their satellites) which are further away from the Sun than Earth have a surface temperature too cold for

liquid water to exist today. However, there is now evidence that Mars had liquid surface water in the past,[8] now present only as ice.[9]

Earth is the only planet in the solar system which has both a mass permitting retention of an oxidising atmosphere, and a distance from the Sun at which the temperature permits liquid water to exist on its surface. It is difficult to see how there could be life as we know it anywhere in the solar system outside the small parallelogram in Figure 1.2. However, an environment similar to that of the earth may well exist on some planets of the 10^{22} other sun-like stars in the universe.

ORIGIN OF LIFE AND THE DEVELOPMENT OF PHOTOSYNTHESIS

Amino acids and a wide range of organic compounds are found in a type of meteorite known as carbonaceous chondrites.[4] Therefore, whether or not such compounds were actually synthesised on the early Earth, as Stanley Miller had proposed,[6] it is highly likely that a wide range of organic compounds were available on the pre-biotic Earth when liquid oceans were formed.

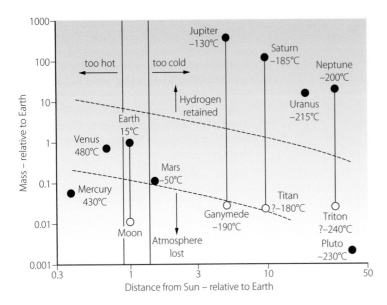

Fig. 1.2 The planets and some of their larger satellites, plotted according to distance from the Sun (abscissa), and mass (ordinate), both scales being logarithmic and relative to Earth. Mean surface temperatures are shown. Potential for life as we know it exists only within the parallelogram surrounding the Earth.

It is less easy to explain the next stage in the evolution of life. An essential feature of all life is the synthesis of proteins using a ribonucleic acid (RNA) template, usually transcribed from the genetic code carried on deoxyribonucleic acid (DNA). There would appear to have been a classical 'chicken and egg' situation. Useful proteins could not be formed without the appropriate sequences in RNA or DNA: RNA and DNA could not be polymerised without appropriate enzymes which are normally proteins. Nevertheless, life did appear, perhaps in the first instance with the genetic code carried only on RNA, or even the much simpler peptide nucleic acid (PNA).[10]

An essential requirement for life is the availability of bio-usable forms of energy. The forms of available energy and their location at the dawn of life remain a mystery. However, one cannot ignore the possibility of hydrothermal vents, such as the black smokers along the mid-ocean ridges at great depths, which still support very simple life forms on the basis of chemoautotrophy. They are totally independent of sunlight, and exploit the profound chemical disequilibrium between the emerging hot, reducing and acid water, containing hydrogen sulphide, methane, ammonia, phosphorus and a range of metals, and the surrounding sea water.[11] It is likely that there have been hydrothermal vents

on Earth for as long as surface water has coexisted with volcanic activity. Chemoautothrophs might, therefore, have appeared as early as 3800 Ma ago.

Hydrothermal vents provide an extremely constrained and hazardous environment for life, dependent on the continued existence of the energy supply. A much more attractive alternative was to utilise the limitless availability of energy in the form of solar visible light. The most familiar of such reactions is the oxygenic photosynthesis of glucose summarised as follows:

$$6CO_2 + 6H_2O + energy = C_6H_{12}O_6 + 6O_2$$

The biochemical adaptation from thermal detection in hydrothermal vents to photosynthesis does not seem to have been insuperable,[12] and it was thought that photosynthesising cyanobacteria (blue-green algae) may have existed 2700 Ma ago.[13] However, it has recently been suggested that this crucial development may have occurred later, closer to 2400 Ma ago when oxygen first appeared in the atmosphere.[14] At a later date, cyanobacteria underwent symbiotic incorporation into the cells of certain eukaryotes to become chloroplasts, which then conferred the biochemical benefits of photosynthesis on their hosts, which include all plants.

THE APPEARANCE OF OXYGEN IN THE ATMOSPHERE

Oxygenic photosynthesis releases oxygen, apparently as a waste product. Initially it accumulated in the surface waters of the oceans, where it oxidised soluble ferrous iron (Fe^{2+}), leached from basalt, which was then deposited as insoluble ferric iron oxide (Fe^{3+}) in the vast so-called banded iron formations. This process prevented concentrations of oxygen in the atmosphere reaching 10^{-5} bar until about 2320 Ma ago.[15] After the atmosphere attained a higher but critical level of oxygen about 1800 Ma ago, banded iron formations seldom appeared, and iron was thereafter deposited in red (ferric) beds.[2]

Oxygen continued to accumulate in the oceans and atmosphere, probably reaching a peak of 25–35% of an atmosphere 300 Ma ago[16] (Figure 1.3). It then decreased to about 14%, contributing to the end-Permian mass extinction at the end of the Palaeozoic Era, about 250 Ma ago.[2] Thereafter it rose slightly above the present atmospheric level for about 100 Ma.

BIOLOGICAL CONSEQUENCES OF AN OXIDISING ENVIRONMENT

It seems likely that the appearance of molecular oxygen in their environment would have been unwelcome to anaerobic organisms. Chapter 26 describes the toxicity of oxygen and its derived free radicals, against which primitive anaerobes would probably have had no defences. Three lines of response can be identified. Some anaerobes sought an anaerobic micro-environment in which to remain and survive. Others developed defences in depth against oxygen and its derived reactive species (page 385). The best response was the development of aerobic metabolism, which gave enormous energetic advantages over organisms relying on anaerobic metabolism (page 200). This required the symbiotic incorporation of purple bacteria which became mitochondria, and the increased availability of biological energy was essential for the evolution of all forms of life more complex than micro-organisms.

Photosynthesis and aerobic metabolism eventually established a cycle of energy exchange between plants and animals, with its ultimate energy input in the form of solar visible light, which was interrupted only under exceptional circumstances. Such circumstances included major meteor strikes and exceptional volcanic activity, both of which can throw vast

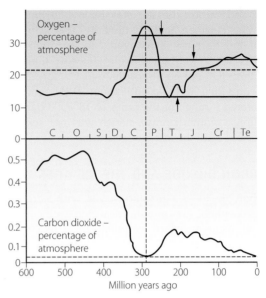

Fig. 1.3 Long-term changes in oxygen and carbon dioxide concentrations during the last 600 Ma. Broken horizontal lines show present atmospheric levels. The vertical broken line shows the Carboniferous/Permian boundary. The continuous horizontal lines with arrows show some oxygen limits suggested by the geological record of forest fires.[2] Geological periods shown by their capital letters are: Cambrian, Ordovician, Silurian, Devonian, Carboniferous and Permian (Palaeozoic Era), and Triassic, Jurassic, Cretaceous (Mesozoic Era) and Tertiary. Recent research suggests levels of carbon dioxide may be slightly less than shown, but the nature of the changes is not in doubt. (From Nunn,[2] reproduced by permission of the Geologists' Association).

quantities of persistent dust into the atmosphere and cause extinctions by blocking photosynthesis.

CHANGES IN CARBON DIOXIDE LEVELS

After the major outgassing phase of the newly formed earth, the concentration of carbon dioxide in the atmosphere probably exceeded 90% of an atmosphere.[17] It declined rapidly, due to weathering ($CO_2 + CaSiO_3 \rightarrow SiO_2 + CaCO_3$) and photosynthesis, reaching about 0.5% at the time of the beginning of the overt fossil record, the Palaeozoic Era, from 570 Ma ago (Figure 1.3). A secondary major decline to near the present atmospheric level occurred during the Carboniferous Period, when the coal-forming forests involved photosynthesis and carbon burial on a massive scale. A sharp increase occurred at the end of the Permian Period (the last Period of the Palaeozoic Era) about 250 Ma ago, and carbon dioxide may have contributed to the end-Permian mass extinction. This coincided with the decrease in oxygen concentration mentioned above. Carbon dioxide concentrations rose to about 0.2% of an atmosphere just before 200 Ma ago, and then declined until about 20 Ma ago, when it entered a range of the order of 180–300 parts per million, volume (ppmv), which was not seriously exceeded until the last few decades.[18]

CARBON DIOXIDE AND THE ICE AGES

Carbon dioxide is a greenhouse gas, with a doubling of atmospheric concentration causing an increase in global average surface temperature '… likely to be in the range 2 to 4.5°C … values substantially higher than 4.5°C cannot be excluded.'[19] DeConto cites the carbon dioxide threshold for Antarctic glaciation as 750 ppmv and for the northern hemisphere as 280 ppmv.[18] However, there is also a periodicity in solar insolation (Milankovitch cycles) which initiates glacial and interglacial cycles. For the last 500 ka, the dominant cycle has been the degree of ellipticity of the Earth's orbit, with a periodicity of about 100 ka,

and its effect is very clear in the mean global temperature record for the last 420 ka derived from Antarctic ice cores (Figure 1.4).[20]

Figure 1.4 also shows a remarkably close correlation between temperature and the atmospheric concentration of carbon dioxide. Detailed analysis of time relations shows that the start of end-glacial warming usually preceded the start of the increase in carbon dioxide by a few thousand years. The initial warming released carbon dioxide from stores and then the increased carbon dioxide concentration provided powerful positive feed-back to temperature. The resultant warming is far greater than can be accounted for simply by the change in insolation.

Casual inspection of Figure 1.4 suggests that the next glacial period is overdue. However, it appears that the rhythmic changes in global mean temperature shown for the last 420 ka will not continue, as we now enter a long phase when the Earth's orbit will remain almost circular. The 100 ka cycle will be in virtual abeyance for about 50 ka, during which there will be a prolonged interglacial.[22] However, it is highly unlikely that mean global temperature will

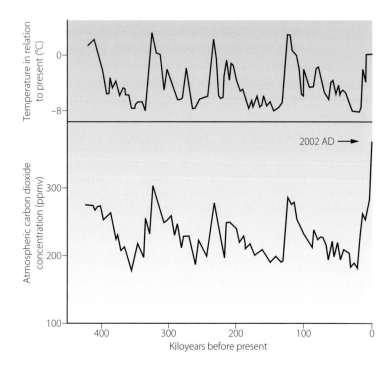

Fig. 1.4 General trends for temperature and atmospheric carbon dioxide concentration, obtained from ice cores from Vostok, Antarctica, for the last 420 000 years. In 2009 the atmospheric carbon dioxide concentration is expected to reach 387 ppmv (see Table 1.3). (Data from Petit et al.[20] and reproduced in part from reference 21, with the permission of the Editor of the Optimum Population Trust Journal.)

remain constant, due to the current increase in the atmospheric carbon dioxide concentration, unprecedented in the last 20 Ma.

RECENT CHANGES IN CARBON DIOXIDE LEVELS

Atmospheric carbon dioxide remained close to 280 ppmv from the beginning of the current interglacial until the start of the industrial revolution (AD 1750). In the next 200 years it increased to 310 ppmv which averaged 0.155 ppmv/yr (Table 1.3). The annual rate of increase rose progressively and, from AD 2000 to 2009, reached 1.89 ppmv/yr, which is nearly 200 times the rate during the rapid rewarming after the last glacial period (Figure 1.4).

On this basis, extrapolation of trends from AD 1750 to the present suggests that the concentration might reach 1000 ppmv by the year AD 2100. This prediction is similar to computed predictions based on analysis of the many primary factors governing atmospheric CO_2 concentrations.[23] Thus we may expect to reach the highest concentration since 24 Ma ago, and above the threshold for Antarctic glaciations.[18] Whether the rate of change continues its present exponential course is critically dependent on the continued efficiency of the global carbon sinks, and attempts to control emissions with all its current political uncertainty. The only certain limitation on emissions would seem to be exhaustion of the world's fossil fuels. Global warming may have disturbing short term effects on ocean currents, particularly a weakening of the north Atlantic conveyor (including the Gulf Stream).[24] This could result in a substantial cooling of north-western Europe.

Table 1.3 Recent changes in atmospheric carbon dioxide concentrations

DATE	ATMOSPHERIC CO_2 MASS IN Gt	ppmv	RATE OF CHANGE ppmv PER YEAR
18 ka ago	420	200	
10 ka ago	588	280	0.01
1750 AD	588	280	0
1950 AD	651	310	0.15
2000 AD	777	370	1.20
2009 AD	813	387	1.89

Gt, gigatonne; ka, thousand years; ppmv, parts per million, volume. Data are from various sources. (Reproduced from Nunn[2] by permission of the Geologists' Association) and most recently from Mauna Loa directly.

THE GREENHOUSE EFFECT

The balance of heat gain from solar radiation is the difference between incoming radiation, mainly in the visible wave lengths, and outgoing radiation which is largely infra-red. The latter is partially trapped in the troposphere, mainly by water vapour (60%) and carbon dioxide (25%). Atmospheric water vapour concentration increases with rising global temperature and therefore provides positive feed-back to global warming. It is estimated that the present greenhouse effect raises the mean surface temperature of the Earth by some 30°C. Carbon dioxide makes a major contribution to the very high surface temperature of Venus (480°C), hotter than Mercury but further from the Sun.

OTHER GREENHOUSE GASES

There are no infra-red absorption bands for water vapour and carbon dioxide between 7 and 13 μm wavelength, and heat loss in this band is considerable. It follows that any gas or vapour with strong infra-red absorption in this range will have a disproportionate greenhouse effect. Such a gas could be considered not so much as thickening the panes in the greenhouse as replacing a missing pane.

After water and carbon dioxide, the most important greenhouse gases are ozone (8% of total effect) and methane (3% of total effect) which is present in the atmosphere at a concentration of only 2 ppmv, but rapidly increasing: it absorbs infra-red some 25 times as effectively as carbon dioxide. Dissolved methane is currently escaping from lakes in the melting tundra, but of greater concern is the vast quantity of buried methane held at high pressure and low temperature in cages of water molecules, known as hydrates or clathrates. Massive escape from hydrates is thought to have been a major factor in the Palaeocene/Eocene Thermal Maximum, 55 Ma before present, with temperature rises of 5–6°C.[25] Fortunately the half-life of methane in the atmosphere is only about six years. The chlorofluorocarbons (2% of total effect) absorb infra-red some 10 000 times as effectively as carbon dioxide, but present atmospheric concentrations are only of the order of 0.003 ppmv. However, with their long half life, they cannot be ignored. Nitrous oxide, mainly of biological origin, also makes a small contribution.

With Earth in an approximately circular orbit for the next 50 ka and solar gain likely to remain reasonably constant,[22] greenhouse gases are now the major factors governing global temperature. Carbon dioxide is rising rapidly towards the highest levels in the last 24 Ma and water vapour will increase with rising temperature. The mean global temperature is predicted to increase to within 90% confidence limits of 1.5–4.5°C by AD 2100. Temperature has already increased by 0.6°C in the last century, mostly since 1950.[26] Not the least serious consequence will be melting of polar ice which has the ultimate potential to raise sea level by 67 m. Sea level has been rising at about 1.8 mm/year since AD 1850 but, since 2004, there have been several reports of increased sea level rise up to 3.0 mm/year and predictions for 2100 indicate a total sea level rise for this century of 0.35–0.5 m.[27]

TURNOVER RATES OF ATMOSPHERIC GASES

Biological and geological turnover rates of carbon dioxide are quantitatively totally different.[2] Living organisms, the atmosphere and surface waters of the oceans contain about 2200 Gt (gigatonnes) of carbon. The annual exchange between photosynthesis and aerobic metabolism is approximately 100 Gt annually, with anthropogenic burning of fossil fuels and deforestation currently releasing about 8 Gt/year in 2002 as shown in Figure 1.5. The total release of carbon from burning and flaring of fossil fuels has now risen from 5 Gt/yr in 1983 to 7.7 Gt/yr in 2005, most of the increase since AD 2002 being attributable to China.

In stark contrast, geological stores (ocean depths, organic biomass and limestone) have a carbon content in excess of 30 000 000 Gt, but with an annual turnover (volcanoes, weathering, etc.) of less than 0.1 Gt per year. Thus, long term changes are governed by the geological stores, while very rapid atmospheric changes can occur as a result of anthropogenic activity. Fossil fuels were buried over the course of 350 Ma, and probably all that is recoverable will be burned in 300 years.

Atmospheric stores of oxygen are almost 600 times greater than those for carbon dioxide. If oxygen decreases at the same rate as the current increase in carbon dioxide, it would take 40 000

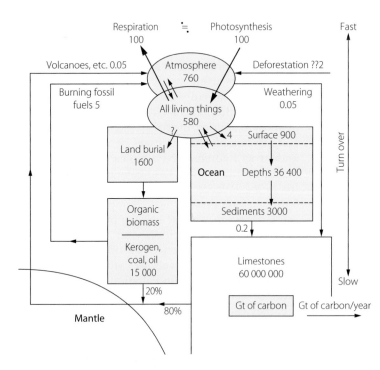

Fig. 1.5 Stores and turnover of carbon dioxide. Stores are in Gt (gigatonnes) and turnover in Gt per year. For recent increases in the burning of fossil fuels see text. (After reference 2, where sources are cited. Reproduced by permission of the Geologists' Association.)

years for sea level Po_2 to fall to the level which pertains in Denver today.

OXYGEN, OZONE AND ULTRAVIOLET SCREENING

In addition to its toxicity and potential for more efficient metabolism, oxygen had a profound effect on evolution by ultraviolet screening. Oxygen itself absorbs ultraviolet radiation to a certain extent, but ozone (O_3) is far more effective. It is formed in the stratosphere from oxygen which undergoes photo-dissociation producing free oxygen atoms. The oxygen atoms then rapidly combine with oxygen molecules to form ozone thus:

$$O_2 \rightleftharpoons 2O$$
$$\downarrow$$
$$O + O_2 \rightleftharpoons O_3$$

The absolute quantity is very small, being the equivalent of a layer of pure ozone only a few millimetres thick. A Dobson unit of ozone is defined as the equivalent of a layer of pure ozone 0.01 mm thick. About 10% of the total atmospheric ozone is in the troposphere, mainly as a pollutant. This also acts as an ultraviolet screen and may become relatively more important in the years to come.

Life evolved in water which provided adequate screening from ultraviolet radiation. The first colonisation of dry land by plants and animals was in the late Silurian Period about 400 Ma years ago, and it has been suggested that this coincided with oxygen and ozone reaching concentrations at which the degree of ultraviolet shielding first permitted organisms to leave the shelter of an aqueous environment.

Ozone is in a state of dynamic equilibrium in the stratosphere and its concentration varies markedly from year to year, in addition to displaying a pronounced annual cycle. Ozone can be removed by the action of many free radicals including chlorine and nitric oxide. Highly reactive chlorine radicals cannot normally pass through the troposphere to reach the stratosphere, but the situation was disturbed by the manufacture of chlorofluorocarbons (e.g. CF_2Cl_2) for use as propellants and refrigerants. These compounds are highly stable in the troposphere with a half-life of the order of 100 years. This permits their diffusion through the troposphere to reach the stratosphere, where they undergo photodissociation to release chlorine radicals, which then react with ozone as follows:

$$Cl + O_3 \rightarrow ClO + O_2$$
$$\uparrow \qquad\qquad \downarrow$$
$$Cl + O_2 \leftarrow ClO + O$$

Chlorine is recycled and it has been estimated that a single chlorine radical will destroy 10000 molecules of ozone before it combines with hydrogen to form the relatively harmless hydrochloric acid. The Antarctic 'hole' in the ozone layer forms in October of each year, when spring sunlight initiates photochemical reactions. Minimal levels fell from 300 Dobson Units in 1960 to a lowest point (88) in 1995.[28] Slight recovery to reach 100 had occurred by 2004.

EVOLUTION AND ADAPTATION

This chapter has outlined the environmental conditions and biological factors under which the atmosphere has evolved to its present composition. In the past, nothing has been permanent, and we can expect a continuation of the interaction between organisms and their environment. What is new is that one species now has the power to cause major changes in the environment, and the atmosphere in particular. These changes will affect a wide range of organisms, and result in the extinction of certain species.

References

1. Taylor SR. *Solar system evolution*. Cambridge: Cambridge University Press; 1992.

*2. Nunn JF. Evolution of the atmosphere. *Proc Geol Assoc*. 1998;109:1–13.

3. Nisbet EG, Sleep NH. The habitat and nature of early life. *Nature*. 2001;409:1083–1091.

4. Oró J. Early chemical stages in the origin of life. In: Bengston S, ed. *Early Life on Earth. Nobel Symposium No. 84*. New York: Columbia University Press; 1994:48-59.

5. MacDonald GA, Hubbard DH. *Volcanoes of the National Parks in Hawaii*. 6th ed. Honolulu: Hawaii Natural History Association; 1972.

6. Miller SL. A production of amino acids under possible primitive earth conditions. *Science.* 1953;117:528–529.

7. Chapman CR, Morrison D. *Cosmic catastrophies.* London: Plenum Press; 1989;97.

8. Malin MC, Edgett KS. Evidence of persistent flow and aqueous sedimentation on early Mars. *Science.* 2003;302:1931–1934.

9. Schorghofer N. Dynamics of ice ages on Mars. *Nature.* 2007;449:192–194.

10. Böhler C, Nielsen PE, Orgel LE. Template switching between PNA and RNA oligonucleotides. *Nature.* 1995;376:578–581.

11. Nisbet EG. Archaean ecology. In: Coward MP, Reis AC, eds. *Early Precambrian Processes.* London: Geological Society; 1995:27–51.

12. Nisbet EG. Origins of photosynthesis. *Nature.* 1995;373: 479–480.

13. Kasting JF. The rise of atmospheric oxygen. *Science.* 2001;293:819–820.

*14. Rasmussen B, Fletcher IR, Brocks JJ, Kilburn MR. Reassessing the first appearance of eukaryotes and cyanobacteria. *Nature.* 2008;455:1101–1104.

15. Bekker A, Holland HD, Wang PL, et al. Dating the rise of atmospheric oxygen. *Nature.* 2004;427:117–120.

*16. Berner RA, Van den Brooks JM, Ward PD. Oxygen and evolution. *Science.* 2007;316:557–558.

17. Kaufman AJ, Xiao S. High CO_2 levels in the Proterozoic atmosphere estimated from analyses of individual microfossils. *Nature.* 2003;425:279–282.

18. DeConto RM, Pollard D, Wilson PA, Pälike H, Lear CH, Pagani M. Thresholds for Cenozoic bipolar glaciation. *Nature.* 2008;455:652–656.

19. Christensen JH, Hewitson B, Busuioc A, et al. Regional climate projections, Climate Change, 2007: The Physical Science Basis. Contribution of Working group I to the Fourth Assessment Report of the Intergovernmental Panel on Climate Change. Cambridge: Cambridge University Press, 2007.

20. Petit JR, Jouzel J, Raynaud D, et al. Climate and atmospheric history of the past 420,000 years from the Vostok ice core, Antarctica. *Nature.* 1999;399:429–436.

21. Nunn JF. Climate change and sea level in relation to overpopulation. *J Optimal Population Trust.* 2004;4:3–9.

22. Loutre MF, Berger A. Future climatic changes: are we entering an exceptionally long interglacial? *Climatic Change.* 2000;46:61–90.

23. Jones CD. Meteorological Office, personal communication. 2005.

24. Broecker WS. Thermohaline circulation, the Achilles heel of our climate system: will man-made CO_2 upset the current balance? *Science.* 1997;278:1582–1588.

25. Story M, Duncan RA, Swisher CC. Paleocene-Eocene thermal maximum and opening of the northeast Atlantic. *Science.* 2007;316:587–589.

26. Karl TR, Trenberth KE. Modern global climate change. *Science.* 2003;302:1719–1723.

27. Nunn JF. Climate change and rising sea level. *Optimum Population Trust Journal.* 2006;6:14–19.

28. Jones AE, Shanklin JD. Continued decline of total ozone over Halley, Antarctica, since 1985. *Nature.* 1995;376:409–411.

Chapter 2

Functional anatomy of the respiratory tract

KEY POINTS

- In addition to conducting air to and from the lungs, the nose, mouth and pharynx have other important functions including speech, swallowing and airway protection.
- Starting at the trachea, the airway divides about 23 times, terminating in an estimated 30 000 pulmonary acini, each containing more than 10 000 alveoli.
- The alveolar wall is ideally designed to provide the minimal physical barrier to gas transfer, whilst also being structurally strong enough to resist the large mechanical forces applied to the lung.

This chapter is not a comprehensive account of respiratory anatomy but concentrates on those aspects that are most relevant to an understanding of function. The respiratory muscles are considered in Chapter 6.

MOUTH, NOSE AND PHARYNX

Breathing is normally possible through either the nose or the mouth, the two alternative air passages converging in the oro-pharynx. Nasal breathing is the norm and has two major advantages over mouth breathing – filtration of particulate matter by the vibrissae hairs and humidification of inspired gas. Humidification by the nose is highly efficient because the nasal septum and turbinates greatly increase the surface area of mucosa available for evaporation and produce turbulent flow so increasing contact between the mucosa and air. However, the nose may offer more resistance to air flow than the mouth, particularly when obstructed by polyps,

adenoids or congestion of the nasal mucosa. Nasal resistance may make oral breathing obligatory and many children and adults breathe only or partly through their mouths at rest. With increasing levels of exercise in normal adults, the respiratory minute volume increases and at a level of about 35l.min^{-1} the oral airway comes into play. Deflection of gas into either the nasal or the oral route is under voluntary control and accomplished with the soft palate, tongue and lips. These functions are best considered in relation to a midline sagittal section (Figure 2.1).

Part (A) shows the normal position for nose breathing, with the mouth closed by occlusion of the lips, and the tongue lying against the hard palate. The soft palate is clear of the posterior pharyngeal wall.

Part (B) shows forced mouth breathing, as for instance when blowing through the mouth, without pinching the nose. The soft palate becomes rigid and is arched upwards and backwards by contraction of tensor and levator palati to lie against a band of the superior constrictor of the pharynx known as Passavant's ridge which, together with the soft palate, forms the palatopharyngeal sphincter. Note also that the orifice of the pharyngotympanic (Eustachian) tube lies above the palatopharyngeal sphincter and the tubes can therefore be inflated by the subject only when the nose is pinched. As the mouth pressure is raised, this tends to force the soft palate against the posterior pharyngeal wall to act as a valve. The combined palatopharyngeal sphincter and valvular action of the soft palate is very strong and can easily withstand mouth pressures in excess of 10 kPa (100 cmH$_2$O).

Part (C) shows the occlusion of the respiratory tract during a Valsalva manoeuvre. The airway is

DOI: 10.1016/B978-0-7020-2996-7.00002-7

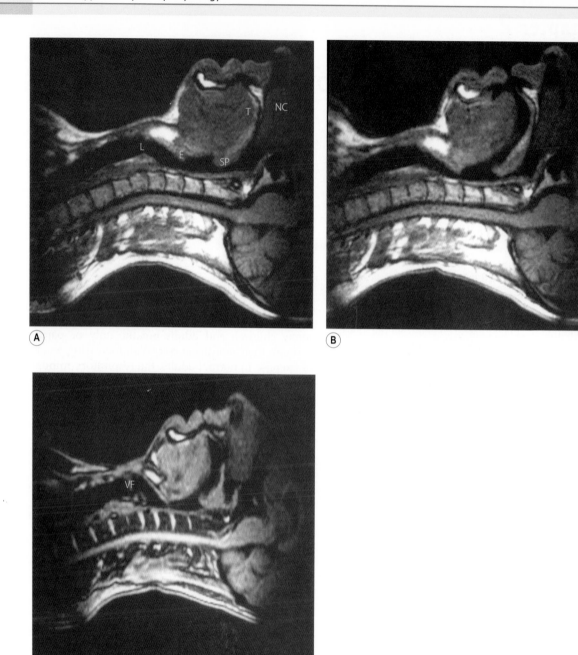

Fig. 2.1 Magnetic resonance imaging scans showing median sagittal sections of the pharynx in a normal subject. (A) Normal nasal breathing with the oral airway occluded by lips and tongue. (B) Deliberate oral breathing with the nasal airway occluded by elevation and backward movement of the soft palate. (C) A Valsalva manoeuvre in which the subject deliberately tries to exhale against a closed airway. Data acquisition for scans (A) and (B) took 45 seconds so anatomical differences between inspiration and expiration will not be visible. I am indebted to Prof M. Bellamy for being the subject. NC, nasal cavity; T, tongue; SP, soft palate; E, epiglottis; VF, vocal fold; L, larynx.

occluded at many sites: the lips are closed, the tongue is in contact with the hard palate anteriorly, the palatopharyngeal sphincter is tightly closed, the epiglottis is in contact with the posterior pharyngeal wall, and the vocal folds are closed so becoming visible in the midline in the figure.

During swallowing the nasopharynx is occluded by contraction of both tensor and levator palati. The larynx is elevated 2–3 cm by contraction of the infrahyoid muscles, stylopharyngeus and palatopharyngeus, coming to lie under the epiglottis. In addition, the aryepiglottic folds are approximated causing total occlusion of the entrance to the larynx. This extremely effective protection of the larynx is capable of withstanding pharyngeal pressures as high as 80 kPa (600 mmHg) which may be generated during swallowing.

Upper airway cross-sectional areas can be estimated from conventional radiographs, magnetic resonance imaging (MRI) as in Figure 2.1, or acoustic pharyngometry. In the latter technique, a single sound pulse of 100 μs duration is generated within the apparatus and passes along the airway of the subject. Recording of the timing and frequency of sound waves reflected back from the airway allows calculation of cross-sectional area which is then presented as a function of the distance travelled along the airway[1] (Figure 2.2). Acoustic pharyngometry measurements correlate well with MRI scans of the airway,[2] and the technique is now sufficiently developed for use in clinical situations with real-time results. For example, acoustic pharyngometry has been used following the placement of a tracheal tube to differentiate between oesophageal and tracheal intubation,[3] and to estimate airway size in patients with sleep disordered breathing (Chapter 16).[4]

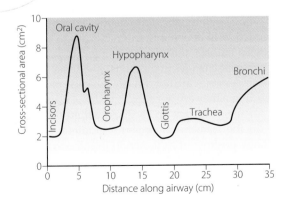

Fig. 2.2 Normal acoustic reflectometry pattern of airway cross-sectional area during mouth breathing.[1,2]

THE LARYNX

The larynx evolved in the lungfish for the protection of the airway during such activities as feeding and perfusion of the gills with water. While protection of the airway remains important, the larynx now has many other functions, all involving varying degrees of laryngeal occlusion.

Speech.[5] Phonation, the laryngeal component of speech, requires a combination of changes in position, tension and mass of the vocal folds (cords). Rotation of the arytenoid cartilages by the posterior cricoarytenoid muscles opens the vocal folds, while contraction of the lateral cricoarytenoid and oblique arytenoid muscles opposes this. With the vocal folds almost closed, the respiratory muscles generate a positive pressure of 5–35 cmH$_2$O which may then be released by slight opening of the vocal folds to produce sound waves. The cricothyroid muscle tilts the cricoid and arytenoid cartilages backwards and also moves them posteriorly in relation to the thyroid cartilage. This produces up to 50% elongation and therefore tensioning of the vocal folds, an action opposed by the thyroarytenoid muscles, which draw the arytenoid cartilages forwards toward the thyroid and so shorten and relax the vocal folds. Tensioning of the cords results in both transverse and longitudinal resonance of the vocal fold allowing the formation of complex sound waves. The deeper fibres of the thyroarytenoids comprise the vocales muscles, which exert fine control over pitch of the voice by slight variations in both the tension and mass of the vocal folds. A more dramatic example of the effect of vocal fold mass on voice production occurs with inflammation of the laryngeal mucosa and the resulting hoarse voice or complete inability to phonate.

Effort closure. Tighter occlusion of the larynx, known as effort closure, is required for making expulsive efforts. It is also needed to lock the thoracic cage and so to secure the origin of the muscles of the upper arm arising from the rib cage, thus increasing the power which can be transmitted to the arm. In addition to simple apposition of the vocal folds described above, the aryepiglottic muscles and their continuation, the oblique and transverse arytenoids, act as a powerful sphincter capable of closing the inlet of the larynx, by bringing the aryepiglottic folds tightly together. The full process enables the larynx to withstand the highest pressures which can be generated in the thorax, usually at least 12 kPa (120 cmH$_2$O) and often more. Sudden release of the obstruction is essential for effective coughing, when the linear velocity of air through the larynx is said to approach the speed of sound.

Laryngeal muscles are involved in controlling airways resistance, particularly during expiration, and this aspect of vocal fold function is described in Chapter 6.

THE TRACHEOBRONCHIAL TREE

An accurate and complete model of the branching pattern of the human bronchial tree remains elusive, though several different models have been described.[6] The most useful and widely accepted approach remains that of Weibel[7] who numbered successive generations of air passages from the trachea (generation 0) down to alveolar sacs (generation 23). This 'regular dichotomy' model assumes that each bronchus regularly divides into two approximately equal size daughter bronchi. As a rough approximation it may therefore be assumed that the number of passages in each generation is double that in the previous generation, and the number of air passages in each generation is approximately indicated by the number 2 raised to the power of the generation number. This formula indicates one trachea, two main bronchi, four lobar bronchi, sixteen segmental bronchi, etc. However, this mathematical relationship is unlikely to be true in practice where bronchus length is variable, pairs of daughter bronchi are often unequal in size, and trifurcations may occur.

Work using computerised tomography to reconstruct, in three dimensions, the branching pattern of the airways has shown that a regular dichotomy system does occur for at least the first six generations.[8] Beyond this point, the same study demonstrated trifurcation of some bronchi, and airways that terminated at generation 8. Table 2.1 traces the characteristics of progressive generations of airways in the respiratory tract.

TRACHEA (GENERATION 0)

The adult trachea has a mean diameter of 1.8 cm and length of 11 cm. It is supported by U-shaped cartilages which are joined posteriorly by smooth muscle bands. The part of the trachea in the neck is not subjected to intrathoracic pressure changes, but it is very vulnerable to pressures arising in the neck due, for example, to tumours or haematoma formation. An external

pressure of the order of 4 kPa (40 cmH$_2$O) is sufficient to occlude the trachea. Within the chest, the trachea can be compressed by raised intrathoracic pressure during, for example, a cough, when the decreased diameter increases the linear velocity of gas flow and therefore the efficiency of removal of secretions.

MAIN, LOBAR AND SEGMENTAL BRONCHI (GENERATIONS 1–4)

The trachea bifurcates asymmetrically, with the right bronchus being wider and making a smaller angle with the long axis of the trachea. Foreign bodies therefore tend to enter the right bronchus in preference to the left. Main, lobar and segmental bronchi have firm cartilaginous support in their walls, U-shaped in the main bronchi, but in the form of irregularly shaped and helical plates lower down with bronchial muscle between. Bronchi in this group (down to generation 4) are sufficiently regular to be individually named (Figure 2.3). Total cross-sectional area of the respiratory tract is minimal at the third generation (Figure 2.4).

These bronchi are subjected to the full effect of changes in intrathoracic pressure and will collapse when the intrathoracic pressure exceeds the intraluminar pressure by about 5 kPa (50 cmH$_2$O). This occurs in the larger bronchi during a forced expiration so limiting peak expiratory flow rate (see Figure 4.7).

SMALL BRONCHI (GENERATIONS 5–11)

The small bronchi extend through about seven generations with their diameter progressively falling from 3.5 to 1 mm. Down to the level of the smallest true bronchi, air passages lie in close proximity to branches of the pulmonary artery in a sheath containing pulmonary lymphatics, which can be distended with oedema fluid giving rise to the characteristic 'cuffing' that is responsible for the earliest radiographic changes in pulmonary oedema. Because these air passages are not directly attached to the lung parenchyma they are not subject to direct traction and rely for their patency on cartilage within their walls and on the transmural pressure gradient, which is normally positive from lumen to intrathoracic space. In the normal subject this pressure gradient is seldom reversed and, even during a forced expiration, the intraluminar pressure in the small bronchi rapidly rises to more than 80% of the alveolar pressure, which is more than the extramural (intrathoracic) pressure.

Table 2.1 Structural characteristics of the air passages[9]

	GENERATION	NUMBER	MEAN DIAMETER (mm)	AREA SUPPLIED	CARTILAGE	MUSCLE	NUTRITION	EMPLACEMENT	EPITHELIUM
Trachea	0	1	18	Both lungs	U-Shaped	Links open end of cartilage			
Main bronchi	1	2	12	Individual lungs				Within connective tissue sheath alongside arterial vessels	Columnar ciliated epithelium
Lobar bronchi	2 → 3	4 → 8	8 → 5	Lobes					
Segmental bronchi	4	16	4	Segments	Irregular shaped	Helical bands	From the bronchial circulation		
Small bronchi	5 → 11	32 → 2000	3 → 1	Secondary lobules					
Bronchioles Terminal bronchioles	12 → 14	4000 → 16000	1 → 0.7		Absent	Strong helical muscle bands		Embedded directly in the lung parenchyma	Cuboidal
Respiratory bronchioles	15 → 18	32000 → 260000	0.4	Pulmonary acinus		Muscle bands between alveoli	From the pulmonary circulation		Cuboidal to flat between alveoli
Alveolar ducts	19 → 22	520000 → 4000000	0.3			Thin bands in alveolar septa		Form the lung parenchyma	
Alveoli	23	8000000	0.2						Alveolar epithelium

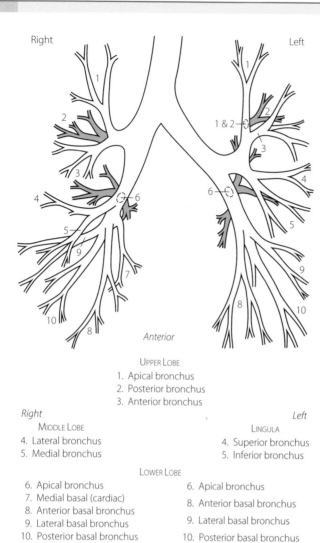

Right   Left

Anterior

Fig. 2.3 Named branches of the tracheobronchial tree, viewed from the front. (Reproduced by permission of the editors of Thorax.)

UPPER LOBE
1. Apical bronchus
2. Posterior bronchus
3. Anterior bronchus

Right   *Left*

MIDDLE LOBE   LINGULA
4. Lateral bronchus   4. Superior bronchus
5. Medial bronchus   5. Inferior bronchus

LOWER LOBE
6. Apical bronchus   6. Apical bronchus
7. Medial basal (cardiac)
8. Anterior basal bronchus   8. Anterior basal bronchus
9. Lateral basal bronchus   9. Lateral basal bronchus
10. Posterior basal bronchus   10. Posterior basal bronchus

BRONCHIOLES (GENERATIONS 12–14)

An important change occurs at about the eleventh generation where the internal diameter is approximately 1 mm. Cartilage disappears from the wall below this level and ceases to be a factor in maintaining patency. However, beyond this level the air passages are directly embedded in the lung parenchyma, the elastic recoil of which holds the air passages open like the guy ropes of a tent. Therefore the calibre of the airways beyond the eleventh generation is mainly influenced by lung volume, since the forces holding their lumina open are stronger at higher lung volumes. The converse of this factor causes airway closure at reduced lung volume (see Chapter 4). In

succeeding generations, the number of bronchioles increases far more rapidly than the calibre diminishes (Table 2.1). Therefore the total cross-sectional area increases until, in the terminal bronchioles, it is about 100 times the area at the level of the large bronchi (Figure 2.4). Thus the flow resistance of these smaller air passages (less than 2 mm diameter) is negligible under normal conditions. However, the resistance of the bronchioles can increase to very high values when their strong helical muscular bands are contracted by the mechanisms described in Chapters 4 and 28. Down to the terminal bronchiole, the air passages derive their nutrition from the bronchial circulation and are thus influenced by systemic arterial blood gas

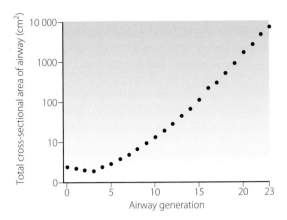

Fig. 2.4 The total cross-sectional area of the air passages at different generations of the airways. Note that the minimum cross-sectional area is at generation 3 (lobar to segmental bronchi). The total cross-sectional area becomes very large in the smaller air passages, approaching a square metre in the alveolar ducts.

levels. Beyond this point the smaller air passages rely upon the pulmonary circulation for their nutrition.

RESPIRATORY BRONCHIOLES (GENERATIONS 15–18)

Down to the smallest bronchioles, the functions of the air passages are solely conduction and humidification. Beyond this point there is a gradual transition from conduction to gas exchange. In the four generations of respiratory bronchioles there is a gradual increase in the number of alveoli in their walls. Like the bronchioles, the respiratory bronchioles are embedded in lung parenchyma, however, they have a well defined muscle layer with bands which loop over the opening of the alveolar ducts and the mouths of the mural alveoli. There is no significant change in calibre of advancing generations of respiratory bronchioles (approximately 0.4 mm diameter).

ALVEOLAR DUCTS (GENERATIONS 19–22)

Alveolar ducts arise from the terminal respiratory bronchiole, from which they differ by having no walls other than the mouths of mural alveoli (about 20 in number). The alveolar septa comprise a series of rings forming the walls of the alveolar ducts and containing smooth muscle. Some 35% of the alveolar gas resides in the alveolar ducts and the alveoli that arise directly from them.

ALVEOLAR SACS (GENERATION 23)

The last generation of the air passages differ from alveolar ducts solely in the fact that they are blind. It is estimated that about 17 alveoli arise from each alveolar sac and account for about half of the total number of alveoli.

PULMONARY ACINUS

A pulmonary acinus is usually defined as the region of lung supplied by a first order respiratory bronchiole and includes the respiratory bronchioles, alveolar ducts and alveolar sacs distal to a single terminal bronchiole (Figure 2.5). This represents generations 15–23 above, but in practice the number of generations within a single acinus is quite variable being between 6 and 12 divisions beyond the terminal bronchiole. A human lung contains about 30 000 acini,[9] each with a diameter of about 3.5 mm and containing in excess of 10 000 alveoli. A single pulmonary acinus is probably the equivalent of the alveolus when it is considered from a functional standpoint as gas movement within the acinus is by diffusion rather than tidal ventilation. Acinar morphometry therefore becomes crucial,[10] in particular the path length between the start of the acinus and the most distal alveolus which in man is between 5 and 12 mm.[9]

RESPIRATORY EPITHELIUM[11,12]

Before inspired air reaches the alveoli it must be humidified, and airborne particles, pathogens and irritant chemicals removed. These tasks are undertaken by the respiratory epithelium and its overlying layer of airway lining fluid, and are described in Chapter 12. To facilitate these functions the respiratory epithelium contains numerous cell types.

Ciliated epithelial cells. These are the most abundant cell type in the respiratory epithelium. In the nose, pharynx and larger airways the epithelial cells are pseudo-stratified, gradually changing to a single layer of columnar cells in bronchi, cuboidal cells in bronchioles, and finally thinning further to merge with the Type I alveolar epithelial cells (see below). They are differentiated from either basal or secretory cells (see below) and are characterised by the presence of around 300 cilia per cell (page 218).

Goblet cells.[13] These are present at a density of about 6000 per mm^2 (in the trachea) and are responsible for producing the thick layer of mucus that lines all but the smallest conducting airways (page 218).

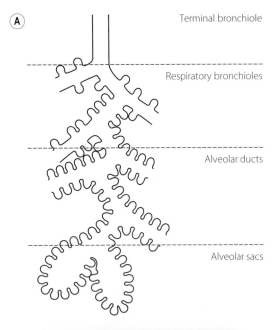

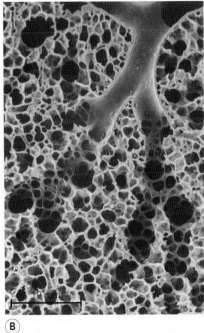

Fig. 2.5 (A) Schematic diagram of a single pulmonary acinus showing four generations between the terminal bronchiole and the alveolar sacs. The average number of generations in human lung is eight, but may be as many as 12. (B) Section of rabbit lung showing respiratory bronchioles leading to alveolar ducts and sacs. Human alveoli would be considerably larger. The scale bar is 0.5 mm. (Photograph kindly supplied by Professor E. R. Weibel.)

Submucosal secretory cells. Submucosal glands occur in the larger bronchi and in the trachea; in the latter there are about 10 submucosal openings per mm^2. The glands comprise both serous cells and mucous cells, with serous cells occurring in the gland acinus, while mucous cells are found closer to the collecting duct. The serous cells have the highest levels of membrane-bound cystic fibrosis transmembrane conductance regulator (CFTR) in the lung (Chapter 28).

Basal cells. These cells lie underneath the columnar cells giving rise to the pseudo-stratified appearance, and are absent in the bronchioles and beyond. They are probably the stem cell responsible for producing new epithelial and goblet cells.

Mast cells. The lungs contain numerous mast cells which are located underneath the epithelial cells of the airways as well as in the alveolar septa. Some also lie free in the lumen of the airways and may be recovered by bronchial lavage. Their important role in bronchoconstriction is described in Chapter 28.

Non-ciliated bronchiolar epithelial (Clara) cells. These cells are found in the mucosa of the terminal bronchioles where they may be the precursor of epithelial cells in the absence of basal cells. They are metabolically active,[14] secreting surfactant proteins A, B and D (page 29), antiprotease enzymes and a variety of other proteins whose functions are mostly unknown though some are involved in the metabolism of chemical toxins.

Neuro-epithelial cells. These cells are found throughout the bronchial tree, but occur in larger numbers in the intrapulmonary and terminal bronchioles. They may be found individually or in clusters as neuro-epithelial bodies, and are of uncertain function in the adult lung.[15] Present in fetal lung tissue in a greater number they may be responsible for controlling lung development. Similar cells elsewhere in the body secrete a variety of amines and peptides with diverse effects such as calcitonin, gastrin releasing peptide, calcitonin gene related peptide and serotonin.

THE ALVEOLI

The mean total number of alveoli has been estimated as 480 million, but ranges from about 270 million to 790 million, correlating with the height of the subject and total lung volume.[16] The size of the alveoli is proportional to lung volume but due to gravity they are normally larger in the upper part of the lung except at maximal inflation when the vertical gradient in size disappears. At functional residual capacity the mean diameter is 0.2 mm.

THE ALVEOLAR SEPTA

The septa are under tension generated partly by collagen and elastin fibres, but more by surface tension at the air–fluid interface (page 28). They are therefore generally flat, making the alveoli polyhedral rather than spherical. The septa are perforated by small fenestrations known as the pores of Kohn (Figure 2.6), which provide collateral ventilation between alveoli. Collateral ventilation also occurs between small bronchioles and neighbouring alveoli, adjacent pulmonary acini and occasionally intersegmental communications,[17] and is more pronounced in patients with emphysema (page 410).[18]

On one side of the alveolar wall the capillary endothelium and the alveolar epithelium are closely apposed, with almost no interstitial space, such that the total thickness from gas to blood is about 0.3 μm (Figures 2.7 and 2.8). This may be considered the 'active' side of the capillary and gas exchange must be more efficient on this side. The other side of the capillary, which may be considered the 'service' side, is usually more than 1–2 μm thick and contains a recognisable interstitial space containing elastin and collagen fibres, nerve endings and occasional migrant polymorphs and macrophages. The distinction between the two sides of the capillary has considerable pathophysiological significance as the active side tends to be spared in the accumulation of both oedema fluid and fibrous tissue (Chapter 29).

The fibre scaffold. The alveolar septum contains a network of fibres which forms a continuum between the peripheral fibres and the axial spiral fibres of the bronchioles. The septal fibre is in the form of a network, through which are threaded the pulmonary capillaries, which are themselves a network. Thus the capillaries pass repeatedly from one side of the fibre scaffold to the other (Figure 2.6), the fibre always residing on the thick (or 'service') side of the capillary allowing the other side to bulge into the lumen of the alveolus. The left side of the capillary in Figure 2.7 is the side with the fibres. Structural integrity of the fibre scaffold is believed to be maintained by the individual fibres being under tension, such that when any fibres are damaged, the alveolar septum disintegrates and adjacent alveoli change shape, ultimately leading to emphysema (page 410).[21]

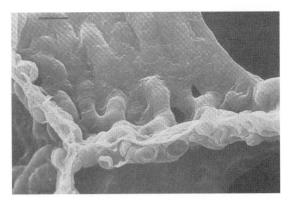

Fig. 2.6 Scanning electron micrograph of the junction of three alveolar septa which are shown in both surface view and section showing the polyhedral structure. Two pores of Kohn are seen to the right of centre. Red blood cells are seen in the cut ends of the capillaries. The scale bar is 10 μm. (Reproduced from reference 19 by permission of the author and the publishers; © Harvard University Press.)

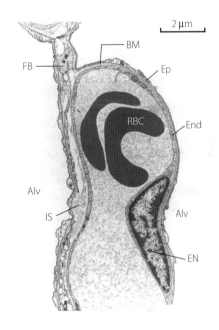

Fig. 2.7 Details of the interstitial space, the capillary endothelium and alveolar epithelium. Thickening of the interstitial space is confined to the left of the capillary (the 'service' side) while the total alveolar/capillary membrane remains thin on the right (the 'active' side) except where it is thickened by the endothelial nucleus. Alv, alveolus; BM, basement membrane; EN endothelial nucleus; End, endothelium; Ep, epithelium; IS, interstitial space; RBC, red blood cell; FB, fibroblast process. (Electron micrograph kindly supplied by Professor E. R. Weibel.)

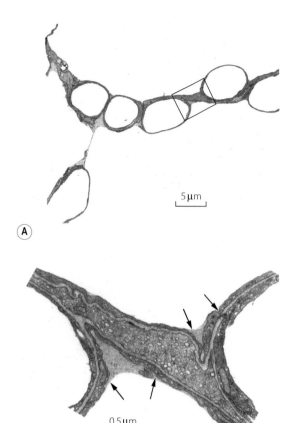

5 μm

(A)

0.5 μm

(B)

Fig. 2.8 (A) Transmission electron micrograph of alveolar septum with lung inflated to 40% of total lung capacity. The section in the box is enlarged in (B) to show alveolar lining fluid, which has pooled in two concavities of the alveolar epithelium and has also spanned the pore of Kohn in (A). There is a thin film of osmophilic material (arrows), probably surfactant, at the interface between air and the alveolar lining fluid. (Reproduced from reference 20 by permission of the authors and the Editors of Journal of Applied Physiology.)

At the cellular level, the scaffolding for the alveolar septa is provided by the basement membrane, which provides the blood–gas barrier with enough strength to withstand the enormous forces applied to lung tissue.[22,23] At the centre of the basement membrane is a layer of type IV collagen, the lamina densa, approximately 50 nm thick and made up of many layers of a diamond-shaped matrix of collagen molecules. On each side of the lamina densa, the collagen layer is attached to the alveolar or endothelial cells by a series of proteins collectively known as laminins, of which seven sub-types are now known. The laminins

are more than simple structural molecules, having complex interactions with membrane proteins and the intracellular cytoskeleton[24] to help regulate cell shape and permeability etc. These aspects of the function of the basement membrane are important. It has been shown that increases in the capillary transmural pressure gradient above about 3 kPa (30 cmH₂O) may cause disruption of endothelium and/or epithelium, while the basement membrane tends to remain intact, sometimes as the only remaining separation between blood and gas.[25]

ALVEOLAR CELL TYPES

Capillary endothelial cells. These cells are continuous with the endothelium of the general circulation and, in the pulmonary capillary bed, have a thickness of only 0.1 μm except where expanded to contain nuclei (Figure 2.7). Electron microscopy shows the flat parts of the cytoplasm to be devoid of all organelles except for small vacuoles (caveolae or plasmalemmal vesicles) which may open onto the basement membrane or the lumen of the capillary or be entirely contained within the cytoplasm (see Figure 2.8). The endothelial cells abut against one another at fairly loose junctions which are of the order of 5 nm wide.[26] These junctions permit the passage of quite large molecules, and the pulmonary lymph contains albumin at about half the concentration in plasma. Macrophages pass freely through these junctions under normal conditions, and polymorphs can also pass in response to chemotaxis (page 455).

Alveolar epithelial cells – type I. These cells line the alveoli and also exist as a thin sheet approximately 0.1 μm in thickness, except where expanded to contain nuclei. Like the endothelium, the flat part of the cytoplasm is devoid of organelles except for small vacuoles. Epithelial cells each cover several capillaries and are joined into a continuous sheet by tight junctions with a gap of only about 1 nm.[26] These junctions may be seen as narrow lines snaking across the septa in Figure 2.6. The tightness of these junctions is crucial for prevention of the escape of large molecules, such as albumin, into the alveoli, thus preserving the oncotic pressure gradient essential for the avoidance of pulmonary oedema (see page 420). Nevertheless, these junctions permit the free passage of macrophages and polymorphs may also pass in response to a chemotactic stimulus. Figure 2.8 shows the type I cell covered with a film of alveolar lining fluid. Type I cells are end cells and do not divide in

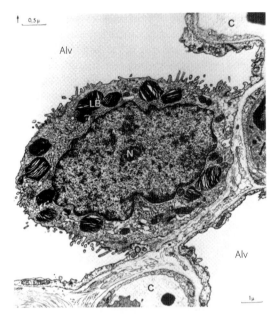

Fig. 2.9 Electron micrograph of a type II alveolar epithelial cell of a dog. Note the large nucleus, the microvilli and the osmiophilic lamellar bodies thought to release surfactant. Alv, alveolus; C, capillary; LB, lamellar bodies; N, nucleus. (Reproduced from reference 29 by permission of Professor E. R. Weibel and the Editors of Physiological Reviews.)

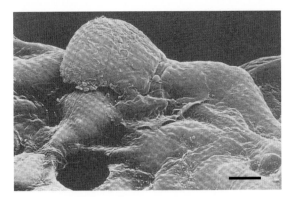

Fig. 2.10 Scanning electron micrograph of an alveolar macrophage advancing to the right over epithelial type I cells. The scale bar is $3\,\mu m$. (Reproduced from reference 19 by permission of the author and the publishers; © Harvard University Press.)

vivo. Their position in the lung means alveolar epithelial cells are exposed to the highest concentrations of oxygen of any mammalian cell, and they are sensitive to damage from high concentrations of oxygen (Chapter 26), but recent work suggests they may have active systems for preventing oxidative stress.[27]

Alveolar epithelial cells – type II. These are the stem cells from which type I cells arise.[28] They do not function as gas exchange membranes, and are rounded in shape and situated at the junction of septa. They have large nuclei and microvilli (Figure 2.9). The cytoplasm contains characteristic striated osmiophilic organelles that contain stored surfactant (page 29). Type II cells are also involved in pulmonary defence mechanisms in that they may secrete cytokines and contribute to pulmonary inflammation. They are resistant to oxygen toxicity, tending to replace type I cells after prolonged exposure to high concentrations of oxygen (Chapter 26).

Alveolar macrophages. The lung is richly endowed with these phagocytes which pass freely from the circulation, through the interstitial space and thence through the gaps between alveolar epithelial cells to lie on their surface within the alveolar lining fluid (Figure 2.10). They can re-enter the body but are remarkable for their ability to live and function outside the body. Macrophages form the major component of host defence within the alveoli, being active in combating infection and scavenging foreign bodies such as small dust particles. They contain a variety of destructive enzymes but are also capable of generating reactive oxygen species (Chapter 26). These are highly effective bactericidal agents but their presence in lung tissue may rebound to damage the host. Dead macrophages release the enzyme trypsin, which may cause tissue damage in patients who are deficient in the protein α_1-antitrypsin.

THE PULMONARY VASCULATURE

PULMONARY ARTERIES

Although the pulmonary circulation carries roughly the same flow as the systemic circulation, the arterial pressure and the vascular resistance are normally only one-sixth as great. The media of the pulmonary arteries is about half as thick as in systemic arteries of corresponding size. In the larger vessels it consists mainly of elastic tissue but in the smaller vessels it is mainly muscular, the transition being in vessels of about 1 mm diameter. Pulmonary arteries lie close to the corresponding air passages in connective tissue sheaths. Table 2.2 shows a scheme for consideration of the branching of the pulmonary arterial tree.[30] This may be compared with Weibel's scheme for the airways (Table 2.1).

Table 2.2 Dimensions of the branches of the human pulmonary artery

ORDERS	NUMBERS	MEAN DIAMETER (mm)	CUMULATIVE VOLUME (ml)
17	1	30	64
16	3	15	81
15	8	8.1	85
14	20	5.8	96
13	66	3.7	108
12	203	2.1	116
11	675	1.3	122
10	2300	0.85	128
9	5900	0.53	132
8	18 000	0.35	136
7	53 000	0.22	138
6	160 000	0.14	141
5	470 000	0.086	142
4	1 400 000	0.054	144
3	4 200 000	0.034	145
2	13 000 000	0.021	146
1	300 000 000	0.013	151

In contrast to the airways (Table 2.1), the branching is asymmetrical and not dichotomous. Singhal et al.[30] therefore grouped the vessels according to orders and not generation as in Table 2.1.

PULMONARY ARTERIOLES

The transition to arterioles occurs at an internal diameter of 100 μm. These vessels differ radically from their counterparts in the systemic circulation, being virtually devoid of muscular tissue. There is a thin media of elastic tissue separated from the blood by endothelium. Structurally there is no real difference between pulmonary arterioles and venules.

PULMONARY CAPILLARIES

Pulmonary capillaries tend to arise abruptly from much larger vessels, the pulmonary metarterioles. The capillaries form a dense network over the walls of one or more alveoli and the spaces between the capillaries are similar in size to the capillaries themselves (Figure 2.6). In the resting state, about 75% of the capillary bed is filled but the percentage is higher in the dependent parts of the lungs. Inflation of the alveoli reduces the cross-sectional area of the capillary bed and increases resistance to blood flow (Chapter 7). One capillary network is not confined to one alveolus but passes from one alveolus to another and blood traverses a number of alveolar

septa before reaching a venule. This clearly has a bearing on the efficiency of gas exchange. From the functional standpoint it is often more convenient to consider the pulmonary microcirculation rather than just the capillaries. The microcirculation is defined as the vessels that are devoid of a muscular layer and it commences with arterioles of diameter 75 μm and continues through the capillary bed as far as venules of diameter 200 μm. Special roles of the microcirculation are considered in Chapters 12 and 29.

PULMONARY VENULES AND VEINS

Pulmonary capillary blood is collected into venules that are structurally almost identical to the arterioles. In fact, Duke[31] obtained satisfactory gas exchange when an isolated cat lung was perfused in reverse. The pulmonary veins do not run alongside the pulmonary arteries but lie some distance away, close to the septa which separate the segments of the lung.

BRONCHIAL CIRCULATION[32]

Down to the terminal bronchioles, the air passages and the accompanying blood vessels receive their nutrition from the bronchial vessels which arise from the systemic circulation. The bronchial circulation therefore provides the heat required for warming and humidification of inspired air, and cooling of the respiratory epithelium causes vasodilation and an increase in the bronchial artery blood flow. About one-third of the bronchial circulation returns to the systemic venous system, the remainder draining into the pulmonary veins, thereby constituting a physiological shunt (page 132).

The bronchial circulation also differs from the pulmonary circulation in its capacity for angiogenesis.[33] Pulmonary vessels have very limited ability to remodel themselves in response to pathological changes while bronchial vessels, like other systemic arteries, can undergo prolific angiogenesis. As a result, the blood supply to most lung cancers (Chapter 30) is derived from the bronchial circulation.

PULMONARY LYMPHATICS

There are no lymphatics visible in the interalveolar septa, but small lymph vessels commence at the junction between alveolar and extra-alveolar spaces. There is a well developed lymphatic system around the bronchi and pulmonary vessels, capable of containing up to 500 ml of lymph, and draining towards the hilum. Down to airway generation 11 the lymphatics lie in a potential space around the air passages and vessels, separating them from the lung parenchyma. This space becomes distended with lymph in pulmonary oedema and accounts for the characteristic butterfly shadow of the chest radiograph. In the hilum of the lung, the lymphatic drainage passes through several groups of tracheobronchial lymph glands, where they receive tributaries from the superficial subpleural plexus. Most of the lymph from the left lung usually enters the thoracic duct whilst the right side drains into the right lymphatic duct. However, the pulmonary lymphatics often cross the midline and pass independently into the junction of the internal jugular and subclavian veins on the corresponding sides of the body.

References

1. Hoffstein V, Fredberg JJ. The acoustic reflection technique for non-invasive assessment of upper airway area. *Eur Respir J.* 1991;4:602–611.

2. Marshall I, Maran NJ, Martin S, et al. Acoustic reflectometry for airway measurements in man: implementation and validation. *Physiol Meas.* 1993;14:157–169.

3. Raphael DT. Acoustic reflectometry profiles of endotracheal and esophageal intubation. *Anesthesiology.* 2000;92:1293–1299.

4. Patel SR, Frame JM, Larkin EK, Redline S. Heritability of upper airway dimensions derived using acoustic pharyngometry. *Eur Respir J.* 2008;32:1304–1308.

5. Bannister LH. Anatomy of speech. In: Williams PL, ed. *Gray's Anatomy.* London: Churchill-Livingstone; 1995:1651–1652.

6. Phillips CG, Kaye SR, Schroter RC. A diameter-based reconstruction of the branching pattern of the human bronchial tree. Part I. Description and application. *Respir Physiol.* 1994;98:193–217.

7. Weibel ER. Why measure lung structure? *Am J Respir Crit Care Med.* 2001;163:314–315.

8. Sauret V, Halson PM, Brown IW, Fleming JS, Bailey AG. Study of the three-dimensional geometry of the central conducting airways in man using computed tomographic (CT) images. *J Anat.* 2002;200:123–134.

9. Haefeli-Bleuer B, Weibel ER. Morphometry of the human pulmonary acinus. *Anat Rec.* 1988;220:401–414.

10. Sapoval B, Filoche M, Weibel ER. Smaller is better – but not too small: A physical scale for the design of the mammalian pulmonary acinus. *Proc Natl Acad Sci USA.* 2002;99:10411–10416.

11. Jeffery PK. Microscopic structure of normal lung. In: Brewis RAL, Corrin B, Geddes DM, Gibson GJ, eds, *Respiratory Medicine.* London: WB Saunders Company Ltd; 1995:54–72.

12. Knight DA, Holgate ST. The airway epithelium: structural and functional properties in health and disease. *Respirology.* 2003;8:432–436.

13. Rogers DF. Airway goblet cells: responsive and adaptable frontline defenders. *Eur Respir J.* 1994;7:1690–1706.

14. Singh G, Katyal SL. Clara cell proteins. *Ann N Y Acad Sci.* 2000;923:43–58.

15. Gosney J. Pulmonary neuro-endocrine cell system in pediatric and adult lung disease. *Micros Res Tech.* 1997;37:107–113.

16. Ochs M, Nyengaard JR, Jung L, et al. The number of alveoli in the human lung. *Am J Respir Crit Care Med.* 2004;169:120–124.

17. Topol M. Collateral respiratory pathways of pulmonary acini in man. *Folia Morphol.* 1995;54:61–66.

18. Cetti EJ, Moore AJ, Geddes DM. Collateral ventilation. *Thorax.* 2006;61:371–373.

19. Weibel ER. *The pathway for oxygen.* Cambridge, Mass.: Harvard University Press; 1984.

20. Gil J, Bachofen H, Gehr P, Weibel ER. Alveolar volume-surface area relation in air and saline filled lungs fixed by vascular perfusion. *J Appl Physiol.* 1979;47:990–995.

*21. Weibel ER. How to make an alveolus. *Eur Respir J.* 2008;31:483–485.

22. Suki B, Ito S, Stamenovic D, Lutchen KR, Ingenito EP. Biomechanics of the lung parenchyma: critical roles of collagen and mechanical forces. *J Appl Physiol.* 2005;98:1892–1899.

23. Maina JN, West JB. Thin and strong! The bioengineering dilemma in the structural and functional design of the blood-gas barrier. *Physiol Rev.* 2005;85:811–844.

*24. Dudek SM, Garcia JGN. Cytoskeletal regulation of pulmonary vascular permeability. *J Appl Physiol.* 2001;91:1487–1500.

25. Tsukimoto K, Mathieu-Costello O, Prediletto R, Elliott AR, West JB. Ultrastructural appearances of pulmonary capillaries at high transmural pressures. *J Appl Physiol.* 1991;71:573–582.

26. DeFouw DO. Ultrastructural features of alveolar epithelial transport. *Am Rev Respir Dis.* 1983;127:S9–S11.

27. Berthiaume Y, Voisin G, Dagenais A. The alveolar type I cells: the new knight of the alveolus? *J Physiol.* 2006;572:609–610.

28. Uhal BD. Cell cycle kinetics in the alveolar epithelium. *Am J Physiol.* 1997;272:L1031–L1045.

29. Weibel ER. Morphological basis of alveolar-capillary gas exchange. *Physiol Rev*. 1973;53:419.

30. Singhal S, Henderson R, Horsfield K, Harding K, Cumming G. Morphometry of the human pulmonary arterial tree. *Circ Res*. 1973;33:190–197.

31. Duke HN. The site of action of anoxia on the pulmonary blood vessels of the cat. *J Physiol*. 1954;125:373.

32. Paredi P, Barnes PJ. The airway vasculature: recent advances and clinical implications. *Thorax*. 2009;64:444–450.

33. Mitzner W, Wagner EM. Vascular remodeling in the circulations of the lung. *J Appl Physiol*. 2004;97:1999–2004.

Chapter 3

Elastic forces and lung volumes

KEY POINTS

- Inward elastic recoil of the lung opposes outward elastic recoil of the chest wall, and the balance of these forces determines static lung volumes.
- Surface tension within the alveoli contributes significantly to lung recoil, and is reduced by the presence of surfactant, though the mechanism by which this occurs is poorly understood.
- Compliance is defined as the change in lung volume per unit change in pressure gradient, and may be measured for lung, thoracic cage or both.
- Various static lung volumes may be measured, and the volumes obtained are affected by a variety of physiological and pathological factors.

An isolated lung will tend to contract until eventually all the contained air is expelled. In contrast, when the thoracic cage is opened it tends to expand to a volume about 1 litre greater than functional residual capacity (FRC). Thus in a relaxed subject with an open airway and no air flowing, for example at the end of expiration or inspiration, the inward elastic recoil of the lungs is exactly balanced by the outward recoil of the thoracic cage.

The movements of the lungs are entirely passive and result from forces external to the lungs. In the case of spontaneous breathing the external forces are the respiratory muscles, while artificial ventilation is usually in response to a pressure gradient that is developed between the airway and the environment. In each case, the pattern of response by the lung is governed by the physical impedance of the respiratory system. This impedance, or hindrance, has numerous origins, the most important of which are:

- Elastic resistance of lung tissue and chest wall
- Resistance from surface forces at the alveolar gas/liquid interface
- Frictional resistance to gas flow through the airways
- Frictional resistance from deformation of thoracic tissues (viscoelastic tissue resistance)
- Inertia associated with movement of gas and tissue.

The last three may be grouped together as non-elastic resistance or respiratory system resistance; they are discussed in Chapter 4. They are measured while gas is flowing within the airways, and work performed in overcoming this 'frictional' resistance is dissipated as heat and lost.

The first two forms of impedance may be grouped together as 'elastic' resistance. These are measured when gas is not flowing within the lung. Work performed in overcoming elastic resistance is stored as potential energy, and elastic deformation during inspiration is the usual source of energy for expiration during both spontaneous and artificial breathing.

This chapter is concerned with the elastic resistance afforded by lungs (including the alveoli) and chest wall, which will be considered separately and then together. When the respiratory muscles are totally relaxed, these factors govern the resting end-expiratory lung volume or FRC, and therefore lung volumes will also be considered in this chapter.

DOI: 10.1016/B978-0-7020-2996-7.00003-9

ELASTIC RECOIL OF THE LUNGS

Lung compliance is defined as the change in lung volume per unit change in transmural pressure gradient (i.e. between the alveolus and pleural space). Compliance is usually expressed in litres (or millilitres) per kilopascal (or centimetres of water) with a normal value of 1.5 l.kPa^{-1} (150 ml.cmH$_2$O^{-1}). Stiff lungs have a low compliance.

Compliance may be described as static or dynamic depending on the method of measurement (page 38). Static compliance is measured after a lung volume has been held at a fixed volume for as long as is practicable, while dynamic compliance is usually measured in the course of normal rhythmic breathing. Elastance is the reciprocal of compliance and is expressed in kilopascals per litre. Stiff lungs have a high elastance.

THE NATURE OF THE FORCES CAUSING RECOIL OF THE LUNG

For many years it was thought that the recoil of the lung was due entirely to stretching of the yellow elastin fibres present in the lung parenchyma. In 1929, von Neergaard (page 243) showed that a lung completely filled with and immersed in water had an elastance that was much less than the normal value obtained when the lung was filled with air. He correctly concluded that much of the 'elastic recoil' was due to surface tension acting throughout the vast air/water interface lining the alveoli.

Surface tension at an air/water interface produces forces that tend to reduce the area of the interface. Thus the gas pressure within a bubble is always higher than the surrounding gas pressure because the surface of the bubble is in a state of tension. Alveoli resemble bubbles in this respect, although the alveolar gas is connected to the exterior by the air passages. The pressure inside a bubble is higher than the surrounding pressure by an amount depending on the surface tension of the liquid and the radius of curvature of the bubble according to the Laplace equation:

$$P = \frac{2T}{R}$$

where P is the pressure within the bubble (dyn. cm^{-2}), T is the surface tension of the liquid (dyn. cm^{-1}) and R is the radius of the bubble (cm). In coherent SI units (see Appendix A), the appropriate units would be pressure in pascals (Pa), surface tension in newtons/metre (N.m^{-1}) and radius in metres (m).

On the left of Figure 3.1A is shown a typical alveolus of radius 0.1 mm. Assuming that the alveolar lining fluid has a normal surface tension of 20 mN.m^{-1} (= 20 dyn.cm^{-1}), the pressure within the alveolus will be 0.4 kPa (4 cmH$_2$O), which is rather less than the normal transmural pressure at FRC. If the alveolar lining fluid had the same surface tension as water (72 mN.m^{-1}), the lungs would be very stiff.

The alveolus on the right of Figure 3.1A has a radius of only 0.05 mm and the Laplace equation indicates that, if the surface tension of the alveolus is the same, its pressure should be double the pressure in the left-hand alveolus. Thus gas would tend to flow from smaller alveoli into larger alveoli and the lung would be unstable which, of course, is not the case. Similarly, the retractive forces of the alveolar lining fluid would increase at low lung volumes and decrease at high lung volumes, which is exactly the reverse of what is observed. These paradoxes were clear to von Neergaard and he concluded that the surface tension of the alveolar lining fluid must be considerably less than would be expected from the properties of simple liquids and, furthermore, that its value must be variable. Observations 30 years later confirmed this when alveolar extracts were shown to have a surface tension much lower than water and which varied in proportion to the area of the interface.[1] Figure 3.1B shows an experiment in which a floating bar is moved in a trough containing an alveolar extract. As the bar is moved to the right, the surface film is concentrated and the surface tension changes as shown in the graph on the right of the figure. During expansion, the surface tension increases to 40 mN.m^{-1}, a value which is close to that of plasma but, during contraction, the surface tension falls to 19 mN.m^{-1}, a lower value than any other body fluid. The course of the relationship between pressure and area is different during expansion and contraction, and a loop is described.

The consequences of these changes are very important. In contrast to a bubble of soap solution, the pressure within an alveolus tends to decrease as the radius of curvature is decreased. This is illustrated in Figure 3.1C where the right-hand alveolus has a smaller diameter and a much lower surface tension than the left-hand alveolus. Gas tends to flow from the larger to the smaller alveolus and stability is maintained.

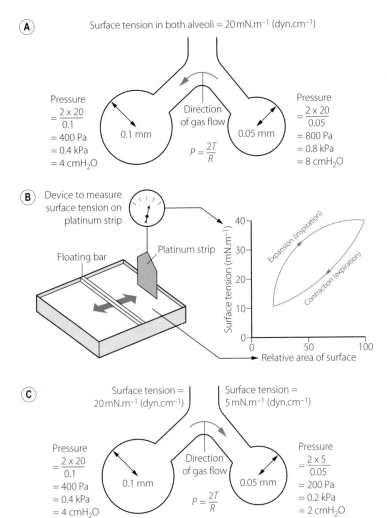

(A) Surface tension in both alveoli = 20 mN.m^{-1} (dyn.cm^{-1})

Pressure
$= \dfrac{2 \times 20}{0.1}$
$= 400$ Pa
$= 0.4$ kPa
$= 4$ cmH$_2$O

0.1 mm

Direction of gas flow

$P = \dfrac{2T}{R}$

0.05 mm

Pressure
$= \dfrac{2 \times 20}{0.05}$
$= 800$ Pa
$= 0.8$ kPa
$= 8$ cmH$_2$O

(B) Device to measure surface tension on platinum strip

Floating bar

Platinum strip

Surface tension (mN.m^{-1})

40 —
30 —
20 —
10 —
0 —

Expansion (inspiration)

Contraction (expiration)

0   50   100
Relative area of surface

(C) Surface tension = 20 mN.m^{-1} (dyn.cm^{-1})   Surface tension = 5 mN.m^{-1} (dyn.cm^{-1})

Pressure
$= \dfrac{2 \times 20}{0.1}$
$= 400$ Pa
$= 0.4$ kPa
$= 4$ cmH$_2$O

0.1 mm

Direction of gas flow

$P = \dfrac{2T}{R}$

0.05 mm

Pressure
$= \dfrac{2 \times 5}{0.05}$
$= 200$ Pa
$= 0.2$ kPa
$= 2$ cmH$_2$O

Fig. 3.1 Surface tension and alveolar transmural pressure. (A) Pressure relations in two alveoli of different size but with the same surface tension of their lining fluids. (B) The changes in surface tension in relation to the area of the alveolar lining film. (C) Pressure relations of two alveoli of different size when allowance is made for the probable changes in surface tension.

THE ALVEOLAR SURFACTANT

The low surface tension of the alveolar lining fluid and its dependence on alveolar radius are due to the presence of a surface-active material known as the surfactant.[2] Some 90% of surfactant consists of lipids, the remainder being proteins and small amounts of carbohydrate. Most of the lipid is phospholipid, of which 70–80% is dipalmitoyl phosphatidyl choline (DPPC), the main constituent responsible for the effect on surface tension. The fatty acids are hydrophobic and generally straight, lying parallel to each other and projecting into the gas phase. The other end of the molecule is hydrophilic and lies within the alveolar lining fluid. The molecule is thus confined to the surface where, being detergents, they lower surface tension in proportion to the concentration at the interface.

Around 10% of surfactant obtained from bronchio-alveolar lavage is protein, most of which are contaminating serum proteins such as albumin and globulin. Approximately 2% of surfactant by weight consists of surfactant proteins (SP), of which there are four types labelled A–D.[3,4] SP-B and SP-C are small proteins that are vital to the stabilisation of the surfactant monolayer (see below); a congenital lack of SP-B results in severe and progressive respiratory failure.[4,5] SP-A, and to a lesser extent SP-D, are involved in the control of surfactant release and possibly in preventing pulmonary infection (see below).[6]

Synthesis of surfactant. Surfactant is both formed in and liberated from the alveolar epithelial type II cell (page 23). The lamellar bodies (see Figure 2.10) contain stored surfactant that is released into the alveolus by exocytosis in response to high volume lung inflation, increased ventilation rate or endocrine stimulation. After release surfactant initially forms areas of a lattice structure termed tubular myelin, which is then reorganised into mono- or multi-layered surface films. This conversion into the functionally active form of surfactant is believed to be critically dependent on surfactant proteins B and C (see below).[4,6] The alveolar half life of surfactant is 15–30 hours with most of its components being recycled by type II alveolar cells. Surfactant protein-A is intimately involved in controlling the surfactant present in the alveolus with type II alveolar cells having SP-A surface receptors, stimulation of which exerts a negative feedback on surfactant secretion and increases re-uptake of surfactant components into the cell.

Action of surfactant. To maintain the stability of alveoli as shown in Figure 3.1, surfactant must alter the surface tension in the alveoli as their size varies with inspiration and expiration. A simple explanation of how this occurs is that during expiration, as the surface area of the alveolus diminishes, the surfactant molecules are packed more densely and so exert a greater effect on the surface tension, which then decreases as shown in Figure 3.1b. In reality, the situation is considerably more complex, and at present poorly elucidated.[4] The classical explanation, referred to as the 'squeeze out' hypothesis, is that as a surfactant monolayer is compressed, the less stable phospholipids are squeezed out of the layer, increasing the amount of stable DPPC molecules which have the greatest effect in reducing surface tension.[7] Surfactant phospholipid is also known to exist in vivo in both monolayer and multilayer forms,[3] and it is possible that in some areas of the alveoli the surfactant layer alternates between these two forms as alveolar size changes during the respiratory cycle. This aspect of surfactant function is entirely dependent on the presence of SP-B, a small hydrophobic protein, which can be incorporated into a phospholipid monolayer, and SP-C, a larger protein with a hydrophobic central portion allowing it to span a lipid bilayer.[4] When alveolar size reduces and the surface film is compressed, SP-B molecules may be squeezed out of the lipid layer so changing its surface properties, while SP-C may serve to stabilise bilayers of lipid to act as a reservoir from which the surface film re-forms when alveolar size increases.

Other effects of surfactant. Pulmonary transudation is also affected by surface forces. Surface tension causes the pressure within the alveolar lining fluid to be less than the alveolar pressure. Since the pulmonary capillary pressure in most of the lung is greater than the alveolar pressure (page 420), both factors encourage transudation, a tendency that is checked by the oncotic pressure of the plasma proteins. Thus the surfactant, by reducing surface tension, diminishes one component of the pressure gradient and helps to prevent transudation.

Surfactant also plays an important part in the immunology of the lung.[2,8,9] The lipid component of surfactant has anti-oxidant activity, so may attenuate lung damage from a variety of causes, and also suppresses some groups of lymphocytes so theoretically protecting the lungs from auto-immune damage. In-vitro studies have shown that SP-A or SP-D can bind to a wide range of pulmonary pathogens including viruses, bacteria, fungi, *Pneumocystis carinii*, and *Mycobacterium tuberculosis*. Acting via specific surface receptors, both SP-A and SP-D activate alveolar neutrophils and macrophages, and enhance the phagocytic actions of the latter during lung inflammation.[9]

ALTERNATIVE MODELS TO EXPLAIN LUNG RECOIL

Treating surfactant-lined alveoli as bubbles that obey Laplace's law has aided the understanding of lung recoil in health and disease for many decades (page 243). This 'bubble model' of alveolar stability is not universally accepted,[10,11] and evidence is mounting that the real situation is more complex. Arguments against the bubble model include:

- in theory, differing surface tensions in adjacent alveoli cannot occur if the liquid lining the alveoli is connected by a continuous liquid layer
- when surfactant layers are compressed at 37°C multilayered 'rafts' of dry surfactant form, though inclusion of surfactant proteins reduces this physico-chemical change
- alveoli are not shaped like perfect spheres with a single entrance point – they are variable polyhedrons with convex bulges in their walls where pulmonary capillaries bulge into them (Figure 2.7).

Two quite different alternative models have been proposed:

Morphological model. Hills has for many years claimed that the surfactant lining alveoli results in a 'discontinuous' liquid lining.[12,13] Based on knowledge of the physical chemistry of surfactants, Hills's

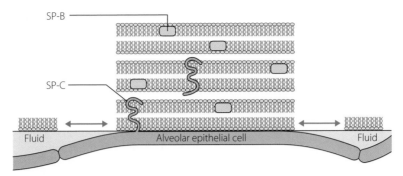

Fig. 3.2 Morphological model of alveolar surfactant. Multilayered, less wettable, 'rafts' of surfactant are interspersed with fluid pools. Surfactant proteins lie within (SP-B) or across (SP-C) the lipid bilayers, facilitating the formation and dispersion of the rafts with each breath to modify the surface forces within the alveolus. (Reproduced with permission from Webster NR, Galley HF. Anaesthesia Science. Oxford: Blackwell Publishing, 2006.)

model shows that surfactant phospholipids are adsorbed directly onto the epithelial cell surface, forming multilayered 'rafts' of surfactant (Figure 3.2). These rafts cause patches of the surface to become less wettable, these areas being interspersed with fluid pools. Surface forces generated by the interaction between the 'dry' areas of surfactant and the areas of liquid are theoretically large enough to maintain alveolar stability. The rafts of surfactant may be many layers thick, and are believed to form and disperse with each breath, their function almost certainly being dependent on both SP-B and SP-C.

Foam model. Scarpelli has developed new techniques for preparing lung tissue for microscopy.[14] By maintaining tissue in a more natural state than previous studies, including keeping lung volume close to normal, he has described a 'new anatomy' for alveoli. Scarpelli's findings seem to show that in vivo alveoli have bubble films across their entrances, with similar lipid bilayer films also existing across alveolar ducts and respiratory bronchioles (Figure 3.3). In this model, each acinus may be considered as a series of interconnected, but closed, bubbles so forming a stable 'foam'. The bubble films are estimated to be less than 7 nm thick[15] so will offer little resistance to gas diffusion, the normal mechanism by which gas movement occurs in a single pulmonary acinus (page 19).

More research is clearly needed to either confirm or refute these models. It would therefore be premature to consign the well-established bubble model of alveolar recoil to the history books, but physiologists should be aware that cracks have begun to appear in a longstanding physiological concept.

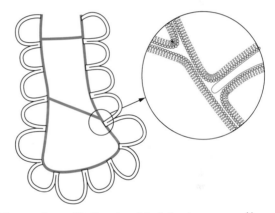

Fig. 3.3 Scarpelli's 'foam' model of alveolar structure.[14] Surfactant (blue) lines the alveoli, and forms films that span both the alveolar openings and the alveolar ducts. Inset: detail of the surfactant layer showing connection between phospholipid monolayer and bilayer (not to scale).

THE TRANSMURAL PRESSURE GRADIENT AND INTRATHORACIC PRESSURE

The transmural pressure gradient is the difference between intrathoracic (or 'intrapleural') and alveolar pressure. The pressure within an alveolus is always greater than the pressure to the surrounding interstitial tissue except when the volume has been reduced to zero. With increasing lung volume, the transmural pressure gradient steadily increases as shown for the whole lung in Figure 3.4. If an appreciable pneumothorax is present, the pressure gradient from alveolus to pleural cavity provides a measure of the overall transmural pressure gradient. Otherwise, the oesophageal pressure may be used to indicate the

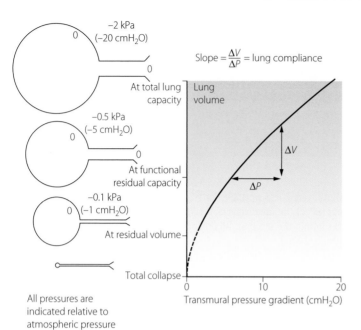

Slope $= \dfrac{\Delta V}{\Delta P} =$ lung compliance

Fig. 3.4 Relationship between lung volume and the difference in pressure between the alveoli and the intrathoracic space (transmural pressure gradient). The relationship is almost linear over the normal tidal volume range. The calibre of small air passages decreases in parallel with alveolar volume. Airways begin to close at the closing capacity and there is widespread airway closure at residual volume. Values in the diagram relate to the upright position and to *decreasing* pressure. The opening pressure of a closed alveolus is not shown.

pleural pressure, but there are conceptual and technical difficulties. The technical difficulties are considered at the end of this chapter while some of the conceptual difficulties are indicated in Figure 3.5.

The alveoli in the upper part of the lung have a larger volume than those in the dependent part except at total lung capacity. The greater degree of expansion of the alveoli in the upper part results in a greater transmural pressure gradient, which decreases steadily down the lung at about 0.1 kPa (or 1 cmH$_2$O) per 3 cm of vertical height; such a difference is indicated in Figure 3.5A. Since the pleural cavity is normally empty, it is not strictly correct to speak of an intrapleural pressure and, furthermore, it would not be constant throughout the pleural 'cavity'. One should think rather of the relationship shown in Figure 3.4 as applying to various horizontal strata of the lung, each with its own volume and therefore its own transmural pressure gradient on which its own 'intrapleural' pressure would depend. The transmural pressure gradient has an important influence on many aspects of pulmonary function and so its horizontal stratification confers a regional difference on many features of pulmonary function, including airway closure, ventilation/perfusion ratios, and therefore gas exchange. These matters are considered in detail in the appropriate chapters of this book.

At first sight it might be thought that the subatmospheric intrapleural pressure would result in the accumulation of gas evolved from solution in blood

and tissues. In fact the total of the partial pressures of gases dissolved in blood, and therefore tissues, is always less than one atmosphere (see Table 26.2), and this factor keeps the pleural cavity free of gas.

TIME DEPENDENCE OF PULMONARY ELASTIC BEHAVIOUR

If an excised lung is rapidly inflated and then held at the new volume, the inflation pressure falls exponentially from its initial value to reach a lower level that is attained after a few seconds. This also occurs in the intact subject, and is readily observed during an inspiratory pause in a patient receiving artificial ventilation (page 39). It is broadly true to say that the volume change divided by the initial change in transmural pressure gradient corresponds to the dynamic compliance while the volume change divided by the ultimate change in transmural pressure gradient (i.e. measured after it has become steady) corresponds to the static compliance. Static compliance will thus be greater than the dynamic compliance by an amount determined by the degree of time dependence in the elastic behaviour of a particular lung. The respiratory frequency has been shown to influence dynamic pulmonary compliance in the normal subject but frequency dependence is much more pronounced in the presence of pulmonary disease.

Hysteresis. If the lungs are slowly inflated and then slowly deflated, the pressure/volume curve

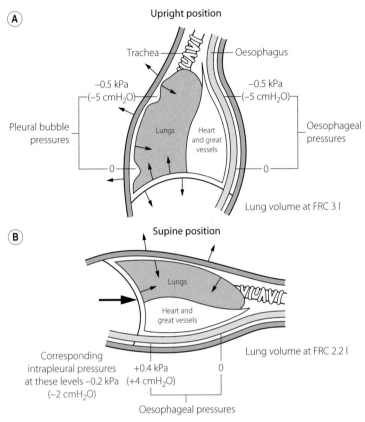

(A) Upright position

Trachea

Oesophagus

−0.5 kPa
(−5 cmH₂O)

−0.5 kPa
(−5 cmH₂O)

Pleural bubble pressures

Lungs   Heart and great vessels

Oesophageal pressures

0   0

Lung volume at FRC 3 l

(B) Supine position

Lungs

Heart and great vessels

Lung volume at FRC 2.2 l

Corresponding intrapleural pressures at these levels −0.2 kPa
(−2 cmH₂O)   +0.4 kPa
(+4 cmH₂O)   0

Oesophageal pressures

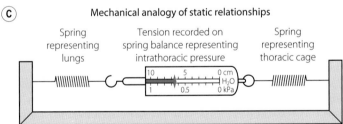

(C) Mechanical analogy of static relationships

Spring representing lungs

Tension recorded on spring balance representing intrathoracic pressure

Spring representing thoracic cage

10   5   0 cm
H₂O
1   0.5   0 kPa

Fig. 3.5 Intrathoracic pressures: static relationships in the resting end-expiratory position. The lung volume corresponds to the functional residual capacity (FRC). The figures in (A) and (B) indicate the pressure relative to ambient (atmospheric). The arrows show the direction of elastic forces. The heavy arrow in (B) indicates displacement by the abdominal viscera. In (C) the tension in the two springs is the same and will be indicated on the spring balance. In the supine position: (1) the FRC is reduced; (2) the intrathoracic pressure is raised; (3) the weight of the heart raises the oesophageal pressure above the intrapleural pressure.

for static points during inflation differs from that obtained during deflation. The two curves form a loop, which becomes progressively broader as the tidal volume is increased (Figure 3.6). Expressed in words, the loop in Figure 3.6 means that rather more than the expected pressure is required during inflation and rather less than the expected recoil pressure is available during deflation. This resembles the behaviour of perished rubber or polyvinyl chloride, both of which are reluctant to accept deformation under stress but, once deformed, are again reluctant to assume their original shape. This phenomenon is present to a greater or lesser extent in all elastic bodies and is known as elastic hysteresis.

CAUSES OF TIME DEPENDENCE OF PULMONARY ELASTIC BEHAVIOUR

There are many possible explanations of the time dependence of pulmonary elastic behaviour, the relative importance of which may vary in different circumstances.

Changes in surfactant activity. It has been explained above that the surface tension of the alveolar lining fluid is greater at larger lung volume and also during inspiration than at the same lung volume during expiration (Figure 3.1B). This is probably the most important cause of the observed hysteresis in the intact lung (Figure 3.6).

Stress relaxation. If a spring is pulled out to a fixed increase in its length, the resultant tension is

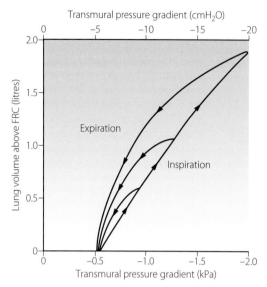

Fig. 3.6 Static plot of lung volume against transmural pressure gradient (intra-oesophageal pressure relative to atmospheric at zero air flow). Note that inspiratory and expiratory curves form a loop that gets wider the greater the tidal volume. These loops are typical of elastic hysteresis. For a particular lung volume, the elastic recoil of the lung during expiration is always less than the distending transmural pressure gradient required during inspiration at the same lung volume.

maximal at first and then declines exponentially to a constant value. This is an inherent property of elastic bodies, known as stress relaxation. Thoracic tissues display stress relaxation and these 'visco-elastic' properties contribute significantly to the difference between static and dynamic compliance as well as forming a component of pulmonary resistance (page 46). The crinkled structure of collagen in the lung is likely to favour stress relaxation and excised strips of human lung show stress relaxation when stretched.

Redistribution of gas. In a lung consisting of functional units with identical time constants[*] of inflation, the distribution of gas should be independent of the rate of inflation, and there should be no redistribution when the lungs are held inflated. However, if different parts of the lungs have different time constants,

the distribution of inspired gas will be dependent on the rate of inflation and redistribution ('pendel-luft') will occur when inflation is held. This problem is discussed in greater detail on page 121 but for the time being we can distinguish 'fast' and 'slow' alveoli (the term 'alveoli' here referring to functional units rather than the anatomical entity). The 'fast' alveolus has a low airway resistance and/or low compliance (or both) while the 'slow' alveolus has a high airway resistance and/or a high compliance (Figure 3.7B). These properties give the fast alveolus a shorter time constant and are preferentially filled during a short inflation. This preferential filling of alveoli with low compliance gives an overall higher pulmonary transmural pressure gradient. A slow or sustained inflation permits increased distribution of gas to slow alveoli and so tends to distribute gas in accord with the compliance of the different functional units. There should then be a lower overall transmural pressure and no redistribution of gas when inflation is held. The extreme difference between fast and slow alveoli shown in Figure 3.7B applies to diseased lungs and no such differences exist in normal lungs. Gas redistribution is therefore unlikely to be a major factor in healthy subjects, but it can be important in patients with airways disease.

Recruitment of alveoli. Below a certain lung volume, some alveoli tend to close and only reopen at a considerably greater lung volume and in response to a much higher transmural pressure gradient than that at which they closed. Recruitment of closed alveoli appears at first sight to be a plausible explanation of all the time-dependent phenomena described above, but there are two reasons why this is unlikely. First, the pressure required for reopening a closed unit is very high and is unlikely to be achieved during normal breathing. Secondly, there is no histological evidence for collapsed alveoli in normal lungs at functional residual capacity. In the presence of pathological lung collapse, a sustained deep inflation may well cause re-expansion and an increased compliance, e.g. during anaesthesia (page 336). Cyclical opening and closing of alveoli during a normal respiratory cycle is unlikely in normal lungs but does occur in injured lungs (page 482).

FACTORS AFFECTING LUNG COMPLIANCE

Lung volume. It is important to remember that compliance is related to lung volume. This factor may be excluded by relating compliance to FRC to yield the specific compliance (i.e. compliance/FRC), which in

---

[*] Time constants are used to describe the exponential filling and emptying of a lung unit. One time constant is the time taken to achieve 63% of maximal inflation or deflation of the lung unit. See Appendix E for details.

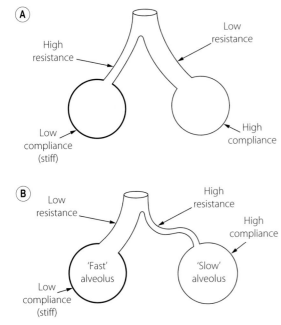

Fig. 3.7 Schematic diagrams of alveoli to illustrate conditions under which static and dynamic compliance may differ. (A) Represents a theoretically ideal state in which there is a reciprocal relationship between resistance and compliance resulting in gas flow being preferentially delivered to the most compliant regions, regardless of the state of inflation. Static and dynamic compliance are equal. This situation is probably never realised even in the normal subject. (B) Illustrates a state that is typical of many patients with respiratory disease. The alveoli can conveniently be divided into 'fast' and 'slow' groups. The direct relationship between compliance and resistance results in inspired gas being preferentially delivered to the stiff alveoli if the rate of inflation is rapid. An end-inspiratory pause then permits redistribution from the fast alveoli to the slow alveoli.

humans is almost constant for both sexes and all ages down to neonatal. The relationship between compliance and lung volume is true not only within an individual lung but also between species. Larger animal species have thicker alveolar septae containing increased amounts of collagen and elastin resulting in larger alveolar diameters,[16] so reducing the pressure needed to expand them. An elephant therefore has larger alveoli and so a higher compliance than a mouse.

Posture. Lung volume, and therefore compliance, changes with posture (page 37). There are however problems in the measurement of intrapleural pressure in the supine position and when this is taken into account it seems unlikely that changes of posture have any significant effect on the specific compliance.

Pulmonary blood volume. The pulmonary blood vessels probably make an appreciable contribution to the stiffness of the lung. Pulmonary venous congestion from whatever cause is associated with reduced compliance.

Age. One would have expected age to influence the elasticity of the lung as of other tissues in the body. However, no correlation has ever been found between age and compliance, even after allowing for predicted changes in lung volume. This accords with the concept of lung 'elasticity' being largely determined by surface forces.

Bronchial smooth muscle tone. Animal studies[17] have shown that an infusion of methacholine sufficient to result in a doubling of airway resistance decreases dynamic compliance by 50%. The airways might contribute to overall compliance or, alternatively, bronchoconstriction could enhance time-dependence and so reduce dynamic, but perhaps not static compliance (Figure 3.7).

Disease. Important changes in lung pressure/volume relationships are found in some lung diseases, and these are described in the relevant chapters in Part 3.

ELASTIC RECOIL OF THE THORACIC CAGE

The thoracic cage comprises the ribcage and the diaphragm. Each is a muscular structure and can be considered as an elastic structure only when the muscles are relaxed, and that is not easy to achieve except under the conditions of paralysis. Relaxation curves have been prepared relating pressure and volumes in the supposedly relaxed subject, but it is now doubted whether total relaxation was ever achieved. For example, in the supine position the diaphragm is not fully relaxed at the end of expiration but maintains a resting tone to prevent the abdominal contents pushing the diaphragm cephalad.

Compliance of the thoracic cage is defined as change in lung volume per unit change in the pressure gradient between atmosphere and the intrapleural space. The units are the same as for pulmonary compliance. The measurement is seldom made but the value is of the order of $2 \, \mathrm{l.kPa}^{-1}$ ($200 \, \mathrm{ml.cmH_2O}^{-1}$).

FACTORS INFLUENCING COMPLIANCE OF THE THORACIC CAGE

Anatomical factors include the ribs and the state of ossification of the costal cartilages. Obesity and even pathological skin conditions may have an appreciable effect. In particular, scarring of the skin overlying the front of the chest may result from scalding in children and this may embarrass the breathing.

In terms of compliance, a relaxed diaphragm simply transmits pressure from the abdomen that may be increased in obesity and abdominal distension. Posture clearly has a major effect and this is considered below in relation to FRC. Compared with the supine position, thoracic cage compliance is 30% greater in the seated subject and the total static compliance of the respiratory system is reduced by 60% in the prone position due to the diminished elasticity of the ribcage and diaphragm when prone.

PRESSURE/VOLUME RELATIONSHIPS OF THE LUNG PLUS THORACIC CAGE

Compliance is analogous to electrical capacitance, and in the respiratory system the compliances of lungs and thoracic cage are in series. Therefore the total compliance of the system obeys the same relationship as for capacitances in series, in which reciprocals are added to obtain the reciprocal of the total value, thus:

$$\cfrac{1}{\text{total compliance}} = \cfrac{1}{\text{lung compliance}} + \cfrac{1}{\text{thoracic cage compliance}}$$

typical static values ($l.kPa^{-1}$) for the supine paralysed patient being:

$$\frac{1}{0.85} = \frac{1}{1.5} + \frac{1}{2}$$

Instead of compliance, we may consider its reciprocal, elastance. The relationship is then much simpler:

Total elastance =
       lung elastance + thoracic cage elastance

corresponding values ($kPa.l^{-1}$) are then:

$$1.17 = 0.67 + 0.5$$

RELATIONSHIP BETWEEN ALVEOLAR, INTRATHORACIC AND AMBIENT PRESSURES

At all times the alveolar/ambient pressure gradient is the sum of the alveolar/intrathoracic (or transmural)

and intrathoracic/ambient pressure gradients. This relationship is independent of whether the patient is breathing spontaneously or being ventilated by intermittent positive pressure. Actual values depend on compliances, lung volume and posture and typical values are shown for the upright conscious relaxed subject in Figure 3.8. The values in the illustration are static and relate to conditions when no gas is flowing.

LUNG VOLUMES

Certain lung volumes, particularly the FRC, are determined by elastic forces. This is therefore a convenient point at which to consider the various lung volumes and their subdivision (Figure 3.9).

Total lung capacity (TLC). This is the volume of gas in the lungs at the end of a maximal inspiration. TLC is achieved when the maximal force generated by the inspiratory muscles is balanced by the forces opposing expansion. It is rather surprising that expiratory muscles are also contracting strongly at the end of a maximal inspiration.

Residual volume (RV). This is the volume remaining after a maximal expiration. In the young, RV is governed by the balance between the maximal force generated by expiratory muscles and the elastic forces opposing reduction of lung volume. However, in older subjects closure of small airways may prevent further expiration.

Functional residual capacity. This is the lung volume at the end of a normal expiration.

Within the framework of TLC, RV and FRC, the other capacities and volumes shown in Figure 3.9 are self-explanatory.

FACTORS AFFECTING THE FRC

So many factors affect the FRC that they require a special section of this chapter. The actual volume of the FRC has particular importance because of its relationship to the closing capacity (see below).

Sex. For the same body height, females have an FRC about 10% less than males.

Age. FRC increases slightly with age, increasing by around 16 ml per year.

Body size. FRC is linearly related to height. Obesity causes a marked reduction in FRC compared with lean subjects of the same height.

Taking these factors into account equations can be used to calculate a normal value for FRC in any individual, for example in white male adults aged between 25–65 years:[18]

Spontaneous respiration

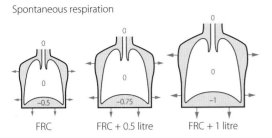

Intermittent positive-pressure ventilation

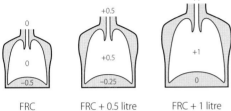

Figures denote pressure relative to atmosphere (kPa)

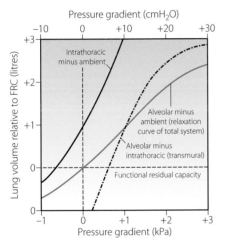

Fig. 3.8 Static pressure/volume relations for the intact thorax for the conscious subject in the upright position. The transmural pressure gradient bears the same relationship to lung volume during both intermittent positive pressure ventilation and spontaneous breathing. The intrathoracic-to-ambient pressure difference, however, differs in the two types of ventilation due to muscle action during spontaneous respiration. At all times: alveolar/ambient pressure difference = alveolar/intrathoracic pressure difference + intrathoracic/ambient pressure difference (due attention being paid to the sign of the pressure difference).

$$FRC = (5.95 \times height) + (0.019 \times age) - (0.086 \times BMI) - 5.3$$

Where FRC is in litres, height in meters, age in years, and BMI (body mass index) in $kg.m^{-2}$.

Diaphragmatic muscle tone. FRC has in the past been considered to be simply the volume at which there is a balance between the elastic forces represented by the inward retraction of the lungs and the outward expansion of the thoracic cage. However, as explained above, it now appears that residual end-expiratory muscle tone is a major factor in the supine position, maintaining the FRC about 400 ml above the volume in the totally relaxed subject, which in practice means paralysed during anaesthesia.

Posture. Figures 3.5 and 3.10 show the reduction in FRC in the supine position, which may be attributed to the increased pressure of the abdominal contents on the diaphragm. Values of FRC in these figures and Table 3.1 are typical for a subject of 1.68–1.70 m height, and reported mean differences between supine and upright positions range from 500 to 1000 ml. Values for FRC in other positions are shown in Table 3.1.

Lung disease. The FRC will be reduced by increased elastic recoil of the lungs, thoracic cage or both. Possible causes include lung fibrosis, pleural thickening, kyphoscoliosis, obesity and scarring of the thorax following burns. Conversely, elastic recoil of the lungs is diminished in emphysema and asthma and the FRC is usually increased (Chapter 28). This is beneficial since airway resistance decreases as the lung volume increases.

FRC IN RELATION TO CLOSING CAPACITY

In Chapter 4 it is explained how reduction in lung volume below a certain level results in airway closure with relative or total underventilation in the dependent parts of the lung. The lung volume below which this effect becomes apparent is known as the closing capacity (CC). With increasing age, CC rises until it equals FRC at around 70–75 years in the upright position but only 44 in the supine position (Figure 3.11). This is a major factor in the decrease of arterial Po_2 with age (page 194).

PRINCIPLES OF MEASUREMENT OF COMPLIANCE

Compliance is measured as the change in lung volume divided by the corresponding change in the appropriate pressure gradient, there being no gas flow when the two measurements are made. For lung compliance the appropriate pressure gradient is alveolar/intrapleural (or intrathoracic) and for the

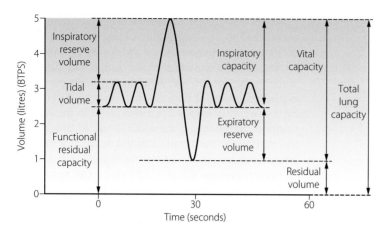

Fig. 3.9 Static lung volumes of Dr Nunn in 1990. The 'spirometer curve' indicates the lung volumes that can be measured by simple spirometry. These are tidal volume, inspiratory reserve volume, inspiratory capacity, expiratory reserve volume and vital capacity. The residual volume, total lung capacity and functional residual capacity cannot be measured by observation of a spirometer without further elaboration of methods. BTPS, body temperature and pressure, saturated.

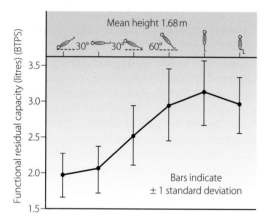

Fig. 3.10 Studies by Dr Nunn and his co-workers of the functional residual capacity in various body positions.

Table 3.1 Effect of posture on some aspects of respiratory function[19]

POSITION	FRC (LITRES) (BTPS)	RIBCAGE BREATHING* (%)	FORCED EXPIRATORY VOLUME IN 1 SECOND (LITRES) (BTPS)
Sitting	2.91	69.7	3.79
Supine	2.10	32.3	3.70
Supine (arms up)	2.36	33.0	3.27
Prone	2.45	32.6	3.49
Lateral	2.44	36.5	3.67

Data for 13 healthy males aged 24–64.
*Proportion of breathing accounted for by movement of the ribcage.

total compliance alveolar/ambient. Measurement of compliance of the thoracic cage is seldom undertaken but the appropriate pressure gradient would then be intrapleural/ambient, measured when the respiratory muscles are totally relaxed.

Volume may be measured with a spirometer, a body plethysmograph or by integration of a flow rate obtained from a pneumotachogram. Points of zero air flow are best indicated by a pneumotachogram. Static pressures can be measured with a simple water manometer but electrical transducers are now more usual. Intrathoracic pressure is normally measured as oesophageal pressure which, in the upright subject, is different at different levels. The pressure rises as the balloon descends, the change being roughly in accord with the specific gravity of the lung $(0.3\,g.ml^{-1})$. It is convention to measure the pressure

32–35 cm beyond the nares, the highest point at which the measurement is free from artefacts due to mouth pressure and tracheal and neck movements. Alveolar pressure equals mouth pressure when no gas is flowing: it cannot be measured directly.

Static compliance. In the conscious subject, a known volume of air is inhaled from FRC and the subject then relaxes against a closed airway. The various pressure gradients are then measured and compared with the resting values at FRC. It is, in fact, very difficult to ensure that the respiratory muscles are relaxed, but the measurement of lung compliance is valid since the static alveolar/intrathoracic pressure difference is unaffected by any muscle activity.

In the paralysed subject there are no difficulties about muscular relaxation and it is very easy to measure static compliance of the whole respiratory

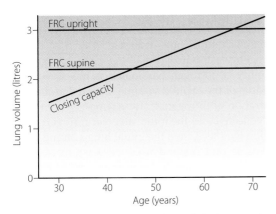

Fig. 3.11 Functional residual capacity and closing capacity as a function of age. (Data from reference 20.)

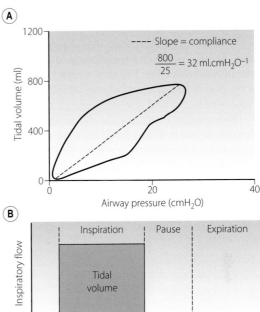

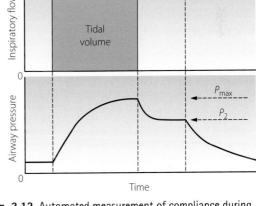

Fig. 3.12 Automated measurement of compliance during intermittent positive pressure ventilation. (A) Dynamic compliance. Simultaneous measurement of tidal volume and airway pressure creates a pressure/volume loop. End-expiratory and end-inspiratory 'no-flow' points occur when the trace is horizontal. At this point, airway pressure and alveolar pressure are equal, so the pressure gradient is the difference between alveolar and atmospheric pressure. Total respiratory system compliance is therefore the slope of the line between these points. Note that in this patient compliance is markedly reduced. (B) Static compliance. Following an end-inspiratory pause the plateau pressure is recorded (P_2) and along with tidal volume the static compliance easily derived. This manoeuvre also provides an assessment of respiratory system resistance by recording the pressure drop ($P_{max} - P_2$) and the inspiratory flow immediately before the inspiratory pause (see page 57).

system simply using recordings of airway pressure and respiratory volumes. However, due to the uncertainties about interpretation of the oesophageal pressure in the supine position (Figure 3.5), there is usually some uncertainty about the pulmonary compliance. For static compliance it is therefore easier to measure *lung* compliance in the upright position, and *total* compliance in the anaesthetised paralysed patient who will usually be in the supine position.

Dynamic compliance. These measurements are made during rhythmic breathing, but compliance is calculated from pressure and volume measurements made when no gas is flowing, usually at end-inspiratory and end-expiratory 'no-flow' points. The usual method involves creation of a pressure–volume loop by displaying simultaneously as *x* and *y* coordinates the required pressure gradient and the respired volume. In the resultant loop, as in Figure 3.12A, the 'no-flow' points are where the trace is horizontal and the dynamic compliance is the slope of the line joining these points.

AUTOMATED MEASUREMENT OF COMPLIANCE

In a spontaneously breathing awake patient lung compliance measurement is difficult because of the requirement to place an oesophageal balloon. However, in anaesthetised patients or those patients receiving intermittent positive pressure ventilation (IPPV) in intensive care the measurement of compliance is considerably easier. Many ventilators and anaesthetic monitoring systems now routinely measure airway pressure and tidal volume. This enables a pressure volume loop to be displayed (Figure 3.12A), from which the dynamic compliance of the respiratory system may be calculated on a continuous breath-by-breath basis. When no gas is flowing during IPPV (at the end of inspiration and expiration) the airway pressure equals alveolar pressure. At this point, the airway pressure recorded by the ventilator therefore equals the difference between alveolar and atmospheric pressure, allowing derivation of the total compliance.

Some ventilators will also measure static compliance. The ventilator will inflate the lung with the patient's usual tidal volume and then pause at end-inspiration for between 0.5 and 2 seconds, until the airway pressure falls to a plateau lasting 300 msec (Figure 3.12B). Static compliance is then calculated from the volume delivered and pressure recorded during the plateau and may be easily compared with dynamic compliance.

PRINCIPLES OF MEASUREMENT OF LUNG VOLUMES

Vital capacity, tidal volume, inspiratory reserve and expiratory reserve can all be measured with a simple spirometer (see Figure 3.9). Total lung capacity, FRC and RV all contain a fraction (the RV) that cannot be measured by simple spirometry. However, if one of these volumes is measured (most commonly the FRC), the others may easily be derived.

MEASUREMENT OF FRC[21]

Three techniques are available. The first employs nitrogen wash-out by breathing 100% oxygen. Total quantity of nitrogen eliminated is measured as the product of the expired volume collected and the concentration of nitrogen. If, for example, 4 l of nitrogen are collected and the initial alveolar nitrogen concentration was 80%, then the initial lung volume was 5 l.

The second method uses the wash-in of a tracer gas such as helium. If, for example, 50 ml of helium are introduced into the lungs and the helium concentration is then found to be 1%, the lung volume is 5 l. Helium is used for this method because of its low solubility in blood. For the technique to be accurate the measurement must be made rapidly or helium dissolving in the tissues and blood will introduce errors.

The third method uses the body plethysmograph. The subject is totally contained within a gas-tight box and he attempts to breathe against an occluded airway. Changes in alveolar pressure are recorded at the mouth and compared with the small changes in lung volume, derived from pressure changes within the plethysmograph. Application of Boyle's law then permits calculation of lung volume.

The last method is the only technique for FRC measurement that includes gas trapped within the lung distal to closed airways.

References

1. Brown ES, Johnson RP, Clements JA. Pulmonary surface tension. *J Appl Physiol*. 1959;14:717–720.

2. Hamm H, Kroegel C, Hohlfeld J. Surfactant: a review of its functions and relevance in adult respiratory disorders. *Respir Med*. 1996;90:251–270.

*3. Whitsett JA, Weaver TE. Hydrophobic surfactant proteins in lung function and disease. *N Engl J Med*. 2002;347:2141–2148.

*4. Weaver TE, Conkright JJ. Functions of surfactant proteins B and C. *Annu Rev Physiol*. 2001;63:555–578.

5. Whitsett J. Hereditary disorders of surfactant homeostasis cause acute and chronic lung disease in infancy. *Thorax*. 2008;63:295–296.

6. Hawgood S, Poulain FR. The pulmonary collectins and surfactant metabolism. *Annu Rev Physiol*. 2001;63:495–519.

*7. Zuo YY, Possmayer F. How does pulmonary surfactant reduce surface tension to very low values? *J Appl Physiol*. 2007;102:1733–1734.

8. Jain D, Atochina-Vasserman EN, Tomer Y, Kadire H, Beers MF. Surfactant protein D protects against acute hyperoxic lung injury. *Am J Respir Crit Care Med*. 2008;178:805–813.

9. Janssen WJ, McPhillips KA, Dickinson MG, et al. Surfactant proteins A and D suppress alveolar macrophage phagocytosis via interaction with SIRPa. *Am J Respir Crit Care Med*. 2008;178:158–167.

10. Dorrington KL, Young JD. Development of the concept of a liquid pulmonary alveolar lining layer. *Br J Anaesth*. 2001;86:614–617.

*11. Scarpelli EM, Hills BA. Opposing views on the alveolar surface, alveolar models, and the role of surfactant. *J Appl Physiol*. 2000;89:408–412.

12. Hills BA. What forces keep the airspaces of the lung dry? *Thorax*. 1982;37:713–717.

13. Hills BA. An alternative view of the role(s) of surfactant and the alveolar model. *J Appl Physiol*. 1999;87:1567–1583.

14. Scarpelli EM. The alveolar surface network: A new anatomy and its physiological significance. *Anat Rec*. 1998;251:491–527.

15. Pal SK, Lechuga J, Drikakis D. On the controversy of the alveolar structure: a molecular dynamics study. *Br J Anaes*. 2008;100. 578P.

16. Mercer RE, Russell ML, Crapo JD. Alveolar septal structure in different species. *J Appl Physiol*. 1994;77:1060–1066.

17. Mitzner W, Blosser S, Yager D, Wagner E. Effect of bronchial smooth muscle contraction on lung compliance. *J Appl Physiol*. 1992;72:158–167.

18. Cotes JE, Chinn DJ, Miller MR. *Lung function. Physiology, measurement and application in medicine*. Oxford: Blackwell Publishing; 2006.

19. Lumb AB, Nunn JF. Respiratory function and ribcage contribution to ventilation in body positions commonly used during anesthesia. *Anesth Analg*. 1991;73:422–426.

20. Leblanc P, Ruff F, Milic-Emili J. Effects of age and body position on 'airway closure' in man. *J Appl Physiol*. 1970;28:448–453.

21. Wanger J, Clausen JL, Coates A, et al. Standardisation of the measurement of lung volumes. *Eur Respir J*. 2005;26:511–522.

Chapter 4

Respiratory system resistance

KEY POINTS

- Gas flow in the airway is a mixture of laminar and turbulent flow, becoming more laminar in smaller airways.
- Respiratory system resistance is a combination of resistance to gas flow in the airways and resistance to deformation of tissues of both the lung and chest wall.
- In smaller airways smooth muscle controls airway diameter under the influence of neural, humoral and cellular mechanisms.
- The respiratory system can rapidly compensate for increases in either inspiratory or expiratory resistance.

Elastic resistance, which occurs when no gas is flowing, results from only two of the numerous causes of impedance to inflation of the lung (listed in the previous chapter). This chapter considers the remaining components, which together are referred to as non-elastic resistance or respiratory system resistance. Most non-elastic resistance is provided by frictional resistance to airflow and thoracic tissue deformation (both lung and chest wall), with small contributions from the inertia of gas and tissue, and compression of intrathoracic gas.[1] Unlike elastic resistance, work performed against non-elastic resistance is not stored as potential energy (and therefore recoverable), but is lost and dissipated as heat.

PHYSICAL PRINCIPLES OF GAS FLOW AND RESISTANCE

Gas flows from a region of high pressure to one of lower pressure. The rate at which it does so is a function of the pressure difference and the resistance to gas flow, thus being analogous to the flow of an electrical current (Figure 4.1). The precise relationship between pressure difference and flow rate depends on the nature of the flow which may be laminar, turbulent or a mixture of the two. It is useful to consider laminar and turbulent flow as two separate entities but mixed patterns of flow

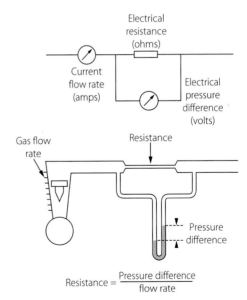

$$\text{Resistance} = \frac{\text{Pressure difference}}{\text{flow rate}}$$

Fig. 4.1 Electrical analogy of gas flow. Resistance is pressure difference per unit flow rate. Resistance to gas flow is analogous to electrical resistance (provided that flow is laminar). Gas flow corresponds to electrical current (amps); gas pressure to potential difference (volts); gas flow resistance to electrical resistance (ohms); and Poiseuille's law corresponds to Ohm's law.

DOI: 10.1016/B978-0-7020-2996-7.00004-0

usually occur in the respiratory tract. With a number of important caveats, similar basic considerations apply to the flow of liquids through tubes, which is considered in Chapter 7.

LAMINAR FLOW

With laminar flow, gas flows along a straight unbranched tube as a series of concentric cylinders that slide over one another, with the peripheral cylinder stationary and the central cylinder moving fastest, the advancing cone forming a parabola (Figure 4.2A).

The advancing cone front means that some fresh gas will reach the end of a tube while the volume entering the tube is still less than the volume of the tube. In the context of the respiratory tract, this is to say that there may be significant alveolar ventilation when the tidal volume is less than the volume of the airways (the anatomical dead space), a fact that is very relevant to high frequency ventilation (page 473).

For the same reason, laminar flow is relatively inefficient for purging the contents of a tube.

In theory, gas adjacent to the tube wall is stationary, so friction between fluid and the tube wall is negligible. The physical characteristics of the airway or vessel wall should therefore not affect resistance to laminar flow. Similarly, the composition of gas sampled from the periphery of a tube during laminar flow may not be representative of the gas advancing down the centre of the tube. To complicate matters further, laminar flow requires a critical length of tubing before the characteristic advancing cone pattern can be established. This is known as the entrance length and is related to the diameter of the tube and the Reynolds' number of the fluid (see below).

Quantitative relationships. With laminar flow the gas flow rate is directly proportional to the pressure gradient along the tube (Figure 4.2B), the constant being thus defined as resistance to gas flow:

$$\Delta P = \text{flow rate} \times \text{resistance}$$

Where ΔP = pressure gradient.

In a straight unbranched tube, the Hagen–Poiseuille equation allows gas flow to be quantified:

$$\text{Flow rate} = \frac{\Delta P \times \pi \times (\text{radius})^4}{8 \times \text{length} \times \text{viscosity}}$$

By combining these two equations:

$$\text{Resistance} = \frac{8 \times \text{length} \times \text{viscosity}}{\pi \times (\text{radius})^4}$$

In this equation the fourth power of the radius of the tube explains the critical importance of narrowing of air passages. With constant tube dimensions, viscosity is the only property of a gas that is relevant under conditions of laminar flow. Helium has a low density but a viscosity close to that of air and will not therefore improve gas flow if the flow is laminar (page 46).

In the Hagen–Poiseuille equation, the units must be coherent. In CGS units, dyn.cm^{-2} (pressure), ml.s^{-1} (flow) and cm (length and radius) are compatible with the unit of poise for viscosity (dyn.sec.cm^{-2}). In SI units, with pressure in kilopascals, the unit of viscosity is newton second.metre^{-2} (see Appendix A). However, in practice it is still customary to express gas pressure in cmH_2O and flow in l.s^{-1}. Resistance therefore continues to usually be expressed as cmH_2O per litre per second ($cmH_2O.l^{-1}.s$).

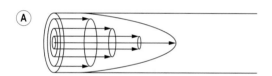

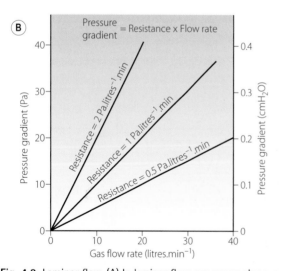

Fig. 4.2 Laminar flow. (A) In laminar flow gas moves along a straight tube as a series of concentric cylinders of gas with the central cylinder moving fastest and the outside cylinder theoretically stationary. This gives rise to a 'cone front' of gas velocity across the tube. (B) The linear relationship between gas flow rate and pressure gradient. The slope of the lines indicates the resistance (1 Pa = 0.01 cmH₂0).

TURBULENT FLOW

High flow rates, particularly through branched or irregular tubes, result in a breakdown of the orderly flow of gas described above. An irregular movement is superimposed on the general progression along the tube (Figure 4.3A), with a square front replacing the cone front of laminar flow. Turbulent flow is almost invariably present when high resistance to gas flow is a problem.

The square front means that no fresh gas can reach the end of a tube until the amount of gas entering the tube is almost equal to the volume of the tube. Turbulent flow is more effective than laminar flow in purging the contents of a tube, and also provides the best conditions for drawing a representative sample of gas from the periphery of a tube. Frictional forces between the tube wall and fluid become more important in turbulent flow.

Quantitative relationships. The relationship between driving pressure and flow rate differs from the relationship described above for laminar flow in three important respects:

1. The driving pressure is proportional to the square of the gas flow rate.
2. The driving pressure is proportional to the density of the gas and is independent of its viscosity.
3. The required driving pressure is, in theory, inversely proportional to the fifth power of the radius of the tube (Fanning equation).

The square law relating driving pressure and flow rate is shown in Figure 4.3B. Resistance, defined as pressure gradient divided by flow rate, is not constant as in laminar flow but increases in proportion to the flow rate. Units such as $cmH_2O.l^{-1}.s$ should therefore be used only when flow is entirely laminar. The following methods of quantification of 'resistance' should be used when flow is totally or partially turbulent.

(a) Two constants. This method considers resistance as comprising two components, one for laminar flow and one for turbulent flow. The simple relationship for laminar flow given above would then be extended as follows:

$$Pressure\ gradient = k_1\ (flow) + k_2\ (flow)^2$$

k_1 contains the factors of the Hagen–Poiseuille equation and represents the laminar flow component while k_2 includes factors in the corresponding equation for turbulent flow. Mead & Agostoni[2] summarised studies of normal human subjects in the following equation:

$$Pressure\ gradient\ (kPa) = 0.24\ (flow) + 0.03\ (flow)^2$$

(b) The exponent n. Over a surprisingly wide range of flow rates, the equation above may be condensed into the following single-term expression with little loss of precision:

$$Pressure\ gradient = \acute{K}\ (flow)^n$$

In this equation n has a value ranging from 1 with purely laminar flow, to 2 with purely turbulent flow, the value of n being a useful indication of the nature of the flow. The constants for the normal human respiratory tract are:

$$Pressure\ gradient\ (kPa) = 0.24\ (flow)^{1.3}$$

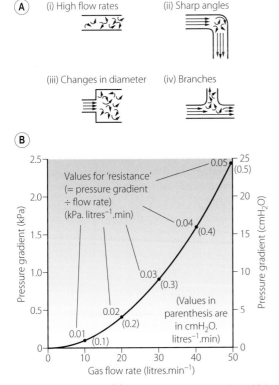

Fig. 4.3 Turbulent flow. (A) Four circumstances under which gas flow tends to be turbulent. (B) The square law relationship between gas flow rate and pressure gradient when flow is turbulent. Note that the value for 'resistance', calculated as for laminar flow, is quite meaningless during turbulent flow.

(c) The graphical method. It is often convenient to represent 'resistance' as a graph of pressure difference against gas flow rate, on either linear or logarithmic coordinates. Logarithmic coordinates have the advantage that the plot is usually a straight line whether flow is laminar, turbulent or mixed, and the slope of the line indicates the value of n in the equation above.

REYNOLDS' NUMBER

In the case of long straight unbranched tubes, the nature of the gas flow may be predicted from the value of Reynolds' number, which is a non-dimensional quantity derived from the following expression:

$$\frac{\text{Linear velocity of gas} \times \text{tube diameter} \times \text{gas density}}{\text{Gas viscosity}}$$

The property of the gas that affects Reynolds' number is the ratio of density to viscosity. When Reynolds' number is less than 2000, flow is predominantly laminar, whereas above a value of 4000, flow is mainly turbulent.[3] Between these values, both types of flow coexist. Reynolds' number also affects the entrance length, that is the distance required for laminar flow to become established, which is derived from:

$$\text{Entrance length} = 0.03 \times \text{tube diameter} \times \text{Reynolds' number}$$

Thus for gases with a low Reynolds' number not only will resistance be less during turbulent flow but laminar flow will become established more quickly after bifurcations, corners and obstructions.

Values for some gas mixtures that a patient may inhale are shown relative to air in Table 4.1. Viscosities of respirable gases do not differ greatly but there may be very large differences in density.

RESPIRATORY SYSTEM RESISTANCE

AIRWAY RESISTANCE

This results from frictional resistance in the airways. In the healthy subject, the small airways make only a small contribution to total airway resistance because their aggregate cross-sectional area increases to very large values after about the eighth generation (see Figure 2.4). Overall airway resistance is therefore dominated by the resistance of the larger airways.

Gas flow along pulmonary airways is very complex when compared to the theoretical tubes described above, and consists of a varying mixture of both laminar and turbulent flow. Both the velocity of gas flow and airway diameter (and therefore Reynolds' number) decrease in successive airway generations from a maximum in the trachea to almost zero at the start of the pulmonary acinus (generation 15). In addition, there are frequent divisions with variable lengths of approximately straight airway between. Finally, in large diameter airways entrance length is normally greater than the length of the individual airway. As a result of these purely physical factors laminar flow cannot become established until approximately the 11th airway generation. Predominantly turbulent flow in the conducting airways has two practical implications. First, the physical characteristics of the airway lining will influence frictional resistance more with turbulent than with laminar flow, so changes in airway lining fluid consistency (page 218) will have a significant effect. Second, gas mixtures containing helium (low Reynolds' number) are more beneficial in overcoming increased resistance in large airways and of less benefit in small airway disease such as asthma.

TISSUE RESISTANCE

In 1955 Mount identified a component of the work of breathing which he attributed to the resistance caused by tissue deformation.[4] D'Angelo et al[5] subsequently described how, in anaesthetised and paralysed subjects, the viscoelastic 'tissue' component of respiratory resistance may be measured.

Figure 4.4 shows the 'spring and dashpot' model, which D'Angelo et al[5] used to illustrate this component of respiratory resistance. Dashpots here represent resistance, and springs elastance (reciprocal of compliance). Upward movement of the upper

Table 4.1 Physical properties of clinically used gas mixtures relating to gas flow

	VISCOSITY RELATIVE TO AIR	DENSITY RELATIVE TO AIR	DENSITY VISCOSITY
Oxygen	1.11	1.11	1.00
70% N_2O/30% O_2	0.89	1.41	1.59
80% He/20% O_2	1.08	0.33	0.31

bar represents an increase in lung volume, caused by contraction of the inspiratory muscles or the application of inflation pressure as shown in the diagram. There is good evidence that, in humans, the left hand dashpot represents predominantly airway resistance. The spring in the middle represents the static elastance of the respiratory system. On the right there is a spring and dashpot arranged in series. With a rapid change in lung volume, the spring is extended while the piston is more slowly rising in the dashpot. In due course (approx 2–3 seconds) the spring returns to its original length and so ceases to exert any influence on pressure/volume relationships. This spring therefore represents the time dependent element of elastance. While it is still under tension at end-inspiration, the combined effect of the two springs results in a high elastance of which the reciprocal is the dynamic compliance. If inflation is held for a few seconds and movement of the piston through the right hand dashpot is completed, the right hand spring ceases to exert any tension and the total elastance is reduced to that caused by the spring in the middle. The reciprocal of this elastance is the static compliance, which is therefore greater than the dynamic compliance. D'Angelo et al[5] stress that the system shown in Figure 4.4 is only a simplified scheme to which many further components could be added; nevertheless the model accords well with experimental findings.

The time dependent change in compliance represented by the spring and dashpot in series could be due to many factors. Redistribution of gas makes only a negligible contribution in normal man, the major component being due to viscoelastic flow resistance in tissue.[1,5] In anaesthetised healthy subjects tissue

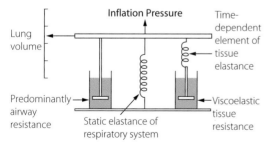

Fig. 4.4 The spring and dashpot model of D'Angelo et al.[5] Inflation of the lungs is represented by the bar moving upwards. The springs represent elastance (reciprocal of compliance) and the dashpots resistance. The spring and dashpot in series on the right confers time dependence which is due to viscoelastic tissue resistance.

resistance is of the order of half of the respiratory system resistance,[5] and seems to be largely unaffected by end-expiratory pressure or tidal volume.[6] Tissue resistance originates from both lung and chest wall tissues with a significant proportion originating in the chest wall.[6,7,8] The magnitude and importance of this component, particularly in lung disease, has often been underestimated and it is clearly important to distinguish airway resistance from that afforded by the total respiratory system. Separate measurement of tissue resistance is described below.

INERTANCE AS A COMPONENT OF RESPIRATORY SYSTEM RESISTANCE

Respired gases, the lungs and the thoracic cage all have appreciable mass and therefore inertia, which must offer an impedance to change in direction of gas flow, analogous to electrical inductance. This component, termed inertance, is extremely difficult to measure, but inductance and inertance offer an impedance that increases with frequency. Therefore, although inertance is generally believed to be negligible at normal respiratory frequencies, it may become appreciable during high frequency ventilation (Chapter 32).

FACTORS AFFECTING RESPIRATORY RESISTANCE

In normal lungs respiratory resistance is controlled by changes in airway diameter mainly in small airways and bronchioles. This would be expected to alter only the airway component of respiratory resistance but animal studies suggest that contraction of bronchial smooth muscle also causes changes in tissue resistance. It is thought that airway constriction distorts the surrounding tissue sufficiently to alter its viscoelastic properties.[9] Airway calibre may be reduced by either physical compression (due to a reversal of the normal transluminal pressure leading to airway collapse) or by contraction of the smooth muscle in the airway wall.

VOLUME–RELATED AIRWAY COLLAPSE

Effect of lung volume on resistance to breathing. When the lung volume is reduced, there is a proportional reduction in the volume of all air-containing components, including the air passages. Thus, if other factors (such as bronchomotor tone) remain constant, airway resistance is an inverse function of lung volume (Figure 4.5) and there is a direct relationship between lung volume and the maximum expiratory flow rate that can be attained (see below). Quantifying airway diameter is difficult from these curves. It is therefore more convenient to refer to conductance, which is the reciprocal of resistance and usually expressed as litres per second per cmH$_2$O. Specific airway conductance (sG$_{aw}$) is the airway conductance relative to lung volume

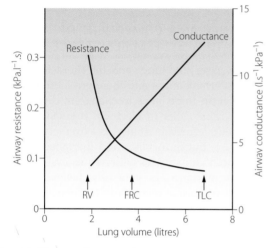

Fig. 4.5 Airway resistance and conductance as a function of lung volume (upright posture). The resistance curve is a hyperbola. Specific conductance (sG$_{aw}$) is the gradient of the conductance line. RV, residual volume; FRC, functional residual capacity; TLC, total lung capacity.

or the gradient of the line showing conductance as a function of lung volume (Figure 4.5). Because it takes into account the important effect of lung volume on airway resistance, it is a useful index of bronchomotor tone.

Gas trapping. At low lung volumes, flow-related airway collapse (see below) occurs more readily because airway calibre and the transmural pressure are less. Expiratory airway collapse gives rise to a 'valve' effect and gas becomes trapped distal to the collapsed airway, leading to an increase in residual volume and FRC. Thus, in general, increasing lung volume reduces airway resistance and helps to prevent gas trapping. This is most conveniently achieved by the application of continuous positive airway pressure (CPAP) to the spontaneously breathing subject or positive end-expiratory pressure (PEEP) to the paralysed ventilated patient (Chapter 32). Many patients with obstructive airways disease acquire the habit of increasing their expiratory resistance by exhaling through pursed lips. Alternatively, premature termination of expiration keeps the lung volume above FRC (intrinsic PEEP, page 476). Both manoeuvres have the effect of enhancing airway transmural pressure gradient and so reducing airway resistance and preventing trapping.

The closing capacity.[10,11] In addition to the overall effect on airway resistance shown in Figure 4.5, there are important regional differences. This is because the airways and alveoli in the dependent parts of the lungs are always smaller than those at

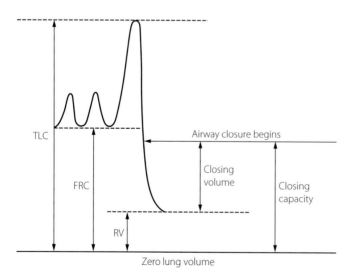

Fig. 4.6 Spirogram to illustrate the relationship between closing volume and closing capacity. This example would be in a young adult with closing capacity less than functional residual capacity (FRC). RV, residual volume; TLC, total lung capacity.

the top of the lung, except at total lung capacity or at zero gravity when all are the same size. As the lung volume is reduced towards residual volume, there is a point at which dependent airways begin to close, and the lung volume at which this occurs is known as the closing capacity (CC). The alternative term, closing volume (CV), equals the closing capacity minus the residual volume (RV) (Figure 4.6). Closing capacity increases linearly with age and is less than FRC in young adults but increases to become equal to FRC at a mean age of 44 years in the supine position and 75 years in the upright position (see Figure 3.11). The closing capacity seems to be independent of body position but the FRC changes markedly with position (see Figure 3.10).

When the FRC is less than the closing capacity, some of the pulmonary blood flow will be distributed to alveoli with closed airways, usually in the dependent parts of the lungs. This will constitute a shunt (page 132), and must increase the alveolar/arterial Po_2 gradient. If the alveolar Po_2 remains the same, the arterial Po_2 must be decreased. This can be seen when volunteers breathe below their FRC, and is particularly marked in older subjects who have a greater closing capacity. Shunting of blood through areas of the lung with closed airways is an important cause of decreasing arterial Po_2 with increasing age (page 194) and changes of position (page 335). Reduction in FRC is closely related to the increased alveolar/arterial Po_2 gradient seen during anaesthesia (page 334).

FLOW–RELATED AIRWAY COLLAPSE

All the airways can be compressed by reversal of the normal transmural pressure gradient to a sufficiently high level. The cartilaginous airways have considerable structural resistance to collapse but even the trachea may be compressed with an external pressure in the range 5–7 kPa (50–70 cmH$_2$O) or when the gas velocity through it becomes suitably high.[12] Airways beyond generation 11 have no structural rigidity (see Table 2.1) and rely instead on the traction on their walls from elastic recoil of the lung tissue in which they are embedded. They can be collapsed by a reversed transmural pressure gradient that is considerably less than that which closes the cartilaginous airways.

Reversal of the transmural pressure gradient may be caused by high levels of air flow during expiration. During all phases of normal breathing, the pressure in the lumen of the air passages should always remain well above the subatmospheric pressure in the thorax, so the airways remain patent. During a maximal forced expiration, the intrathoracic pressure rises to well above atmospheric, resulting in high gas flow rates. Pressure drops as gas flows along the airways and there will therefore be a point at which airway pressure equals the intrathoracic pressure. At that point (the equal pressure point) the smaller air passages are held open only by the elastic recoil of the lung parenchyma in which they are embedded or, if it occurs in the larger airways, by their structural rigidity. Downstream of the equal pressure point, the transmural pressure gradient is reversed and at some point may overcome the forces holding the airways open, resulting in airway collapse. This effect is also influenced by lung volume (see above) and the equal pressure point moves progressively down towards the smaller airways as lung volume is decreased.

Flow related collapse is best demonstrated on a flow/volume plot. Figure 4.7 shows the normal relationship between lung volume on the abscissa and instantaneous respiratory flow rate on the ordinate. Time is not directly indicated. In part (A) of the figure the small loop shows a normal tidal excursion above FRC and with air flow rate either side of zero. Arrows show the direction of the trace. At the end of a maximal expiration the black square indicates residual volume. The lower part of the large curve then shows the course of a maximal inspiration to TLC (black circle). There follow four expiratory curves, each with different expiratory effort and each attaining a different peak expiratory flow rate. Within limits, the greater the effort, the greater is the resultant peak flow rate. However, all the expiratory curves terminate in a final common pathway, which is independent of effort. In this part of the curves, the flow rate is limited by airway collapse and the maximal air flow rate is governed by the lung volume (abscissa). The greater the effort the greater the degree of airway collapse and the resultant gas flow rate remains the same. Figure 4.7B shows the importance of a maximal inspiration before measurement of peak expiratory flow rate.

MUSCULAR CONTROL OF AIRWAY DIAMETER

Small airways are the site of most of the important causes of obstruction in a range of pathological

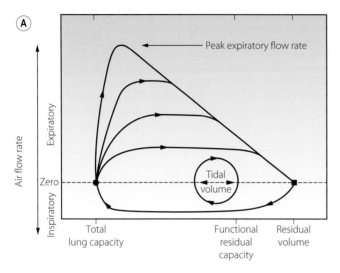

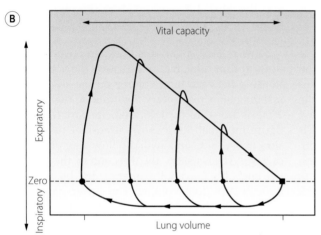

Fig. 4.7 Normal flow/volume curves. Instantaneous air flow rate (ordinate) is plotted against lung volume (abscissa). (A) The normal tidal excursion is shown as the small loop. In addition, expiration from total lung capacity at four levels of expiratory effort are shown. Within limits, peak expiratory flow rate is dependent on effort but, during the latter part of expiration, all curves converge on an effort-independent section where flow rate is limited by airway collapse. (B) The effect of forced expirations from different lung volumes. The pips above the effort-independent section probably represent air expelled from collapsed airways.

conditions described in Chapter 28. Four pathways are involved in controlling muscle tone in small bronchi and bronchioles:

1. Neural pathways
2. Humoral (via blood) control
3. Direct physical and chemical effects
4. Local cellular mechanisms.

These may conveniently be considered as discrete mechanisms but in practice there is considerable interaction between them, particularly in disease. Neural control is the most important in normal lung, with direct stimulation and humoral control contributing under some circumstances. Cellular mechanisms, particularly mast cells, have little influence under normal conditions but are important in airway disease (Chapter 28).

NEURAL PATHWAYS[13,14]

Parasympathetic system.[3] This system is of major importance in the control of bronchomotor tone and when activated can completely obliterate the lumen of small airways.[13] Both afferent and efferent fibres travel to the lung in the vagus nerve with efferent ganglia in the walls of small bronchi. Afferents arise from receptors under the tight junctions of the bronchial epithelium and respond either to noxious stimuli acting directly on the receptors (see below) or from cytokines released by cellular mechanisms such as mast cell degranulation. Efferent nerves release acetylcholine (ACh), which acts at M_3 muscarinic receptors to cause contraction of bronchial smooth muscle, whilst also stimulating M_2 pre-junctional muscarinic receptors to exert negative feedback on ACh release.[3] A complex series of second messengers is involved in bringing about smooth muscle contraction in response to ACh (see below). Stimulation of any part of the reflex arc results in bronchoconstriction. Some degree of resting tone is normally present[14] and may therefore permit some degree of bronchodilation when vagal tone is reduced in a similar fashion to vagal control of heart rate.

Sympathetic system. In contrast to the parasympathetic system, the sympathetic system is poorly represented in the lung and not yet proven to be of major importance in humans. Indeed it appears unlikely that there is any direct sympathetic innervation of the airway smooth muscle, although there may be an inhibitory effect on cholinergic neurotransmission in some species.

Non-cholinergic parasympathetic nerves.[14,15] The airways are provided with a third autonomic control which is neither adrenergic nor cholinergic. This is the only potential bronchodilator nervous pathway in man, though the exact role of these nerves in humans remains uncertain. The efferent fibres run in the vagus nerve and pass to the smooth muscle of the airway where they cause slow (several minutes) and prolonged relaxation of bronchi. The neurotransmitter is vasoactive intestinal peptide (VIP), which produces airway smooth muscle relaxation by promoting the production of nitric oxide (NO). How NO brings about smooth muscle relaxation in the airway is not as fully understood as its effect on vascular smooth muscle. It seems likely that NO has its effect without having to cross the cell membrane by some form of cell surface interaction that produces activation of guanylate cyclase to produce cyclic GMP and muscle relaxation.[16] Resting airway tone does involve bronchodilation by NO, but whether this is from local cellular production of NO or non-cholinergic parasympathetic nerves and VIP-mediated release of NO is not clear.[13]

HUMORAL CONTROL[3,17]

In spite of the minimal significance of sympathetic innervation, bronchial smooth muscle has plentiful β_2-adrenergic receptors, which are highly sensitive to circulating adrenaline, and once again act via complex second messenger systems described below.[18] Basal levels of adrenaline probably do not contribute to bronchial muscle tone, but this mechanism is brought into play during exercise or during the sympathetic 'stress response'. There are a few α-adrenergic receptors which are bronchoconstrictor but unlikely to be of clinical significance.

PHYSICAL AND CHEMICAL EFFECTS

Direct stimulation of the respiratory epithelium activates the parasympathetic reflex described above causing bronchoconstriction. Physical factors known to produce bronchoconstriction include mechanical stimulation of the upper air passages by laryngoscopy and the presence of foreign bodies in the trachea or bronchi. Inhalation of particulate matter, an aerosol of water or just cold air may cause bronchoconstriction, the latter being used as a simple provocation test. Many chemical stimuli result in bronchoconstriction including liquids with low pH such as gastric acid and gases such as sulphur dioxide, ammonia, ozone and nitrogen dioxide.

LOCAL CELLULAR MECHANISMS

Inflammatory cells in the lung include mast cells, eosinophils, neutrophils, macrophages and lymphocytes and the role of these cells in lung infection and inflammation is described in Chapters 28, 30 and 31. These inflammatory cells are all stimulated by a variety of pathogens, but some may also be activated by the direct physical factors described in the previous paragraph. Once activated, cytokine production causes amplification of the response, and a variety of mediators are released that can cause bronchoconstriction (Table 4.2). These mediators are produced in normal individuals, but patients with airway disease are usually 'hyper-responsive' and so develop symptoms of bronchospasm more easily.

DRUG EFFECTS ON AIRWAY SMOOTH MUSCLE

β_2 AGONISTS

Non-specific β-adrenoreceptor agonists (e.g. isoprenaline) were the first bronchodilator drugs to be widely used for treating asthma. However, cardiac effects from β_1 receptor stimulation in the heart were believed to be responsible for an increase in mortality during acute asthma, and the development

Table 4.2 Mediators involved in alteration of bronchial smooth muscle tone during airway inflammation[19,20]

SOURCE	BRONCHOCONSTRICTION		BRONCHODILATATION	
	MEDIATOR	RECEPTOR	MEDIATOR	RECEPTOR
Mast cells & other pro-inflammatory cells	Histamine	H_1	Prostaglandin E_2	EP
	Prostaglandin D_2	TP	Prostacyclin (PGI$_2$)	EP
	Prostaglandin $F_{2\alpha}$	TP		
	Leukotrienes $C_4 D_4 E_4$	CysLT$_1$		
	PAF	PAF		
	Bradykinin	B_2		
C–fibres	Substance P	NK$_2$		
	Neurokinin A	NK$_2$		
	CGRP	CGRP		
Endothelial & epithelial cells	Endothelin	ET$_B$		

PAF, platelet activating factor; CGRP, calcitonin gene-related peptide.

of β_2 specific drugs (e.g. salbutamol, terbutaline) soon followed. Later, long-acting β_2-agonists (e.g. salmeterol) were developed and are now widely used for treating asthma. The therapeutic effect of β_2-agonists is more complex than simple relaxation of airway smooth muscle as they are also known to inhibit the secretion of inflammatory cytokines and most of the bronchoconstrictor mediators shown in Table 4.2,[21] and even to increase surfactant release.[22] Controversy associated with β_2-agonists still continues today – their effect on inflammatory cells and ability to down-regulate β_2 receptors are both potentially harmful,[23] and concerns now exist about the mortality of some groups of patients taking long-acting β_2-agonists.[24] These observations have contributed to the gradual move away from β_2-agonists in asthma therapy (page 409).

The β_2 receptor. The molecular basis of the functional characteristics of the β adrenoceptor are now clearly elucidated.[25] It contains 413 amino acids and has seven transmembrane helices (Figure 4.8). The agonist binding site is within this hydrophobic core of the protein, which sits within the lipid bilayer of the cell membrane. This affects the interaction of drugs at the binding site in that more lipophilic drugs form a depot in the lipid bilayer from which they can repeatedly interact with the binding site of the receptor, producing a much longer duration of action than hydrophilic drugs. Receptors exist in either activated or inactivated form, the former state

occurring when the 3rd intracellular loop (Figure 4.8) is bound to GTP and the α-subunit of the Gs-protein. β_2 receptor agonists probably do not induce a significant conformational change in the protein structure but simply stabilise the activated form allowing this to predominate.

Activation of the G-protein by the β_2 receptor in turn activates adenylate cyclase to convert adenosine triphosphate to cyclic adenosine monophosphate (cAMP).[25] Cyclic-AMP causes relaxation of the muscle cell by inhibition of calcium release from intracellular stores and probably also activates protein kinase A to phosphorylate some of the regulatory proteins involved in the actin–myosin interaction.

Two β_2 receptor genes are present in humans, with a total of 18 polymorphisms described,[26] giving rise to a large number of possible phenotypes. Studies of these phenotypes continue, with some clinical differences being observed between individuals,[25] but the contribution that different β_2 receptor phenotypes make to the overall prevalence of asthma appears to be minimal.[26,27]

PHOSPHODIESTERASE INHIBITORS[28]

After its production following β_2 receptor stimulation, cAMP is rapidly hydrolysed by the intracellular enzyme phosphodiesterase (PDE), inhibition of which will therefore prolong the smooth muscle relaxant effect of β_2 receptor stimulation. Seven

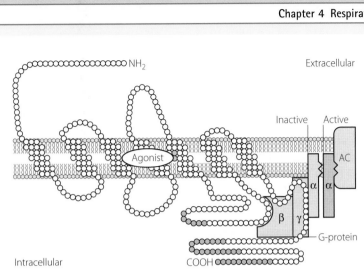

Fig. 4.8 Molecular mechanisms of β_2-adrenoceptor stimulation. The receptor exists in activated and inactivated states according to whether or not the α subunit of the G-protein is bound to adenyl cyclase (AC). The agonist binds to three amino acid residues on the third and fifth transmembrane domains, and by doing so stabilises the receptor G-protein complex in the activated state. The intracellular C-terminal region of the protein (blue) is the area susceptible to phosphorylation by intracellular kinases causing inactivation of the receptor and down-regulation.

subgroups of PDE have now been identified, with subgroups PDE3 and PDE4 occurring in airway smooth muscle, but the PDE inhibitors currently used in asthma such as theophylline are non-specific for the different subgroups.[19] This lack of specificity of currently used PDE inhibitors accounts for their wide ranging side effects, which continue to limit their therapeutic use.

ANTICHOLINERGIC DRUGS

The ACh receptor. Stimulation of M_3 ACh receptors also activates a G-protein, characterised as Gq. This in turn activates phospholipase C to stimulate the production of inositol triphosphate (IP$_3$), which then binds to sarcoplasmic reticulum receptors causing release of calcium from intracellular stores. The elevation of intracellular calcium activates myosin light chain kinase, which phosphorylates part of the myosin chain to activate myosin ATPase and initiate crossbridging between actin and myosin.[19] IP$_3$ is converted into the inactive inositol diphosphate by IP$_3$ kinase. Tachykinin, histamine and leukotriene receptors responsible for broncho-constriction from other mediators (Table 4.2) act by a very similar mechanism, being linked to G-protein–phospholipase C complexes, which lead to IP$_3$ formation.[29]

There are now believed to be many molecular interactions between the IP$_3$ and cAMP signalling pathways. Activation of phospholipase C by protein Gq also liberates intracellular diacylglycerol that activates another membrane-bound enzyme protein kinase C. This enzyme is able to phosphorylate a variety of proteins including G-proteins and the β_2 receptor itself (Figure 4.8) causing uncoupling of the receptor from the G-protein and down-regulation of the transduction pathway.[19,25]

Anticholinergic drugs used in the airway are classified into short acting (e.g. ipratropium) or long acting (e.g. tiotropium) types. They are more useful in treating chronic obstructive pulmonary disease than asthma (Chapter 28), because only in the former disease is increased parasympathetic activity thought to contribute to symptoms. These drugs have similar binding affinities for both M_2 and M_3 receptors, giving rise to opposing effects on the degree of stimulation of airway smooth muscle. Differences in relative numbers of M_2 and M_3 receptors between individuals and in different disease states[13] will therefore explain the variability in response seen with inhaled anticholinergic drugs.

LEUKOTRIENE ANTAGONISTS[30]

Even in non-asthmatic individuals, leukotrienes are potent bronchoconstrictors, so the therapeutic potential of leukotriene antagonists has been extensively investigated. Activation of phospholipase A_2 by inflammatory cells initiates the pathway, which ultimately produces three leukotrienes (Table 4.2, Figure 4.9). In the lung, these all act via a single receptor ($CysLT_1$) on airway smooth muscle cells to cause contraction via the G-protein–IP_3 system described above. Leukotrienes have a wide range of activities apart from bronchoconstriction, in particular amplification of the inflammatory response by chemotaxis of eosinophils.

As may be predicted from their actions, antagonists of the $CysLT_1$ receptor (e.g. montelukast, zafirlukast) are not effective in treating acute bronchoconstriction, but are useful in situations when the leukotriene pathway has been activated by stimulation of inflammatory cells. They are therefore most likely to be of benefit in prevention of bronchospasm in chronic asthma, but their place in asthma therapy remains uncertain.

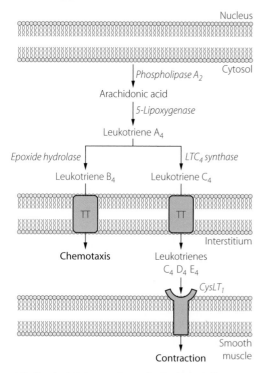

Fig. 4.9 The leukotriene pathway in the lung. Inflammatory mediators stimulate phospholipase A_2 to produce arachidonic acid from the phospholipid of the nuclear membrane. Leukotrienes B_4 and C_4 leave the cell via a specific transmembrane transporter (TT) protein. Non-specific peptidases in the interstitium convert leukotriene C_4 into D_4 and E_4, all of which stimulate the $CysLT_1$ receptor to cause intense broncho-constriction. (After reference 30.)

COMPENSATION FOR INCREASED RESISTANCE TO BREATHING

In animals, very little compensation for resistive loading occurs until Pco_2 increases, which stimulates ventilation and overcomes the resistance. In humans the response is more complex.

Inspiratory resistance. The normal response to increased inspiratory resistance is increased inspiratory muscle effort with little change in the FRC. Accessory muscles may be brought into play according to the degree of resistance.

There are two principal mechanisms of compensation for increased inspiratory resistance. The first operates immediately and even during the first breath in which resistance is applied. It seems probable that the muscle spindles indicate that the inspiratory muscles have failed to shorten by the intended amount and their afferent discharge then augments the activity in the motoneurone pool of the anterior horn. This is the typical servo operation of the spindle system with which the intercostal muscles are richly endowed (page 89). This reflex, mediated at the spinal level, is preserved during general anaesthesia (page 345).

In awake humans, the spinal response is accompanied by a further stimulus to ventilation mediated in suprapontine areas of the brain, possibly in the cerebral cortex.[31] This 'behavioural' response defends ventilation even in the face of significant inspiratory loading, preventing any change in Pco_2. If the response does indeed depend on cortical activity, this would explain why resistive loading during physiological sleep can be problematic (Chapter 16).

Expiratory resistance. Expiration against a pressure of up to 1 kPa (10 cmH$_2$O) does not usually result in activation of the expiratory muscles in conscious or anaesthetised subjects. The additional work to overcome this resistance is, in fact, performed by the inspiratory muscles. The subject augments his inspiratory force until he achieves a lung volume (FRC) at which the additional elastic recoil is sufficient to overcome the expiratory resistance (Figure 4.10). The mechanism for resetting the FRC at a higher level probably requires accommodation of the intrafusal fibres of the spindles to allow for an altered length of diaphragmatic muscle fibres due to the obstructed expiration. This would reset the developed inspiratory tension in accord with the increased FRC.[32] The conscious subject normally uses his expiratory muscles to overcome expiratory pressures in excess of about 1 kPa (10 cmH$_2$O).

Patients show a remarkable capacity to compensate for acutely increased resistance such that arterial P_{CO_2} is usually normal. However, the efficiency of these mechanisms in maintaining alveolar ventilation carries severe physiological consequences. In common with other muscles, the respiratory muscles can become fatigued and this is a major factor in the onset of respiratory failure. A raised P_{CO_2} in a patient with increased respiratory resistance is therefore always serious. Also, intrathoracic pressure will rise during acutely increased expiratory resistance and so impede venous return and reduce cardiac output (page 479) to the point that syncope may occur.

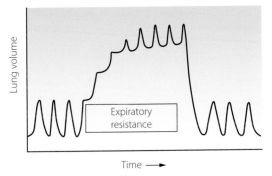

Fig. 4.10 Spirogram showing the response of an anaesthetised patient to the sudden imposition of an expiratory resistance. Note that there is an immediate augmentation of the force of contraction of the inspiratory muscles. This continues with successive breaths until the elastic recoil is sufficient to overcome the expiratory resistance.[32]

PRINCIPLES OF MEASUREMENT OF RESPIRATORY RESISTANCE AND CLOSING CAPACITY

RESPIRATORY SYSTEM RESISTANCE

Resistance is determined by the simultaneous measurement of gas flow rate and the driving pressure gradient. In the case of the respiratory tract, the difficulty centres around the measurement of the pressure gradient between mouth and alveolus. Problems also arise because of varying nomenclature and different methods for measuring different components of respiratory system resistance (Table 4.3).[33,34] In all cases, apparatus resistance must be measured separately and subtracted from the value obtained in the subject.

Normal values for total respiratory system resistance are variable because of the large changes with lung volume and methodological differences, but typical values for a healthy male subject are shown in Table 4.3.

Pressure–flow technique. In Chapter 3 it was shown how simultaneous measurement of tidal volume and intrathoracic (oesophageal) pressure yielded the dynamic compliance of the lung (see Figure 3.12). For this purpose, pressures were selected at the times of zero air flow when pressures were uninfluenced by air flow resistance. The same apparatus may be employed for the determination of flow resistance by subtracting the pressure component used in overcoming elastic forces (Figure 4.11). The shaded areas in the pressure trace indicate the components of the pressure required to overcome flow resistance and these may be related to the concurrent gas flow rates.

Table 4.3 Components of respiratory system resistance[33]

	MOUTH AND PHARYNX	LARYNX AND LARGE AIRWAYS	SMALL AIRWAYS < 3 mm DIAMETER	ALVEOLI AND LUNG TISSUE	CHEST WALL	TOTAL
Contribution (kPa. l^{-1}.s)	0.05	0.05	0.02	0.02	0.12	0.26
Airway resistance		Body plethysmograph Interrupter technique				0.12
Pulmonary resistance		Pressure flow technique				0.14
Respiratory system resistance		Oscillating air flow technique End-inspiratory interruption				0.26

Shaded areas indicate which components contribute to each form of resistance, whilst the text in the shaded boxes states the methodology used to measure each form of resistance.

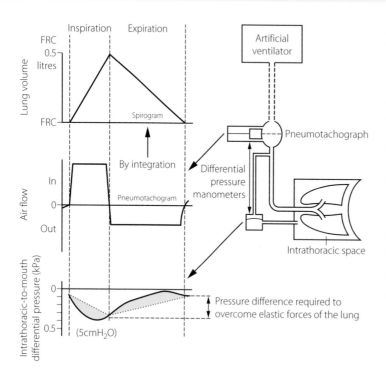

Fig. 4.11 The measurement of pulmonary resistance and dynamic compliance by simultaneous measurement of air flow and intrathoracic-to-mouth differential pressure. The spirogram is conveniently obtained by integration of the pneumotachogram. In the pressure trace, the dotted line shows the pressure changes that would be expected in a hypothetical patient with no pulmonary resistance. Compliance is derived as shown in Figure 3.12. Pulmonary resistance is derived as the difference between the measured pressure differential and that which is required for elastic forces (shaded area) compared with the flow rate shown in the pneumotachograph. Note that the pneumotachogram is a much more sensitive indicator of the no-flow points than the spirogram.

Alternatively, the intrathoracic to mouth pressure gradient and respired volume may be displayed as *x* and *y* coordinates of a loop. Figure 3.12 showed how dynamic compliance could be derived from the no-flow points of such a loop. The area of the loop is a function of the work performed against flow resistance.

The use of an oesophageal balloon makes the method a little invasive, but it does allow continuous measurement of resistance. By measuring intrathoracic pressure, the chest wall component of resistance is excluded so providing a measure of pulmonary resistance, which is airways resistance plus the lung component of tissue resistance.

Oscillating air flow. In this technique, a high frequency oscillating air flow is applied to the airways, with measurement of the resultant pressure and air flow changes. By application of alternating current theory it is possible to derive a continuous measurement of airway resistance.[35] The technique measures total respiratory resistance, and may be used throughout a vital capacity manoeuvre and so to display resistance as a function of lung volume and derive specific airway conductance.

The body plethysmograph. During inspiration, alveolar pressure falls below ambient as a function of airway resistance and the alveolar gas expands in accord with Boyle's law. The increased displacement of the body is then recorded as an increase in pressure in the body plethysmograph. Airway resistance may be derived directly from measurements of air flow and pressure changes, and the method requires the subject to perform either a 'panting' respiratory manoeuvre or to breathe with a small tidal volume. Despite these requirements plethysmography is generally non-invasive and allows FRC to be measured at the same time,[33] but results for airway resistance may be inconsistent.[36]

The interrupter technique. A single manometer may be used to measure both mouth and alveolar pressure if the air passages distal to the manometer are momentarily interrupted with a shutter. The method is based on the assumption that, while the airway is interrupted, the mouth pressure comes to equal the alveolar pressure. Resistance is then determined from the relationship between flow rate (measured before interruption) and the pressure

difference between mouth (measured before interruption) and alveoli (measured at the end of the
interruption). Interruption duration must be short
enough to avoid disturbing the subject's breathing
pattern but long enough to allow equilibration of
pressure along the airway. In practice, interruption
is for 50–100 ms occurring repeatedly throughout
the respiratory cycle. The technique is adequate
for measuring resistance in normal lungs but it is
doubtful if equilibration occurs fully in subjects
with diseased airways. The interrupter method
measures airway resistance and excludes tissue
resistance.

End-inspiratory interruption. This method is now
widely used for measuring the tissue component of
respiratory system resistance.[5–8,37] The method may
only be used in anaesthetised paralysed subjects
receiving artificial ventilation with accurate control
of the respiratory cycle. Following a constant flow
inflation of the lung, the airway is occluded for
0.5–3 s before a passive exhalation occurs. To prevent artefacts during the inspiratory pause, numerous successive breaths may be averaged.[7] Figure
4.12 shows the changes in gas flow, transpulmonary pressure (P_L), oesophageal pressure and lung
volume averaged over 33 breaths. Immediately
before occlusion, P_L reaches a value of P_{max}, which
is governed by both elastic and non-elastic resistance. The fall in pressure following occlusion is
biphasic. Immediately after airway occlusion, the
P_L falls rapidly to P_1 and $P_{max} - P_1$ is referred to
as interrupter resistance and believed to reflect airway resistance as in the interrupter method already
described.

In the second phase, a slower decay in pressure
occurs from P_1 to P_2, which represents the loss of
the time-dependent element of tissue compliance
(due to visco-elastic behaviour) and therefore represents tissue resistance:

$$\text{Tissue resistance} = \frac{P_1 - P_2}{\text{Flow rate of inflation}}$$

In practice, the pressure signal may be converted
into digital form and computer analysis calculates
the three pressures.[7]

Where these pressures are recorded determines
which component of tissue resistance is measured.
In Figure 4.12, transpulmonary pressure (tracheal
minus oesophageal pressure) is recorded so allowing

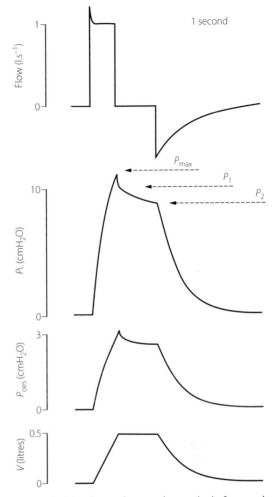

Fig. 4.12 End-inspiratory interruption method of measuring
resistance. Following a constant flow positive pressure breath,
there is an end-inspiratory pause of almost one second
before passive exhalation. The peak airway pressure (P_{max})
falls initially very quickly to P_1 and thereafter more slowly to
a plateau P_2. Tissue resistance, airway resistance and total
resistance can then all be calculated (see text for details). In
this example, showing the average of 33 consecutive breaths,
both transpulmonary (tracheal minus oesophageal) pressure
and oesophageal pressure relative to atmosphere have been
measured, allowing lung and chest wall components of tissue
resistance to be calculated separately. Flow, airway flow rate;
P_L, transpulmonary pressure; P_{oes}, oesophageal pressure; V,
change in lung volume. (After reference 7.)

calculation of the tissue resistance of the lung alone.
Oesophageal pressure is also recorded, so allowing
calculation of the thoracic cage component of tissue
resistance.

Finally, measurement of tracheal to atmospheric pressure gradient allows calculation of total respiratory resistance:

$$\text{Respiratory system resistance} = \frac{P_{\max} - P_2}{\text{Flow rate of inflation}}$$

This technique is utilised by the current generation of ventilators to calculate respiratory system resistance. The same static respiratory manoeuvre described in the previous chapter for calculation of static compliance (Figure 3.12B) also allows measurement of $P_{\max}$ and P_2 from which respiratory system resistance is calculated (Figure 4.12).

MEASUREMENT OF CLOSING CAPACITY[10,33]

This is perhaps the most convenient place to outline the measurement of closing capacity. It is the maximal lung volume at which airway closure can be detected in the dependent parts of the lungs

(page 48). The measurement is made during expiration and is based on having different concentrations of a tracer gas in the upper and lower parts of the lung. This may be achieved by inspiration of a bolus of tracer gas at the commencement of an inspiration from residual volume, at which time airways are closed in the dependent part of the lungs (Figure 4.13). The tracer gas will then be preferentially distributed to the upper parts of the lungs. After a maximal inspiration to total lung capacity, the patient slowly exhales while the concentration of the tracer gas is measured at the mouth. When lung volume reaches the closing capacity and airways begin to close in the dependent parts, the concentration of the tracer gas will rise (phase IV) above the alveolar plateau (phase III). Suitable tracers are ^{133}Xe or 100% oxygen (measured as a fall in nitrogen concentration). The technique can be undertaken in the conscious subject who performs the ventilatory manoeuvres spontaneously or in the paralysed subject in whom ventilation is artificially controlled.

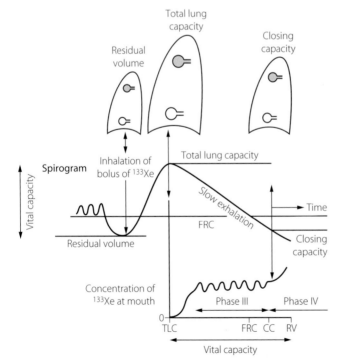

Fig. 4.13 Measurement of closing capacity by the use of a tracer gas such as ^{133}Xe. The bolus of tracer gas is inhaled near residual volume and, due to airway closure, is distributed only to those alveoli whose air passages are still open (shown shaded in the diagram). During expiration, the concentration of the tracer gas becomes constant after the dead space is washed out. This plateau (phase III) gives way to a rising concentration of tracer gas (phase IV) when there is closure of airways leading to alveoli which did not receive the tracer gas.

References

*1. Milic-Emili J, Robatto FM, Bates JHT. Respiratory mechanics in anaesthesia. *Br J Anaesth.* 1990;65:4–12.

2. Mead J, Agostini E. Dynamics of Breathing. Handbook of Physiology, Section 3 1964:1:1.

3. Burwell DR, Jones JG. The airways and anaesthesia – 1: Anatomy, physiology and fluid mechanics. *Anaesthesia.* 1996;51:849–857.

4. Mount LE. The ventilation flow-resistance and compliance of rat lungs. *J Physiol.* 1955;127:157–167.

5. D'Angelo E, Calderini E, Torri G, Robatto FM, Bonon D, Milic-Emili J. Respiratory mechanics in anaesthetised paralysed humans: effects of flow, volume and time. *J Appl Physiol.* 1989;67:2556–2564.

6. D'Angelo E, Tavola M, Milic-Emili J. Volume and time dependence of respiratory system mechanics in normal anaesthetised paralysed humans. *Eur Respir J.* 2000;16:665–672.

7. D'Angelo E, Prandi E, Tavola M, Calderini E, Milic-Emili J. Chest wall interrupter resistance in anaesthetised paralysed humans. *J Appl Physiol.* 1994;77:883–887.

*8. D'Angelo E, Robatto FM, Calderini E, et al. Pulmonary and chest wall mechanics in anaesthetised paralysed humans. *J Appl Physiol.* 1991;70:2602–2610.

9. Kimmel E, Seri M, Fredberg JJ. Lung tissue resistance and hysteretic modelling of lung parenchyma. *J Appl Physiol.* 1995;79:461–466.

*10. Milic-Emili J, Torchio R, D'Angelo E. Closing volume: a reappraisal (1967–2007). *Eur J Appl Physiol.* 2007;99:567–583.

11. Drummond GB, Milic-Emili J. Forty years of closing volume. *Br J Anaesth.* 2007;99:772–774.

12. Aljuri N, Venegas JG, Freitag L. Viscoelasticity of the trachea and its effects on flow limitation. *J Appl Physiol.* 2006;100:384–389.

13. Canning BJ, Fischer A. Neural regulation of airway smooth muscle tone. *Respir Physiol.* 2001;125:113–127.

*14. Canning BJ. Reflex regulation of airway smooth muscle tone. *J Appl Physiol.* 2006;101:971–985.

15. Widdicombe JG. Autonomic regulation: i-NANC/e-NANC. *Am J Respir Crit Care Med.* 1998;158:S171–S175.

16. Drazen JM, Gaston B, Shore SA. Chemical regulation of pulmonary airway tone. *Annu Rev Physiol.* 1995;57:151–170.

17. Thomson NC, Dagg KD, Ramsay SG. Humoral control of airway tone. *Thorax.* 1996;51:461–464.

18. Hakonarson H, Grunstein MM. Regulation of second messengers associated with airway smooth muscle contraction and relaxation. *Am J Respir Crit Care Med.* 1998;158:S115–S122.

*19. Barnes PJ. Pharmacology of airway smooth muscle. *Am J Respir Crit Care Med.* 1998;158:S123–S132.

20. Thirstrup S. Control of airway smooth muscle tone. I – Electrophysiology and contractile mediators. *Respir Med.* 2000;94:328–336.

21. Barnes PJ. Effect of β-agonists on inflammatory cells. *J Allergy Clin Immunol.* 1999;104:S10–S17.

22. Enhorning G. Surfactant in airway disease. *Chest.* 2008;133:975–980.

23. Bernstein IL. β₂-agonists: Déjà vu all over again. The second generation controversy. *Chest.* 2002;122:763–765.

24. O'Byrne PM, Ädelroth E. β₂ déjà vu. *Chest.* 2006;129:3–5.

*25. Johnson M. The β-adrenoceptor. *Am J Respir Crit Care Med.* 1998;158:S146–S153.

26. Hall IP, Sayers I. Pharmacogenetics and asthma: false hope or new dawn?. *Eur Respir J.* 2007;29:1239–1245.

27. Wjst M. β₂-adrenoreceptor polymorphisms and asthma. *Lancet.* 2006;368:710–711.

28. Barnes PJ. Theophylline. New perspectives for an old drug. *Am J Respir Crit Care Med.* 2003;167:813–818.

29. Reynolds PN, Holmes MD, Scicchitano R. Role of tachykinins in bronchial hyper-responsiveness. *Clin Exp Pharmacol Physiol.* 1997;24:273–280.

30. Drazen JM, Isreal E, O'Byrne PM. Treatment of asthma with drugs modifying the leukotriene pathway. *N Engl J Med.* 1999;340:197–206.

31. Raux M, Straus C, Redolfi S, et al. Electroencephalographic evidence for pre-motor cortex activation during inspiratory loading in humans. *J Physiol.* 2007;578:569–578.

32. Nunn JF, Ezi-Ashi TI. The respiratory effects of resistance to breathing in anaesthetised man. *Anesthesiology.* 1961;22:174–185.

33. Cotes JE, Chinn DJ, Miller MR. *Lung function. Physiology, measurement and application in medicine.* Oxford: Blackwell Publishing; 2006.

34. Phagoo SB, Watson RA, Silverman M, Pride NB. Comparison of four methods of assessing airflow resistance before and after induced airway narrowing. *J Appl Physiol.* 1995;79:518–525.

35. Goldman M, Knudson RJ, Mead J, Paterson N, Schwaber JR, Wohl ME. A simplified measurement of respiratory resistance by forced oscillation. *J Appl Physiol.* 1970;28:113–116.

36. Bar-Yishay E. Whole-body plethysmography. The human factor. *Chest.* 2009;135:1412–1414.

37. Jonson B, Beydon L, Brauer K, Mansson C, Valind S, Grytzell H. Mechanics of the respiratory system in healthy anesthetised humans with an emphasis on viscoelastic properties. *J Appl Physiol.* 1993;75:132–140.

Chapter 5

Control of breathing

KEY POINTS

- The respiratory centre in the medulla generates the respiratory rhythm using an oscillating network of six groups of interconnecting neurones.
- Many other diverse areas of the central nervous system influence respiratory control, these connections being coordinated by the pons.
- Irritant and stretch receptors in the lungs and diaphragm are involved in a series of reflex actions on the respiratory centre to influence respiratory activity.
- Central chemoreceptors respond to changes in pH caused by alterations in carbon dioxide partial pressure, rapidly increasing ventilation in response to elevated arterial P_{CO_2}.
- Peripheral chemoreceptors, principally in the carotid body, increase ventilation in response to reduced arterial P_{O_2}.

Early in pregnancy the fetal brainstem develops a 'respiratory centre', which produces uninterrupted rhythmic breathing activity for many years.[1] Throughout life the subject is mostly unaware of this action, which is closely controlled by a combination of chemical and physical reflexes. In addition, when required, breathing may (within limits) be completely over-ridden by voluntary control or interrupted by swallowing and involuntary nonrhythmic acts such as sneezing, vomiting, hiccuping or coughing. The control system is highly complex, with its automatic ability to adapt the action of the respiratory muscles to the changing demands of posture, speech, voluntary movement, exercise and innumerable other circumstances which alter the respiratory requirement or influence the performance of the respiratory muscles.

THE ORIGIN OF THE RESPIRATORY RHYTHM[2]

Early attempts to find the site of respiratory control used an anatomical approach involving the removal or stimulation of specific areas of the brainstem in animals (page 244). Subsequent development of precise imaging techniques allowed localisation of respiratory regions in normal human subjects, and these studies confirm that much of the historical animal work does apply to humans.[3] The anatomical approach to understanding respiratory control has also been succeeded by a biochemical approach as new research methods and the possibility of therapeutic intervention have led to an explosion of interest in the chemical interactions between and within respiratory neurones.

ANATOMICAL LOCATION OF THE 'RESPIRATORY CENTRE'

The medulla is accepted as the area of brain where the respiratory pattern is generated and where the various voluntary and involuntary demands on respiratory activity are coordinated. There are many neuronal connections both into and out of the medulla, as summarised in Figure 5.1, the functions of which are described below.

Respiratory neurones in the medulla are mainly concentrated in two anatomical areas, the ventral and dorsal respiratory groups, which have numerous interconnections (Figure 5.2).

DOI: 10.1016/B978-0-7020-2996-7.00001-5

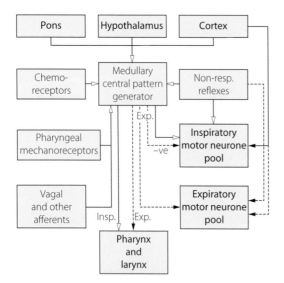

Fig. 5.1 Afferent and efferent connections to and from the medullary central pattern generator. The broken lines are expiratory pathways, which normally remain silent during quiet breathing.

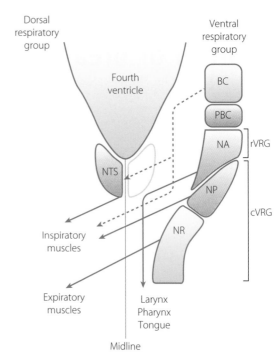

Fig. 5.2 Dorsal view of the organisation of respiratory neurones in the medulla. For clarity, the dorsal respiratory group (nucleus tractus solitarius, NTS) is shown only on the left and the ventral respiratory group (VRG) is shown only on the right. The VRG consists of the Bötzinger (BC) and Pre-Bötzinger (PBC) complexes, the rostral VRG area (rVRG) including the nucleus ambiguous (NA), and the caudal VRG area including the nucleus para-ambigualis (NP) and nucleus retroambigualis (NR). Areas with predominantly expiratory activity are shaded blue, and those with inspiratory activity shaded grey. Fibres that decussate are shown crossing the midline. The broken lines are expiratory pathways that inhibit inspiratory neurones.

The *dorsal* respiratory group lies in close relation to the nucleus tractus solitarius, where visceral afferents from cranial nerves IX and X terminate (Figure 5.2). It is predominantly composed of inspiratory neurones with upper motor neurones passing to the inspiratory anterior horn cells of the opposite side. The dorsal group is primarily concerned with timing of the respiratory cycle.

The *ventral* respiratory group comprises a column of respiratory neurones:[4]

- caudal ventral respiratory group, including the nucleus retroambigualis, which is predominantly expiratory with upper motor neurones passing to the contralateral expiratory muscles, and the mainly inspiratory nucleus para-ambigualis that controls the force of contraction of the contralateral inspiratory muscles.

- rostral ventral respiratory group, mostly made up of the nucleus ambiguous, which is involved in airway dilator functions of the larynx, pharynx and tongue.

- Pre-Bötzinger complex, believed to be the anatomical location of the central pattern generator (CPG).

- Bötzinger complex (within the nucleus retrofacialis) which has widespread expiratory functions.

CENTRAL PATTERN GENERATOR[2,5]

Unlike in the heart, there is no single 'pacemaker' neurone responsible for initiating breathing. Instead, a group-pacemaker hypothesis is proposed in which groups of associated neurones generate regular bursts of neuronal activity.[6] For breathing, the group-pacemaker involves a complex interaction of at least six groups of neurones with identifiable firing patterns spread throughout the medulla, though concentrated in the region of the pre-Bötzinger complex. Groups of neurones include early inspiratory, inspiratory augmenting (Iaug), late-inspiratory interneurones (putative 'off-switch' neurones), early expiratory decrementing, expiratory

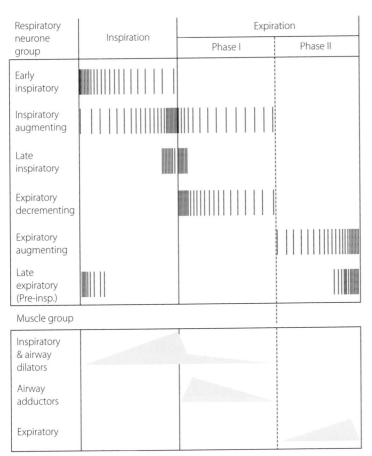

Respiratory neurone group	Inspiration	Expiration	
		Phase I	Phase II
Early inspiratory			
Inspiratory augmenting			
Late inspiratory			
Expiratory decrementing			
Expiratory augmenting			
Late expiratory (Pre-insp.)			
Muscle group			
Inspiratory & airway dilators			
Airway adductors			
Expiratory			

Fig. 5.3 Firing patterns of the respiratory neurone groups involved in central pattern generation and the corresponding respiratory muscle group activity. Note that expiration is divided into two phases representing passive (phase I) and active (phase II) expiration. See text for details.

augmenting, and late expiratory pre-inspiratory neurones. Typical firing patterns and the resulting muscle group activity are shown schematically in Figure 5.3. The resultant respiratory cycle may be divided into three phases:

1. Inspiratory phase. A sudden onset is followed by ramp increase in Iaug neurones resulting in motor discharge to the inspiratory muscles, including the pharyngeal dilator muscles. Pharyngeal dilator muscles start to contract shortly before the start of inspiration, possibly by activation of late expiratory (pre-inspiratory) neurones.

2. Post-inspiratory or expiratory phase I. This is characterised by declining discharge of the Iaug neurones and therefore motor discharge to the inspiratory muscles. Early expiratory decrementing neurones also produce declining activity in the laryngeal adductor muscles. This phase therefore represents passive expiration with a gradual let down of inspiratory muscle tone and an initial braking

of the expiratory gas flow rate (page 84) by the larynx.

3. Expiratory phase II. The inspiratory muscles are now silent and if required, expiratory augmenting neurones will be activated to produce a gradual increase in expiratory muscle activity.

Alterations in the rate at which spontaneous neuronal activity increases or decreases and the point at which the next group of neurones are activated allow an infinite variation of respiratory patterns. For example, during quiet breathing in the supine position, early expiratory neurones will reduce activity slowly and expiratory augmenting neurones will be active only briefly, resulting in almost totally passive exhalation. The converse situation will arise following exercise or at a minute volume in excess of about $40\,\mathrm{l.min^{-1}}$ when expiration will be immediately and almost totally active.

In practice, many such rhythm-generating networks are represented in parallel, so it is difficult to abolish the respiratory rhythm even with extensive brainstem damage.

Cellular mechanisms of central pattern generation.[2] Respiratory neurones that exhibit spontaneous activity achieve this by a combination of intrinsic membrane properties and excitatory and inhibitory feedback mechanisms requiring neurotransmitters. In practice, neurotransmitters (both inhibitory and excitatory) have a dual effect – they recruit other cells by direct activation and modulate the spontaneous activity of a single cell by effects on its own membrane ion channels, for example slowing the rate at which an action potential travels along a dendrite.

In a similar fashion to rhythm generation in cardiac tissue, a combination of potassium and calcium ion channels are involved. For instance, in a single Iaug neurone slow membrane depolarisation occurs so producing a spontaneous discharge. These cells then 'recruit' other Iaug cells by excitatory postsynaptic potentials (EPSPs) and a crescendo of Iaug activity develops. Calcium-dependent potassium channels then begin to be activated and repolarise the cells so 'switching off' the Iaug respiratory group. Activation of other cell groups, for instance expiratory augmenting neurones, will result in activation of inhibitory postsynaptic potentials (IPSPs) on the Iaug neurones to hyperpolarise the neurone and inhibit the next wave of inspiratory activity. Similar membrane effects occur in all the respiratory neurone groups shown in Figure 5.3.

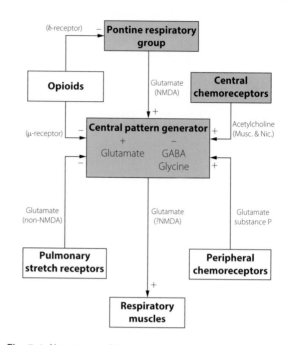

Fig. 5.4 Neurotransmitters and neuromodulators in the respiratory centre. Boxes indicate functional neuronal groups and bold type represents other influences on the respiratory centre. Substances involved in neurotransmission are shown with the most likely receptor subtype, in parentheses, if known. + indicates excitatory effect increasing respiratory activity; − indicates inhibitory activity decreasing respiration. Many of the connections shown may not be active during normal resting conditions.

NEUROTRANSMITTERS INVOLVED IN CPG AND RESPIRATORY CONTROL[2,7]

These are summarised in Figure 5.4. Central pattern generation requires a combination of excitatory and inhibitory neurotransmitters. Excitatory amino acids (usually glutamate) activate several different receptors. These are divided into two groups; *N*-methyl-D-aspartate (NMDA) receptors, which are fast acting ion channels and non-NMDA receptors, which are slower reacting receptors involving G-protein mediated effects. Inhibitory neurotransmitters include glycine and γ-aminobutyric acid (GABA) acting via specific glycine receptors and $GABA_A$ receptors respectively to hyperpolarise the neurone and thereby inhibit its activity. These two inhibitory transmitters act quite independently during different phases of CPG.

Neuromodulators are substances that can influence the CPG output, but are not themselves involved in rhythm generation. There are numerous neuromodulators of respiration, many of which have several subtypes of receptors. Their exact role in normal human respiration remains unclear, but they are of undoubted relevance in both normal and abnormal breathing. For example, exogenous opioids are known to have a profound depressant effect on respiratory activity in humans (page 77), indicating the presence of opioid receptors in the respiratory centre, but administration of the opioid antagonist naloxone has no effect on respiration in resting normal subjects. Other neuromodulators include acetylcholine, which acts via both muscarinic and nicotinic receptors to mediate the effect of central chemoreceptors on respiration. Serotonin (5-hydroxytryptamine, 5HT) has many conflicting effects on respiration as a result of the numerous receptor subtypes present. Glutamate acts as a neuromodulator via both NMDA and non-NMDA receptors to mediate the pontine influence on CPG and is also involved in the influence of pulmonary stretch receptors and peripheral chemoreceptors on the respiratory pattern. Substance P also has an excitatory influence resulting in an increase in tidal volume in response to peripheral chemoreceptor activity. This diverse collection of neuromodulators probably all ultimately act via a common intracellular signalling pathway within CPG neurones, involving protein kinases A and C that in turn influence the activity of GABA, glycine and glutamate linked potassium and chloride channels.[8]

EFFERENT PATHWAYS FROM THE RESPIRATORY CENTRE

Respiratory motor neurones in the brainstem are pooled into two separate areas, corresponding to inspiratory and expiratory muscle activity (see Figure 5.1). The complex integration of respiratory control seen in the CPG neurones continues to take place at the junction of the upper motor neurone with the anterior horn cell of the lower motor neurone. Three groups of upper motor neurones converge on the anterior horn cells supplying the respiratory muscles. The first group of upper motor neurones is from the dorsal and ventral respiratory groups of the medulla and are concerned with both inspiratory and expiratory output from the CPG. The second group is concerned with voluntary control of breathing (speech, respiratory gymnastics, etc.) and the third group with involuntary non-rhythmic respiratory control (swallowing, cough, hiccup, etc.). Each group of upper motor neurones occupies a specific anatomical location within the spinal cord. Neuronal control of the respiratory muscles is described in Chapter 6.

CENTRAL NERVOUS SYSTEM CONNECTIONS TO THE RESPIRATORY CENTRE

THE PONS[2]

There is no doubt of the existence of pontine neurones firing in synchrony with different phases of respiration, now referred to as the pontine respiratory group (PRG). Previously known as the pneumotaxic centre, three groups of neurones were identified (inspiratory, expiratory and phase-spanning) that were believed to be involved in controlling the timing of the respiratory cycle. The PRG is no longer considered to be essential for the generation of the respiratory rhythm, but does nevertheless influence the medullary respiratory neurones via a multisynaptic pathway contributing to fine control of the respiratory rhythm as, for example, in setting the lung volume at which inspiration is terminated. There are many central afferent pathways into the PRG, including connections to the hypothalamus, the cortex and the nucleus tractus solitarius. These connections suggest that the pons coordinates the respiratory effects of numerous CNS activities including cortical control, peripheral sensory information (odour, temperature), and visceral/cardiovascular inputs.

CEREBRAL CORTEX[9]

Breathing can be voluntarily interrupted and the pattern of respiratory movements altered within limits determined mainly by changes in arterial blood gas tensions. This is essential for such acts as speech, singing, sniffing, coughing, expulsive efforts and the performance of tests of ventilatory function. The neurones involved in this cortical 'over-ride' of respiration may completely bypass the respiratory centre and act directly on the respiratory muscle lower motoneurones.[10]

Volitional changes in respiration are common, and under some circumstances overcome the usual chemical control of respiration. For example, conscious respiratory drive may well maintain breathing in subjects following voluntary hyperventilation when the P_{CO_2} is below the apnoeic threshold (page 70). There are usually minor changes in the respiratory pattern when subjects focus their attention on their breathing as when physiological mouth pieces or breathing masks are used.[11]

In addition to volitional changes in the pattern of breathing, there are numerous other suprapontine reflex interferences with respiration such as sneezing, mastication, swallowing and coughing.[12] Reflex control of respiration during speech is complex.[13] During prolonged conversation, respiratory rate and tidal volume must be maintained approximately normal to prevent biochemical disturbance. In addition, for speech to be easily understood, pauses to allow inspiration must occur at appropriate boundaries in the text – for example between sentences. To achieve this, the brain performs complex assessments of the forthcoming speech to select appropriate size breaths to prevent cumbersome interruptions. This is easier to achieve during reading aloud when 88% of breaths are taken at appropriate boundaries in the text, compared with a figure of only 63% during spontaneous speech.[13]

ONDINE'S CURSE (PRIMARY ALVEOLAR HYPOVENTILATION SYNDROME)

In 1962 Severinghaus & Mitchell[14] described three patients who exhibited long periods of apnoea, even when awake, but who breathed on command. They termed the condition 'Ondine's curse' from its first description in German legend. The water nymph, Ondine, having been jilted by her mortal husband, took from him all automatic functions, requiring him to remember to breathe. When he finally fell asleep, he died. The condition is seen in adults with primary alveolar hypoventilation occurring as a feature of many different diseases, including chronic poliomyelitis and stroke.[15] Characteristics include a raised P_{CO_2} in the absence of pulmonary pathology, a flat CO_2/ventilation response curve and periods of apnoea which may be central or obstructive. A similar condition is also produced by overdosage with opioids.

Ondine's curse is also used to describe the rare condition of congenital central hypoventilation syndrome in which babies are born with a permanent defect in automatic respiratory control, leading to apnoea and hypoventilation during sleep.[16] In addition, these children have abnormal respiratory responses to exercise and in keeping with the German legend also have abnormalities of cardiac control.[17] In spite of such severe abnormalities, noninvasive methods of nocturnal ventilation and diaphragmatic pacing have led to almost normal lives for many of these children.[16]

PERIPHERAL INPUT TO THE RESPIRATORY CENTRE AND NON-CHEMICAL REFLEXES

REFLEXES ARISING FROM THE UPPER RESPIRATORY TRACT[18,19]

Nose. Water and stimulants such as ammonia or cigarette smoke may cause apnoea as part of the diving reflex (page 313). Irritants can initiate sneezing which, unlike coughing, cannot be undertaken voluntarily.

Pharynx. Mechanoreceptors that respond to pressure play a major role in activation of the pharyngeal dilator muscles (page 83). There is ample evidence that local anaesthesia of the pharynx impairs their action. Irritants may cause bronchodilatation, hypertension, tachycardia, and secretion of mucus in the lower airway.

Larynx. The larynx has a dense sensory innervation with fibres from the subglottic region in the recurrent laryngeal nerve and those from the supraglottic region in the internal branch of the superior laryngeal nerve. Most reflexes arise from the supraglottic area, as section of the latter nerve abolishes almost all reflex activity. There are three groups of receptors. Mechanoreceptors respond to changes in transmural pressure or laryngeal motion and result in increased pharyngeal dilator muscle activity, particularly during airway obstruction. Cold receptors are found superficially on the vocal folds and activation generally results in depression of ventilation. The importance of this reflex in adult humans is uncertain, but these receptors may also produce bronchoconstriction in susceptible individuals (Chapter 28). Irritant receptors respond to many substances such as distilled water, cigarette smoke and inhaled anaesthetics, and, in a similar fashion to direct mechanical stimulation of the larynx, cause cough, laryngeal closure and bronchoconstriction.

The cough reflex.[20] This may be elicited by chemical or mechanical stimuli arising in the larynx, trachea, carina or main bronchi. Which of these sites is responsible for the initiation of a cough is difficult to determine. For chemical stimuli the larynx may be of less importance as superior laryngeal nerve block has little effect on cough stimulated by citric acid inhalation,[21] and in patients following heart–lung transplant inhalation of the normally potent stimulant distilled water results in little or no cough (page 505). Coughing can be initiated or partially inhibited voluntarily but the reflex is complex and comprises three main stages:

1. Inspiratory phase, which takes into the lungs a volume of air sufficient for the expiratory activity.
2. Compressive phase, involving a forced expiration against a closed glottis. Transient changes of pressure up to 40 kPa (300 mmHg) may occur in the thorax, arterial blood and the cerebrospinal fluid (CSF) during the act of coughing.
3. Expulsive phase, in which the glottis opens allowing rapid expiratory flow throughout the

respiratory tract. During this phase the linear velocity of gas flow will be greatest in the narrowest section of the airway, usually the large bronchi, trachea and larynx (see Figure 2.4), an area referred to as the 'choke point'. This high velocity gas, with its turbulent flow, increases the shear forces between the gas and airway lining fluid, which is dragged from the airway wall and swept up towards the pharynx.

Expiration reflex.[20,22] Similar to a cough, this reflex originates in the larynx and is believed to exist in order to prevent material being aspirated into the upper airway. It differs from a cough by the absence of an inspiratory phase, the compressive and expulsive phases occurring immediately and from the lung volume present at the time the larynx is irritated. The distinction between the cough and expiration reflexes is important – a large inspiration as seen at the start of a cough would not be helpful in the presence of solid or liquid at the laryngeal inlet.

REFLEXES ARISING IN THE LUNG

Pulmonary stretch receptors and their associated reflexes.[23] There are many different types of receptors in the lungs sensitive to inflation, deflation, mechanical and chemical stimulation, afferents from which are mostly conducted by the vagus, although some fibres may be carried in the sympathetic nerves. Slowly adapting stretch receptors (SARs) are found predominantly in the airways rather than in the alveoli, and are closely associated with the tracheobronchial smooth muscle. Lung inflation stimulates the SARs, which are named 'slowly adapting' due to their ability to maintain their firing rate when lung inflation is maintained, thus acting as a form of lung volume sensor. Conversely, rapidly adapting stretch receptors (RARs) are located in the superficial mucosal layer,[18] and are stimulated by changes in tidal volume, respiratory frequency or changes in lung compliance.[23] The RARs also differ from SARs in being nociceptive and chemosensitive, responding to a wide range of chemical irritants, mechanical stimuli and inflammatory mediators.

How these receptors transduce a mechanical change in the tissue into an action potential is unknown. Hypotheses include the release of mediators from nearby associated cells that activate a receptor on the neurone, or ion channels may exist that respond directly to an alteration in their physical shape.[24] Afferent nerves from all these receptors converge on the nucleus tractus solitarius (NTS) of the medulla, where their signals are modulated and coordinated before further polysynaptic pathways communicate with the other regions of the respiratory centre. This processing of the afferent inputs by the NTS is believed to be capable of neuronal plasticity, which means the modulation can be altered by prolonged changes in external environment that influence the afferent inputs.[25]

The reflexes associated with pulmonary stretch receptors have attracted much attention since the associated inflation and deflation reflexes were described by Hering & Breuer in 1868.[26] Breuer was a clinical assistant to Professor Hering but apparently the work was at his own instigation. However, Hering, who was a corresponding member of the Vienna Academy of Science, published Breuer's work under his own name, in accord with the custom of the time. Breuer's role was clearly stated in Hering's paper but he was not a co-author. Later the same year, Breuer published a much fuller account of his work under his own name.

The inflation reflex consists of inhibition of inspiration in response to an increased pulmonary transmural pressure gradient (as in sustained inflation of the lung). An exactly similar effect may be obtained by obstructing expiration so that an inspiration is retained in the lungs.

The significance of the Hering–Breuer reflex in humans is controversial.[27,28] There appears to be an important species difference between laboratory animals, in which the reflex is easy to demonstrate, and humans in whom the reflex is very weak.[29] Pragmatic evidence that the Hering–Breuer reflex is unimportant in awake humans comes from studies showing normal breathing patterns in volunteers following bilateral vagal nerve block[30] and in patients who have had bilateral lung transplants, when both lungs must be totally denervated (Chapter 33). Conversely, studies in which conscious perception of chest wall position is suppressed by applying imperceptible amounts of assisted ventilation have demonstrated that respiratory pattern is altered within the physiological range, demonstrating the presence of a vagal feedback mechanism.[28,31] Although the Hering–Breuer inflation reflex therefore appears to exist but have minimal functional significance in adults, it is widely accepted as being present in neonates and infants.[32]

The deflation reflex consists of an augmentation of inspiration in response to deflation of the lung and can be demonstrated in man.[33] These results are consistent with the hypothesis that lung deflation has a reflex excitatory effect on breathing, but that the threshold is higher in man than for other mammalian species.

Head's paradoxical reflex. Head, working in Professor Hering's laboratory, described a reversal of the inflation reflex.[34] Many authors have reported that, with normal vagal conduction, sudden inflation of the lungs of many species may cause a transient inspiratory effort before the onset of apnoea due to the inflation reflex.[29] A similar response may also be elicited in new-born infants,[35] but it has not been established whether this 'gasp reflex' is analogous to Head's paradoxical reflex. All anaesthetists are aware that, after administration of respiratory depressants, transient increases in airway pressure often cause an immediate deep gasping type of inspiration.

OTHER PULMONARY AFFERENTS

C-fibre endings lie in close relationship to the capillaries, one group is in relation to the bronchial circulation and the other to the pulmonary microcirculation. The latter correspond to Paintal's juxtapulmonary capillary receptors (J receptors, for short).[18,36]

These receptors are relatively silent during normal breathing but are stimulated under various pathological conditions. They are similar to RARs described above, being nociceptive and activated by reactive oxygen species,[37] tissue damage, accumulation of interstitial fluid and release of various mediators. In the laboratory they can be activated by intravascular injection of capsaicin to produce the so-called pulmonary chemoreflex which comprises bradycardia, hypotension, apnoea or shallow breathing, bronchoconstriction and increased mucus secretion.[18,28] They may well be concerned in the dyspnoea of pulmonary vascular congestion and the ventilatory response to exercise and pulmonary embolisation. C-fibre endings have been characterised in physiological studies but have never been identified histologically, although non-myelinated nerve fibres are seen in the alveolar walls.

REFLEXES ARISING FROM OUTSIDE THE AIRWAY AND LUNGS

Phrenic nerve afferents.[38] Approximately one-third of neurones in the phrenic nerve are afferent, with the majority arising from muscle spindles and tendon organs forming the spinal reflex arc described on page 89. However, some afferent neurones continue through the ipsilateral spinal cord to the brainstem and somatosensory cortex. Experimental stimulation of phrenic afferent fibres results in a reduction of respiratory efferent activity, but stimulation of some smaller afferent fibres has the opposite effect. Thus the physiological role of phrenic afferents remains obscure, but it is unlikely that they have any influence on normal breathing. The sensory information provided by phrenic afferents is believed to be important in the perception of, and compensation for, increased inspiratory loads and these afferents are important in the 'breaking point' following a breath hold (page 76).

Baroreceptor reflexes. The most important groups of arterial baroreceptors are in the carotid sinus and around the aortic arch. These receptors are primarily concerned with regulation of the circulation, but a large decrease in arterial pressure produces hyperventilation, while in animals a substantial rise in arterial pressure causes respiratory depression and, ultimately, apnoea.

Afferents from the musculoskeletal system. These probably do not contribute to normal resting ventilation but have an important role in the hyperventilation of exercise (Chapter 15).

THE INFLUENCE OF CARBON DIOXIDE ON RESPIRATORY CONTROL[39,40]

For many years it was believed that the respiratory centre itself was sensitive to carbon dioxide. However, it is now known that both central and peripheral chemoreceptors are responsible for the effect of carbon dioxide on breathing, the latter accounting for about 80% of the total ventilatory response.[39] Because of their reliance on extra-cellular pH (see below) the central chemoreceptors are regarded as monitors of steady-state arterial $P\text{CO}_2$ and tissue perfusion in the brain, while the peripheral chemoreceptors respond more to short term and rapid changes in arterial $P\text{CO}_2$.[41]

LOCALISATION OF THE CENTRAL CHEMORECEPTORS

Studies in animals indicate that central chemosensitive areas are located within 0.2 mm of the ventrolateral surface of the medulla, in a region now referred to as the retrotrapezoid nucleus (RTN).[42] Neurones of the RTN are glutaminergic, and have selective connections to the nearby CPG.[40] Many other areas of the CNS display increased neural activity with carbon dioxide stimulation including other areas of the medulla, the midline pons, small areas in the cerebellum, and the limbic system,[3] though the contribution of these areas to respiratory control is unclear.

MECHANISM OF ACTION

An elevation of arterial P_{CO_2} causes an approximately equal rise of extracellular fluid, CSF, cerebral tissue and jugular venous P_{CO_2}, which are all about 1.3 kPa (10 mmHg) more than the arterial P_{CO_2}. Over the short term, and without change in CSF bicarbonate, a rise in CSF P_{CO_2} causes a fall in CSF pH. The blood–brain barrier (operative between blood and CSF) is permeable to carbon dioxide but not hydrogen ions, and in this respect resembles the membrane of a P_{CO_2}-sensitive electrode (page 174). In both cases, carbon dioxide crosses the barrier and hydrates to carbonic acid, which then ionises to give a pH inversely proportional to the log of the P_{CO_2}. A hydrogen ion sensor is thus made to respond to P_{CO_2}.

The mechanism by which a change in pH causes stimulation of chemoreceptor neurones remains disputed: the RTN may contain pH sensitive potassium channels, and release of adenosine triphosphate (ATP) has been proposed.[39]

Compensatory bicarbonate shift in the CSF. If the P_{CO_2} of CSF is maintained at an abnormal level, the CSF pH gradually returns towards normal over the course of many hours as a result of changes in the CSF bicarbonate concentration. This is analogous to, and proceeds in parallel with, the partial restoration of blood pH in patients with chronic hyper- or hypocapnia. Compensatory changes in bicarbonate concentrations are similar in both CSF and blood, suggesting a common mechanism.[43] Bicarbonate shift in CSF could therefore result simply from passive ion distribution, although the possibility of active ion transfer cannot be completely excluded. Examples of situations when this normalisation of CSF pH may occur include prolonged periods of hypocapnic artificial ventilation and the hypocapnia that occurs in response to hypoxia at altitude (page 282). Once the hypocapnia is reversed, for example when the artificial ventilation is no longer required, hyperventilation may follow for several hours. Compensatory changes in CSF pH are not confined to respiratory alkalosis, but are also found in chronic respiratory acidosis and metabolic acidosis and alkalosis. In a study of patients with a variety of pathological acid-base disturbances, values of CSF pH did not differ by more than 0.011 units from the normal value (7.326) in spite of mean arterial pH values ranging from 7.334 to 7.523.[44] If the bicarbonate concentration in CSF is itself altered by pathological factors, the pH is changed and ventilatory disturbances follow. For example, after intracranial haemorrhage patients may spontaneously hyperventilate,[45] and in these patients the CSF pH and bicarbonate have been shown to be below the normal values.

THE P_{CO_2}/VENTILATION RESPONSE CURVE

Following a rise in arterial P_{CO_2}, respiratory depth and rate increase until a steady state of hyperventilation is achieved after a few minutes. The response is linear over the range that is usually studied and may therefore be defined in terms of two parameters, slope and intercept (see Appendix E):

$$\text{ventilation} = S(P_{CO_2} - B)$$

where S is the slope (l.min^{-1}.kPa^{-1} or l.min^{-1}.mmHg^{-1}), and B is the intercept at zero ventilation (kPa or mmHg). The blue line in Figure 5.5 is a typical normal curve with an intercept (B) of about 4.8 kPa (36 mmHg) and a slope (S) of about 15 l.min^{-1}.kPa^{-1} (2 l.min^{-1}.mmHg^{-1}). There is in fact a very wide individual variation in P_{CO_2}/ventilation response curves, including a circadian variation within individuals,[46] and the response may be decreased by normal hormonal changes, disease or drugs. The dashed curve in Figure 5.5 shows the effect of changing ventilation on arterial P_{CO_2} when the inspired carbon dioxide concentration is negligible, and is a section of a rectangular hyperbola. The normal resting P_{CO_2} and ventilation are indicated by the intersection of this curve with the normal P_{CO_2}/ventilation response curve, which is usually obtained by varying the carbon dioxide concentration in the inspired gas.

When subjects hyperventilate voluntarily and reduce their P_{CO_2} below the threshold for CO_2 stimulation of respiration a variety of responses are seen, varying from apnoea to normal respiration

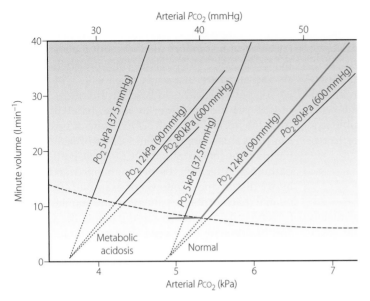

Fig. 5.5 Two fans of P_{CO_2}/ventilation response curves at different values of P_{O_2}. The right-hand fan is at normal metabolic acid–base state (zero base excess). The left-hand fan represents metabolic acidosis. The broken line represents the P_{CO_2} produced by the indicated ventilation for zero inspired P_{CO_2}, at basal metabolic rate. The intersection of the broken curve and any response curve indicates the resting P_{CO_2} and ventilation for the relevant metabolic acid–base state and P_{O_2}. The blue curve is the normal response. See text for details.

or even hyperventilation.[47] Figure 5.5 shows two possible extensions to the normal response curve (in blue) below the threshold for CO_2 stimulation (dashed line). The first is an extrapolation of the curve to intersect the x axis (zero ventilation) at a P_{CO_2} known as the apnoeic threshold (dotted lines in Figure 5.5). If P_{CO_2} is depressed below this point, apnoea may result, and this is seen in some subjects. The second type of extension (shown on the blue line) is horizontal and to the left, like a hockey stick, representing the response of a subject who continues to breathe regardless of the fact that his P_{CO_2} has been reduced. The resting arterial point at resting ventilation is normally approximately 0.3 kPa to the left of the extrapolated response curve,[48] supporting the idea of a hockey stick shaped response curve. When breathing below this threshold for the onset of CO_2 stimulated ventilation (the angle of the hockey stick) hypoxia seems to have no influence.[47] This variable ventilatory response to low P_{CO_2} almost certainly arises from the cortical control of respiration maintaining breathing despite a lack of chemical drive, particularly when awake.

As P_{CO_2} is raised, a point of maximal ventilatory stimulation is reached, probably within the range 13.3–26.7 kPa (100–200 mmHg), beyond which respiratory fatigue and CO_2 narcosis intervene

(Chapter 23). The ventilatory stimulation is reduced until, at very high P_{CO_2}, the ventilation is actually depressed below the control value and finally apnoea results, at least in animals and almost certainly in humans as well.

The P_{CO_2}/ventilation response curve is the response of the entire respiratory system to the challenge of a raised P_{CO_2}. Apart from reduced sensitivity of the central chemoreceptors, the overall response may be blunted by partial neuromuscular blockade or by obstructive or restrictive lung disease. These factors must be taken into account in drawing conclusions from a reduced response, and diffuse airway obstruction is a most important consideration. Nevertheless the slope of the P_{CO_2}/ventilation response curve remains one of the most valuable parameters in the assessment of the responsiveness of the respiratory system to carbon dioxide and its depression by drugs.

Time course of P_{CO_2}/ventilation response.[49] As described above, the initial ventilatory response to elevated P_{CO_2} is extremely rapid occurring within just a few minutes, at which time about 75% of the final ventilatory response has occurred. With sustained hypercapnia, the minute ventilation continues to increase for a further hour before reaching a plateau, which is sustained for at least 8 hours in healthy subjects.

THE INFLUENCE OF OXYGEN ON RESPIRATORY CONTROL

As for carbon dioxide, it was initially thought that hypoxia stimulated respiration by a direct effect on the respiratory centre. However, around 1930 the histological studies of de Castro[50] led him to suggest a chemoreceptor function for the carotid bodies, and the respiratory role of the peripheral chemoreceptors was established by Heymans[51] who received a Nobel prize for his work.

PERIPHERAL CHEMORECEPTORS[52]

The peripheral chemoreceptors are fast-responding monitors of the arterial blood, responding to a fall in Pa_{O_2}, a rise in Pa_{CO_2} or H^+ concentration, or a fall in their perfusion rate. An increase in ventilation is the result of stimulation. The bilaterally paired carotid bodies, rather than the aortic bodies, are almost exclusively responsible for the respiratory response. Each is only about $6 mm^3$ in volume and they are located close to the bifurcation of the common carotid artery. The carotid bodies undergo hypertrophy and hyperplasia under conditions of chronic hypoxia and are usually lost in the operation of carotid endarterectomy (see below).

Histology. The carotid bodies contain large sinusoids with a very high rate of perfusion – about 10 times the level that would be proportional to their metabolic rate, which is itself very high. Therefore the arterial/venous Po_2 difference is small. This accords with their role as a sensor of arterial blood gas tensions, and their rapid response, which is within the range 1–3 seconds.

At the cellular level, the main feature is the glomus or type I cell, which is in synaptic contact with nerve endings derived from an axon with its cell body in the petrosal ganglion of the glossopharyngeal nerve. Type I cells are partly encircled by type II cells whose function is still uncertain, but they may be dormant stem cells that can be activated by hypoxia to generate new type I cells.[52] Efferent nerves, which are known to modulate receptor afferent discharge, include preganglionic sympathetic fibres from the superior cervical ganglion, amounting to 5% of the nerve endings on the glomus cell.

Discharge rate in the afferent nerves from the carotid body increases in response to the following forms of stimulation:

Decrease of arterial Po_2. Stimulation is by decreased Po_2 and not by reduced oxygen content (at least down to about half the normal value). Thus there is little stimulation in anaemia, carboxyhaemoglobinaemia or methaemoglobinaemia. Quantitative aspects of the hypoxic ventilatory response are described in detail below.

Decrease of arterial pH. Acidaemia of perfusing blood causes stimulation, the magnitude of which is the same whether it is due to respiratory or metabolic acidosis. Quantitatively, the change produced by elevated Pco_2 on the peripheral chemoreceptors is only about one-sixth of that caused by the action on the central chemosensitive areas (see below). This response does however occur very rapidly,[41,49] and only develops when a 'threshold' value of arterial Pco_2 is exceeded.[47]

Hypoperfusion of peripheral chemoreceptors causes stimulation, possibly by causing a 'stagnant hypoxia' of the chemoreceptor cells (see below). Hypoperfusion may result from severe systemic hypotension.

Blood temperature elevation causes stimulation of breathing via the peripheral chemoreceptors. In addition, the ventilatory responses to both hypoxia and CO_2 are enhanced by a modest (1.4°C) rise in body temperature.

Chemical stimulation by a wide range of substances is known to cause increased ventilation through the medium of the peripheral chemoreceptors. These substances fall into two groups. The first comprises agents such as nicotine and acetylcholine that stimulate sympathetic ganglia. The second group of chemical stimulants comprises substances such as cyanide and carbon monoxide which block the cytochrome system and so prevent oxidative metabolism. Drugs which stimulate respiration via the peripheral chemoreceptors are described below.

MECHANISM OF ACTION OF PERIPHERAL CHEMORECEPTORS[52,53,54]

There is now general agreement that oxygen-sensitive potassium channels are responsible for the hypoxic response of Type I cells, similar channels being found in most cells of the body that respond to hypoxia.[54] Many different oxygen-sensitive potassium channels exist, with varying types occurring in different species, different tissues and under different circumstances within a species. Hypoxia inhibits the activity of the potassium channel, which alters the membrane potential of the cell and stimulates calcium channels to open, allowing an influx of extracellular calcium which stimulates transmitter release. The molecular mechanism by which potassium channels respond to Po_2 is unknown, including whether or not there is a direct effect on the channel itself or whether other, hypoxia induced, molecules are responsible. Contenders for this role include reactive oxygen species (Chapter 26) produced either from mitochondria or from reduced nicotinamide adenine dinucleotide phosphate (NADPH) oxidase, or possibly even carbon monoxide produced by haemoxygenase, an antioxidant enzyme constitutively expressed in most cells and closely associated with the potassium channels in Type I cells. These potential molecular messengers of hypoxia are probably not essential for the glomus cells to respond to low Po_2, but they may be important in modulating the response, for example when perfusion of the carotid body is poor.

Stimulation of the chemoreceptors by an increased arterial Pco_2 is dependent on carbonic anhydrase (present in the Type I cell) and there is therefore the possibility of both raised Pco_2 and decreased arterial pH acting through an increase in intracellular hydrogen ion concentration, as in the central chemoreceptors.

Various neurotransmitters have been identified within the carotid body with dopamine, acetylcholine and adenosine triphosphate (ATP) being the most prominent, though noradrenaline, angiotensin II, substance P and enkephalins have also been identified, though the role of each is uncertain. Acetylcholine and ATP are most likely to be the neurotransmitters involved between the Type I cell and the afferent nerves.[55] The other molecules seem to have an autocrine rather than neurotransmitter role, in that their release into the carotid body tissues modulates the response of the cells to the various stimuli.[55] For example, dopamine is abundant in Type I cells and released in response to hypoxia, its presence causing inhibition of calcium channels so effectively 'damping' the acute response. Similarly, the α_2 adrenoceptor agonist clonidine reduces the ventilatory response to acute hypoxia indicating that noradrenaline also has an inhibitory effect.[56] Angiotensin II increases the sensitivity of the potassium channels to hypoxia, and may be produced locally within the carotid body in response to long term hypoxia or poor carotid body perfusion, as seen in heart failure.[57]

The gain of the carotid bodies is under nervous control. There is an efferent pathway in the sinus nerve which, on excitation, decreases chemoreceptor activity. Excitation of the sympathetic nerve supply to the carotid body causes an increase in activity.

Other effects of stimulation. Apart from the well known increase in depth and rate of breathing, peripheral chemoreceptor stimulation causes a number of other effects, including bradycardia, hypertension, increase in bronchiolar tone and adrenal secretion. Stimulation of the carotid bodies has predominantly respiratory effects, whilst the aortic bodies have a greater influence on the circulation.

TIME COURSE OF THE VENTILATORY RESPONSE TO SUSTAINED HYPOXIA[58]

By controlling the concentration of inhaled oxygen, arterial oxygen saturation can be reduced and then maintained at a constant level of hypoxia, usually with a Sa_{O_2} of about 80%. In order to separate the effects on ventilation of hypoxia and Pco_2 most studies use isocapnic conditions, where the subject's alveolar Pco_2 is maintained at their control (resting ventilation) level by addition of CO_2 to the inspired gas. The interaction of Pco_2 and hypoxia in ventilatory control is discussed below. With a moderate degree of sustained hypoxia the ventilatory response is triphasic as shown in Figure 5.6. The three phases are described separately.

Acute hypoxic response. This is the first immediate and rapid increase in ventilation. Sudden imposition of hypoxia results in stimulation of ventilation within the lung-to-carotid body circulation time (about 6 s), but in most studies the response appears slower due to the delay between reducing inspired oxygen and the reduction in alveolar and then arterial Po_2. Ventilation continues to increase for between 5 and 10 minutes, rapidly reaching high levels.

Many factors affect the acute ventilatory response. There are wide variations between individuals, within an individual on different days, between male and female subjects, and with the hormonal changes of the menstrual cycle. A small number of otherwise normal subjects lack a measurable ventilatory response to hypoxia when studied at normal Pco_2. This is of little importance under

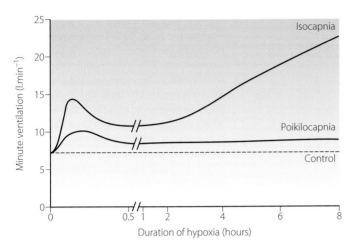

Fig. 5.6 Time course of the ventilatory response to hypoxia ($Sa_{O_2} \approx 80\%$). Practical problems prevent the continuous and rapid measurement of minute volume and respiratory gases for 8 hours, so the curves are produced from combining the data from three studies. When arterial P_{CO_2} is maintained at normal levels (isocapnia) the response is triphasic. When arterial P_{CO_2} is not controlled (poikilocapnia) the magnitude of the response is damped because the hypoxia induced hyperventilation reduces P_{CO_2} and therefore respiratory drive. See Figure 17.3 for respiratory effects of prolonged hypoxia. (After references 59, 60 and 61.)

normal circumstances, because the P_{CO_2} drive from the central chemoreceptors will normally ensure a safe level of P_{O_2}. However, in certain therapeutic and abnormal environmental circumstances, such as at high altitude, it could be dangerous.

Hypoxic ventilatory decline (HVD). Shortly after the acute hypoxic response reaches a peak, minute ventilation begins to decline reaching a plateau level, still above the resting ventilation, after 20–30 minutes (Figure 5.6). The degree of HVD in an individual correlates with the acute hypoxic response – the greater the initial increase in ventilation the greater the subsequent decline.[60] Though not completely elucidated yet, the mechanism of HVD appears to have a significant centrally mediated component,[62] and represents a change in ventilatory drive rather than a decline in the sensitivity of the receptors to hypoxia.[63] In animals, central glutamate release is involved in the acute hypoxic response, whilst GABA is implicated in producing HVD.[64]

Ventilatory response to sustained hypoxia. Once HVD is complete, continued isocapnic hypoxia results in a second, more slow, rise in ventilation over several hours (Figure 5.6). Ventilation continues to increase for at least 8 hours,[62] and reaches a plateau by 24 hours.[65] Species differences in this response again make elucidation of the mechanism in humans difficult, but the most likely explanation is a direct effect of hypoxia on the carotid bodies, possibly mediated by angiotensin II (page 223).

Hypoxia for more than 2–3 days only occurs following ascent to altitude, and the effects of this are described in Chapter 17.

VENTILATORY RESPONSE TO PROGRESSIVE HYPOXIA

Instead of maintaining a constant degree of hypoxia, ventilation may be measured during a progressive reduction in P_{O_2}. Once again, by controlling inspired gas concentrations, alveolar P_{O_2} may be reduced from 16 to 5 kPa (120 to 40 mmHg) over 15 minutes,[66] and ventilation increases progressively throughout this period. The response under these circumstances probably equates to the acute hypoxic response. If alveolar P_{O_2} is plotted against minute ventilation a P_{O_2}/ventilation response curve is produced (Figure 5.7). A P_{O_2}/ventilation response curve approximates to a rectangular hyperbola (see Appendix E), asymptotic to the ventilation at high Pa_{O_2} (zero hypoxic drive) and to the Pa_{O_2} at which ventilation theoretically becomes infinite (known as 'C' and about 4.3 kPa). Figure 5.7 shows a typical example but there are very wide individual variations. Note that there is a small but measurable difference in ventilation between normal and very high P_{O_2}.

The initial ventilatory response to P_{O_2} may be expressed as:

$$\frac{W}{Pa_{O_2} - C}$$

where W is a multiplier (i.e. the gain of the system) and partly dependent upon the P_{CO_2}. The ventilatory response here is the difference between the actual ventilation and the ventilation at high P_{O_2}, P_{CO_2} being unchanged.

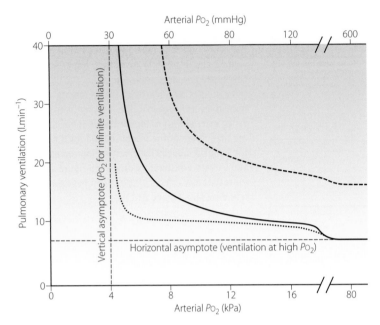

Fig. 5.7 Ventilatory response to progressive hypoxia. The heavy curve represents the normal P_{O_2}/ventilation response under isocapnic conditions, that is with P_{CO_2} maintained at the resting value. It has the form of a rectangular hyperbola asymptotic to the ventilation at high P_{O_2} and the P_{O_2} at which ventilation becomes infinite. The curve is displaced upwards by both hypercapnia and exercise at normal P_{CO_2} (dashed line). Hypocapnia displaces the curve downwards (dotted line) regardless of whether the hypocapnia results from not controlling P_{CO_2} (poikilocapnia) or by deliberately reducing P_{CO_2}. (Data from references 66, 67 and 68.)

The inconvenience of the non-linear relationship between ventilation and P_{O_2} may be overcome by plotting ventilation against oxygen saturation. The relationship is then linear with a negative slope, at least down to a saturation of 70%.[69] This approach is the basis of a simple non-invasive method of measurement of the hypoxic ventilatory response (see below).

IATROGENIC LOSS OF PERIPHERAL CHEMORECEPTOR SENSITIVITY[70]

Nerves from the carotid bodies are usually divided during bilateral carotid endarterectomy, which provides evidence that the carotid bodies are not essential for the maintenance of reasonably normal breathing under conditions of rest and mild exercise. Indeed, there is some evidence that the common finding of atheromatous disease at the carotid bifurcation may itself reduce chemoreceptor function and that a careful, 'nerve sparing', carotid endarterectomy can increase the ventilatory response to hypoxia.[71] Deliberate abolition of the hypoxic ventilatory response by carotid endarterectomy has been advocated as a treatment for incapacitating dyspnoea in severe respiratory disease.[72]

CENTRAL HYPOXIC DEPRESSION OF BREATHING

In addition to its effects on peripheral chemoreceptors, hypoxia also has a direct effect on the respiratory centre. Central respiratory neurone activity is depressed by hypoxia, and apnoea follows severe medullary hypoxia whether due to ischaemia or to hypoxaemia. With denervated peripheral chemoreceptors, phrenic motor activity becomes silent when the medullary P_{O_2} falls to about 1.7 kPa (13 mmHg).[73] More intense hypoxia causes a resumption of breathing with an abnormal pattern, possibly driven by a 'gasping' centre. This pattern of central hypoxic depression appears to be particularly marked in neonates and may be the relic of a mechanism to prevent the fetus from attempting to breathe in utero.

Mechanisms of hypoxic depression of ventilation. Medullary P_{CO_2}, and therefore ventilation, may be reduced by increased cerebral blood flow induced by hypoxia, and severe hypoxia causes depletion of high-energy phosphates. However, it has also been shown that neonatal hypoxia results in decreased levels of excitatory neurotransmitters (glutamate and aspartate) and increased levels of inhibitory substances, particularly GABA and endogenous opioids, both powerful respiratory depressants.

INTEGRATION OF THE CHEMICAL CONTROL OF BREATHING

The two main systems contributing to chemical control of breathing have been described quite separately, but in the intact subject this is not possible. For example, the peripheral chemoreceptors respond (slightly) to changes in P_{CO_2}, and hypoxia affects the respiratory centre directly as well as via the carotid body receptors. An overall view of the chemical control of breathing is shown schematically in Figure 5.8.

It was originally thought that the various factors interacted according to the algebraic sum of the individual effects caused by changes of P_{CO_2}, P_{O_2}, pH, etc. Hypoxia and hypercapnia were, for example, thought to be simply additive in their effects, but it is now realised that this was a very simplistic view of a complex system.

EFFECTS OF P_{CO_2} AND pH ON THE HYPOXIC VENTILATORY RESPONSE[66]

The acute hypoxic response is enhanced at elevated P_{CO_2} as shown by the upper dashed curve in Figure 5.7, the mechanism being indicated by broken line B in Figure 5.8. This interaction contributes to the ventilatory response in asphyxia being greater than the sum of the response to be expected from the rise in P_{CO_2} and the fall in P_{O_2} if considered separately.

Responses to both acute and prolonged hypoxia are depressed by hypocapnia, as shown in the lower dotted curve in Figure 5.7. This results from opposing effects on the CPG of increased chemoreceptor input and decreased central chemoreceptor drive. On prolonged exposure to hypoxia at altitude, this effect continues until acclimatisation takes place (page 282).

Poikilocapnic conditions occur when no attempt is made to control P_{CO_2} during hypoxic ventilation, and the hypoxia induced hyperventilation immediately gives rise to hypocapnia. Though rarely studied, this situation is important as poikilocapnia will occur in clinical situations. Early studies of the effects of P_{CO_2} on hypoxic ventilation showed that without control of P_{CO_2} the hypoxia driven increase in ventilation is almost exactly counteracted by the P_{CO_2} driven depression of ventilation resulting in no change in minute volume until breathing less than 10% oxygen.[67,68] Many earlier studies were, however, performed before technology allowed elucidation

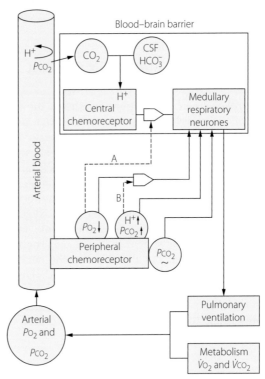

Fig. 5.8 Scheme of connections between individual aspects of chemical control of breathing. See text for details.

of the time course of hypoxic ventilation, and may have been measuring the plateau of ventilation after hypoxic ventilatory decline rather than the acute hypoxic response. More recent studies have shown that poikilocapnic conditions attenuate, but do not abolish, the first two phases of the ventilatory response to constant hypoxia (Figures 5.7 and 5.8).[59,60] Increased ventilation with sustained (over 1 hour) hypoxia is abolished during poikilocapnia but the minute volume does remain above resting levels (Figure 5.6).[61]

Exercise enhances the response to hypoxia even if the P_{CO_2} is not raised,[74] possibly due to lactic acidosis, oscillations of arterial P_{CO_2}, afferent input from muscle, or perhaps to catecholamine secretion. The upper broken curve in Figure 5.7 would also correspond to the response during exercise at an oxygen consumption of about $800\,ml.min^{-1}$. It is important to note that the slope of the curve at normal P_{O_2} is considerably increased in both these circumstances, so there will then be an appreciable 'hypoxic' drive to ventilation at normal P_{O_2}. Enhanced response to P_{O_2} during exercise seems to be an important component in the overall ventilatory response to exercise (Chapter 15).

EFFECTS OF Pa_{O_2} AND pH ON CENTRAL CHEMORECEPTOR RESPONSE[47]

The broken line (A) in Figure 5.8 shows the influence of the peripheral chemoreceptor drive on the gain of the central ventilatory response to P_{CO_2}. Typical quantitative relationships are shown in Figure 5.5, with hypoxia at the left of each fan and hyperoxia on the right. The curve marked P_{O_2} 80 kPa represents total abolition of chemoreceptor drive obtained by the inhalation of 100% oxygen.

Metabolic acidosis displaces the whole fan of curves to the left as shown in Figure 5.5. The intercept (B) is reduced but the slope of the curves at each value of P_{O_2} is virtually unaltered. Display of the fan of P_{CO_2}/ventilation response curves at different P_{O_2} is a particularly complete method of representing the state of respiratory control in a patient, but is impractical to determine.

PERIODIC BREATHING

This term describes a respiratory pattern in which ventilation waxes and wanes in a regular pattern. It is normal in neonates (page 254), but seen only during sleep in adults, occurring more frequently in the elderly[75] and in all ages when sleeping at altitude (page 287). The cause of periodic breathing is unknown, but is likely to involve an abnormality of the chemical control of breathing, possibly a poorly responsive or over-damped control system.[74] Cheyne–Stokes respiration is an extreme form of periodic breathing in which apnoea occurs during the hypoventilation phase, and is seen most commonly in patients with heart failure. In the case of Cheyne–Stokes respiration abnormalities of respiratory control and lung function contribute, but the slow circulation time seen in patients with heart failure introduces further periodicity into the breathing pattern.[76]

BREATH HOLDING

INFLUENCE OF P_{CO_2} AND P_{O_2}

When the breath is held after air breathing, the arterial and alveolar P_{CO_2} are remarkably constant at the breaking point and values are normally close to 6.7 kPa (50 mmHg). This does not mean that P_{CO_2}

is the sole or dominant factor and concomitant hypoxia is probably more important. Preliminary oxygen breathing delays the onset of hypoxia, and breath-holding times may be greatly prolonged with consequent elevation of P_{CO_2} at the breaking point. The relationship between P_{CO_2} and P_{O_2} at breaking point, after starting from different levels of oxygenation, is shown in Figure 5.9.

On the basis of changing blood gas tensions and the great variability of individuals' responses it might be predicted that subjects with 'flat' ventilatory responses to oxygen and carbon dioxide would be able to hold their breath longer. Elite breath-hold divers (page 297) have been shown to have a blunted response to carbon dioxide but not to hypoxia.[77]

EFFECT OF LUNG VOLUME

Breath-holding time is directly proportional to the lung volume at the onset of breath holding, partly because this has a major influence on oxygen stores. There are, however, other effects of lung volume and its change, which are mediated by afferents arising from the chest wall, diaphragm and the lung itself. Prolongation of breath-holding times are seen after bilateral vagal and glossopharyngeal nerve block,[78] and following complete muscular paralysis of conscious subjects.[79] These studies suggest that much of the distress leading to the termination of breath-holding is caused by frustration of the involuntary contractions of the respiratory muscles, which increase progressively during breath-holding. Fowler's experiment in 1954 easily demonstrates the importance of frustration of involuntary respiratory movements.[80] After normal air breathing, the breath is held until breaking point. If the expirate is then exhaled into a bag and immediately reinhaled, there is a marked sense of relief although it may be shown that the rise of P_{CO_2} and fall of P_{O_2} are uninfluenced.

Extreme durations of breath holding may be attained after hyperventilation and preoxygenation. Times of 14 minutes have been reached and the limiting factor is then reduction of lung volume to residual volume, as oxygen is removed from the alveolar gas.

DRUG EFFECTS ON THE CONTROL OF BREATHING

Considering the therapeutic potential of drugs that could specifically influence respiratory drive, it is

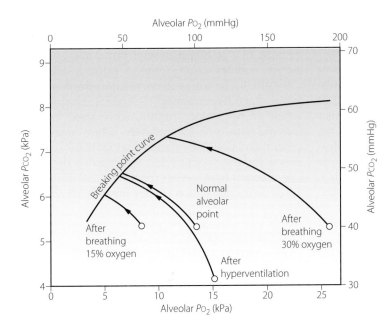

Fig. 5.9 The 'breaking point' curve defines the coexisting values of alveolar P_{O_2} and P_{CO_2}, at the breaking point of breath holding, starting from various states. The normal alveolar point is shown and the curved arrow shows the changes in alveolar gas tensions that occur during breath holding. Starting points are displaced to the right by preliminary breathing of oxygen enriched gases, and to the left by breathing mixtures containing less than 21% oxygen. Hyperventilation displaces the point representing alveolar gas to the right and downwards. The length of arrows from starting point to the breaking point curve gives an approximate indication of the duration of breath hold. This can clearly be prolonged by oxygen breathing or by hyperventilation, maximal duration occurring after hyperventilation with 100% oxygen.

surprising that so few drugs affecting respiratory control have been developed. Elucidation of the mechanisms for the control of breathing described in this chapter is a relatively recent event, particularly when considering the neurotransmitters and neuromodulators involved. The large number of different receptors involved in normal respiratory control (Figure 5.4) means that drugs affecting a single receptor may have little effect, or unpredictable effects, on respiration and so be of little clinical use. In addition, the neurotransmitters and neuromodulators involved are widely distributed throughout the central nervous system (CNS), so agonists or antagonists of their receptors are likely to have diverse effects resulting in unacceptable adverse effects.

Many other factors apart from the drug itself affect respiratory activity, so the effect that a drug exerts on the respiration of an individual patient is complex and unpredictable. For example in a healthy patient recovering from surgery under general anaesthesia, pain, anxiety, stress and changes in blood chemistry will be stimulating breathing whilst sedation, sleep and residual anaesthetic or analgesic agents will all be tending to depress respiration.

RESPIRATORY DEPRESSANTS

Any drug that depresses CNS activity may depress respiration, either individually or in combination with other CNS depressants such as alcohol. Almost all general anaesthetic agents reduce ventilation in a dose-dependent fashion, and are described in detail on page 327. Two specific groups of drugs that have well documented depressant effects on ventilation are opioid analgesics and benzodiazepines.

Opioids[81,82,83] Figure 5.4 shows that both μ- and δ-opioid receptors are present in the respiratory centre. As indicated above, the role of these receptors in normal respiratory control is unknown. Animal studies suggest that μ-receptors in the pre-Bötzinger complex (Figure 5.2) may be involved in normal respiratory control.[83] In humans, the evidence is less clear. In healthy subjects, administration of the non-specific opioid receptor antagonist naloxone has no effect on respiration.[81]

Agonists of μ-opioid receptors, such as morphine, cause dose-dependent depression of respiration normally characterised by a slow respiratory rate, but tidal volume is also commonly reduced. Female subjects show a greater susceptibility to the respiratory depression seen with opioids.[83] Ventilatory responses to hypoxia and hypercapnia are also severely impaired, removing the physiological safety mechanism for patients. Partial agonists at the μ-receptor, such as nalbuphine and buprenorphine, have a ceiling effect for their analgesic efficacy that is associated with a lesser effect on ventilation than full agonists. Most of the analgesic effects of clinically used opioids are also mediated by the μ-receptor, so the respiratory depressant effect of opioid drugs is currently inseparable from their therapeutic effect. Equi-analgesic doses of different opioids show similar degrees of respiratory depression, but the speed of onset of the drug does affect the clinical pattern of respiratory depression that occurs. With rapidly acting opioids such as fentanyl, apnoea normally follows its intravenous administration, but when an equi-analgesic dose of the slower acting morphine is administered, apnoea is unusual, because hypercapnia develops to counteract the respiratory depression.[84]

Benzodiazepines. Benzodiazepines exert their effect by binding directly to $GABA_A$ receptors, and increasing the inhibitory effect of endogenous GABA. Figure 5.4 shows that GABA is involved in respiratory central pattern generation so it is unsurprising that benzodiazepines affect respiration. Parenterally administered benzodiazepine drugs, such as midazolam or diazepam, cause a dose-dependent reduction in resting ventilation and reduce the ventilatory response to hypoxia[85] and hypercapnia.[81] The degree of respiratory impairment seen correlates well with their effect on consciousness. Reduced resting ventilation with midazolam can be reversed with the benzodiazepine antagonist flumazenil, though the responses to hypoxia and hypercapnia may still be abnormal despite the subjects no longer being sedated.[86] Unlike for opioids, the respiratory depressant effects of benzodiazepines seem to have a ceiling effect, with massive overdoses of these drugs rarely causing life-threatening respiratory depression unless other CNS depressants, commonly alcohol, are ingested simultaneously.

RESPIRATORY STIMULANTS

Non-specific CNS stimulant drugs have existed for many years, and, as part of their general stimulant effects, also increase respiratory drive. Early drugs of this type such as nikethamide and almitrine were used as respiratory stimulants, but at doses effective for stimulating respiration they had an unacceptably high incidence of CNS toxicity such as headache, agitation, muscle spasms or convulsions.

Doxapram is the only currently used respiratory stimulant, and seems to be more specific for respiratory stimulation than its predecessors, though still has a high incidence of CNS side effects. Doxapram works by stimulating the peripheral chemoreceptors to increase respiratory drive,[87] this effect

occurring at lower doses than those causing more generalised CNS stimulation. In healthy subjects, infusion of a standard dose of doxapram approximately doubles resting minute volume, and also substantially increases the ventilatory responses to hypoxia and hypercapnia.[88] Despite this impressive action on respiratory control, when used to treat patients with type 2 ventilatory failure (page 393) generalised CNS stimulation undoubtedly contributes to the therapeutic effect by reversing the sedative effects of hypercapnia (page 357) and increasing the patient's perception of their breathlessness.[89]

METHODS FOR ASSESSMENT OF BREATHING CONTROL

In assessing the control of breathing under ideal conditions, arterial blood gas tensions would be measured continuously. In practice, this is invasive and rapid measurements are impossible, so in almost all cases end-tidal gas concentration is mea-sured and converted to partial pressure. In normal healthy subjects with reasonable slow respiratory rates, these measurements will equate well to alveolar and therefore arterial tension, but this may not be the case in patients.

SENSITIVITY TO CARBON DIOXIDE

A lack of ventilatory response to carbon dioxide may result from impaired function of the respiratory system anywhere between the medullary neurones and the mechanical properties of the lung (see Figure 27.2). Thus it cannot be assumed that a decreased ventilation/P_{CO_2} response is necessarily due to failure of the central chemoreceptor mechanism.

Steady state method. This technique requires the simultaneous measurement of minute volume and P_{CO_2} after P_{CO_2} has been raised by increasing the concentration of carbon dioxide in the inspired gas. The ventilation is usually reasonably stable after 5 minutes of inhaling a fixed concentration of carbon dioxide. Severinghaus's pseudo steady state method[90] measures ventilation after 4 minutes and is a useful compromise giving highly repeatable results.[48] Several points are needed to define the P_{CO_2}/ventilation response curve and it is a time-consuming process, which may be distressing to some patients.

Rebreathing method. Introduced by Read in 1967, this technique greatly simplified determination of the slope of the Pco_2/ventilation response curve.[91] The subject rebreathes for up to four minutes from a 6-litre bag originally containing 7% carbon dioxide and about 50% oxygen, the remainder being nitrogen. The carbon dioxide concentration rises steadily during rebreathing while the oxygen concentration should remain above 30%. Thus there should be no appreciable hypoxic drive and ventilation is driven solely by the rising arterial Pco_2, which should be very close to the Pco_2 of the gas in the bag. Ventilation is measured by any convenient means and plotted against the Pco_2 of the gas in the bag. The Pco_2/ventilation response curve measured by the rebreathing technique is displaced to the right by about 0.7 kPa (5 mmHg) compared with the steady state method, but the slope agrees closely with the steady state method,[48,91] and is much easier to perform.

SENSITIVITY TO HYPOXIA[92]

There is often some reluctance to test sensitivity to hypoxia because of the reduced Po_2 to which the patient is exposed. Various approaches to the problem have been described, of which three are used (albeit rarely) in practice.

Steady state method. This is the classical technique and is best undertaken by preparing Pco_2/ventilation response curves at different levels of Po_2, which are presented as a fan (Figure 5.5). The spread of the fan is an indication of peripheral chemoreceptor sensitivity but it is also possible to present the data in the form of the rectangular hyperbola (see Figure 5.7) by plotting the ventilatory response for different values of Po_2 at the same Pco_2.

Rebreathing method. Read's rebreathing method is described above and has been adapted to measure the response to hypoxia.[69] The oxygen concentration of the rebreathed gas is reduced by the oxygen consumption of the subject, but active steps have to be taken to maintain the Pco_2 at a constant level. Calculation of the response is greatly simplified by measuring the oxygen saturation (usually non-invasively by means of a pulse oximeter) and plotting the response as ventilation against saturation. This normally approximates to a straight line and the slope is a function of the chemoreceptor sensitivity. However, even if Pco_2 is held constant, the response is directly influenced by the patient's sensitivity to Pco_2.

Intermittent inhalation of high oxygen concentration. This method avoids exposing subjects to hypoxia. Temporary withdrawal of peripheral chemoreceptor drive by inhalation of oxygen should reduce ventilation by about 15%. This may be used as an indication of the existence of carotid body activity but clearly it is much less sensitive than the steady state method.

References

1. Blanco CE. Maturation of fetal breathing activity. *Biol Neonate.* 1994;65:182–188.

2. Bianchi AL, Denavit-Saubie M, Champagnat J. Central control of breathing in mammals: Neuronal circuitry, membrane properties, and neurotransmitters. *Physiol Rev.* 1995;75:1–31.

3. Corfield DR, Fink GR, Ramsay SC, et al. Evidence for limbic system activation during CO₂-stimulated breathing in man. *J Physiol.* 1995;488:77–84.

4. Rekling JC, Feldman JL. Pre-Bötzinger complex and pacemaker neurones: hypothesised site and kernel for respiratory rhythm generation. *Annu Rev Physiol.* 1998;60:385–405.

5. Richter DW, Ballanyi K, Schwarzacher S. Mechanisms of respiratory rhythm generation. *Curr Opin Neurobiol.* 1992;2:788–793.

6. Del Negro CA, Hayes JA. A 'group pacemaker' mechanism for respiratory rhythm generation. *J Physiol.* 2008;586:2245–2246.

*7. Ramirez JM, Telgkamp P, Elsen FP, Quellmalz UJA, Richter DW. Respiratory rhythm generation in mammals: synaptic and membrane properties. *Respir Physiol.* 1997;110:71–85.

8. Richter DW, Lalley PM, Pierrefiche O, et al. Intracellular signal pathways controlling respiratory neurons. *Respir Physiol.* 1997;110:113–123.

9. Horn EM, Waldrop TG. Suprapontine control of respiration. *Respir Physiol.* 1998;114:201–211.

10. Corfield DR, Murphy K, Guz A. Does the motor cortical control of the diaphragm 'bypass' the brain stem respiratory centres in man? *Respir Physiol.* 1998;114:109–117.

11. Western PJ, Patrick JM. Effects of focussing attention on breathing with and without apparatus on the face. *Respir Physiol.* 1988;72:123–130.

12. Matsuo K, Hiiemae KM, Gonzalez-Fernandez M, Palmer JB. Respiration during feeding on solid food: alterations in breathing during mastication, pharyngeal bolus aggregation, and swallowing. *J Appl Physiol.* 2008;104:674–681.

13. Winkworth AL, Davis PJ, Adams RD, Ellis E. Breathing patterns during spontaneous speech. *J Speech Hear Res*. 1995;38:124–144.

14. Severinghaus JW, Mitchell RA. Ondine's curse: failure of respiratory centre automaticity while asleep. *Clin Res*. 1962;10:122.

15. Vingerhoets F, Bogousslavsky J. Respiratory dysfunction in stroke. *Clin Chest Med*. 1994;15:729–737.

16. Weese-Mayer DE, Silvestri JM, Menzies LJ, Morrow-Kenny AS, Hunt CE, Hauptman SA. Congenital central hypoventilation syndrome: diagnosis, management, and long-term outcome in thirty-two children. *J Pediatr*. 1992;120:381–387.

17. Woo MS, Woo MA, Gozal D, Jansen MT, Keens TG, Harper RM. Heart rate variability in congenital central hypoventilation syndrome. *Pediatr Res*. 1992;31:291–296.

*18. Widdicombe JG. Afferent receptors in the airways and cough. *Respir Physiol*. 1998;114:5–15.

19. Sant'Ambrogio G, Tsubone H, Sant'Ambrogio FB. Sensory information from the upper airway: Role in the control of breathing. *Respir Physiol*. 1995;102:1–16.

20. Widdicombe J, Fontana G. Cough: what's in a name? *Eur Respir J*. 2006;28:10–15.

21. Stockwell M, Lang S, Yip R, Zintel T, White C, Gallagher CG. Lack of importance of the superior laryngeal nerves in citric acid cough in humans. *J Appl Physiol*. 1993;75:613–617.

22. Tatar M, Hanacek J, Widdicombe J. The expiration reflex from the trachea and bronchi. *Eur Respir J*. 2008;31:385–390.

23. Widdicombe J. Airway receptors. *Respir Physiol*. 2001;125:3–15.

24. Taylor-Clark T, Undem BJ. Transduction mechanisms in airway sensory nerves. *J Appl Physiol*. 2006;101:950–959.

25. Bonham AC, Chen C-Y, Sekizawa S, Joad JP. Plasticity in the nucleus tractus solitarius and its influence on lung and airway reflexes. *J Appl Physiol*. 2006;101:322–327.

26. Ullman E. About Hering and Breuer. In: Porter R, ed. *Breathing: Hering–Breuer Centenary Symposium*. Edinburgh and London: Churchill Livingstone; 1970:3.

27. Gaudy JH. The Hering–Breuer reflex in man? *Br J Anaesth*. 1991;66:627–628.

28. Kubin L, Alheid GF, Zuperku EJ, McCrimmon DR. Central pathways of pulmonary and lower airway vagal afferents. *J Appl Physiol*. 2006;101:618–627.

29. Widdicombe JG. Respiratory reflexes in man and other mammalian species. *Clin Sci*. 1961;21:163–170.

30. Guz A, Noble MIM, Trenchard D, Cochrane HL, Makey AR. Studies on the vagus nerves in man: their role in respiratory and circulatory control. *Clin Sci*. 1964;27:293–304.

31. BuSha BF, Stella MH, Manning HL, Leiter JC. Termination of inspiration by phase dependent respiratory vagal feedback in awake normal humans. *J Appl Physiol*. 2002;93:903–910.

32. Rabbette PS, Fletcher ME, Dezateux CA, Soriano-Brucher H, Stocks J. Hering–Breuer reflex and respiratory system compliance in the first year of life: a longitudinal study. *J Appl Physiol*. 1994;76:650–656.

33. Guz A, Noble MIM, Eisle JH, Trenchard D. The effect of lung deflation on breathing in man. *Clin Sci*. 1971;40:451–461.

34. Head H. On the regulation of respiration. *J Physiol (Lond)*. 1889;10:1–70.

35. Cross KW, Klaus M, Tooley WH, Weisser K. The response of the new-born baby to inflation of the lungs. *J Physiol (Lond)*. 1960;151:551–565.

36. Paintal AS. Some recent advances in studies on J receptors. *Adv Exp Med Biol*. 1995;381:15–25.

37. Gerhold KA, Bautista DM. TRPA1: irritant detector of the airways. *J Physiol*. 2008;586:14.

38. Frazier DT, Revelette WR. Role of phrenic nerve afferents in the control of breathing. *J Appl Physiol*. 1991;70:491–496.

39. Gourine AV. On the peripheral and central chemoreception and control of breathing: an emerging role of ATP. *J Physiol*. 2005;568:715–724.

40. Guyenet PG, Stornetta RL, Bayliss DA. Retrotrapezoid nucleus and central chemoreception. *J Physiol*. 2008;586:2043–2048.

41. Nattie E. Why do we have both peripheral and central chemoreceptors? *J Appl Physiol*. 2006;100:9–10.

42. Sato M, Severinghaus JW, Basbaum AI. Medullary CO_2 chemoreceptor neuron identification by c-fos immunochemistry. *FASEB J*. 1991;5:A1120.

43. Forster HV, Dempsey JA, Chosy LW. Incomplete compensation of CSF [H^+] in man during acclimatisation to high altitude. *J Appl Physiol*. 1975;38:1067–1072.

44. Mitchell RA, Carman CT, Severinghaus JW, Richardson BW, Singer MM, Snider S. Stability of cerebrospinal fluid pH in chronic acid-base disturbances in blood. *J Appl Physiol*. 1965;20:443–452.

45. Froman C, Crampton-Smith A. Hyperventilation associated with low pH of cerebrospinal fluid after intracranial haemorrhage. *Lancet*. 1966;1:780–782.

46. Spengler CM, Czeisler CA, Shea SA. An endogenous circadian rhythm of respiratory control in humans. *J Physiol*. 2000;526:683–694.

*47. Mohan R, Duffin J. The effect of hypoxia on the ventilatory response to carbon dioxide in man. *Respir Physiol*. 1997;108:101–115.

48. Lumb AB, Nunn JF. Ribcage contributions to CO_2 response during rebreathing and steady state methods. *Respir Physiol.* 1991;85:97–110.

49. Tansley JG, Pedersen MEF, Clar C, Robbins PA. Human ventilatory response to 8h of euoxic hypercapnia. *J Appl Physiol.* 1998;84:431–434.

50. de Castro F. Sur la structure et l'innervation de la glande intercarotidienne. *Trab Lab Invest Biol Univ Madrid.* 1926;26:365.

51. Heymans C, Bouckaert JJ, Dautrebande L. Sinus carotidien et réflexes respiratoire. *Arch Int Pharmacodyn Ther.* 1930;39:400.

*52. López-Barneo J, Ortega-Sáenz P, Pardal R, Pascual A, Piruat JI. Carotid body oxygen sensing. *Eur Respir J.* 2008;32:1386–1398.

53. Prabhakar NR. Oxygen sensing by the carotid body chemoreceptors. *J Appl Physiol.* 2000;88:2287–2295.

54. Weir K, López-Barneo J, Buckler KJ, Archer SL. Acute oxygen-sensing mechanisms. *N Engl J Med.* 2005;353:2042–2055.

55. Nurse CA. Neurotransmission and neuromodulation in the chemosensory carotid body. *Auton Neurosci.* 2005;120:1–99.

56. Foo IT, Warren PM, Drummond GB. Influence of oral clonidine on the ventilatory response to acute and sustained isocapnic hypoxia in human males. *Br J Anaesth.* 1996;76:214–220.

57. Leung PS. Novel roles of a local angiotensin-generating system in the carotid body. *J Physiol.* 2006;575:4.

58. Powell FL, Milsom WK, Mitchell GS. Time domains of the hypoxic ventilatory response. *Respir Physiol.* 1998;112:123–134.

59. Huang SY, Alexander JK, Grover RF, et al. Hypocapnia and sustained hypoxia blunt ventilation on arrival at high altitude. *J Appl Physiol.* 1984;56:602–606.

60. Easton PA, Slykerman LJ, Anthonisen NR. Ventilatory response to sustained hypoxia in normal adults. *J Appl Physiol.* 1986;61:906–911.

61. Howard LSGE, Robbins PA. Ventilatory response to 8h of isocapnic and poikilocapnic hypoxia in humans. *J Appl Physiol.* 1995;78:1092–1097.

62. Robbins PA. Hypoxic ventilatory decline: site of action. *J Appl Physiol.* 1995;78:373–374.

63. Garcia N, Hopkins SR, Elliott AR, Aaron EA, Weinger MB, Powell FL. Ventilatory response to 2-h sustained hypoxia in humans. *Respir Physiol.* 2000;124:11–22.

64. Soto-Arape I, Burton MD, Kazemi H. Central amino acid neurotransmitters and the hypoxic ventilatory response. *Am J Respir Crit Care Med.* 1995;151:1113–1120.

65. Cruz JC, Reeves JT, Grover RF, et al. Ventilatory acclimatisation to high altitude is prevented by CO_2 breathing. *Respiration.* 1980;39:121–130.

66. Weil JV, Byrne-Quinn E, Sodal IE, et al. Hypoxic ventilatory drive in normal man. *J Clin Invest.* 1970;49:1061–1072.

67. Dripps RD, Comroe JH. The effect of the inhalation of high and low oxygen concentrations on respiration, pulse rate, ballistocardiogram and arterial oxygen saturation (oximeter) of normal individuals. *Am J Physiol.* 1947;149:277–291.

68. Cormack RS, Cunningham DJC, Gee JBL. The effect of carbon dioxide on the respiratory response to want of oxygen in man. *Q J Exp Physiol.* 1957;42:303–316.

69. Rebuck AS, Campbell EJM. A clinical method for assessing the ventilatory response to hypoxia. *Am Rev Respir Dis.* 1974;109:345–350.

*70. Timmers HJLM, Wieling W, Karemaker JM. Lenders JWM. Denervation of carotid and baro-chemoreceptors in humans. *J Physiol.* 2003;553:3–11.

71. Vanmaele RG, De Backer WA, Willeman MJ, et al. Hypoxic ventilatory response to carotid endarterectomy. *Eur J Vasc Surg.* 1992;6:241–244.

72. Vanmaele RG. De Leersnijder, Bal J, Van Kerkhoven W, Bongaerts P, Vaerenberg C. One year follow-up after bilateral carotid body resection for COPD. *Eur J Respir Dis.* 1983;64(suppl 126):470.

73. Edelman NH, Neubauer JA. Hypoxic depression of breathing. In: Crystal RG, West JB, eds *The lung, scientific foundations.* New York: Raven; 1991:1341.

74. Weil JVW, Byrne-Quinn E, Sodal IE, Kline JS, McCullough RE, Filley GF. Augmentation of chemosensitivity during mild exercise in normal man. *J Appl Physiol.* 1972;33:813–819.

75. Wellman A, Malhotra A, Jordan AS, Schory K, Gautam S, White DP. Chemical control stability in the elderly. *J Physiol.* 2007;581:291–298.

76. Lorenzi-Filho G, Genta PR. A new straw in the genesis of Cheyne-Stokes respiration. *Chest.* 2008;134:7–9.

77. Grassi B, Ferretti G, Costa M, et al. Ventilatory responses to hypercapnia and hypoxia in elite breath-hold divers. *Respir Physiol.* 1994;97:323–332.

78. Guz A, Noble MIM, Widdicombe JG, Trenchard D, Mushin WW, Makey AR. The role of the vagal and glossopharyngeal afferent nerves in respiratory sensation, control of breathing and arterial pressure regulation in conscious man. *Clin Sci.* 1966;30:161–170.

79. Campbell EJM, Godfrey S, Clark TJH, Freedman S, Norman J. The effect of muscular paralysis induced by tubocurarine on the duration and sensation of breath holding during hypercapnia. *Clin Sci.* 1969;36:323–328.

80. Fowler WS. Breaking point of breath-holding. *J Appl Physiol*. 1954;6:539–545.

81. Shook J, Watkins WD, Camporesi EM. Differential roles of opioid receptors in respiration, respiratory disease, and opiate-induced respiratory depression. *Am Rev Respir Dis*. 1990;142:895–909.

82. Dahan A, Teppema LJ. Influence of anaesthesia and analgesia on the control of breathing. *Br J Anaesth*. 2003;91:40–49.

*83. Pattinson KTS. Opioids and the control of respiration. *Br J Anaesth*. 2008;100:747–758.

84. Gross JB. When you breathe in you inspire, when you don't breathe, you ... expire. *Anesthesiol*. 2003;99:767–770.

85. Alexander CM, Gross JB. Sedative doses of midazolam depress hypoxic ventilatory response in humans. *Anesth Analg*. 1988;67:377–382.

86. Gross JB, Blouin RT, Zandsberg S, Conard PF, Häussler J. Effect of flumazenil on ventilatory drive during sedation with midazolam and alfentanil. *Anesthesiology*. 1996;85:713–720.

87. Scott RM, Whitwam JG, Chakrabarti MK. Evidence of a role for the peripheral chemoreceptors in the ventilatory response to doxapram in man. *Br J Anaesth*. 1977;49:227–231.

88. Burki NK. Ventilatory effects of doxapram in conscious human subjects. *Chest*. 1984;85:600–604.

89. Ebihara S, Ogawa H, Sasaki H, Hida W, Kikuchi Y. Doxapram and perception of dyspnea. *Chest*. 2002;121:1380–1381.

90. Severinghaus JW. Proposed standard determination of ventilatory responses to hypoxia and hypercapnia in man. *Chest*. 1976;70:129s.

91. Read DJC. A clinical method for assessing the ventilatory response to carbon dioxide. *Australas Ann Med*. 1967;16:20–32.

92. Duffin J. Measuring the ventilatory response to hypoxia. *J Physiol*. 2007;584:285–293.

Chapter 6

Pulmonary ventilation

KEY POINTS

- Pharyngeal and laryngeal muscles display both tonic and phasic contraction to maintain airway patency and to regulate air flow.
- The diaphragm, intercostal, and some neck muscles bring about inspiration by a complex combination of actions, these varying with different postures.
- Expiration is normally passive, except during exercise or at minute volumes several times higher than normal, when intercostal and abdominal wall muscle contraction causes active expiration.
- The 'work of breathing' describes the power needed to overcome both the elastic recoil of the respiratory system and the non-elastic resistance to gas flow, and is normally generated by the respiratory muscles used for inspiration.

Breathing consists of rhythmic changes in lung volume brought about by the medullary respiratory neurones described in Chapter 5. Several muscle groups are involved in effecting the change in lung volume. First, muscles of the pharynx and larynx control upper airway resistance; secondly the diaphragm, ribcage, spine and neck muscles bring about inspiration; and finally, muscles of the abdominal wall, ribcage and spine are used when active expiration is required. Many of these muscle groups have common origins and attachments such that their activity is complex and dependent both on each other and many non-respiratory factors including posture, locomotion and voluntary activity.

UPPER AIRWAY MUSCLES

During inspiration through the nose, the pressure in the pharynx must fall below atmospheric by an amount equal to the product of inspiratory gas flow rate and the flow resistance afforded by the nose (see Figure 4.1). This development of only a few kilopascals of sub-atmospheric pressure in the pharynx tends to cause the pharynx to collapse.

Pharyngeal obstruction in response to these pressure changes during inspiration is opposed by reflex contraction of pharyngeal dilator muscles during inspiration.[1] The afferent side of the reflex arises from mechanoreceptors in the pharynx and larynx. These pressure receptors respond in a graded manner to sub-atmospheric pressure, and have myelinated afferent fibres to facilitate a rapid response.[2,3] Based on the observation that the pharyngeal dilator reflex is less active during sleep (page 270) the reflex pathway is believed to involve higher centres of the brain.[4] Nevertheless, the reflex is extremely rapid with both genioglossus and tensor palati electromyographic (EMG) activity increasing less than 50 ms after a negative pressure is applied to the pharynx. This compares with a reaction time for voluntary tongue movements of 190 ms.[2] The efferent side of the reflex involves most of the pharyngeal dilator muscles, which display tonic contraction and/or phasic inspiratory activity. Airway diameters are well maintained down to pressures of 1.5 kPa (15 cmH$_2$O) below atmospheric, during active but not passive breathing manoeuvres.[5] Pulmonary slowly adapting stretch receptors (page 67) may also be involved in the reflex as the activity of all pharyngeal dilator muscles is inhibited by lung inflation.[6]

There is no significant narrowing of the airway when changing from the erect to the supine posture in the normal subject.[7] Genioglossus EMG activity is increased by 34% in the supine position, presumably to counteract the effect of gravity on the tongue.[8] Anatomical considerations suggest that patency of the nasopharynx in the supine position is maintained by tensor palati, palatoglossus and palatopharyngeus, and tonic but not phasic respiratory activity has been detected in levator palati.[9] The soft palate tends to fall back against the posterior pharyngeal wall in the supine position without contraction of these muscles.

Failure of the various mechanisms that preserve pharyngeal airway patency may occur in sleep, hypoxia or anaesthesia; their occurrence and prevention are discussed in Chapters 16 and 22.

Laryngeal control of airway resistance. During quiet breathing, movement of the vocal folds is used as a choke for fine control of airway resistance. On inspiration, phasic activity of the posterior cricoarytenoid muscles, acting by rotating the arytenoid cartilages, abducts the vocal cords to minimise resistance.[10] A greater effect occurs during expiration, when phasic electrical activity in thyroarytenoid muscles indicates adduction of the vocal cords,[13] and therefore an increase in resistance. This may help to prevent collapse of the lower airways (page 49).

RESPIRATORY MUSCLES OF THE TRUNK

Nomenclature in this area can be confusing with different authors using different terms. The trunk (referred to as chest wall by some studies) may be divided into the ribcage and abdomen. These two compartments are separated by the diaphragm and both are therefore greatly influenced by its activity.

THE DIAPHRAGM

The diaphragm is a membranous muscle separating the abdominal cavity and chest, and in adults has a total surface area[11] of approximately $900 \, cm^2$. It is the most important inspiratory muscle, with motor innervation solely from the phrenic nerves (C3, 4, 5). In comparison with other skeletal muscles, the diaphragm is extremely active. Muscle fibres within the diaphragm can reduce their length by up to 40%

between residual volume and total lung capacity,[11] and spend 45% of each day contracting, compared with only 14% for the soleus muscle.[12] The diaphragm has considerable reserve of function, and unilateral phrenic block causes little decrement of overall ventilatory capacity. Despite the importance of the diaphragm to respiration, bilateral phrenic interruption is still compatible with good ventilatory function.

Mechanics of diaphragmatic function. The origins of the crural part of the diaphragm are the lumbar vertebrae and the arcuate ligaments, whilst the costal parts arise from the lower ribs and xiphisternum. Both parts are inserted into the central tendon. Recent studies of human subjects using MRI scans, illustrated in Figure 6.1, have enabled the in vivo actions of the diaphragm to be better defined.[11,13,14] Under normal circumstances, a zone of apposition exists around the outside of the diaphragm where it is in direct contact with the internal aspect of the ribcage, with no lung in between, but the parietal pleura still allowing free movement of the diaphragm. At upright FRC in humans, approximately 55% of the diaphragm surface area is in the zone of apposition.[11]

There are many ways by which diaphragm contraction may bring about an increase in lung volume,[15] and these are illustrated schematically in Figure 6.2. These may be considered using a 'piston in a cylinder' analogy, the trunk representing the cylinder and the diaphragm the piston (Figure 6.2A). Figure 6.2B illustrates the first possible mechanism, involving downward movement of the diaphragm simply by shortening the zone of apposition around the whole cylinder and leaving the dome shape unchanged. This is a pure 'piston-like' action and has the advantage of very efficient conversion of diaphragm muscle fibre shortening into changes in lung volume. Figure 6.2C illustrates 'non-piston-like' behaviour in which the zone of apposition remains unchanged but an increase in the tension of the diaphragm dome reduces the curvature, so expanding the lung. This is likely to be less efficient than piston-like behaviour because much of the muscle tension developed simply opposes the opposite side of the diaphragm rather than moving the diaphragm downwards, such that in theory, when the diaphragm becomes flat, further contraction will have no effect on lung volume. Finally, Figure 6.2D incorporates both types of behaviour already described but also now includes expansion of the lower ribcage (known as 'piston in an expanding cylinder') that occurs with diaphragmatic contraction,

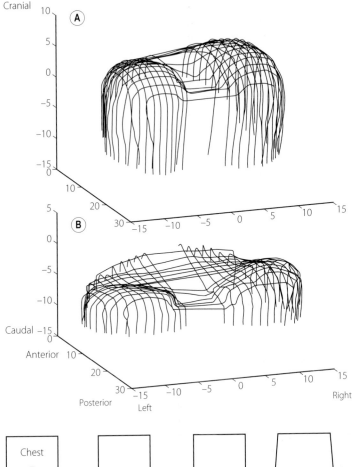

Fig. 6.1 Three-dimensional reconstructions of the human diaphragm at functional residual capacity using fast computed tomography scanning (dimensions in cm). (A) Normal subject showing extensive zone of apposition and normal curvature of the diaphragm domes. (B) Patient with hyperinflated chest as a result of chronic obstructive pulmonary disease (page 411). Note the reduced zone of apposition and the flattened diaphragm domes. (After reference 14 by permission of the authors and the publishers of American Journal of Respiratory and Critical Care Medicine.)

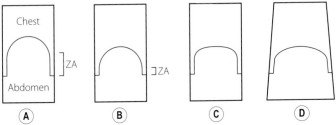

Fig. 6.2 'Piston in a cylinder' analogy of the mechanisms of diaphragm actions on the lung volume. (A) Resting end-expiratory position. (B) Inspiration with pure piston-like behaviour. (C) Inspiration with pure non-piston-like behaviour. (D) Combination of piston-like and non-piston-like behaviour in an expanding cylinder, which equates most closely with inspiration in vivo. ZA, zone of apposition.

particularly in the supine position, and so represents a simple description of the in vivo situation.

In the supine position, diaphragm action is a combination of all the above mechanisms as well as a change in shape involving a tilting and flattening of the diaphragm in the antero-posterior direction.[11]

RIBCAGE MUSCLES[16]

As already described, the ribcage may be regarded as a cylinder with length governed primarily by the diaphragm and secondarily by flexion and extension of the spine. The cross-sectional area of the cylinder

is governed by movement of the ribs. This movement involves mainly rotation of the neck of the rib about the axis of the costovertebral joints, and their shape is such that elevation of the ribs in this way increases both the lateral and anteroposterior diameter of the ribcage. Elevation of the ribs by the intercostal muscles tends to result in a 'bucket handle' action, whilst elevation of the anterior ribcage by, for example, the sternomastoid muscle elevating the sternum results in a 'pump-handle' type of movement. These two actions tend to occur together, and depend also on other requirements such as posture and upper limb movements. Upper ribs are inserted into the sternum and do not necessarily behave in quite the same way as the lower 'floating' ribs, which are inserted into the more flexible costal cartilage.

The intercostal muscles are divided into the external group, fibres of which run in a caudal–ventral direction from their upper rib and are deficient anteriorly, and the less powerful internal group which have fibres running caudal–dorsal from their upper rib and are deficient posteriorly. Internal intercostal muscles of the upper ribcage become thicker anteriorly where they are known as the parasternal intercostal muscles. In 1749, mechanical considerations led Hamberger to suggest that the external intercostals were primarily inspiratory, and the internal intercostals primarily expiratory.[17] Though an oversimplification,[16] this has generally been confirmed by electromyography. The parasternal portion of the internal intercostals are inspiratory in both humans and animals, and the inspiratory activity of external intercostals, though minimal during quiet breathing, becomes increasingly important during stimulated breathing. Posture plays an important role in intercostal activity in humans. For example, during the rather extreme postural challenge of rotating the trunk, which changes the mechanical properties of the ribs, the respiratory activity of internal and external intercostals is reversed with internal intercostals becoming expiratory and vice versa.[18]

Scalene muscles are active in inspiration during quiet breathing in humans[19] particularly when upright. Their role is to elevate the ribcage and this counteracts the tendency of the diaphragm to cause inward displacement of the upper ribs. Innervation is from C1 to C5.

Accessory muscles. These are silent in normal breathing in humans but as ventilation increases, the inspiratory muscles contract more vigorously and accessory muscles are recruited. Considerable hyperventilation (about 50 1.min^{-1}) or severe increases in respiratory loading are usually present before the accessory muscles become active. Accessory muscles include the sternocleidomastoids, extensors of the vertebral column, pectoralis minor, trapezius and the serrati muscles. Many of these muscles, for example the pectorals, reverse their usual origin/insertion and help to expand the chest, provided the arms and shoulder girdle are fixed by grasping a suitable support.

ABDOMINAL MUSCLES

With the exception of gas within the bowel lumen, the abdomen is an incompressible volume held between the diaphragm and the abdominal muscles. Contraction of either will cause a corresponding passive displacement of the other. Thus abdominal muscles are generally expiratory.

Rectus abdominis, external oblique, internal oblique and tranversalis muscles are the most important expiratory muscles, whilst the muscles of the pelvic floor have a supportive role. Contraction of these muscles results in an increase in abdominal pressure displacing the diaphragm in a cephalad direction. In addition, their insertion into the costal margin results in a caudad movement of the ribcage, so assisting expiration by opposing the ribcage muscles. Gastric pressure is a valuable index of their activity because their contraction will always cause an increase in intra-abdominal pressure.

In the supine position, the abdominal muscles are normally inactive during quiet breathing and become active only when the minute volume exceeds about 40 1.min^{-1}, in the face of substantial expiratory resistance, during phonation or when making expulsive efforts. When upright, their use in breathing is complicated by their role in the maintenance of posture.

INTEGRATION OF RESPIRATORY MUSCLE ACTIVITY

BREATHING

Figure 6.3 shows the radiographic appearance of the ribcage at residual volume, the normal expiratory level and at maximal inspiration, and illustrates the enormous range of movement within the semi-rigid ribcage. Expiration normally proceeds passively to the functional residual capacity (FRC), which may be considered as the equilibrium position governed by the balance of elastic forces, unless modified by residual end-expiratory tone in certain muscle groups. Inspiration is the active phase, entering the inspiratory capacity but normally leaving a substantial volume unused (the inspiratory reserve volume). Similarly, there is a substantial volume (the expiratory reserve volume) between FRC and the residual volume (see Figure 3.9). By voluntary effort it is possible to effect a satisfactory tidal exchange anywhere within the vital capacity, but the work of breathing is minimal at FRC.

Although we tend to think of the respiratory muscles individually, it is important to remember that they act together in an extraordinarily complex

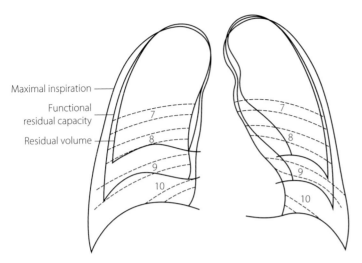

Maximal inspiration

Functional
residual capacity

Residual volume

7   7

8   8

9   9

10   10

Fig. 6.3 Outlines of chest radiographs of a normal subject at various levels of lung inflation. The numbers refer to ribs as seen in the position of maximal inspiration. (With thanks to Dr R. L. Marks who was the subject.)

interaction that is influenced by factors including posture, minute volume, respiratory load, disease and anaesthesia. Figure 6.4 illustrates some features of the interaction.[18,20]

Inspiration. In Figure 6.4 it can be seen that the ribcage inspiratory muscles (external intercostals and scalenes) and diaphragm act in parallel to inflate the lungs, with posture affecting which muscle group is dominant (see below). In either position, diaphragm activity alone results in a widening of the lower ribcage and an indrawing of the upper ribcage (often seen with spontaneous respiration during general anaesthesia), which must be countered by the intercostal and neck muscles contracting simultaneously.

Expiration. Requires no muscular activity during quiet breathing in the supine position, because the elastic recoil of the lungs provides the energy required, aided by the weight of the abdominal contents pushing the diaphragm in a cephalad direction. In the upright posture and during stimulated ventilation the internal intercostal muscles and the abdominal wall muscles are active in returning the ribcage and diaphragm to the resting position. In extreme hyperventilation, for example following exercise, the expiratory muscles become progressively more important until ventilation assumes a quasi sine wave push-pull pattern.

SEPARATION OF VOLUME CONTRIBUTION OF RIBCAGE AND ABDOMEN

Konno & Mead originally proposed that the separate contributions to tidal volume of changes in ribcage (RC) and abdominal (AB) compartments could be measured.[22] Essentially similar results may be obtained by measuring either antero-posterior distance (magnetometers), circumference (strain gauge) or cross-sectional area (respiratory inductance plethysmography, RIP[23]). Once initially calibrated to convert measurements of trunk dimensions into volumes, the sum of RC and AB movements correlates well with tidal volume and provides an excellent non-invasive measure of ventilation. RC/(RC + AB) indicates the proportion of tidal volume that can be attributed to expansion of the ribcage (usually expressed as %RC). However, such is the complexity of the muscular system described above that changes in %RC cannot be attributed to changes in the force of contraction of any particular muscle. Figure 6.5 shows RIP traces during normal breathing in different positions.

EFFECT OF POSTURE ON RESPIRATORY MUSCLES

Upright posture, whether standing or sitting, is associated with greater expansion of the ribcage[23] such that %RC is around 67% (Figure 6.5). To account for this, increased EMG activity has been demonstrated in the both the scalene and the parasternal intercostals muscles.[24]

Supine position. When supine, the weight of the abdominal contents pushes the diaphragm upwards, so that in the supine position the diaphragm tends to lie some 4 cm higher, which accords with the reduction in FRC when supine (see Figure 3.10). With the diaphragm higher in the chest, its fibre length is greater and it can therefore contract more

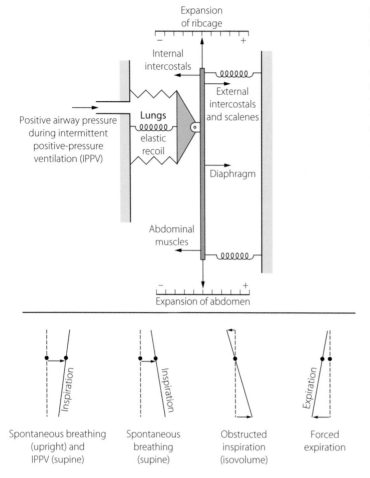

Fig. 6.4 A model of the balance of static and dynamic forces acting on the respiratory system. The central bar, attached to the lungs, is floating freely, held in equilibrium by the elastic forces at the end-expiratory position as shown. It may be displaced by the actions of the various muscles shown, with movement to the right generally indicating inspiration and vice versa. Action of the various inspiratory or expiratory muscles causes changes, not only in the lung volume but also in the inclination of the bar, which represents relative changes in the cross-sectional area of the ribcage and abdomen. See text for details. (Derived from references 20 and 21.)

The broken line represents FRC

effectively, counteracting the tendency to airway closure at the reduced FRC. The dimensions of the ribcage are probably little altered, and the increased diaphragm activity therefore results in a reduced %RC of about 33% in the supine position.[23] In the prone and lateral position, RC contribution does not differ significantly from that in the supine position (Figure 6.5).[23]

Lateral position. In this position (Figure 6.6), only the lower dome of the diaphragm is pushed higher into the chest by the weight of the abdominal contents while the upper dome is flattened. It follows that the lower dome can contract more effectively than the upper, and the ventilation of the lower lung is about twice that of the upper. This is fortunate since gravity causes a preferential perfusion of the lower lung (page 123).

CHEMORECEPTOR ACTIVATION

In animals, clear differences have been demonstrated in the respiratory muscle response to hyperventilation induced either by hypoxia or hypercapnia. For an equivalent minute volume, hypoxia stimulates mostly inspiratory muscles whilst hypercapnia stimulates both inspiratory and expiratory groups. Similar responses occur in humans, with diaphragm EMG activity increasing in response to both hypercapnia and hypoxia, but more rapidly in the latter, and expiratory muscle activity increasing almost exclusively during hypercapnic hyperventilation.[24] Hyperventilation in response to hypercapnia in the supine position results in a small increase in RC contribution (7% per kPa $P\text{CO}_2$ or 1% per mmHg $P\text{CO}_2$).[25]

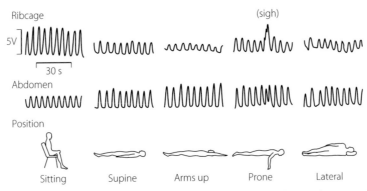

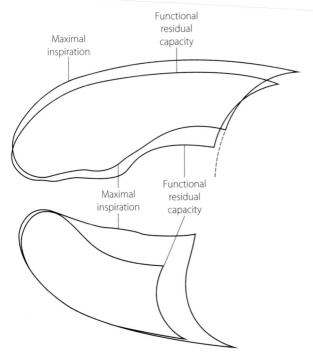

Fig. 6.5 Normal respiratory inductance plethysmography (RIP) traces. The amplitude (in volts) of the RIP signal reflects the cross-sectional area of the rib cage (RC) and abdomen (AB). The sum of the RC and AB signals correlates closely with tidal volume. The figure shows normal breathing in five different positions, demonstrating the predominantly RC contribution when upright and AB contribution in all horizontal positions. Note the spontaneous sigh occurring in the prone position, resulting entirely from rib cage expansion. (After reference 23 by permission of the publishers of Anesthesia and Analgesia.)

Fig. 6.6 Radiographic outlines of the lungs at two levels of lung volume in a conscious subject during spontaneous breathing in the lateral position (right side down). This is the same subject as in Figure 6.3: comparison will show that, in the lateral position at FRC, the lower lung is close to residual volume while the upper lung is close to inspiratory capacity. The diaphragm therefore lies much more cephalad in the lower half of the chest. Both these factors contribute to the greater volume changes that occur in the lower lung during inspiration.

NEURONAL CONTROL OF RESPIRATORY MUSCLES

The respiratory muscles, in common with other skeletal muscles, have their tension controlled by a servo mechanism mediated by muscle spindles. They appear to play a more important role in the intercostal muscles than in the diaphragm but muscle spindles do exist in both. Their function is largely inferred from knowledge of their well established role in other skeletal muscles not concerned with respiration.

Two types of cell can be distinguished in the motor neurone pool of the anterior horn cell. The alpha motoneurone has a thick efferent fibre (12–20 μm diameter) and passes in the ventral root

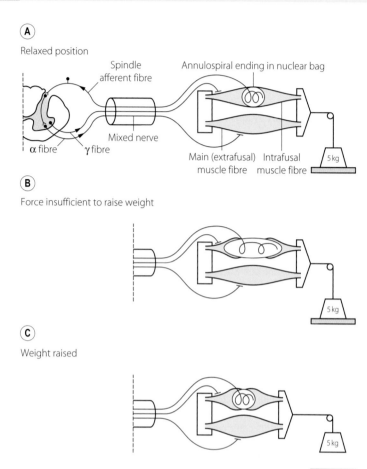

(A)

Relaxed position

Spindle
afferent fibre   Annulospiral ending in nuclear bag

Mixed nerve

α fibre   γ fibre

Main (extrafusal)   Intrafusal
muscle fibre   muscle fibre   5 kg

(B)

Force insufficient to raise weight

5 kg

(C)

Weight raised

5 kg

Fig. 6.7 Diagrammatic representation of the servo mechanism mediated by the muscle spindles. (A) The resting state with muscle and intrafusal fibres of spindle relaxed. (B) The muscle is attempting to lift the weight following discharge of both alpha and gamma systems. The force developed by the muscle is insufficient: the weight is not lifted and the muscle cannot shorten. However, the intrafusal fibres are able to shorten and stretch the annulospiral endings in the nuclear bag of the spindle. Afferent discharge causes increased excitation of the motor neurone pool in the anterior horn. (C) Alpha discharge is augmented and the weight is finally lifted by the more powerful contraction of the muscle. When the weight is lifted, the tension on the nuclear bag is relieved and the afferent discharge from the spindle ceases. This series of diagrams relates to the lifting of a weight but it is thought that similar action of spindles is brought into play when inspiratory muscles contract against increased airways resistance.

directly to the neuromuscular junction of the muscle fibre (Figure 6.7A). The gamma motor neurone has a thin efferent fibre (2–8 μm), which also passes in the ventral root, but terminates in the intrafusal fibres of the muscle spindle. Contraction of the intrafusal fibres alone (without overall shortening of the muscle) increases the tension in the central part of the spindle (the nuclear bag), causing stimulation of the annulospiral endings. Impulses so generated are then transmitted via fibres that lie in the dorsal root to reach the anterior horn where they have an excitatory effect on the alpha motor neurones. Using this system, an efferent impulse transmitted by the gamma system causes reflex contraction of the main muscle mass by means of an arc through the annulospiral afferent and the alpha motor neurone. Thus contraction of the whole muscle may be controlled entirely by efferents travelling in the gamma fibres and this is believed to occur in relation to breathing.[26]

Alternatively, muscle contraction may in the first instance result from discharge of both the alpha and gamma motoneurones. If shortening of the muscle is unopposed, main (extrafusal) and intrafusal fibres will contract together and the tension in the nuclear bag of the spindle will be unchanged. If, however, the shortening of the muscle is opposed, the intrafusal fibres will shorten more than the extrafusal fibres, causing the nuclear bag to be stretched (Figure 6.7B). The consequent stimulation of the annulospiral endings results in afferent activity that raises the excitatory state of the motor neurones, causing the main muscle fibres to increase their tension until the resistance is overcome, allowing the muscle to shorten and the tension in the nuclear bag of the spindle to be reduced (Figure 6.7C).

By this mechanism, fine control of muscle contraction is possible. The message from the upper motor neurone is in the form: 'muscles should contract with whatever force may be found necessary to effect such and such a shortening', and not simply: 'muscles should contract with such and such a force'. The former message is typical of input into a servo system and far more satisfactory when the load is not known in advance.

For respiratory muscles, a servo system is very advantageous. The message conveyed by the efferent tract from the inspiratory neurones of the medulla would be in the form: 'inspiratory muscles should contract with whatever force may be necessary to effect a required change in length (corresponding to a certain tidal volume)' and not simply: 'inspiratory muscles should contract with such and such a force'. A servo system also provides an excellent mechanism for rapid response to sudden changes in airway resistance. The nature and magnitude of the response of the inspiratory muscles to added resistance to breathing is described in Chapter 4, and the immediate effectiveness of the response is easily explicable in terms of muscle spindles.

MUSCLE FIBRE SUBTYPES[27]

Respiratory muscles, like all skeletal muscle, contain different types of muscle fibre classified according to which isoform of myosin heavy chain (MHC) is expressed. Table 6.1 shows the three fibre types known to exist in human respiratory muscles and their contractile and biochemical features. Which isoform of MHC is expressed in a muscle fibre determines the velocity of contraction (Table 6.1). Different isoforms of enzymes involved in muscle relaxation also exist in the different fibre types, and so influence the rate at which relaxation occurs, and therefore the ability of the cell to maintain a tetanic contraction. Type I fibres contract and relax slowly, but can maintain tension for long periods using aerobic metabolic pathways, and are fatigue resistant. In contrast, type IIb fibres rely mainly on glycolytic metabolic pathways for energy supply, contraction is quicker and stronger in bursts of activity, and they fatigue easily. Type IIa fibres have properties intermediate between these two extreme fibre types. The proportions of different fibre types in a muscle therefore reveals the sort of work normally undertaken by the muscle, for example in muscles mainly involved in maintaining posture, type I fibres predominate, whilst in those requiring intermittent activity such as hand muscles type IIa or IIb fibres predominate.

Relative proportions of the different fibre types in human respiratory muscle are shown in Table 6.1,

Table 6.1 Properties of muscle fibre types found in human respiratory muscle, and their relative proportions in normal and pathological situations[27,28,29]

	TYPE I	TYPE IIa	TYPE IIb
Contractile properties:			
Velocity of shortening	+	+ +	+ + + +
Tetanic force	+	+	+ +
Fatigue resistance	+ + + +	+ + +	+
Biochemical properties:			
Mitochondrial density	+ + +	+ + +	+
ATP consumption rate	+	+ +	+ + + +
Oxidative enzymes	+ + +	+ + +	+
Glycolytic enzymes	+	+ +	+ + + +
Glycogen content	+	+ +	+ + +
Relative proportions in:			
Normal subjects	45%	39%	16%
COPD	↑↑	↓	↓↓
Steroid myopathy	↔	↔	↓↓↓
Artificial ventilation[†]	↓	↑	↔

[†]Animal studies only. COPD, chronic obstructive pulmonary disease (Chapter 28); ATP, adenosine triphosphate.

but it is unclear which types of fibre are responsible for different respiratory muscle activities. In animal respiratory muscles, which tend to have less type II fibres than humans, both eupnoeic and stimulated breathing can be achieved solely by using type I fibres, and type II fibres are only required for expulsive efforts such as sneezing and coughing.[12] A high proportion of type I fibres (45% in human diaphragm) indicates that they are probably responsible for both posture and respiration in humans, and that type II fibres are again only required for expulsive efforts and active movements such as running, jumping etc. Respiratory disease, drugs and artificial ventilation all cause changes in the relative proportions of different fibre types in respiratory muscles (Table 6.1).

RESPIRATORY MUSCLE FATIGUE AND DISUSE[27,30]

The diaphragm, like other striated muscles, is subject to fatigue – defined as an inability to sustain tension with repeated activity.[30] For non-respiratory skeletal muscle, fatigue may be 'central' – that is, the subject is not trying hard enough (either consciously or subconsciously) – but this is unlikely to be significant in respiration because subjects with respiratory failure usually have a high central respiratory drive. Peripheral fatigue occurs when the frequency of motor nerve action potentials becomes chronically increased in an attempt to increase muscle tension. Eventually, when working against an unsustainable load, striated muscle shows a progressive loss of the high frequency component of the EMG relative to lower frequencies. Finally, relaxation of the muscle fibre, the energy-requiring part of contraction, becomes excessively prolonged and the muscle is unable to respond to the next action potential in order to generate the required tension. In the diaphragm, resistive loads less than 40% of maximum may be sustained indefinitely, but loads greater than 40% of maximum can only be sustained for a short time.[31]

Blood supply to respiratory muscles may be important in fatigue.[32] Animal studies have shown that increased cardiac output and diaphragmatic blood flow (stimulated with noradrenaline) augment the contractility of fatigued diaphragm. In addition, patients with severe congestive cardiac failure, and therefore low cardiac output, have weakened respiratory muscles compared with matched controls, despite having similar muscle strength in the arms.[33] The high rate of activity of respiratory muscles seems to leave them more susceptible to weakness in the face of reduced oxygen supply when compared with other muscles, a situation that often causes problems in intensive care when trying to wean patients from artificial ventilation before their cardiovascular function is adequate (page 474).

EFFECT OF DISUSE[12,34,35]

The diaphragm may be rested by artificial ventilation with or without neuromuscular blockade, and the effect on diaphragmatic performance is clearly important. After only 18 hours of mechanical ventilation there are histological and gene-expression changes indicating muscle fibre atrophy,[36] and within days diaphragm strength is substantially reduced (Table 6.1).[27] Extrapolating these results to all artificially ventilated patients is difficult, as there are numerous factors affecting respiratory muscle strength in critically ill patients.[35] Even so, it seems safe to assume that complete inactivity of the normally very active respiratory muscles will be detrimental to their function, and recent developments in artificial ventilation have mostly focussed on supporting, rather than replacing, activity of the patient's respiratory muscles (Chapter 32).

THE WORK OF BREATHING

When expiration is passive during quiet breathing, the work of breathing is performed entirely by the inspiratory muscles. Approximately half of this work is dissipated during inspiration as heat in overcoming the frictional forces opposing inspiration. The other half is stored as potential energy in the deformed elastic tissues of lungs and chest wall. This potential energy is thus available as the source of energy for expiration and is then dissipated as heat in overcoming the frictional forces resisting expiration. Energy stored in deformed elastic tissue thus permits the work of *expiration* to be transferred to the *inspiratory* muscles. This remains true with moderate increases of either inspiratory or expiratory resistance, lung volume and therefore elastic recoil being increased in the latter condition (page 54).

The actual work performed by the respiratory muscles is very small in the healthy resting subject. Under these circumstances the oxygen consumption of the respiratory muscles is only about 3 ml.min^{-1} or less than 2% of the metabolic rate. Furthermore, the efficiency of the respiratory muscles is only about 10%. The efficiency is further reduced in many forms of respiratory disease, certain deformities, pregnancy and when the minute volume is increased (Figure 6.8). When maximal ventilation is approached, the efficiency falls to such a low level that additional oxygen made available by further increases in ventilation will be entirely consumed by the respiratory muscles.

UNITS OF MEASUREMENT OF WORK

Work is performed when a force moves its point of application, and the work is equal to the product of force and distance moved. Similarly, work is performed when force is applied to the plunger of a syringe raising the pressure of gas contained therein. In this case the work is equal to the product of the mean pressure and the change in volume, or alternatively the product of the mean volume and the change in pressure. The units of work are identical whether the product is *force × distance* or *pressure × volume*. A multiplicity of units have been used for measuring work and are listed in Appendix A.

Power is a measure of the rate at which work is being (or can be) performed. The term 'work of

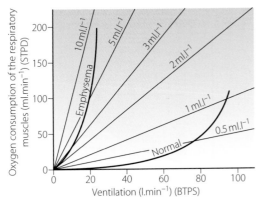

Fig. 6.8 Oxygen consumption of the respiratory muscles plotted against minute volume of respiration. The isopleths indicate the oxygen cost of breathing in millilitres of oxygen consumed per litre of minute volume. The curve obtained from the normal subject shows the low oxygen cost of breathing up to a minute volume of 70 l.min^{-1}. Thereafter the oxygen cost rises steeply. In a patient with chronic obstructive pulmonary disease the oxygen cost of breathing is not only much higher at the resting minute volume but also rises more steeply as ventilation increases. At a minute volume of 20 l.min^{-1}, the respiratory muscles are consuming 200 ml of oxygen per minute, and a further increase of ventilation would consume more oxygen than it would make available to the rest of the body. (After reference 37 by permission of the Journal of Applied Physiology.)

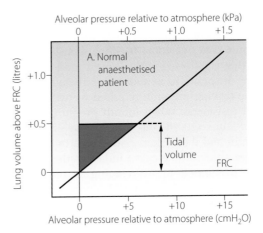

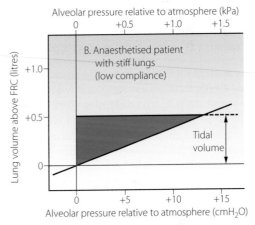

Fig. 6.9 Work of breathing against elastic resistance during passive inflation. The lines show pressure/volume plots of the lungs of anaesthetised patients (conscious subjects are shown in Figure 3.8). The length of the pressure/volume curve covered during inspiration forms the hypotenuse of a right-angled triangle whose area equals the work performed against elastic resistance. Note that the area is greater when the pressure/volume curve is flatter (indicating stiffer or less compliant lungs).

breathing', as it is normally used and when expressed in watts, is thus a misnomer because we are referring to the rate at which work is being performed and *power* is the correct term. 'Work of breathing' would be appropriate for a single event such as one breath, and joules would then be the appropriate units.

DISSIPATION OF THE WORK OF BREATHING

The work of breathing overcomes two main sources of impedance. The first is the elastic recoil of the lungs and chest wall (Chapter 3) and the second is the non-elastic resistance to gas flow (Chapter 4).

Work against elastic recoil. When an elastic body is deformed, no work is dissipated as heat and all work is stored as potential energy. Figure 6.9A shows a section of the alveolar pressure/volume plot for the total respiratory system, showing only the straight part of the curve from near FRC (see Figure 3.7). As the lungs are inflated, the plot forms the hypotenuse of a triangle, whose area represents the work done

against elastic resistance. The area of the triangle (half the base times the height) will thus equal either half the tidal volume times the pressure change or the mean pressure times the volume change. Either product has the units of work or energy (joules) and represents the potential energy available for expiration. In Figure 6.9B, the pressure/volume curve is flatter, indicating stiffer or less compliant lungs. For the same tidal volume, the area of the triangle is increased. This indicates the greater amount of work performed against elastic resistance and the greater potential energy available for expiration.

Work against resistance to gas flow. Frictional resistance was ignored in Figure 6.9. Additional pressure is required to overcome frictional resistance to gas flow that is reflected in the mouth pressure, which, during inspiration, is above the alveolar pressure by the driving pressure required to overcome frictional resistance. When mouth pressure is plotted as in Figure 6.10, the inspiratory curve is bowed to the right and the darker shaded area to the right of the pressure volume curve indicates the additional work performed in overcoming inspiratory frictional resistance. Figure 6.10B represents a patient with increased airway resistance. The expiratory curve, not shown in Figure 6.10, would be bowed to the left as the mouth-to-alveolar pressure gradient is reversed during expiration.

THE MINIMAL WORK OF BREATHING

For a constant minute volume, the work performed against elastic resistance is increased when breathing is slow and deep. Conversely, the work performed against air flow resistance is increased when breathing is rapid and shallow. If the two components are summated and the total work is plotted against respiratory frequency, it will be found that there is an optimal frequency at which the total work of breathing is minimal (Figure 6.11). If there is increased elastic resistance (as in patients with pulmonary fibrosis), the optimal frequency is increased, while in the presence of increased air flow resistance the optimal frequency is decreased. Humans and animals tend to select a respiratory frequency close to that which minimises respiratory work. This applies to different species, different age groups and also to pathological conditions.

MEASUREMENT OF VENTILATION

Volume may be measured either directly or by the continuous integration of instantaneous gas flow rate (Figure 6.12).

DIRECT MEASUREMENT OF RESPIRED VOLUMES[38]

Inspiratory and expiratory tidal volumes (and therefore minute volume) may be markedly different, and the difference is important in calculations of gas exchange. The normal respiratory exchange ratio of about 0.8 means that inspiratory minute

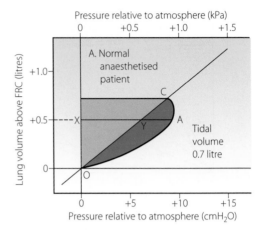

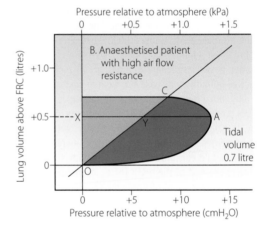

Fig. 6.10 Work of breathing against air flow resistance during passive inflation. The sloping line OYC is the alveolar pressure/volume curve. The curve OAC is the mouth pressure/volume curve during inflation of the lungs. The darker shaded area indicates the work of inspiration performed against air flow resistance. This work is increased in the patient with high resistance (B). At the point when 500 ml gas has entered the patient, XY represents the pressure distending the lungs, while YA represents the pressure overcoming air flow resistance. XA is the inflation pressure at that moment. The lighter shaded areas represent the work done against elastic resistance (see Figure 6.9).

volume is about 50 ml larger than expiratory minute volume in the resting subject. Much larger differences can arise during exercise and during uptake or wash-out of an inert gas such as nitrogen or, to a greater extent, nitrous oxide.

Water-sealed spirometers provide the reference method for the measurement of ventilation (Figure 6.12), and may be precisely calibrated by water displacement. They provide negligible resistance to

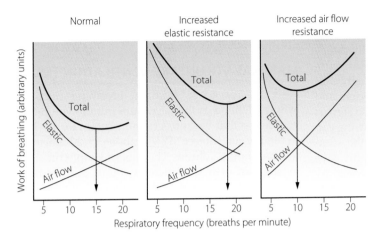

Fig. 6.11 Minimal work of breathing. The diagrams show the work done against elastic and air flow resistance separately and summated to indicate the total work of breathing at different respiratory frequencies. The total work of breathing has a minimum value at about 15 breaths per minute under normal circumstances. For the same minute volume, minimum work is performed at higher frequencies with stiff (less compliant) lungs and at lower frequencies when the air flow resistance is increased.

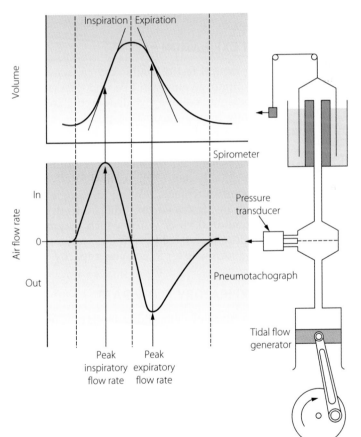

Fig. 6.12 Relationship between volume and flow rate. The upper graph shows volume plotted against time; this type of tracing is obtained from a spirometer. The lower graph shows instantaneous air flow rate plotted against time; this type of tracing is obtained from a pneumotachograph. At any instant, the flow-rate trace indicates the slope of the volume trace, while the volume trace indicates the cumulative area under the flow-rate trace. *Flow* is the differential of volume; *volume* is the integral of flow rate. Differentiation of the spirometer trace gives a 'pneumotachogram'; integration of the pneumotachogram gives a 'spirometer' trace.

breathing and, by suitable design, may have a satisfactory frequency response up to very high respiratory frequencies.

Dry spirometers are hinged bellows, usually with electronic displays of both volume and instantaneous flow rate. Their accuracy approaches that of a water-filled spirometer and they are far more convenient in use.

Impellers and turbines. The best known of these instruments is the respirometer developed by Wright in 1955.[39] The mechanism is entirely mechanical with indication of volume on a dial but the output may be converted to an electrical signal to indicate either tidal volume or minute volume. In general the respirometer is accurate and tends to read low at low minute volumes and high at high minute volumes; departure from normality is thus exaggerated and the instrument is essentially safe.

Respiratory inductance plethysmography. Reference has been made above (page 87) to this method of measurement of cross-sectional area of ribcage and abdominal compartments. The sum of these signals correlates well with lung volume and, following calibration against a spirometer, changes in the summated signals provide a very useful non-invasive method of measuring ventilation, uninfluenced by the presence of a mouthpiece or mask, and feasible during sleep (Figure 6.5).

MEASUREMENT OF VENTILATORY VOLUMES BY INTEGRATION OF INSTANTANEOUS GAS FLOW RATE

Electronics have made measurement of ventilatory volumes by integration of instantaneous flow rate a widespread technique in clinical environments. There are many methods for measuring rapidly changing gas flow rates of which the original was pneumotachography. This employs measurement of the pressure gradient across a laminar resistance, which ensures that the pressure drop is directly proportional to flow rate. This is illustrated in Figure 6.12 where the resistance is a wire mesh screen. It is necessary to take precautions to prevent errors due to different gas composition and temperature, and to prevent condensation of moisture on the screen. The pressure drop need not exceed a few millimetres of water and the volume can be very small. The pneumotachograph should not therefore interfere with respiration.

Most ventilators and anaesthetic machines currently in use can measure respiratory volumes. A pneumotachograph or electronic turbine system is used, normally on the expired limb of the breathing system, and designed to be of very low resistance to allow measurements during spontaneous respiration. In this way, each expired tidal volume may be measured from which respiratory rate and minute volume can be derived, and a useful method of detecting apnoea or disconnection is therefore provided.

MEASUREMENT OF VENTILATORY CAPACITY[38,40]

Measurement of ventilatory capacity is the most commonly performed test of respiratory function. The ratio of ventilatory capacity to actual ventilation is a measure of ventilatory reserve and of the comfort of breathing.

MAXIMAL VOLUNTARY VENTILATION (MVV)

Also referred to as maximal breathing capacity, MBC is defined as the maximum minute volume of ventilation that the subject can maintain for 12–15 s. In the normal subject MVV is about 15–20 times the resting minute volume. The subject simply breathes in and out of a spirometer without the need for removal of carbon dioxide; although simple, the test is exhausting to perform and is now seldom used. The average fit young male adult should have an MBC of about 170 $l.min^{-1}$ but normal values depend upon body size, age and sex.

FORCED EXPIRATION

A more practical test of ventilatory capacity is the forced expiratory volume in 1 second (FEV_1) which is the maximal volume exhaled in the first second starting from a maximal inspiration. A simple spirometer is all that is required. It is far more convenient to perform than the MVV and less exhausting for the patient. It correlates well with the MVV, which is normally about 35 times the FEV_1. A variety of similar measurements relating to a single forced expiration are described, including forced expiratory volume in 0.5 s or 0.75 s, which may be useful in children, or forced expiratory volume in 6 s which is a surrogate for forced vital capacity.[40]

PEAK EXPIRATORY FLOW RATE

Most convenient of all the indirect tests of ventilatory capacity is the peak expiratory flow rate. This can be measured with simple and inexpensive hand-held devices, and is an easy method for assessing large airway calibre. Interpretation of measurements of maximal expirations may be misleading. It should be remembered that these tests measure active expiration, which plays no part in normal breathing. They are most commonly performed as a measure of airway obstruction and are extensively used in patients with asthma and chronic obstructive airway disease. However, the results also depend on many other factors, including chest restriction, motivation and muscular power. The measurements may also be inhibited by pain. A more specific indication of airway resistance is the ratio of FEV_1 to vital capacity, which should exceed 75% in the normal subject.

ASSESSMENT OF THE RESPIRATORY MUSCLES[41]

Severe abnormalities of muscle function may be assessed by simple observation of spontaneous breathing. During inspiration, paradoxical movements of the trunk may occur such as inward displacement of the abdominal wall (diaphragm failure) or inward movement of the upper chest (intercostal failure). Fluoroscopy or ultrasound imaging of the diaphragm provides a more subtle form of observation, and is helpful in detecting phrenic nerve damage, particularly if unilateral when the body surface changes will be less obvious.

Vital capacity (VC, Figure 3.9) is accepted as the best 'bedside' monitor of respiratory muscle function, particularly when performed supine.[41] Performance of a VC manoeuvre requires patient cooperation and coordination, and a single low reading is non-specific. However, repeated measurement allows the observation of a trend in VC to be followed, and a 25% reduction is unequivocally abnormal. In spite of the many causes of a reduced VC, this method of assessing respiratory muscle function is very useful for monitoring the development of progressive muscle weakness in conditions such as myasthenia gravis and Guillain–Barré syndrome (page 395).

Pressure measurements, when breathing against an imposed resistance, are used to assess both inspiratory and expiratory muscle strength. All require some patient compliance and involve a degree of respiratory discomfort so these tests, though more specific than VC for respiratory muscle function, are not widely used. Mouth pressure may be measured whilst a slow inspiration or expiration is performed against a moderate respiratory resistance, or mouth pressure may be measured during a rapid 'sniff' procedure in which the nasal airway acts as the resistance.

References

1. Cheng S, Butler JE, Gandevia SC, Bilston LE. Movement of the tongue during normal breathing in awake healthy humans. *J Physiol.* 2008;586:4283–4294.
2. Horner RL, Innes JA, Guz A. Reflex pharyngeal dilator muscle activation by stimuli of negative airway pressure in awake man. *Sleep.* 1993;16(suppl 8):S85–S86.
*3. Widdicombe J. Airway receptors. *Respir Physiol.* 2001;125:3–15.
4. Remmers JE. Wagging the tongue and guarding the airway. Reflex control of the genioglossus. *Am J Respir Crit Care Med.* 2001;164:2013–2015.
5. Wheatley JR, Kelley WT, Tully A, Engel LA. Pressure-diameter relationships in the upper airway in awake supine subjects. *J Appl Physiol.* 1991;70:2242–2251.
6. Bailey EF, Fregosi RF. Modulation of upper airway muscle activities by bronchopulmonary afferents. *J Appl Physiol.* 2006;101:609–617.

7. Yildirim N, Fitzpatrick MF, Whyte KF, Jalleh R, Wightman AJA, Douglas NJ. The effect of posture on upper airway dimensions in normal subjects and in patients with the sleep apnea/hypopnea syndrome. *Am Rev Respir Dis.* 1991;144:845–847.
8. Douglas NJ, Jan MA, Yildirim N, Warren PM, Drummond GB. Effect of posture and breathing route on genioglossal EMG activity in normal subjects and in patients with the sleep apnea/hypopnea syndrome. *Am Rev Respir Dis.* 1993;148:1341–1345.
9. Tangel DJ, Mezzanotte WS, White DP. Influence of sleep on tensor palatini EMG and upper airway resistance in normal men. *J Appl Physiol.* 1991;70:2574–2581.
10. Brancatisano TP, Dodd DS, Engel LA. Respiratory activity of posterior cricoarytenoid muscle and vocal cords in humans. *J Appl Physiol.* 1984;57:1143–1149.

*11. Gauthier AP, Verbanck S, Estenne M, Segebarth C, Macklem PT, Paiva M. Three-dimensional reconstruction of the in vivo human diaphragm shape at different lung volumes. *J Appl Physiol.* 1994;76:495–506.
12. Sieck GC. Physiological effects of diaphragm muscle denervation and disuse. *Clin Chest Med.* 1994;15:641–659.
13. Loring SH. Invited editorial on "Three-dimensional reconstruction of the in vivo human diaphragm shape at different lung volumes." *J Appl Physiol.* 1994;79:493–4.
14. Cassart M, Pettiaux N, Gevenois PA, Paiva M, Estenne M. Effect of chronic hyperinflation on diaphragm length and surface area. *Am J Respir Crit Care Med.* 1997;156:504–508.
15. Petroll WM, Knight H. Rochester DF. A model approach to assess diaphragmatic volume

displacement. *J Appl Physiol.* 1990;69:2175–2182.

*16. De Troyer A, Kirkwood PA, Wilson TA. Respiratory action of the intercostal muscles. *Physiol Rev.* 2005;85:717–756.

17. Hamberger GE. De Respirirationis Mechanismo et Usu Genuino. Jena: 1749.

18. Rimmer KP, Ford GT, Whitelaw WA. Interaction between postural and respiratory control of human intercostal muscles. *J Appl Physiol.* 1995;79:1556–1561.

19. Hudson AL, Gandevia SC, Butler JE. The effect of lung volume on the co-ordinated recruitment of scalene and sternomastoid muscles in humans. *J Physiol.* 2007;584:261–270.

20. Hillman DR, Finucane KE. A model of the respiratory pump. *J Appl Physiol.* 1987;63:951–961.

21. Drummond GB. Chest wall movements in anaesthesia. *Eur J Anaesthiol.* 1989;6:161–196.

22. Konno K, Mead J. Measurement of the separate volume changes of ribcage and abdomen during breathing. *J Appl Physiol.* 1967;22:407–422.

23. Lumb AB, Nunn JF. Respiratory function and ribcage contribution to ventilation in body positions commonly used during anaesthesia. *Anesth Analg.* 1991;73:422–426.

24. Xie S, Takasaki Y, Popkin J, Orr D, Bradley TD. Chemical and postural influence on scalene and diaphragmatic activation in humans. *J Appl Physiol.* 1991;70:658–664.

25. Lumb AB, Nunn JF. Ribcage contribution to CO_2 response during rebreathing and steady state methods. *Respir Physiol.* 1991;85:97–110.

26. Robson JG. The respiratory centres and their responses. In: Evans FT, Gray TC, eds, *Modern Trends in Anaesthesia – 3*. London: Butterworths; 1967.

*27. Laghi F, Tobin MJ. Disorders of the respiratory muscles. *Am J Respir Crit Care Med.* 2003;168:10–48.

28. Gayan-Ramirez G, Decramer M. Effects of mechanical ventilation on diaphragm function and biology. *Eur Respir J.* 2002;20:1579–1586.

29. Levine S, Kaiser L, Leferovich J, Tikunov B. Cellular adaptations in the diaphragm in chronic obstructive pulmonary disease. *N Engl J Med.* 1997;337:1799–1806.

30. Moxham J. Respiratory muscle fatigue: mechanisms, evaluation and therapy. *Br J Anaesth.* 1990;65:43–53.

31. Roussos C, Macklem PT. Diaphragmatic fatigue in man. *J Appl Physiol.* 1977;43: 189–197.

32. Fujii Y, Toyooka H, Amaha K. Diaphragmatic fatigue and its recovery are influenced by cardiac output. *J Anaesth.* 1991;5:17–23.

33. Hammond MD, Bauer KA, Sharp JT, Rocha RD. Respiratory muscle strength in congestive cardiac failure. *Chest.* 1990;98: 1091–1094.

34. Sieck GC, Mantilla CB. Effect of mechanical ventilation on the diaphragm. *N Engl J Med.* 2009;358:1392–1394.

35. Callahan LA. Invited editorial on "Acquired respiratory muscle weakness in critically ill patients: what is the role of mechanical ventilation-induced diaphragm dysfunction?" *J Appl Physiol.* 2009;106:360–361.

36. Levine S, Nguyen T, Taylor N, et al. Rapid disuse atrophy of diaphragm fibers in mechanically ventilated humans. *N Engl J Med.* 2008;358:1327–1335.

37. Campbell EJM, Westlake EK, Cherniak RM. Simple methods of estimating oxygen consumption and the efficiency of the muscles of breathing. *J Appl Physiol.* 1957;11:303–308.

38. Miller MR, Hankinson J, Brusasco V, et al. Standardisation of spirometry. *Eur Respir J.* 2005;26:319–338.

39. Wright BM. A respiratory anemometer. *J Physiol.* 1955;127:25P.

40. Cotes JE, Chinn DJ, Miller MR. *Lung function. Physiology, measurement and application in medicine*. Oxford: Blackwell Publishing; 2006.

41. Polkey MI, Green M, Moxham J. Measurement of respiratory muscle strength. *Thorax.* 1995;50:1131–1135.

Chapter 7

The pulmonary circulation

KEY POINTS

- Pulmonary blood flow approximates to cardiac output, and can increase several-fold with little change in pulmonary arterial pressure.
- Passive distension and recruitment of closed pulmonary capillaries, particularly in the upper zones of the lung, allow pulmonary vascular resistance to fall as blood flow increases.
- Active control of pulmonary vascular resistance has only a minor role in controlling pulmonary vascular resistance and involves intrinsic responses in vascular smooth muscle, modulated by numerous neural and humoral factors.
- Hypoxic pulmonary vasoconstriction of pulmonary arterioles is a fundamental difference from the systemic circulation, though the mechanism of this response to hypoxia remains uncertain.

Evolution first led to the development of a separate pulmonary circulation in amphibians, though in this case both systemic and pulmonary circulations are supplied by a single ventricle and there is therefore a great deal of mixing of blood between the two. The occurrence of warm-blooded animals led to a 10-fold increase in oxygen requirements, which may only be achieved through having a pulmonary circulation almost completely separate from the systemic circulation.[1]

PULMONARY BLOOD FLOW

The flow of blood through the pulmonary circulation is approximately equal to the flow through the whole of the systemic circulation. It therefore varies from about $6l.min^{-1}$ under resting conditions, to as much as $25l.min^{-1}$ in severe exercise. It is remarkable that such an increase can normally be achieved with minimal increase in pressure. Pulmonary vascular pressures and vascular resistance are much less than those of the systemic circulation. Consequently the pulmonary circulation has only limited ability to control the regional distribution of blood flow within the lungs and is markedly affected by gravity, which results in overperfusion of the dependent parts of the lung fields. Maldistribution of the pulmonary blood flow has important consequences for gaseous exchange, and these are considered in Chapter 8.

In fact, the relationship between the inflow and outflow of the pulmonary circulation is much more complicated (Figure 7.1). The lungs receive a significant quantity of blood from the bronchial arteries, which usually arise from the arch of the aorta. Blood from the bronchial circulation returns to the heart in two ways. From a plexus around the hilum, blood from the pleurohilar part of the bronchial circulation returns to the superior vena cava via the azygos veins, and this fraction may thus be regarded as normal systemic flow, neither arising from nor returning to the pulmonary circulation. However, another fraction of the bronchial circulation, distributed more peripherally in the lung, passes through postcapillary anastomoses to join the pulmonary veins, constituting an admixture of venous blood with the arterialised blood from the alveolar capillary networks.

The situation may be further complicated by blood flow through precapillary anastomoses from

DOI: 10.1016/B978-0-7020-2996-7.00007-6

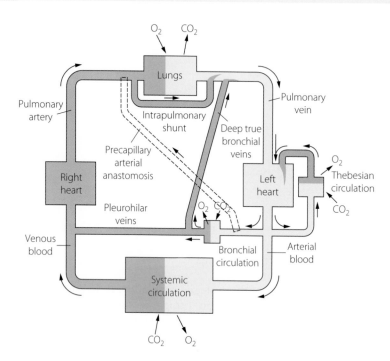

Fig. 7.1 Schema of bronchopulmonary anastomoses and other forms of venous admixture in the normal subject. Part of the bronchial circulation returns venous blood to the systemic venous system while another part returns venous blood to the pulmonary veins and so constitutes venous admixture. Other forms of venous admixture are the Thebesian circulation of the left heart and flow through atelectatic parts of the lungs. It will be clear from this diagram why the output of the left heart must be slightly greater than that of the right heart.

the bronchial arteries to the pulmonary arteries. These communications (so-called 'sperr arteries') have muscular walls and are thought to act as sluice gates, opening when increased pulmonary blood flow is required. Their functional significance in normal subjects is unknown, but in diseased lungs flow through these anastomoses may be crucial. For example, in situations involving pulmonary oligaemia (e.g. pulmonary artery stenosis, pulmonary embolism) blood from the bronchial arteries will flow through the anastomoses to supplement pulmonary arterial flow.[2] It should be noted that a Blalock–Taussig shunt operation achieves the same purpose for palliation of patients with cynanotic congenital heart disease.

PULMONARY BLOOD VOLUME

As a first approximation the right heart pumps blood into the pulmonary circulation, while the left heart pumps away the blood that returns from the lungs. Therefore, provided that the output of the two sides is the same, the pulmonary blood volume will remain constant. However, very small differences in the outputs of the two sides must result in large changes in pulmonary blood volume if they are maintained for more than a few beats.

FACTORS INFLUENCING PULMONARY BLOOD VOLUME

Posture. Change from the supine to the erect position decreases the pulmonary blood volume by almost one-third, which is about the same as the corresponding change in cardiac output. Both changes result from pooling of blood in dependent parts of the systemic circulation.

Systemic vascular tone. Because the systemic circulation has much greater vasomotor activity than the pulmonary circulation, an overall increase in vascular tone will tend to squeeze blood from the systemic into the pulmonary circulation. This may result from the release of endogenous catecholamines, administration of vasoconstrictor drugs, or from passive compression of the body in a G-suit. The magnitude of the resulting volume shift will depend on many factors such as position, overall blood volume and activity of the numerous humoral and nervous mechanisms controlling pulmonary vascular tone at the time (see below). Conversely, it seems likely that pulmonary blood volume would be diminished when systemic tone is diminished, as for example during sepsis or with regional anaesthesia when systemic vascular resistance is decreased with no effect on the autonomic supply to the pulmonary vasculature.

PULMONARY VASCULAR PRESSURES

Pulmonary arterial pressure is only about one-sixth of systemic arterial pressure, although the capillary and venous pressures are not greatly different for the two circulations (Figure 7.2). There is thus only a small pressure drop along the pulmonary arterioles and therefore a reduced potential for active regulation of the distribution of the pulmonary blood flow. This also explains why there is little damping of the arterial pressure wave, and the pulmonary capillary blood flow is markedly pulsatile.

Consideration of pulmonary vascular pressures carries a special difficulty in the selection of the reference pressure. Systemic pressures are customarily measured with reference to ambient atmospheric pressure, but this is not always appropriate when considering the pulmonary arterial pressure, which is relatively small in comparison with the intrathoracic and pulmonary venous pressures. This may be important in two circumstances. First, the extravascular (intrathoracic) pressure may have a major influence on the intravascular pressure and should be taken into account. Secondly, the driving pressure through the pulmonary circulation may be markedly influenced by the pulmonary venous pressure, which must be taken into account when measuring pulmonary vascular resistance. We must therefore distinguish between pressures within the pulmonary circulation expressed in the three different forms listed below. Measurement techniques may be adapted to indicate these pressures directly (Figure 7.3).

Intravascular pressure is the pressure at any point in the circulation relative to atmosphere. This is the customary way of expressing pressures in the systemic circulation, and is also the commonest method of indicating pulmonary vascular pressures.

Transmural pressure is the difference in pressure between the inside of a vessel and the tissue surrounding the vessel. In the case of the larger pulmonary vessels, the outside pressure is the intrathoracic pressure (commonly measured as the oesophageal pressure, as shown in Figure 7.3). This method should be used to exclude the physical effect of major changes in intrathoracic pressure.

Driving pressure is the difference in pressure between one point in the circulation and another point downstream. The driving pressure of the pulmonary circulation as a whole is the pressure difference between pulmonary artery and left atrium. This is the pressure that overcomes the flow resistance and should be used for determination of vascular resistance.

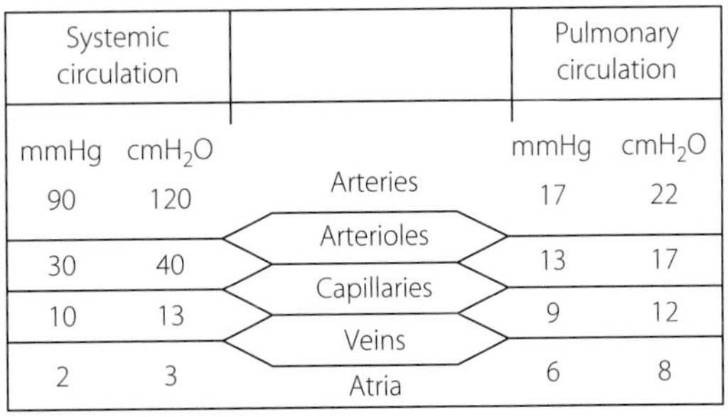

Systemic circulation			Pulmonary circulation	
mmHg	cmH₂O		mmHg	cmH₂O
90	120	Arteries	17	22
		Arterioles		
30	40		13	17
		Capillaries		
10	13		9	12
		Veins		
2	3	Atria	6	8

Fig. 7.2 Comparison of typical mean pressure gradients along the systemic and pulmonary circulations. (Mean pressures relative to atmosphere.)

These differences are far from being solely academic. For example, an increase in intrathoracic pressure due to positive pressure ventilation will increase the pulmonary arterial intravascular pressure, but will also similarly increase pulmonary venous intravascular pressure and therefore driving pressure (and therefore flow) remains unchanged. Similarly, if the primary problem is a raised left atrial pressure, blood will 'back-up' through the pulmonary circulation and pulmonary arterial intravascular pressure will also be raised but the driving pressure will again not be increased. Therefore for assessing pulmonary blood flow (and so resistance) driving pressure is the correct measurement, but this requires pulmonary venous (left atrial) pressure to be recorded, which is difficult to achieve continuously (page 113). Pulmonary arterial intravascular pressure is usually measured and the value must therefore be interpreted with caution.

Typical normal values for pressures within the pulmonary circulation are shown in Figure 7.3. The effect of gravity on the pulmonary vascular pressure may be seen, and it will be clear why pulmonary oedema is most likely to occur in the lower zones of the lungs where the intravascular pressures and the transmural pressure gradients are highest.

EFFECT OF INTRA–ALVEOLAR PRESSURE

Alteration of intra-alveolar pressure causes changes in intrathoracic pressure according to the following relationship:

Intrathoracic pressure =
    alveolar pressure − alveolar transmural pressure

Alveolar transmural pressure is a function of lung volume (Figure 3.8) and, when the lungs are

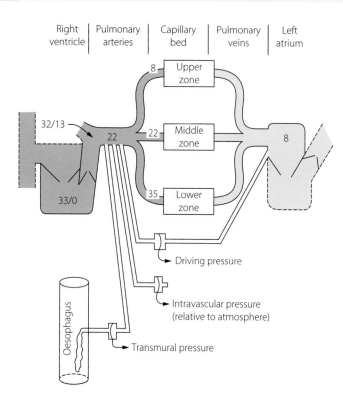

Fig. 7.3 Normal values for pressures in the pulmonary circulation relative to atmospheric (cmH$_2$O). Systolic and diastolic pressures are shown for the right ventricle and pulmonary trunk, and mean pressures elsewhere. Note the effect of gravity on pressures at different levels in the lung fields. Three different manometers are shown connected to indicate driving pressure, intravascular pressure and transmural pressure.

passively inflated, the intrathoracic pressure will normally increase by rather less than half the inflation pressure. The increase will be even less if the lungs are stiff, and thus a low compliance protects the circulation from inflation pressure (page 480). Intravascular pressures are normally increased directly and instantaneously by the effects of changes in intrathoracic pressure, and this explains the initial rise in systemic arterial pressure during a Valsalva manoeuvre (page 478). It also explains the cyclical changes in pulmonary arterial pressure during spontaneous respiration, with pressures greater during expiration than during inspiration. Such changes would not be seen if transmural pressure were measured (Figure 7.3).

In addition to the immediate physical effect of an increase in intrathoracic pressure on intravascular pressures, there is a secondary physiological effect due to interference with venous return. This accounts for the secondary decline in systemic pressure seen in the Valsalva manoeuvre.

PULMONARY VASCULAR RESISTANCE

Vascular resistance is an expression of the relationship between driving pressure and flow, as in the case of resistance to gas flow. It may be expressed in similar terms as follows:

Pulmonary vascular resistance
$$= \frac{\text{pulmonary driving pressure}}{\text{cardiac output}}$$

There are, however, important caveats and the concept of pulmonary vascular resistance is not a simple parallel to Ohm's law, appropriate to laminar flow (page 43). First, the tubes through which the blood flows are not rigid but tend to expand as flow is increased, particularly in the pulmonary circulation with its low vasomotor tone. Consequently the resistance tends to fall as flow increases and the plot of pressure against flow rate is neither linear (see Figure 4.2) nor curved with the concavity upwards (see Figure 4.3) but curved with the concavity downwards. The second complication is that blood is a non-Newtonian fluid (due to the presence of the corpuscles) and its viscosity varies with the shear rate, which is a function of its linear velocity.

Vascular resistance in the lung. Although the relationship between flow and pressure in blood vessels is far removed from simple linearity, there is a widespread convention that pulmonary vascular resistance should be expressed in a form of the equation above. This is directly analogous to electrical resistance, as though there were laminar flow of a Newtonian fluid though rigid pipes. It would, of course, be quite impractical in the clinical situation to measure pulmonary driving pressure at different values of cardiac output to determine the true nature of their relationship.

Vascular resistance is expressed in units derived from those used for expression of pressure and flow rate. Using conventional units, vascular resistance is usually expressed in units of mmHg per litre per minute. In absolute CGS units, vascular resistance is usually expressed in units of dynes/square centimetre per cubic centimetre/second (i.e. dyn.sec. cm^{-5}). The appropriate SI units will probably be $kPa.l^{-1}.minute$. Normal values for the pulmonary circulation in the various units are as follows:

	Driving pressure	Pulmonary blood flow	Pulmonary vascular resistance
SI Units	1.2 kPa	5 l.min^{-1}	0.24 kPa.l^{-1}.min
Conventional units	9 mmHg	5 l.min^{-1}	1.8 mmHg.l^{-1}.min
Absolute CGS units	12 000 dyn. cm^{-2}	83 cm^3.sec^{-1}	144 dyn.sec.cm^{-5}

Localisation of the pulmonary vascular resistance. In the systemic circulation the greatest part of resistance is in the arterioles, along which the pressure falls from a mean value of about 12 kPa (90 mmHg) down to about 4 kPa (30 mmHg) (see Figure 7.2). This pressure drop largely obliterates the pulse pressure wave, and the systemic capillary flow is not pulsatile to any great extent. In the pulmonary circulation, the pressure drop along the arterioles is very much smaller than in the systemic circulation and, as an approximation, the pulmonary vascular resistance is equally divided between arteries, capillaries and veins. Pulmonary arteries and arterioles, with muscular vessel walls, are mostly extra-alveolar and involved in active control of pulmonary vascular resistance by mechanisms such as nervous, humoral or gaseous control. In contrast, pulmonary capillaries are intimately associated with the alveolus (see Figure 2.7) so resistance of these vessels is therefore greatly influenced by alveolar pressure and volume. Thus in the pulmonary circulation, vessels without the power of active vasoconstriction play a major role in governing total vascular resistance and the distribution of the pulmonary blood flow.

PASSIVE CHANGES IN PULMONARY VASCULAR RESISTANCE

EFFECT OF PULMONARY BLOOD FLOW (CARDIAC OUTPUT)

The pulmonary circulation can adapt to large changes in cardiac output with only small increases in pulmonary arterial pressure. Thus pulmonary vascular resistance must decrease as flow increases. Reduced resistance implies an increase in the total cross-sectional area of the pulmonary vascular bed and particularly the capillaries. These adaptations to increased flow occur partly by passive distension of vessels and partly by recruitment of collapsed vessels, the former being the most important factor.

Recruitment of previously unperfused pulmonary vessels occurs in response to increased pulmonary flow. This is particularly true of the capillary bed, which is devoid of any vasomotor control, so allowing the opening of new passages in the network of capillaries lying in the alveolar septa, and is most likely to occur in the upper part of the lung where capillary pressure is lowest (zone 1, see below). Capillary recruitment was first described in histological studies involving sections cut in lungs rapidly frozen while perfused with blood, which showed that the number of open capillaries increased with rising pulmonary arterial pressure, particularly in the mid-zone of the lung.[3] Recruitment of capillaries in the intact lung remains poorly understood. Studies using colloidal gold particles in the circulation demonstrate that there is perfusion in all pulmonary capillaries, including in zone 1, during normal ventilation.[4] A similar study, this time with airway pressure increased above pulmonary capillary pressure, showed no flow in almost two-thirds of capillaries in zone 1.[5] It therefore seems that with increased alveolar pressure unperfused capillaries are available for recruitment but that under normal circumstances, with low airway pressures, there is flow in all capillaries. However, these studies using colloidal particles cannot discriminate between plasma or blood flow and have led to speculation that some, *almost* collapsed, capillaries may contain only plasma ('plasma skimming') or even blood flow from the bronchial circulation.[6]

Distension in the entire pulmonary vasculature occurs in response to increased transmural pressure gradient, and is again most likely to occur in capillaries devoid of muscular control. In one study, capillary diameter increased from 5 to 10 μm as the transmural pressure increased from 0.5 to 2.5 kPa (5 to 25 cmH₂O).[7] As described in the previous section it now seems likely that capillaries never collapse completely and therefore passive distension is clearly the more important adaptation to increased flow.

A striking example of the ability of the pulmonary vasculature to adapt to changing flow occurs after pneumonectomy (page 494), when the remaining lung will normally take the entire resting pulmonary blood flow without a rise in pulmonary arterial pressure. There is, inevitably, a limit to the flow that can be accommodated without an increase in pressure, and this will be less if the pulmonary vascular bed is affected by disease or surgery. The most important pathological cause of increased pulmonary blood flow is left-to-right shunting through a patent ductus arteriosus or through atrial or ventricular septal defects. Under these circumstances the pulmonary blood flow may be several-fold greater than the systemic flow before pulmonary hypertension develops. Despite this, remodelling of the pulmonary vessels commonly results in an increase in vascular resistance, causing an earlier and more severe rise in pulmonary arterial pressure.

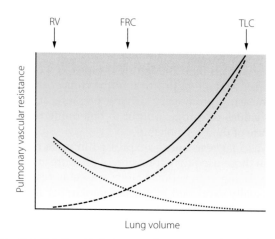

Fig. 7.4 Relationship between pulmonary vascular resistance (PVR) and lung volume. The solid line represents total PVR and is minimal at the functional residual capacity (FRC). Compression of alveolar capillaries (dashed line) is responsible for the increased PVR as lung volume approaches total lung capacity (TLC). Increasing PVR as lung volume approaches residual volume (RV) may result from either compression of corner capillaries (dotted line) or extra-alveolar vessels, or hypoxia-induced vasoconstriction in collapsed lung units. It should be noted that this graph is derived from studies mainly involving isolated animal lungs and may not be applicable to the intact subject.

EFFECT OF LUNG INFLATION

Reference has been made above to the effect of alveolar pressure on pulmonary vascular pressures. The effect on pulmonary vascular resistance is complex. Confusion has arisen in the past because of failure to appreciate that pulmonary vascular resistance must be derived from driving pressure and not from pulmonary arterial or transmural pressure (Figure 7.3). This is important because inflation of the lungs normally influences the pressure in the oesophagus, pulmonary artery and left atrium and so can easily conceal the true effect on vascular resistance.

When pulmonary vascular resistance is correctly calculated from the driving pressure, there is reasonable agreement that the pulmonary vascular resistance is minimal at FRC and that changes in lung volume in either direction cause a small increase in resistance, particularly at high lung volumes (Figure 7.4). These observations may be explained by considering pulmonary capillaries as belonging to three distinct groups:[8]

Alveolar capillaries are sandwiched between two adjacent alveolar walls, usually bulging into one alveolus (see Figure 2.7), and supported from collapse only by the pressure in the capillary and flimsy septal fibrous tissue. Expansion of the alveolus will therefore compress these capillaries and increase their contribution to pulmonary vascular resistance. If the lung consisted entirely of alveolar capillaries then pulmonary vascular resistance would be directly related to lung volume.

Corner capillaries lie within the junction between three or more alveoli, and are not therefore sandwiched between alveolar walls. In this area, the alveolar wall is believed to form 'pleats' during lung deflation, which are then stretched out longitudinally (rather than expanded outwards) during inspiration and so have little effect on the blood vessels nearby. Indeed, blood vessels in this area are generally uninfluenced by alveolar pressure but may expand at high lung volume and constrict at very small lung volumes, possibly secondary to local hypoxia surrounding the collapsed alveoli.

Extra-alveolar vessels provide an additional explanation for the increased pulmonary vascular resistance at small lung volumes. Compression of larger pulmonary vessels at low lung volumes may result

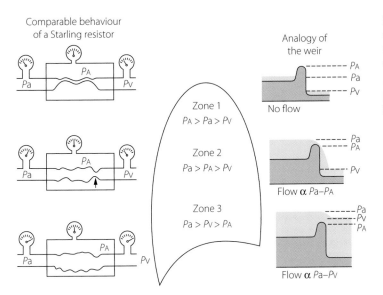

Comparable behaviour of a Starling resistor

Analogy of the weir

Fig. 7.5 The effect of gravity on pulmonary vascular resistance is shown by comparison with a Starling resistor (left) and with a weir (right). *Pa*, pulmonary artery pressure; *P*A, alveolar pressure; *P*v, pulmonary venous pressure (all pressures relative to atmosphere). See text for full discussion.

in reduced flow in dependent parts of the lung (page 123), and this is likely to contribute to the overall change in pulmonary vascular resistance.

The anatomical difference between these capillaries is undoubted, whilst the effect of the anatomical features on physiology are unproven. Much of the work has involved mathematical modelling based on animal studies in the open-chested or isolated preparation, and the relevance of these to the intact human remains uncertain.

EFFECT OF GRAVITY ON ALVEOLAR AND VASCULAR PRESSURES

The vascular weir. The interplay of alveolar pressure, flow rate and vascular resistance is best considered by dividing the lung field into three zones.[9] Figure 7.5 shows behaviour as a Starling resistor and also the analogy of a weir. A Starling, or threshold, resistor can be visualised as a length of compressible tubing within a rigid chamber, such that flow occurs only when the upstream pressure (left gauges in Figure 7.5) exceeds the pressure within the chamber (middle gauges) and a reduction in the downstream pressure (right gauges) cannot initiate flow. In zone 1 of Figure 7.5, the pressure within the arterial end of the collapsible vessels is less than the alveolar pressure, and therefore insufficient to open the vessels that remain collapsed as in a Starling resistor. The upstream water is below the top of the weir and so there can be no flow. The downstream (venous) pressure is irrelevant. Zone 1

corresponds to conditions that may apply in the uppermost parts of the lungs.

In the mid-zone of the lungs (zone 2 of Figure 7.5), the pressure at the arterial end of the collapsible vessels exceeds the alveolar pressure and, under these conditions, a collapsible vessel, behaving like a Starling resistor, permits flow in such a way that the flow rate depends on the arterial/alveolar pressure difference. Resistance in the Starling resistor is concentrated at the point marked with the arrow in Figure 7.5. The greater the difference between arterial and alveolar pressure, the more widely the collapsible vessels will open and the greater will be the flow. Note that the venous pressure is still not a factor that affects flow or vascular resistance. This condition is still analogous to a weir, the upstream depth (head of pressure) corresponding to the arterial pressure, and the height of the weir corresponding to alveolar pressure. Flow depends solely on the difference in height between the upstream water level and the top of the weir. The depth of water below the weir (analogous to venous pressure) cannot influence the flow of water over the weir unless it rises above the height of the weir.

In the lower zone of the lungs (zone 3 of Figure 7.5), the pressure in the venous end of the capillaries is above the alveolar pressure, and under these conditions a collapsible vessel behaving like a Starling resistor will be held wide open and the flow rate will, as a first approximation, be governed by the arterial/venous pressure difference (the driving pressure) in the normal manner for the systemic

Table 7.1 Receptors and agonists involved in active control of pulmonary vascular tone

RECEPTOR GROUP	SUBTYPES	PRINCIPAL AGONISTS	RESPONSES	ENDOTHELIUM DEPENDENT?
Adrenergic	α_1	noradrenaline	constriction	no
	α_2	noradrenaline	dilatation	yes
	β_2	adrenaline	dilatation	yes
Cholinergic	M_3	acetylcholine	dilatation	yes
Amines	H_1	histamine	variable	yes
	H_2	histamine	dilatation	no
	$5\text{-}HT_1$	5-HT	variable	variable
Purines	P_{2x}	ATP	constriction	no
	P_{2y}	ATP	dilatation	yes
	A_1	Adenosine	constriction	no
	A_2	Adenosine	dilatation	no
Eicosanoids	TP	thromboxane A_2	constriction	no
	?	prostacyclin (PGI_2)	dilatation	?
Peptides	NK_1	Substance P	dilatation	yes
	NK_2	Neurokinin A	constriction	no
	?	VIP	relaxation	variable
	AT	angiotensin	constriction	no
	ANP	ANP	dilatation	no
	B_2	bradykinin	dilatation	yes
	ET_A	endothelin	constriction	no
	ET_B	endothelin	dilatation	yes
	?	adrenomedullin	dilatation	?
	V_1	vasopressin	dilatation	yes

The existence of many of the substances listed is at present only established in animals, and their physiological or pathological relevance in humans therefore remains uncertain. From references 11 and 12. 5-HT, 5-hydroxytryptamine; ATP, adenosine triphosphate; VIP, vasoactive intestinal peptide; ANP, atrial natriuretic peptide.

circulation. However, as the intravascular pressure increases in relation to the alveolar pressure, the collapsible vessels will be further distended and their resistance will be correspondingly reduced. Returning to the analogy of the weir, the situation is now one in which the downstream water level has risen until the weir is completely submerged and offers little resistance to the flow of water, which is largely governed by the difference in the water level above and below the weir. However, as the levels rise further, the weir is progressively more and more submerged and what little resistance it offers to water flow is diminished still further.

ACTIVE CONTROL OF PULMONARY VASCULAR RESISTANCE

In addition to the passive mechanisms described, pulmonary blood vessels are also able to control vascular resistance by active vasoconstriction and

vasodilatation, and there is now evidence that the pulmonary vasculature is normally kept in a state of active vasodilatation.[10]

CELLULAR MECHANISMS CONTROLLING PULMONARY VASCULAR TONE[11,12,13]

There are many mechanisms by which pulmonary vascular tone may be controlled (Table 7.1), but the role of many of these in the human lung is uncertain. Some of the receptor-agonist systems in Table 7.1 have only been demonstrated in vitro using animal tissue, but may eventually emerge as important in humans either for normal maintenance of pulmonary vascular tone or during lung injury (Chapter 31). Activity of some, though not all, of the mechanisms listed in Table 7.1 are dependent on the endothelial lining of the pulmonary blood vessels. It seems likely that many basic control mechanisms occur within the smooth muscle cell whilst the endothelium acts as a modulator of the response. Some control mechanisms such as the autonomic nervous system and hypoxic pulmonary vasoconstriction have been extensively investigated in humans and are described separately below.

Receptors. Endothelial and smooth muscle cells of the pulmonary vasculature each have numerous receptor types, and the agonists for these receptors may originate from nerve endings (e.g. acetylcholine, noradrenaline), be produced locally (e.g. eicosanoids, endothelin), or arrive via the blood (e.g. peptides). In addition, many similar or identical compounds produce opposing effects by their actions on differing sub-groups of receptors for example α_1 (vasoconstrictor) and β_2 (vasodilator) adrenergic receptors. There remains therefore a large number of poorly understood systems acting together to bring about control of pulmonary vascular smooth muscle.

Second messengers. Pulmonary vasodilators that act directly on the smooth muscle such as prostaglandins, vasoactive intestinal peptide and under some circumstances β_2 agonists, mostly activate adenyl cyclase to produce cyclic adenosine 3',5' monophosphate (cAMP) as a second messenger. In turn, cAMP causes a host of intracellular activity via activation of protein kinase enzymes that reduce both the phosphorylation of myosin and intracellular calcium levels to bring about relaxation of the muscle cell.

Receptors that cause contraction of pulmonary vascular smooth muscle are usually G-protein coupled. Activation produces a second messenger, inositol 1,4,5-triphosphate (IP_3), which releases calcium from intracellular stores and activates myosin phophorylation to produce contraction.

Role of the endothelium and nitric oxide.[11] Furchgott & Zawadzki in 1980 were the first to demonstrate that endothelial cells were required for acetylcholine (ACh) induced relaxation in isolated aortic tissue, the messenger passing between the endothelium and smooth muscle cells being termed endothelium-derived relaxing factor,[14] the major part of which was subsequently shown to be nitric oxide (NO). Many pulmonary vasodilator mechanisms have been shown to be endothelium dependent (Table 7.1) and it is likely that NO is a common pathway for producing relaxation of vascular smooth muscle from a variety of stimuli.

Nitric oxide synthase (NOS) produces NO by the conversion of L-arginine to L-citrulline, via a highly reactive hydroxy-arginine intermediate (Figure 7.6). NOS is involved in both stages, and requires many cofactors including calmodulin and NADPH, and probably other flavine derived factors

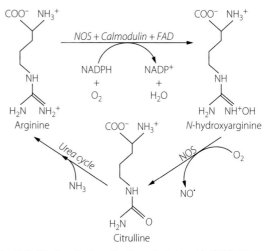

Fig. 7.6 Biochemical production of nitric oxide (NO). Nitric oxide synthase (NOS) acts as a catalyst for a two stage reaction to convert arginine to citrulline. Oxygen is required at both stages, and NADPH, calmodulin and flavine adenine dinucleotide (FAD) are required as cofactors for the first stage and are believed to control the rate of NO production. Citrulline produced in this reaction may then enter the urea cycle, and using ammonia derived from amino acid metabolism, is converted back into arginine.

such as flavine adenine dinucleotide. Control of NOS activity depends on the availability of the substrate, arginine, and the concentrations of the various cofactors. Citrulline produced by NOS enters the urea cycle and is converted back into arginine (Figure 7.6). This pathway utilises ammonia derived from the conversion of amino acids into energy-producing substrates such as pyruvate, and provides a mechanism by which ammonium ions may be converted into relatively harmless nitrates (via NO). The biological disposal of nitric oxide is described on page 194.

Nitric oxide synthase exists in two forms known as constitutive and inducible. Inducible NO synthase (iNOS) is produced in many cells but only in response to activation by inflammatory mediators and other cytokines, and once activated can produce large amounts of NO for long periods. Constitutive NO synthase (cNOS) is permanently present in some cells, including pulmonary endothelium, and produces short bursts of low levels of NO in response to changes in calcium and calmodulin levels. In systemic vessels, sheer stress of the blood vessel wall may directly activate calcium-dependent potassium channels to activate cNOS,

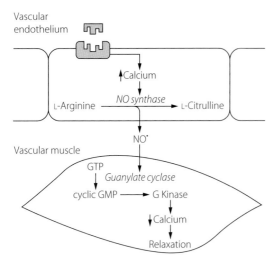

Fig. 7.7 Schematic pathway for the activation of constitutive nitric oxide synthase and the action of nitric oxide in the pulmonary vasculature. There are many different receptors thought to act via this mechanism to bring about vasodilatation. See text for details.

but in the pulmonary circulation receptor stimulation is the usual source of altered calcium levels and cNOS activation.

The mechanism by which receptor activation leads to muscle relaxation is illustrated in Figure 7.7. Nitric oxide diffuses from the site of production to the smooth muscle cell where it activates guanylate cyclase to produce cyclic guanosine 3′,5′ monophosphate (cGMP), which in turn activates a protein kinase enzyme. This system is similar to the cAMP pathway described above and causes relaxation by a combination of effects on cytosolic calcium levels and the activity of enzymes controlling myosin activity.

There is now good evidence that basal production of NO occurs in normal human lungs and contributes to the maintenance of low pulmonary vascular resistance.[10,15] Both of these studies have used N^G-monomethyl-L-arginine (L-NMMA), a NOS inhibitor, to demonstrate reduced global or regional pulmonary blood flow.

HYPOXIC PULMONARY VASOCONSTRICTION

When vasoconstriction occurs in response to hypoxia, pulmonary blood vessels are displaying their fundamental difference from systemic vessels. Hypoxic pulmonary vasoconstriction (HPV) is mediated both by mixed venous (pulmonary arterial) P_{O_2} and alveolar P_{O_2} (Figure 7.8), the greater

influence being from the alveolus. The overall response to P_{O_2} is non-linear. This may be deduced from Figure 7.8 by noting the pressure response for different values of the isobaric P_{O_2} (the broken line), and it will be seen that the general shape of the response curve resembles an oxyhaemoglobin dissociation curve with a P_{50} of about 4 kPa (30 mmHg). The combined effect of hypoxia in alveolar gas and mixed venous blood may be considered as acting at a single point,[16] which exerts a 'stimulus' P_{O_2} as follows:

$$P(\text{stimulus})_{O_2} = P\bar{v}_{O_2}{}^{0.375} \times P_{A_{O_2}}{}^{0.626}$$

In addition to the effect of mixed venous and alveolar P_{O_2}, the bronchial arterial P_{O_2} influences tone in the larger pulmonary arteries via the vasa vasorum.[17]

Regional hypoxic pulmonary vasoconstriction is beneficial as a means of diverting the pulmonary blood flow away from regions in which the oxygen tension is low and is an important factor in the optimisation of ventilation/perfusion relationships (Chapter 8). It is also important in the fetus to minimise perfusion of the unventilated lung. However, long term continuous or intermittent HPV leads to remodelling of the pulmonary vasculature and pulmonary hypertension, and this response is disadvantageous in a range of clinical conditions (see Chapter 29).

The pressor response to hypoxia results from constriction of small arterioles of 30–200 μm in diameter and begins within a few seconds of the P_{O_2} decreasing. In humans, hypoxia in a single lobe of the lung results in a rapid decline in perfusion of the lobe such that after 5 minutes regional blood flow is half that during normoxia.[19] With prolonged hypoxia HPV is biphasic: the initial rapid response reaches a plateau after about 5 minutes, with the second phase occurring around 40 minutes later[20] (Figure 7.9) and reaching a maximal response 2–4 hours after the onset of hypoxia.[21]

MECHANISM OF HPV[22-26]

Neural connections to the lung are not required as HPV occurs in isolated lung preparations and in humans following lung transplantation.[27] Attempts to elucidate the mechanism of HPV have been hampered by species differences, the multitude of systems affecting pulmonary vascular tone and a lack of

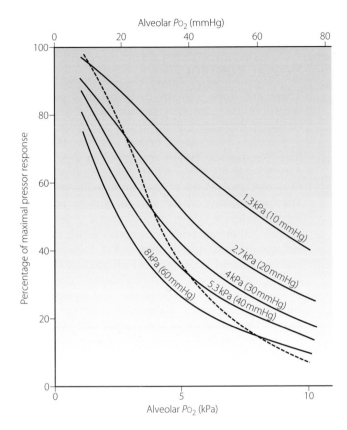

Fig. 7.8 Pulmonary vasoconstriction (ordinate) as a function of alveolar Po_2 (abscissa) for different values of mixed venous Po_2 (indicated for each curve). The broken line shows the response when the alveolar and mixed venous Po_2 are identical. (Data from reference 18.)

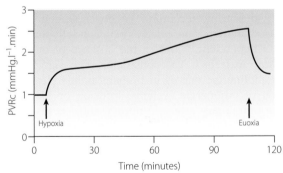

Fig. 7.9 Time course of the hypoxic pulmonary vasoconstriction response to prolonged isocapnic hypoxia in humans (end-tidal Po_2 6.7 kPa, 50 mmHg). Phase 1 of the response is complete within a few minutes, then the phase 2 response occurs around 40 minutes later PVRc, pulmonary vascular resistance corrected for cardiac output. Note that after prolonged hypoxia PVRc does not return to baseline immediately. (After reference 20.)

appreciation of the biphasic nature of the response. Uncertainties remain on the cellular mechanism of HPV, but there is now agreement that contraction of pulmonary artery smooth muscle cells (PASMC) in response to hypoxia is an inherent property of these cells, and that pulmonary endothelial cells only act to modulate the PASMC response.[23]

Oxygen sensing in PASMC is similar to that already described for glomus cells in the carotid body (page 71). Hypoxia leads to a small increase in intracellular calcium concentration, and also a rho kinase-mediated increase in the calcium sensitivity of the contractile proteins of the cell.[26] These changes in calcium activity result from opening of voltage-dependent L-type calcium channels, stimulated in turn by hypoxia-induced inhibition of voltage gated potassium (Kv) channels. As in the carotid body, the molecular oxygen sensor that affects the Kv channel remains controversial. This may be an inherent property of the Kv channel itself[28] though mitochondria, nicotinamide adenine dinucleotide phosphate oxidases and reactive oxygen species (Chapter 26) are also involved.[24,29]

Modulation by the endothelial cell of the PASMC response to hypoxia may either enhance or inhibit HPV.[23] Inhibitors of HPV include prostacyclin (PGI_2) and nitric oxide (NO), both of which may exist to maintain some perfusion of hypoxic lung regions,[22] though their role in normal lung is uncertain.

For example, prostacyclin is a potent pulmonary vasodilator but cyclo-oxygenase, which is required for its production, is inhibited by hypoxia – which may therefore diminish the vasodilator effects.[22] Similarly, basal NO secretion by endothelial cells may act to moderate HPV, but hypoxia also inhibits endothelial NO production and so enhances HPV. Molecules that enhance HPV include thromboxane A_2 (see below) and endothelin. Endothelin is a 21 amino acid peptide released by endothelial cells in response to hypoxia.[30] It is a potent vasoconstrictor peptide which has a prolonged effect on pulmonary vascular tone such that this mechanism is probably involved in the second slow phase of HPV (Figure 7.9). Endothelin is believed to be involved in producing the pulmonary hypertension associated with altitude hypoxia (see Chapter 17), though attempts to enhance HPV with endothelin infusions have not been successful.[21] Two groups of endothelin receptors are described, ET_A and ET_B, and the ratio of these two receptors varies between the central and peripheral vasculature of the lung. Apart from its vasoconstrictor effects, endothelin can also stimulate cellular proliferation of either vascular endothelial cells or pulmonary fibroblasts, and so has an important role in the pulmonary vascular remodelling that accompanies long-term hypoxia.

HPV is therefore a complex and poorly elucidated system. In normal subjects HPV within the lung is inhomogeneous,[31] with intense vasoconstriction in some areas and relative overperfusion elsewhere, the degree to which this occurs varying between individuals which has important implications when travelling to high altitude (page 286). Another fascinating recent finding relates to iron metabolism and HPV. Increased iron availability (achieved by intravenous infusion) attenuates HPV, while reducing iron availability by administration of desferrioxamine enhances the response.[32] These observations may be highly significant for patients given that normal subjects have widely varying iron status, depending on such factors as sex, diet and chronic illness.[33]

EFFECTS OF $P\text{CO}_2$ AND pH ON PULMONARY VASCULAR RESISTANCE

Elevated $P\text{CO}_2$ has a slight pressor effect, for example, hypoventilation of one lobe of a dog's lung reduces perfusion of that lobe, although its ventilation/perfusion ratio is still reduced.[34] Both respiratory and metabolic acidosis augment HPV.[8,35] Alkalosis, whether respiratory (hypocapnia) or metabolic in origin, causes pulmonary vasodilatation[8] and attenuates HPV.[36]

NEURAL CONTROL

There are three systems involved in autonomic control of the pulmonary circulation,[11,12] which are similar to those controlling airway tone (page 50).

Adrenergic sympathetic nerves originate from the first five thoracic nerves and travel to the pulmonary vessels via the cervical ganglia and a plexus of nerves around the trachea and smaller airways. They act mainly on the smooth muscle of arteries and arterioles down to a diameter of less than $60\,\mu\text{m}$.[8,11] There are both α_1 receptors which mediate vasoconstriction, usually in response to noradrenaline release, and β_2 receptors which produce vasodilatation mainly in response to circulating adrenaline. Overall, α_1 effects predominate and sympathetic stimulation increases pulmonary vascular resistance.[11] The influence of the sympathetic system is not as strong as in the systemic circulation and seems to have little influence under resting conditions. There is no obvious disadvantage in this respect in patients with lung transplant (see Chapter 33).

Cholinergic nerves of the parasympathetic system travel in the vagus nerve and cause pulmonary vasodilatation by release of ACh and stimulation of M_3 muscarinic receptors.[11] Acetylcholine-mediated vasodilatation is accepted as being endothelium and NO dependent,[10] and in the absence of endothelium, ACh is a vasoconstrictor. The significance of cholinergic nerves in humans is less clear than that of adrenergic systems. Infusion of ACh into the pulmonary artery in normal subjects results in vasodilatation,[10] so ACh receptors clearly exist, but cholinergic nerve fibres have not been demonstrated histologically around human pulmonary vessels.[11]

Non-adrenergic, non-cholinergic (NANC)[11] nerves are closely related anatomically to the other autonomic mechanisms but with different neurotransmitters and are similar to the NANC nerves controlling airway smooth muscle (page 51). In the lung, most NANC nerves are inhibitory, causing vasodilatation via release of NO, possibly in conjunction with peptides (Table 7.1). The functional significance of this system is unknown.

HUMORAL CONTROL

Pulmonary vascular endothelium is involved in the metabolism of many circulating substances (Chapter 12), some of which cause changes in vascular tone (Table 7.1). Which of these are involved in the control of normal pulmonary vascular resistance is unclear, and it is quite possible that very few are, but some are undoubtedly involved in pulmonary vascular disease (Chapter 29).

Catecholamines. Circulating adrenaline following sympathetic stimulation acts on both α and β receptors and results in a predominantly vasoconstrictor response. Exogenous adrenaline and related inotropes such as dopamine have a similar effect.

Eicosanoids. Arachidonic acid metabolism via the cyclo-oxygenase pathway (to prostaglandins and thromboxane) and lipoxygenase pathway (to leukotrienes) has been demonstrated in pulmonary vessels in animals. The products of arachidonic acid metabolism have diverse biological effects in many physiological systems and the pulmonary vasculature is no exception. Arachidonic acid itself, thromboxane A_2, $PGF_{2\alpha}$, PGD_2, PGE_2 and LTB_4 are all vasoconstrictors whilst PGI_2 (prostacyclin) is usually a vasodilator. These pathways are believed to be involved in pathological pulmonary hypertension resulting from sepsis, reperfusion injury or congenital heart disease.[11]

Amines. Histamine relaxes pulmonary vascular smooth muscle during adrenaline-induced constriction but constricts resting smooth muscle. Constriction is in response to H_1 stimulation on smooth muscle cells whilst relaxation occurs either via H_1 receptors on endothelium (NO dependent) or H_2 receptors on smooth muscle cells. 5-hydroxytryptamine (serotonin) is liberated from activated platelets and is a potent vasoconstrictor. It may be involved in pulmonary hypertension secondary to emboli (page 426).

Peptides. Numerous peptides that are vasoactive in the pulmonary circulation are shown in Table 7.1. Responses are again diverse, many systems producing vasodilatation via endothelium receptors and vasoconstriction via direct effects on smooth muscle (e.g. substance P and neurokinin A).[11]

Purine nucleosides such as adenosine and ATP are highly vasoactive, again with variable responses according to the amount of tone in the pulmonary blood vessel.[11] Adenosine is a pulmonary vasodilator in normal subjects.[37]

DRUG EFFECTS ON THE PULMONARY CIRCULATION

A higher than normal pulmonary arterial pressure occurs rarely as a primary disease but commonly develops as a secondary consequence of chronic hypoxia from a variety of lung diseases (Chapter 29). Considering the wide range of receptor–agonist systems present in the pulmonary vasculature (Table 7.1) it is surprising that there are only a few effective drugs available. One reason for this is the non-specific nature of many of the receptors found in the pulmonary vasculature, such that drugs acting on these receptors have widespread effects elsewhere in the body that make them therapeutically unacceptable. Another problem with pulmonary vasodilators in respiratory disease is that abolishing HPV removes the body's main mechanisms for compensating for poor respiratory function. For example, nifedipine administered sublingually in patients with severe airways disease causes a significant reduction in pulmonary hypertension, but this is associated with a worsening of arterial hypoxaemia.[38] As a way of avoiding both these problems, delivering drugs by inhalation has had some success,[39] particularly if the drug is inactivated before reaching the systemic circulation.

INHALED DRUGS

Nitric oxide. Inhaled NO (iNO) in patients with severe lung disease is a selective pulmonary vasodilator, with the systemic circulation being unaffected due to its rapid inactivation by haemoglobin (page 194). Nitric oxide therefore increases blood flow to well ventilated areas of the lung and so diverts blood flow away from poorly ventilated areas,[40] thereby decreasing ventilation–perfusion mismatch and improving arterial oxygenation. In addition to its role in modulating vascular tone and oxygenation NO may play a significant role as an immunomodulator, for example by reducing leukocyte adhesion and activation[41] it may attenuate lung inflammation (Chapter 31).

Inhaled NO in the presence of oxygen is rapidly oxidised to NO_2, the rate of oxidation being directly related to oxygen concentration and the square of NO concentration. NO_2 can react with water to form highly injurious nitric and nitrous acids that can cause severe pneumonitis and pulmonary oedema. Hence to minimise the production of NO_2 both the concentration of oxygen and NO, and the contact time between the two, should be minimised. Some of the beneficial effects of iNO may be short lived, whilst rapid discontinuation of iNO leads to a rebound phenomenon, probably due to inhibition of endogenous NO, with decreased oxygenation and increased pulmonary artery pressures. Hence iNO should be withdrawn in a slow stepwise fashion. Despite these numerous drawbacks, therapeutic iNO in some groups of patients with acute lung injury does seem to produce improved clinical outcomes.[42]

Prostacyclin.[39,43] Intravenous prostacyclin (PGI$_2$) has been used for some time for treatment of pulmonary hypertension and to reduce PA pressure in critically ill patients, but its lack of selectivity for the pulmonary vasculature causes significant adverse effects. When delivered by inhalation, metabolism of PGI$_2$ by the lung is negligible, so systemic absorption occurs. However, the dose required by inhalation is very small, so despite its systemic absorption clinically significant adverse effects are minimal.

SYSTEMIC DRUGS[44]

Prostacyclin and its analogues may be administered continuously by the intravenous or subcutaneous routes.[43] Prostacyclin has a half-life of less than 5 minutes, so a variety of synthetic analogues have been developed such as iloprost (half life ~30 min) and more recently treprostinil (half life ~4.5 h).

Angiotensin-converting enzyme inhibitors reduce pulmonary vascular resistance in patients with pulmonary hypertension secondary to lung disease, but only with long term treatment. These drugs are also believed to reduce pulmonary vascular remodelling (page 428). Losartan, an angiotensin II receptor antagonist, reduces pulmonary artery pressure within hours of administration, without detriment to the patient's oxygen saturation.[45]

Phosphodiesterase (PDE) inhibitors can inhibit the breakdown of both cAMP and cGMP, and so enhance the activity of these cellular messengers that bring about vascular smooth muscle cell relaxation from a variety of pathways (see above), including all those mediated by NO. These drugs have been used to reduce pulmonary hypertension by both the intravenous and inhaled routes. Of particular interest for the pulmonary circulation are selective inhibitors of type 5 PDE which is specific for pulmonary cGMP breakdown. Sildenafil, more well known for its use as a treatment for impotence, is an oral inhibitor of PDE5 with few side effects that acts as a pulmonary vasodilator by enhancing the effects of endogenous NO.[46]

Calcium antagonists such as nifedipine reduce secondary pulmonary hypertension in a dose dependent fashion by inhibition of the L-type calcium channels on PASMCs described above. However, as already described, in some patient groups hypoxaemia may worsen, and at the large doses often needed to reduce pulmonary hypertension, the negative inotropic effects of calcium antagonists become significant and right heart failure caused by the pulmonary hypertension can deteriorate.

Endothelin receptor antagonists competitively antagonise both ET$_A$ and ET$_B$ receptors, though in the clinical situation ET$_B$ effects seem to predominate and reduce PA pressure. Endothelin has been implicated in vascular remodelling of pulmonary vessels with chronic hypoxia, so these drugs may also slow this process. Bosentan, a non-selective oral endothelin antagonist, is now approved for the treatment of patients with pulmonary hypertension, and more selective ET antagonists such as sitaxsentan continue to be evaluated though currently do not seem to offer any particular advantage over non-selective drugs.[30]

PRINCIPLES OF MEASUREMENT OF THE PULMONARY CIRCULATION

Detailed consideration of haemodynamic measurement techniques lie outside the scope of this book. The following section presents only the broad principles of measurement such as may be required in relation to respiratory physiology.

PULMONARY BLOOD VOLUME

Available methods are based on the technique used for measurement of cardiac output by dye dilution (see below). The flow rate so obtained is multiplied by the interval between the time of the injection of the dye and the mean arrival time of the dye at the sampling point. This product indicates the amount of blood lying between injection and sampling sites and the volume result obtained therefore depends very much on exactly where sampling occurs. Total pulmonary blood volume may be measured by sampling from the proximal pulmonary artery and the pulmonary vein (or left atrium). Typical values are of the order of 0.5–1.0 litres or 10–20% of total blood volume in an adult.

Table 2.2 shows the anatomical distribution of the pulmonary blood volume within the pulmonary arterial tree which has a volume of the order of 150 ml. Pulmonary capillary volume may be calculated from measurements of diffusing capacity (see Chapter 9), and this technique yields values of the order of 80 ml. The pulmonary veins therefore contain over half of the pulmonary blood volume as they possess much less vasomotor tone than the pulmonary arteries.

PULMONARY VASCULAR PRESSURES

Pressure measurements within the pulmonary circulation are almost always made with electronic pressure transducers, which measure instantaneous pressure against time (Figure 7.10). Systolic and diastolic pressures are measured from the peaks and troughs of this trace, and the mean pressure is derived electronically.

Figure 7.3 shows the sites at which pressure must be measured to obtain the various forms of pulmonary vascular pressure (page 101). Driving pressure, the most useful of these, requires measurement of pulmonary arterial and pulmonary venous (left atrial) pressures.

Pulmonary arterial pressure may be measured using a balloon flotation catheter. Following insertion into the right atrium via a central vein, a balloon of <1 ml volume is inflated to encourage the catheter tip to follow the flow of blood through the right ventricle and pulmonary valve into the pulmonary artery (Figure 7.10). The most commonly used catheter is the Swan–Ganz, named after the two cardiologists who devised the catheter after Dr Swan watched sailboats being propelled by the wind in 1967.[47]

Left atrial pressure represents pulmonary venous pressure and is measured in humans by one of three possible techniques, of which only the first is used commonly in clinical practice.

- Pulmonary artery occlusion pressure (PAOP).[48] Occlusion pressures are obtained by advancing the Swan–Ganz catheter into a branch of the pulmonary artery, with the balloon inflated, until the arterial pulsation disappears (Figure 7.10). There should then be no flow in the column of blood between the tip of the catheter and the left atrium, and the manometer will indicate left atrial pressure.
- A left atrial catheter may be sited during cardiac surgery and passed through the chest wall for use postoperatively.
- A catheter may be passed retrogradely from a peripheral systemic artery.

PULMONARY BLOOD FLOW

The method used for measurement of pulmonary blood flow will affect whether or not the result includes venous admixture such as the bronchial circulation and intrapulmonary shunts shown in Figure 7.1. Though of minimal relevance in normal subjects, in patients with lung disease venous admixture may be highly significant. In general, methods involving uptake of an inert gas from the alveoli will exclude venous admixture, and all other methods include it.

The Fick principle states that the amount of oxygen extracted from the respired gases equals the amount added to the blood which flows through the lungs. Thus the oxygen uptake of the subject must equal the product of pulmonary blood flow and arteriovenous oxygen content difference:

$$\dot{V}_{O_2} = \dot{Q}(Ca_{O_2} - C\bar{v}_{O_2})$$

therefore:

$$\dot{Q} = \frac{\dot{V}_{O_2}}{(Ca_{O_2} - C\bar{v}_{O_2})}$$

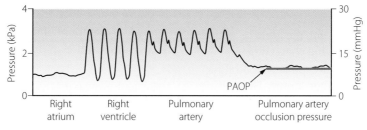

Fig. 7.10 Pressure traces obtained when inserting a balloon flotation catheter in a patient receiving intermittent positive pressure ventilation. With the balloon inflated, the catheter tip follows blood flow through the right atrium, right ventricle, and pulmonary artery until it occludes a branch of the pulmonary artery. The pulmonary artery occlusion pressure (PAOP) is the pressure measured distal to the balloon and equates to pulmonary venous and left atrial pressures. Note the respiratory swings in the trace caused by positive pressure ventilation. PAOP is measured as the mean pressure at end-expiration.

All the quantities on the right-hand side can be measured, although determination of the oxygen content of the mixed venous blood requires catheterisation of the right ventricle or, preferably, the pulmonary artery as described above. Interpretation of the result is less easy. The calculated value includes the intrapulmonary arteriovenous shunt, but the situation is complicated beyond the possibility of easy solution if there is appreciable extrapulmonary admixture of venous blood (see Figure 7.1). The second major problem is that spirometry measures the total oxygen consumption including that of the lung. The Fick equation excludes the lung (see page 212) but the difference is negligible with healthy lungs. There is evidence that the oxygen consumption of infected lungs may be very large (page 212) and therefore the Fick method of measurement of cardiac output would appear to be invalid under such circumstances.

Methods based on uptake of inert tracer gases. A modified Fick method of measurement of cardiac output may be employed with any fairly soluble inert gas. The tracer gas is inhaled either continually or for a single breath and the end-tidal partial pressure of tracer gas then measured. Analysis of volume and composition of expired tracer gas permits measurement of gas uptake. Since the duration of the procedure is short and does not permit recirculation, it may be assumed that the mixed venous concentration of the tracer gas is zero. The Fick equation then simplifies to the following:

Cardiac output =
    tracer gas uptake/arterial tracer gas concentration

The arterial tracer gas concentration equals the product of the arterial gas tension (assumed equal to the alveolar [end-tidal] gas tension) and the solubility coefficient of the tracer gas in blood. Thus arterial blood sampling may be avoided so the method is relatively non-invasive.

All the methods based on the uptake of inert tracer gases have the following characteristics:

- They measure pulmonary capillary blood flow, excluding any flow through shunts. This is in contrast to the Fick and dye methods.
- The assumption that the tension of the tracer gas is the same in end-expiratory gas and arterial blood is invalid in the presence of either alveolar dead space or shunt (see Chapter 8).
- Some of the tracer gas dissolves in the tissues lining the respiratory tract and is carried away

by blood perfusing these tissues. The indicated blood flow is therefore greater than the actual pulmonary capillary blood flow.

The tracer gas used has varied through the years with nitrous oxide and acetylene being used early this century. In the most recent version of the technique, freon is the tracer gas used. In this case, argon (highly insoluble gas) is added to the gas mixture to ensure complete mixing of the freon with alveolar gas, and also to detect subjects with a large respiratory dead space (see Chapter 8) in whom the method is invalid.[49]

Dye or thermal dilution. Currently the most popular technique for measurement of cardiac output is by dye dilution. An indicator substance is introduced as a bolus into a large vein and its concentration is measured continuously at a sampling site in the systemic arterial tree. Figure 7.11A shows the method as it is applied to continuous non-circulating flow as, for example, of fluids through a pipeline. The downstream concentration of dye is displayed on the y axis of the graph against time on the x axis. The dye is injected at time t_1 and is first detected at the sampling point at time t_2. The uppermost curve shows the form of a typical curve. There is a rapid rise to maximum concentration followed by a decay that is an exponential wash-out in form (see Appendix E), reaching insignificant levels at time t_3. The second graph shows the concentration (y axis) on a logarithmic scale when the exponential part of the decay curve becomes a straight line (see Figure E.5). Between times t_2 and t_3, the mean concentration of dye equals the amount of dye injected, divided by the volume of fluid flowing past the sampling point during the interval $t_2 - t_3$, which is the product of the fluid flow rate and the time interval $t_2 - t_3$. The equation may now be rearranged to indicate the flow rate of the fluid as the following expression:

$$\frac{\text{amount of dye injected}}{\text{mean concentration of dye} \times \text{time interval } t_2 - t_3}$$

The amount of dye injected is known and the denominator is the area under the curve.

Figure 7.11B shows the more complicated situation when fluid is flowing round a circuit. Under these conditions, the front of the dye-laden fluid may lap its own tail so that a recirculation peak appears on the graph before the primary peak has decayed to insignificant levels. This commonly

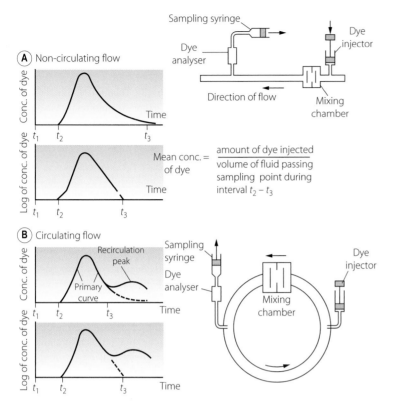

Fig. 7.11 Measurement of flow by dye dilution. (A) The measurement of continuous non-circulating flow rate of fluid in a pipeline. The bolus of dye is injected upstream and its concentration is continuously monitored downstream. The relationship of the relevant quantities is shown in the equation. Mean concentration of dye is determined from the area under the curve. (B) The more complicated situation when recirculation occurs and the front of the circulating dye laps its own tail, giving a recirculation peak. Reconstruction of the primary curve is based on extrapolation of the primary curve before recirculation occurs. This is facilitated by the fact that the down curve is exponential and therefore a straight line on a logarithmic plot.

occurs when cardiac output is determined in humans, and steps must be taken to reconstruct the tail of the primary curve as it would have been had recirculation not taken place. This is done by extrapolating the exponential wash-out which is usually established before the recirculation peak appears. This is shown as the broken lines in the graphs of Figure 7.11B. The calculation of cardiac output then proceeds as described above for non-recirculating flow. This previously laborious procedure is now performed electronically as an integral part of the apparatus for measuring cardiac output.

Many different indicators have been used for the dye dilution technique, but currently the most satisfactory appears to be 'coolth'. A bolus of cold saline is injected and the dip in temperature is recorded downstream with the temperature record corresponding to the dye curve. No blood sampling is required and temperature is measured directly with a thermometer mounted on the catheter. The 'coolth' is dispersed in the systemic circulation and therefore there is no recirculation peak to complicate the calculation. The thermal method is particularly suitable for repeated measurements.

References

1. Harris P. The evolution of the pulmonary circulation. *Thorax*. 1995;49:S5–S8.
2. Hasegawa I, Kobayashi K, Kohda E, Hiramatsu K. Bronchopulmonary arterial anastomosis at the precapillary level in human lung. *Acta Radiol*. 1999;39:578–584.
3. Warrell DA, Evans JW, Clarke RO, Kingaby GP, West JB. Pattern of filling in the pulmonary capillary bed. *J Appl Physiol*. 1972;32:346–356.
4. König MF, Lucocq JM, Weibel ER. Demonstration of pulmonary vascular perfusion by electron and light microscopy. *J Appl Physiol*. 1993;75:1877–1883.
5. Conhaim RL, Harms BA. Perfusion of alveolar septa in

isolated rat lungs in zone 1. *J Appl Physiol.* 1993;75:704–711.

6. Johnson RL, Hsai CCW. Functional recruitment of pulmonary capillaries. *J Appl Physiol.* 1994;76:1405–1407.

7. Sobin SS, Fung YC, Tremer HM, Rosenquist TH. Elasticity of the pulmonary alveolar microvascular sheet in the cat. *Circ Res.* 1972;30:440–450.

8. Fishman AP. Pulmonary circulation. In: Fishman AP, Fisher AB, Geiger SR, eds *Handbook of Physiology, Section 3 – The respiratory system.* Bethesda MD: American Physiological Society; 1987:93–97.

9. West JB, Dollery CT. Distribution of blood flow and the pressure–flow relations of the whole lung. *J Appl Physiol.* 1965;20:175–183.

*10. Cooper CJ, Landzberg MJ, Anderson TJ, et al. Role of nitric oxide in the local regulation of pulmonary vascular resistance in humans. *Circulation.* 1996;93:266–271.

11. Barnes PJ, Liu SF. Regulation of pulmonary vascular tone. *Pharmacol Rev.* 1995;47: 87–131.

12. Kobayashi Y, Amenta F. Neurotransmitter receptors in the pulmonary circulation with particular emphasis on pulmonary endothelium. *J Auton Pharmacol.* 1994;14:137–164.

13. Wilkins MR, Zhao L, Al-Tubuly R. The regulation of pulmonary vascular tone. *Br J Clin Pharmacol.* 1996;42:127–131.

14. Cherry PD, Furchgott RF, Zawadzki JV, Jothianandan D. Role of endothelial cells in relaxation of isolated arteries by bradykinin. *Proc Natl Acad Sci USA.* 1982;79:2106–2110.

15. Stamler JS, Loh E, Roddy M-A, Currie KE, Craeger MA. Nitric oxide regulated basal systemic and pulmonary vascular resistance in healthy humans. *Circulation.* 1994;89:2035–2040.

16. Marshall BE, Marshall C, Frasch HF. Control of the pulmonary circulation. In: Stanley TH, Sperry RJ, eds *Anesthesia and the Lung.* Dordrecht: Kluwer; 1992:9–18.

17. Marshall BE, Marshall C, Magno M, Lilagan P, Pietra GG. Influence of bronchial artery Po_2 on pulmonary vascular resistance. *J Appl Physiol.* 1991;70:405–415.

18. Marshall BE, Marshall C. Anesthesia and the pulmonary circulation. In: Covino BG, Fozzard HA, Rehder K, Strichartz G, eds *Effects of Anesthesia.* Bethesda, MD: American Physiological Society; 1983.

19. Morrell NW, Nijran KS, Biggs T, Seed WA. Magnitude and time course of acute hypoxic pulmonary vasoconstriction in man. *Respir Physiol.* 1995;100:271–281.

20. Talbot NP, Balanos GM, Dorrington KL, Robbins PA. Two temporal components within the human pulmonary vascular response to ~2 h of isocapnic hypoxia. *J Appl Physiol.* 2005;98:1125–1139.

21. Talbot NP, Balanos GM, Robbins PA, Dorrington KL. Can intravenous endothelin-1 be used to enhance hypoxic pulmonary vasoconstriction in healthy humans? *Br J Anaesth.* 2008;101:466–472.

22. Aaronson PI, Robertson TP, Ward JPT. Endothelium-derived mediators and hypoxic pulmonary vasoconstriction. *Respir Physiol Neurobiol.* 2002;132:107–120.

23. Weir K, López-Barneo J, Buckler KJ, Archer SL. Acute oxygen-sensing mechanisms. *N Engl J Med.* 2005;353:2042–2055.

*24. Sommer N, Dietrich A, Schermuly RT, et al. Regulation of hypoxic pulmonary vasoconstriction: basic mechanisms. *Eur Respir J.* 2008;32:1639–1651.

25. Moudgil R, Michelakis ED, Archer SL. Hypoxic pulmonary vasoconstriction. *J Appl Physiol.* 2005;98:390–403.

26. Aaronson PI, Robertson TP, Knock GA, et al. Hypoxic pulmonary vasoconstriction: mechanisms and controversies. *J Physiol.* 2006;570:53–58.

27. Robin ED, Theodore J, Burke CM, et al. Hypoxic pulmonary vasoconstriction persists in the human transplanted lung. *Clin Sci.* 1987;72:283–287.

*28. Coppock EA, Martens JR, Tamkun MM. Molecular basis of hypoxia-induced pulmonary vasoconstriction: role of voltage-gated K^+ channels. *Am J Physiol.* 2001;281:L1–L12.

29. Waypa GB, Schumacker PT. Hypoxic pulmonary vasoconstriction: redox events in oxygen sensing. *J Appl Physiol.* 2005;98:404–414.

30. Dupuis J, Hoeper MM. Endothelin receptor antagonists in pulmonary arterial hypertension. *Eur Respir J.* 2008;31:407–415.

31. Dehnert C, Risse F, Ley S, et al. Magnetic resonance imaging of uneven pulmonary perfusion in hypoxia in humans. *Am J Respir Crit Care Med.* 2006;174: 1132–1138.

32. Smith TG, Balanos GM, Croft QP, et al. The increase in pulmonary arterial pressure caused by hypoxia depends on iron status. *J Physiol.* 2008;586:5999–6005.

33. Joyner MJ, Johnson BD. Iron lung? New ideas about hypoxic pulmonary vasoconstriction. *J Physiol.* 2008;586:5837–5838.

34. Suggett AJ, Barer GR, Mohammed FH, Gill GW. The effects of localised hyperventilation on ventilation/perfusion ($\dot{V}/\dot{Q}$) ratios and gas exchange in the dog lung. *Clin Sci.* 1982;63:497–503.

35. Rudolph AM, Yuan S. Response of the pulmonary vasculature to hypoxia and H^+ ion concentration changes. *J Clin Invest.* 1966;45:399–411.

36. Benumof JL, Wahrenbrock EA. Blunted hypoxic pulmonary vasoconstriction by increased lung

vascular pressures. *J Appl Physiol.* 1975;38:846–850.

37. Reid PG, Fraser A, Watt A, Henderson A, Routledge P. Acute haemodynamic effects of adenosine in conscious man. *Eur Heart J.* 1990;11:1018–1028.

38. Kalra L, Bone MF. Effect of nifedipine on physiologic shunting and oxygenation in chronic obstructive pulmonary disease. *Am J Med.* 1993;94:419–423.

39. Lowson SM. Inhaled alternatives to nitric oxide. *Anesthesiology.* 2002;96:1504–1513.

40. Bigatello LM, Hurford WE, Hess D. Use of inhaled nitric oxide for ARDS. *Respir Care Clin N Am.* 1997;3:437–458.

41. Kavanah BP, Mouchawar A, Goldsmith J, et al. Effects of inhaled NO and inhibition of endogenous NO synthesis in oxidant-induced acute lung injury. *J Appl Physiol.* 1994;76:1324–1329.

42. Malarkkan N, Snook NJ, Lumb AB. New aspects of ventilation in acute lung injury. *Anaesthesia.* 2003;58:647–667.

43. Gomberg-Maitland M, Olschewski H. Prostacyclin therapies for the treatment of pulmonary arterial hypertension. *Eur Respir J.* 2008;31:891–901.

44. Fischer LG, Van Aken H, Bürkle H. Management of pulmonary hypertension: physiological and pharmacological considerations for anesthesiologists. *Anesth Analg.* 2003;96:1603–1616.

45. Kiely DG, Cargill RI, Wheeldon NM, Coutie WJ, Lipworth BJ. Haemodynamic and endocrine effects of type 1 angiotensin II receptor blockade in patients with hypoxaemic cor pulmonale. *Cardiovasc Res.* 1997;33:201–208.

46. Galiè N, Ghofrani HA, Torbicki A, et al. Sildenafil citrate therapy for pulmonary arterial hypertension. *N Engl J Med.* 2005;353:2148–2157.

47. Swan HJC, Ganz W. Hemodynamic monitoring: a personal and historical perspective. *Can Med Assoc J.* 1979;121:868–871.

*48. Pinsky MR. Pulmonary artery occlusion pressure. *Intensive Care Med.* 2003;29:19–22.

49. Winter SM. Clinical non-invasive measurement of effective pulmonary blood flow. *Int J Clin Monit Comput.* 1995;12:121–140.

Chapter 8

Distribution of pulmonary ventilation and perfusion

KEY POINTS

- As a result of gravity, both ventilation and perfusion are distributed preferentially to dependent regions of the lung, and so vary with posture.
- In healthy lungs ventilation and perfusion are closely matched with little variation of the ventilation to perfusion ($\dot{V}/\dot{Q}$) ratio in different lung regions.
- Regions of lung with $\dot{V}/\dot{Q}$ ratio of 0 represent intrapulmonary shunting of mixed venous blood, whilst regions with $\dot{V}/\dot{Q}$ ratio of infinity constitute the alveolar dead space.
- Physiological dead space describes the part of each tidal volume that does not take part in gas exchange, and is made up of alveolar and anatomical dead space components.

The lung may be considered as a simple exchanger with a gas inflow and outflow, and a blood inflow and outflow (Figure 8.1). There is near-equilibrium of oxygen and carbon dioxide tensions between the two outflow streams from the exchanger itself. This theoretical model assumes that gas flow in and out of the alveolus and blood flow through the pulmonary capillary are both continuous. This assumption may be true within alveoli where at normal tidal volumes gas movement is by diffusion (page 19) but pulmonary capillary blood flow is pulsatile (page 101). This model has been deliberately drawn without counter-current flow, which would be far more efficient. Such a system operates in the gills of fishes and the lungs of birds (page 289), and brings the Po_2 of arterial blood close to the Po_2 of their environment.

Gas exchange will clearly be optimal if ventilation and perfusion are distributed in the same proportion to one another throughout the lung. Conversely, to take an extreme example, if ventilation were distributed entirely to one lung and perfusion to the other, there could be no gas exchange, although total ventilation and perfusion might each be normal. This chapter begins with consideration of the spatial and temporal distribution of ventilation, followed by similar treatment for the pulmonary circulation. Distribution of ventilation and perfusion are then considered in relation to one another. Finally the concepts of dead space and shunt are presented.

DISTRIBUTION OF VENTILATION

SPATIAL AND ANATOMICAL DISTRIBUTION OF INSPIRED GAS

Distribution between the two lungs in the normal subject is influenced by posture and by the manner of ventilation. By virtue of its larger size, the right lung normally enjoys a ventilation slightly greater than the left lung in both the upright and the supine position (Table 8.1). In the lateral position, the lower lung is always better ventilated regardless of the side on which the subject is lying although there still remains a bias in favour of the right side.[1] Fortunately, the preferential ventilation of the lower lung accords with increased perfusion of the same lung, so the ventilation/perfusion ratios of the two lungs are not greatly altered on assuming the lateral position. However, the upper lung tends to be better ventilated in the anaesthetised patient in the lateral position, regardless of the mode of ventilation and particularly with an open chest (Table 8.1).

DOI: 10.1016/B978-0-7020-2996-7.00008-8

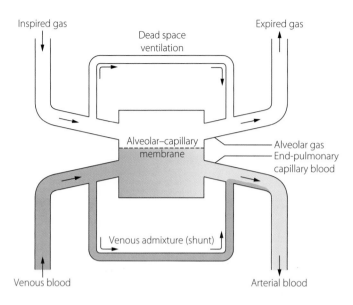

Fig. 8.1 In this functional representation of gas exchange in the lungs, the flow of gas and blood is considered as a continuous process with movement from left to right. Under most circumstances equilibrium is obtained between alveolar gas and end-pulmonary capillary blood, the gas tensions in the two phases being almost identical. However, alveolar gas is mixed with dead space gas to give expired gas, and end-pulmonary capillary blood is mixed with shunted venous blood to give arterial blood. Thus both expired gas and arterial blood have tensions that differ from those in alveolar gas and end-pulmonary capillary blood.

Table 8.1 Distribution of resting lung volume (FRC) and ventilation between the two lungs in humans

	SUPINE		RIGHT LATERAL (LEFT SIDE UP)		LEFT LATERAL (RIGHT SIDE UP)	
	RIGHT LUNG	LEFT LUNG	RIGHT LUNG	LEFT LUNG	RIGHT LUNG	LEFT LUNG
Conscious[1]	1.69	1.39	1.68	2.07	2.19	1.38
	53%	47%	61%	39%	47%	53%
Anaesthetised – spontaneous breathing[2]	1.18	0.91	1.03	1.32	1.71	0.79
	52%	48%	45%	55%	56%	44%
Anaesthetised – artificial ventilation[3]	1.36	1.16	1.33	2.21	2.29	1.12
	52%	48%	44%	56%	60%	40%
Anaesthetised – thoracotomy[4]					–	–
					83%	17%

The first figure is the unilateral FRC (litres) and the second the percentage partition of ventilation. Each study refers to separate subjects or patients.

In addition to causing postural differences between ventilation of the left and right lungs, gravity also influences the distribution of ventilation within each lung. Lung tissue may be considered as a semi-fluid or gel-like substance confined within the chest cavity, and the weight of the tissue above compresses the tissue below such that the density of the lung increases as vertical height reduces.[5,6] Thus in dependent areas lung tissue is less expanded than in non-dependent areas and so is more compliant and receives more ventilation.

Distribution of ventilation to horizontal slices of lung has been studied for many years by inhalation of radioactive isotopes, this technique having the advantage of being easily performed in a variety of postures and the disadvantage of low spatial resolution. In the upright position, with slow vital capacity inspirations, uppermost slices of the lung have a ventilation of around one-third that of slices at the bases. A slow inspiration from functional residual capacity (FRC), as occurs during normal resting ventilation, results in a smaller vertical gradient down the lung with the ratio of basal to apical ventilation being approximately 1.5:1. In any horizontal position the vertical height of the lung is reduced by about 30% and therefore the gravitational force generating maldistribution is much less. A variety of scanning techniques can now be used to quantifying regional ventilation in the supine position,[7,8,9] and have confirmed earlier findings that normal tidal breathing results in preferential ventilation of the posterior slices of the lungs compared with the anterior slices.[10]

Gravity is not the only factor influencing regional ventilation. Scanning techniques with the ability to measure ventilation in areas of lung only a few cubic millimetres in size have demonstrated increased ventilation in central, compared with peripheral, lung regions.[5] This is likely to result from unequal branching patterns of the airways in a similar fashion to that seen in pulmonary blood vessels (see below).[5]

DISTRIBUTION OF INSPIRED GAS IN RELATION TO THE RATE OF ALVEOLAR FILLING

Starting from FRC, preferential ventilation of the dependent parts of the lung is only present at inspiratory flow rates below 1.5 $l.s^{-1}$. At higher flow rates, distribution becomes approximately uniform. Fast inspirations from FRC reverse the distribution of ventilation, with preferential ventilation of the upper parts of the lungs, which is contrary to the distribution of pulmonary blood flow (see below). Normal inspiratory flow rate is however much less than 1.5 $l.s^{-1}$ (approximately 0.5 $l.s^{-1}$), so there will be a small vertical gradient of ventilation during normal breathing.

The rate of inflation of the lung as a whole is a function of inflation pressure, compliance and airway resistance. It is convenient to think in terms of the time constant (explained in Appendix E), which is the product of the compliance and resistance and is:

- the time required for inflation to 63% of the final volume attained if inflation is prolonged indefinitely.

or

- the time that would be required for inflation of the lungs if the initial gas flow rate were maintained throughout inflation (see Appendix E, Figure E.6).

These considerations apply equally to large and small areas of the lungs; Figure 3.6 shows fast and slow alveoli, the former with a short time constant and the latter with a long time constant. Figure 8.2 shows some of the consequences of different *functional units* of the lung having different time constants. For simplicity, Figure 8.2 describes the response to passive inflation of the lungs by development of a constant mouth pressure but the considerations are fundamentally similar for both spontaneous respiration and artificial ventilation.

Figure 8.2A shows two functional units of identical compliance and resistance. If the mouth pressure is increased to a constant level, there will be an increase in volume of each unit equal to the mouth pressure multiplied by the compliance of the unit. The time course of inflation will follow the wash-in type of exponential function (Appendix E), and the time constants will be equal to the product of compliance and resistance of each unit and therefore identical. If the inspiratory phase is terminated at any instant, the pressure and volume of each unit will be identical and no redistribution of gas will occur between the two units.

Figure 8.2B shows two functional units, one of which has half the compliance but twice the resistance of the other. The time constants of the two will thus be equal. If a constant inflation pressure is maintained, the one with the lower compliance will increase in volume by half the volume change of the other. Nevertheless, the pressure build-up within each unit will be identical. Thus, as in the previous example, the relative distribution of gas between the two functional units will be independent of the rate or duration of inflation. If the inspiratory phase is terminated at any point, the pressure in each unit will be identical and no redistribution will occur between the different units.

In Figure 8.2C, the compliances of the two units are identical but the resistance of one is twice that of the other. Therefore, its time constant is double that of its fellow and it will fill more slowly, although the volume increase in both units will be the same if inflation is prolonged indefinitely. Relative distribution between the units is thus dependent on the rate and duration of inflation. If inspiration is checked by closure of the upper airway after 2 seconds (for example), the pressure will be higher in the unit with the lower resistance. Gas will then be redistributed from one unit to the other as shown by the arrow in the diagram.

Figure 8.2D shows a pair of units with identical resistances but the compliance of one being half that of the other. Its time constant is thus half that of its fellow and it has a faster time course of inflation. However, because its compliance is half that of the other, the ultimate volume increase will only be half that of the other unit when inflation is prolonged

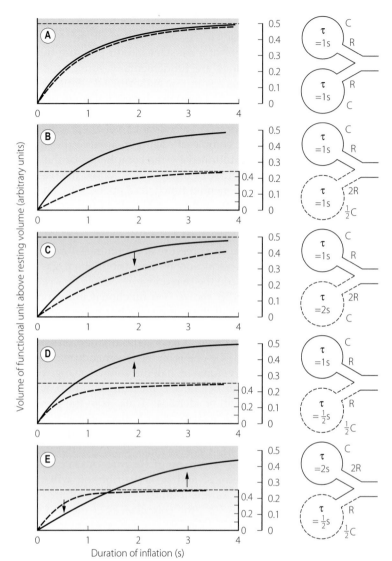

Fig. 8.2 The effect of mechanical characteristics on the time course of inflation of different functional units of the lung when exposed to a sustained constant inflation pressure. The y co-ordinate is volume change, but a scale showing intra-alveolar pressure is shown on the right. Separate pressure scales are necessary when the compliances are different. In each case the continuous curve relates to the upper unit and the broken curve to the lower unit. Arrows show the direction of gas redistribution if inflow is checked by closure of the upper airway at the times indicated. See text for explanation of the changes. τ = time constant.

indefinitely. The relative distribution of gas between the two units is dependent upon the rate and duration of inflation. Pressure rises more rapidly in the unit with the lower compliance, and if inspiration is checked by closure of the upper airway at 2 seconds (for example), gas will be redistributed from one unit to the other as shown by the arrow.

An interesting and complex situation occurs when one unit has an increased resistance and the other a reduced compliance (Figure 8.2E). This combination also features in the presentation of the concept of fast and slow alveoli in Figure 3.6. In the present example the time constant of one unit is four times that of the other, while the ultimate

volume changes are determined by the compliance as in Figure 8.2D. When the inflation pressure is sustained, the unit with the lower resistance (the 'fast alveolus') shows the greater volume change at first, but rapidly approaches its equilibrium volume. Thereafter the other unit (the 'slow alveolus') undergoes the major volume changes, the inflation of the two units being out of phase with one another. Throughout inspiration, the pressure build-up in the unit with the shorter time constant is always greater and, if inspiration is checked by closure of the upper airway, gas will be redistributed from one unit to the other as shown by the arrows in Figure 8.2E.

These complex relationships may be summarised as follows. If the inflation pressure is sustained indefinitely, the volume change in different units of the lungs will depend solely upon their regional compliances. *If their time constants are equal*, the build-up of pressure in the different units will be identical at all times during inflation and therefore:

- Distribution of inspired gas will be independent of the rate, duration or frequency of inspiration.
- Dynamic compliance (so far as it is influenced by considerations discussed in relation to Figure 3.7) will not be affected by changes in frequency and should not differ greatly from static compliance.
- If inspiration is checked by closure of the upper airway, there will be no redistribution of gas within the lungs.

If, however, the time constants of different units are different it follows that:

- Distribution of inspired gas will be dependent on the rate, duration and frequency of inspiration.
- Dynamic compliance will be decreased as respiratory frequency is increased and should differ significantly from static compliance.
- If inspiration is checked by closure of the upper airway, gas will be redistributed within the lungs.

EFFECT OF MALDISTRIBUTION ON THE ALVEOLAR 'PLATEAU'

If different functional units of the lung empty synchronously during expiration, the composition of the expired air will be approximately constant after the gas in the airways (anatomical dead space) has been flushed out. However, this will not occur when there is maldistribution with fast and slow units as shown in Figure 3.7. The slow units are slow both to fill and to empty, and thus are hypoventilated for their volume; therefore they tend to have a high Pco_2 and low Po_2 and are slow to respond to a change in the inspired gas composition. This forms the basis of the single-breath test of maldistribution, in which a single breath of 100% oxygen is used to increase alveolar Po_2 and decrease alveolar Pn_2. The greatest increase of Po_2 will clearly occur in the functional units with the best ventilation per unit volume, which will usually have the shortest time constants. The *slow* units will make the predominant contribution to the *latter* part of exhalation, when the mixed exhaled Po_2 will decline and the Pn_2 will increase. Thus the expired alveolar plateau of nitrogen will be sloping upwards in patients with maldistribution. It

should, however, be stressed that this test will only be positive if maldistribution is accompanied by sequential emptying of units due to differing time constants. For example, Figure 8.2B shows definite maldistribution, due to the different regional compliances that directly influence the regional ventilation. However, because time constants are equal, there will be a constant mix of gas from both units during the course of expiration (i.e. no sequential emptying) and therefore the alveolar plateau would remain flat in spite of Po_2 and Pn_2 being different for the two units. However, maldistribution due to the commoner forms of lung disease is usually associated with different time constants and sequential emptying. Routine continuous monitoring of expired carbon dioxide concentration during anaesthesia allows some assessment of maldistribution of ventilation. As for the single breath nitrogen test, an upward sloping expiratory plateau of carbon dioxide indicates sequential emptying of alveoli with different time constants (page 175), but a level plateau does not indicate normal distribution of ventilation, just equal time constants of lung units.

DISTRIBUTION OF PERFUSION

Since the pulmonary circulation operates at low pressure, it is rarely distributed evenly to all parts of the lung and the degree of non-uniformity is usually greater than for gas.

Distribution between the two lungs. Measuring unilateral pulmonary blood flow in humans is difficult, but indirect methods show that unilateral pulmonary blood flow is similar to the distribution of ventilation observed in the supine position (Table 8.1). In the lateral position, the diameter of the thorax is of the order of 30 cm and so the column of blood in the pulmonary circulation exerts a hydrostatic pressure that is high in relation to the mean pulmonary arterial pressure. A fairly gross maldistribution therefore occurs with much of the upper lung comprising zone 2 and much of the lower lung comprising zone 3 (see Figure 7.5).[11]

GRAVITATIONAL EFFECTS ON REGIONAL PULMONARY BLOOD FLOW

In the previous chapter, it was shown how the pulmonary vascular resistance is mainly in the capillary bed and is governed by the relationship between alveolar, pulmonary arterial and pulmonary venous pressures. Early studies with radioactive tracers in the blood took place at total lung capacity and showed flow increasing progressively down the lung in the upright position. However, Hughes et al. later found that there was a significant reduction of flow in the most dependent parts of the lung, which was termed zone 4, where the reduction in flow appears to be due to compression of larger blood vessels by increased interstitial pressure.[12] This effect becomes progressively more important as lung volume was reduced from total lung capacity towards the residual volume. Figure 8.3 is derived from the work of Hughes' group, and shows that pulmonary perfusion *per alveolus* is, in fact, reasonably uniform at the lung volumes relevant to normal tidal exchange. However, the dependent parts of the lung contain larger numbers of smaller alveoli than the apices at FRC, and the perfusion *per unit lung volume* is therefore increased at the bases.[11]

In the supine position the differences in blood flow between apices and bases are replaced by differences between anterior and posterior regions. Supine subjects can be studied using the same variety of scanning techniques as used for assessing ventilation

(page 138), revealing the same height-dependent gradients in alveolar size and perfusion as seen in earlier observations in upright subjects. Blood flow *per unit lung volume* increases by 11% per cm of descent through the lung,[13] whilst ventilation increases but less dramatically (Figure 8.4),[14] resulting in a smaller ventilation to perfusion ratio in dependent areas.[13] These studies also showed that the number of alveoli per cubic centimetre of lung was approximately 30% greater in the posterior compared with anterior lung (Figure 8.4).[14] Thus the increased perfusion in dependent areas of lung is again mainly caused by an increase in the number of (relatively small) alveoli. Smaller more numerous alveoli in dependent regions result from the weight of lung tissue above, and as blood accounts for two thirds of the weight of lung tissue this provides an automatic matching of ventilation and perfusion.

GRAVITY–INDEPENDENT REGIONAL BLOOD FLOW[5]

It is now accepted that gravity is not the only cause of the variability of regional pulmonary blood flow, though its relative contribution remains controversial.[15,16] Physiological studies in space some years ago showed that at microgravity regional blood flow becomes more uniform than on Earth, but residual non-uniformity still persists (page 308). A variety of

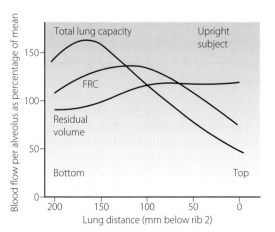

Fig. 8.3 Pulmonary perfusion per alveolus as a percentage of that expected if all alveoli were equally perfused (in the upright position). At total lung capacity, perfusion increases down to 150 mm, below which perfusion is slightly decreased (zone 4). At FRC, zone 4 conditions apply below 100 mm, and at residual volume the perfusion gradient is actually reversed. It should be noted that perfusion has been calculated *per alveolus*. If shown as perfusion *per unit lung volume*, the non-uniformity at total lung capacity would be the same because alveoli are all the same size at total lung capacity. At FRC there are more but smaller alveoli at the bases and the non-uniformity would be greater. (After reference 12.)

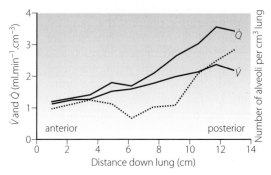

Fig. 8.4 Vertical gradients in ventilation and perfusion in the supine position. Data are mean results from PET scans of 8 subjects during normal breathing, and for each vertical level represent the average value for a horizontal slice of lung. The solid lines relate to the left ordinate and are ventilation ($\dot{V}$) and perfusion ($\dot{Q}$) per cubic centimetre of lung tissue. Ventilation and perfusion both increase on descending through the lung. The dotted line relates to the right ordinate and represents the number of alveoli per unit lung volume, which increases in dependent areas such that the blood flow *per alveolus* remains fairly constant. (After references 13 and 14.)

methods have been used to study pulmonary blood flow in the prone position.[13,14,17] These studies have consistently found that although blood flow becomes more uniform, the flow distribution when prone is not simply a reversal of the supine position, as may be expected if gravity was the only influence.[18]

Some groups estimate that gravity is responsible for only 25% of the regional blood flow variability seen.[5,17] Pulmonary blood flow may vary in a radial fashion, with greater flow to central, compared to peripheral, lung regions in each horizontal slice of lung.[19] Regional flow is believed to be influenced by vascular architecture, with the branching pattern of the pulmonary vasculature being responsible for the observed gravity-independent variation (the fractal hypothesis).[20] Two aspects of vascular structure contribute to the variations in flow. First, bifurcations of pulmonary arteries into two slightly different size vessels will have a large effect on the flow rates in each.[5] Secondly, pulmonary arteries are more numerous than pulmonary airways as a result of small extra branches, often given off at right angles, throughout the pulmonary arterial tree. Mathematical modelling indicates that these 'supernumerary' branches contribute significantly to the heterogeneity of regional perfusion.[21]

VENTILATION IN RELATION TO PERFUSION[22]

It is convenient to consider the relationship between ventilation and perfusion in terms of the ventilation/perfusion ratio (abbreviated to $\dot{V}/\dot{Q}$). Each quantity is measured in litres per minute and taking the lungs as a whole, typical resting values might be $4 \, l.min^{-1}$ for alveolar ventilation and $5 \, l.min^{-1}$ for pulmonary blood flow. Thus the overall ventilation perfusion ratio would be 0.8. If ventilation and perfusion of all alveoli were uniform then each alveolus would have an individual $\dot{V}/\dot{Q}$ ratio of 0.8. In fact, ventilation and perfusion are not uniformly distributed but may range all the way from unventilated alveoli to unperfused alveoli with every gradation in between. Unventilated alveoli will have a $\dot{V}/\dot{Q}$ ratio of zero and the unperfused alveoli a $\dot{V}/\dot{Q}$ ratio of infinity.

Alveoli with no ventilation ($\dot{V}/\dot{Q}$ ratio of zero) will have Po_2 and Pco_2 values that are the same as those of mixed venous blood, because the trapped air in the unventilated alveoli will equilibrate with mixed venous blood. Alveoli with no perfusion ($\dot{V}/\dot{Q}$ ratio of infinity) will have Po_2 and Pco_2 values that are the same as those of the inspired gas, because there is no gas exchange to alter the composition of the inspired gas that is drawn into these alveoli. Alveoli with intermediate values of $\dot{V}/\dot{Q}$ ratio will thus have Po_2 and Pco_2 values that are intermediate between those of mixed venous blood and inspired gas. Figure 8.5 is a Po_2/Pco_2 plot with the thick line joining the mixed venous point to the inspired gas point. This line covers all possible combinations of alveolar Po_2 and Pco_2, with an indication of the $\dot{V}/\dot{Q}$ ratios that determine them.

The inhalation of higher than normal partial pressures of oxygen moves the inspired point of the curve to the right. The mixed venous point also moves to the right but only by a small amount

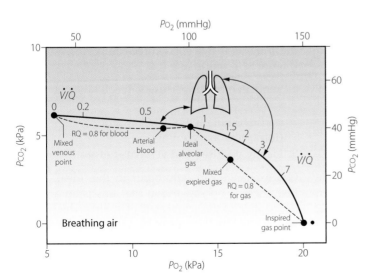

Fig. 8.5 The heavy line indicates all possible values for Po_2 and Pco_2 of alveoli with ventilation perfusion ($\dot{V}/\dot{Q}$) ratios ranging from zero to infinity (subject breathing air). Values for normal alveoli are distributed as shown in accord with their vertical distance up the lung field. Mixed expired gas may be considered as a mixture of 'ideal' alveolar and inspired gas (dead space). Arterial blood may be considered as a mixture of blood with the same gas tensions as 'ideal' alveolar gas and mixed venous blood (shunt).

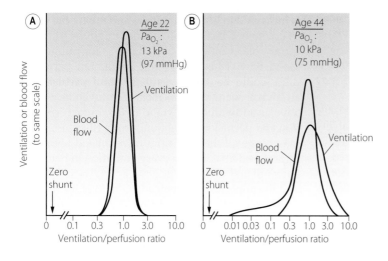

Fig. 8.6 The distribution of ventilation and blood flow in relation to ventilation/perfusion ($\dot{V}/\dot{Q}$) ratios in two normal subjects. (A) A male aged 22 years with typical narrow spread and no measurable intrapulmonary shunt or alveolar dead space. (B) The wider spread of $\dot{V}/\dot{Q}$ ratios in a male aged 44 years. There is still no measurable intrapulmonary shunt or alveolar dead space, but the appreciable distribution of blood flow to underperfused alveoli is sufficient to reduce the arterial Po_2 to 10 kPa (75 mmHg) while breathing air. (After reference 24 by permission of the authors and copyright permission of the American Society for Clinical Investigation.)

for reasons that are explained on page 377. A new curve must be prepared for each combination of values for mixed venous blood and inspired gas. The curve can then be used to demonstrate the gas tensions in the horizontal strata of the lung according to their different $\dot{V}/\dot{Q}$ ratios (Figure 8.5).

All of the techniques described above that measure regional ventilation and perfusion in horizontal strata of the lung only discriminate between functionally large regions of the lung. This limitation was overcome by the multiple inert gas elimination technique (MIGET).[23] The methodology, which is outlined on page 138, permits the plotting of the distribution of pulmonary ventilation and perfusion, not in relation to anatomical location, but in a large number of compartments defined by their $\dot{V}/\dot{Q}$ ratios, expressed on a logarithmic scale.

Figure 8.6 shows typical plots for healthy subjects.[24] For the young adult (Figure 8.6A), both ventilation and perfusion are mainly confined to alveoli with $\dot{V}/\dot{Q}$ ratios in the range 0.5–2.0. There is no measurable distribution to areas of infinite $\dot{V}/\dot{Q}$ (i.e. alveolar dead space) or zero $\dot{V}/\dot{Q}$ ratio (i.e. intrapulmonary shunt), but the method does not detect extrapulmonary shunt which must be present to a small extent (page 132). For the older subject (Figure 8.6B), there is a widening of the distribution of $\dot{V}/\dot{Q}$ ratios, with the main part of the curve now in the range of $\dot{V}/\dot{Q}$ ratios 0.3–5.0. In addition, there is the appearance of a 'shelf' of distribution of blood flow to areas of low $\dot{V}/\dot{Q}$ ratio in the range 0.01–0.3. This probably represents gross underventilation of dependent areas of the lung due to airway closure when the closing capacity exceeds the functional

residual capacity (see Figure 3.11). The effect of increased spread of $\dot{V}/\dot{Q}$ ratios on gas exchange is considered below (page 136).

The pattern of distribution of $\dot{V}/\dot{Q}$ ratios shows characteristic changes in a number of pathological conditions such as pulmonary oedema and pulmonary embolus.[25] Some examples are shown in Figure 8.7.

QUANTIFICATION OF SPREAD OF $\dot{V}/\dot{Q}$ RATIOS AS IF IT WERE DUE TO DEAD SPACE AND SHUNT

The MIGET method of analysis illustrated in Figures 8.6 and 8.7 is technically complex. A less precise but highly practical approach was described in the 1940s by both Fenn et al[26] and Riley & Cournard.[27] The essence of what has generally become known as the Riley approach is to consider the lung as if it were a three-compartment model (Figure 8.8) comprising:

1. ventilated but unperfused alveoli (alveolar dead space)
2. perfused but unventilated alveoli (intrapulmonary shunt)
3. ideally perfused and ventilated alveoli.

Gas exchange can only occur in the 'ideal' alveolus. There is no suggestion that this is an accurate description of the actual state of affairs, which is better depicted by the type of plot shown in Figure 8.6, where the analysis would comprise some 50 compartments in contrast to the three compartments of the Riley model. However, the parameters of the

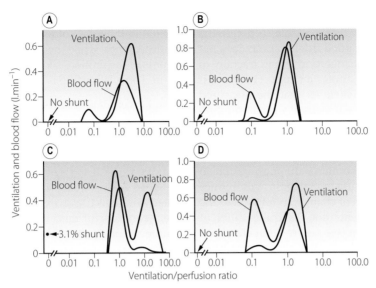

Fig. 8.7 Examples of abnormal patterns of maldistribution of ventilation and perfusion, to be compared with the normal curves in Figure 8.6. (A) Chronic obstructive pulmonary disease. The blood flow to units of very low $\dot{V}/\dot{Q}$ ratio would cause arterial hypoxaemia and simulate a shunt. (B) Asthma, with a more pronounced bimodal distribution of blood flow than the patient shown in (A). (C) Bimodal distribution of ventilation in a 60-year-old patient with chronic obstructive pulmonary disease, predominantly emphysema. A similar pattern is seen after pulmonary embolism. (D) Pronounced bimodal distribution of perfusion after a bronchodilator was administered to the patient shown in (B). (After reference 25 by permission of the author and publishers.)

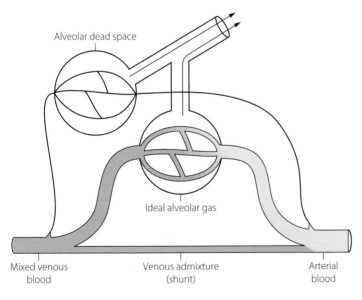

Fig. 8.8 Three-compartment (Riley) model of gas exchange. The lung is imagined to consist of three functional units comprising alveolar dead space, 'ideal' alveoli and venous admixture (shunt). Gas exchange occurs only in the 'ideal' alveoli. The measured alveolar dead space consists of true alveolar dead space together with a component caused by $\dot{V}/\dot{Q}$ scatter. The measured venous admixture consists of true venous admixture (shunt) together with a component caused by $\dot{V}/\dot{Q}$ scatter. Note that 'ideal' alveolar gas is exhaled contaminated with alveolar dead space gas, so it is not possible to sample 'ideal' alveolar gas.

three-compartment model may be easily determined and the values obtained are of direct relevance to therapy. Thus an increased dead space can usually be offset by an increased minute volume, and arterial P_{O_2} can be restored to normal with shunts up to about 30% by an appropriate increase in the inspired oxygen concentration (see Figure 8.11 below).

Methods for calculating dead space and shunt for the three-compartment model are described at the end of the chapter, but no analytical techniques are required beyond measurement of blood and gas Pco_2 and Po_2. It is then possible to determine what fraction of the inspired tidal volume does not participate in gas exchange and what fraction of the cardiac output constitutes a shunt. However, it is most important to remember that the measured value for 'dead space' will include a fraction representing ventilation of *relatively* underperfused alveoli, and the measured value for 'shunt' will include a fraction representing perfusion of *relatively* underventilated alveoli. Furthermore, although perfusion of relatively underventilated alveoli will reduce arterial Po_2, the pattern of change, in relation to the inspired oxygen concentration, is quite different from that of a true shunt (see Figure 8.12 below).

The concept of 'ideal' alveolar gas is considered below (page 139), but it will be clear from Figure 8.8 that ideal alveolar gas cannot be sampled for analysis. There is a convention that ideal alveolar Pco_2 is assumed to be equal to the arterial Pco_2 and that the respiratory exchange ratio of ideal alveolar gas is the same as that of expired air.

DEAD SPACE

It was realised in the nineteenth century that an appreciable part of each inspiration did not penetrate to those regions of the lungs in which gas exchange occurred and was therefore exhaled unchanged. This fraction of the tidal volume has long been known as the dead space, while the effective part of the minute volume of respiration is known as the alveolar ventilation. The relationship is as follows:

alveolar ventilation = respiratory frequency
(tidal volume − dead space)

$$\dot{V}_A = f(V_T - V_D)$$

It is often useful to think of two ratios. The first is the dead space/tidal volume ratio (often abbreviated to Vd/Vt and expressed as a percentage). The second useful ratio is the alveolar ventilation/minute volume ratio. The first ratio indicates the wasted part of the breath, while the second gives the utilised portion of the minute volume. The sum of the two ratios is unity and so one may easily be calculated from the other.

COMPONENTS OF THE DEAD SPACE

The preceding section considers dead space as though it were a single homogeneous component of expired air. The situation is actually more complicated, and Figure 8.9 shows in diagrammatic form the various components of a single expired breath.

The first part to be exhaled will be the *apparatus dead space* if the subject is employing any form of

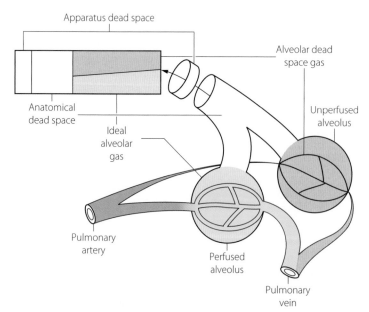

Fig. 8.9 Components of a single breath of expired gas. The rectangle is an idealised representation of a single expired breath. The physiological dead space equals the sum of the anatomical and alveolar dead spaces. The alveolar dead space does not equal the volume of unperfused spaces at alveolar level but only the part of their contents that is exhaled. This varies with tidal volume.

external breathing apparatus. The next component will be from the *anatomical dead space*, which is the volume of the conducting air passages with the qualifications considered below. Thereafter gas is exhaled from the alveolar level and the diagram shows two representative alveoli, corresponding to the two ventilated compartments of the three-compartment lung model shown in Figure 8.8. One alveolus is perfused and, from this, 'ideal' alveolar gas is exhaled. The other alveolus is unperfused and so without gas exchange and, from this alveolus, the exhaled gas therefore approximates in composition to inspired gas. This component of the expirate is known as *alveolar dead space* gas, which is important in many pathological conditions. The *physiological dead space* is the sum of the anatomical and alveolar dead spaces and is defined as the sum of all parts of the tidal volume that do not participate in gas exchange.

In Figure 8.9, the final part of the expirate is called an end-tidal or, preferably, an end-expiratory sample and consists of a mixture of ideal alveolar gas and alveolar dead space gas. The proportion of alveolar dead space gas in an end-expiratory sample is variable. In a healthy resting subject the composition of such a sample will be close to that of ideal alveolar gas. However, in many pathological states (and during anaesthesia), an end-expiratory sample may contain a substantial proportion of alveolar dead space gas and thus be unrepresentative of the alveolar (and therefore arterial) gas tensions. For symbols, the small capital a relates to ideal alveolar gas as in $P_{A_{CO_2}}$, while end-expiratory gas is distinguished by a small capital e, suffixed with a prime (e.g. $P_{E'_{CO_2}}$) and mixed expired gas a small capital e with a bar ($P_{\bar{E}_{CO_2}}$). The term 'alveolar/arterial P_{O_2} difference' always refers to ideal alveolar gas. Unqualified, the term 'alveolar' may mean either end-tidal or ideal alveolar, depending on the context. This is a perennial source of confusion and it is better to specify either ideal alveolar gas or end-expiratory gas.

It must again be stressed that Figure 8.9 is only a model to simplify quantification and there may be an infinite gradation of $\dot{V}/\dot{Q}$ ratios between zero and infinity. However, it is often helpful from the quantitative standpoint, particularly in the clinical field, to consider alveoli *as if* they fell into the three categories shown in Figure 8.8.

ANATOMICAL DEAD SPACE

The anatomical dead space is now generally defined as the volume of gas exhaled before the CO_2 concentration rises to its alveolar plateau, according to the technique of Fowler[28] outlined at the end of this chapter (see Figure 8.16).

The volume of the anatomical dead space, in spite of its name, is not constant and is influenced by many factors, some of which are of considerable clinical importance. Most of these factors influence the anatomical dead space by changing the volume of the conducting airways, except for changes in tidal volume and respiratory rate, which affect the flow pattern of gas passing along the airways.

FACTORS INFLUENCING THE ANATOMICAL DEAD SPACE

Size of the subject must clearly influence the dimensions of the conducting air passages and anatomical dead space increases with body size.

Age. In early infancy, anatomical dead space is approximately $3.3 \, ml.kg^{-1}$, and by the age of 6 years this has decreased to the adult value of approximately $2 \, ml.kg^{-1}$. Throughout this period of development, intrathoracic anatomical dead space remains constant at $1 \, ml.kg^{-1}$ while the volumes of the nose, mouth and pharynx change relative to body weight.[29] From early adulthood, anatomical dead space increases by approximately 1 ml per year.

Posture influences many lung volumes, including the anatomical dead space, with typical values for healthy subjects when supine being a third less than when sitting.

Position of the neck and jaw has a pronounced effect on the anatomical dead space with mean values in conscious subjects of 143 ml with the neck extended and jaw protruded, 119 ml in the normal position, and 73 ml with the neck flexed and chin depressed.[30] It is noteworthy that the first position is the one used by resuscitators and anaesthetists to procure the least possible airway resistance. Unfortunately, it also results in the maximum dead space.

Lung volume at the end of inspiration affects the anatomical dead space, since the volume of the air passages changes in proportion to the lung volume. The increase is of the order of 20 ml additional anatomical dead space for each litre increase in lung volume.[31]

Tracheal intubation, tracheostomy or laryngeal mask airway use will bypass much of the extrathoracic anatomical dead space, which is normally about 70 ml. These methods of airway maintenance bypass approximately half of the total anatomical dead space.[30,32,33] Any advantage gained is usually lost by the addition of further apparatus dead space to the breathing system by, for example, the use of a breathing system filter or a heat and moisture exchanging humidifier.

Drugs acting on the bronchiolar musculature will affect the anatomical dead space, with any bronchodilator drug (page 51) causing a small increase in anatomical dead space.

Tidal volume and respiratory rate. A reduction in tidal volume results in a marked reduction of the anatomical dead space as measured by Fowler's method, and this limits the fall of alveolar ventilation resulting from small tidal volumes. This is important in spontaneously breathing comatose or anaesthetised patients who will often have tidal volumes smaller than the normal anatomical dead space of 150 ml.

Reduced anatomical dead space with small tidal volumes is unlikely to result from changes in the physical dimensions of the airways, and results mostly from changes in the flow patterns and mixing of gases within the airways. First, at low flow rates there is a greater tendency towards laminar flow of gas through the air passages (page 46). Inspired gas advances with a cone front and the tip of the cone penetrates the alveoli before all the gas in the conducting passages has been washed out. Secondly, with a slow respiratory rate and/or a prolonged inspiratory time, there is more time for mixing of gases between the alveoli and the smaller airways. Mixing will occur by simple diffusion, possibly aided by a mixing effect of the heartbeat, which tends to mix all gas lying below the carina. This effect is negligible at normal rates of ventilation, but becomes marked during hypoventilation. For example, in one hypoventilating patient, Nunn and Hill found alveolar gas at the carina at the beginning of expiration.[32] A similar effect occurs during breath holding when alveolar gas mixes with dead space gas as far up as the glottis.

ALVEOLAR DEAD SPACE

Alveolar dead space may be defined as the part of the inspired gas that passes through the anatomical dead space to mix with gas at the alveolar level, but which does not take part in gas exchange. The cause of the failure of gas exchange is lack of effective perfusion of the spaces to which the gas is distributed at the alveolar level. Measured alveolar dead

space must sometimes contain a component due to the ventilation of *relatively* underperfused alveoli, which have a very high (but not infinite) $\dot{V}/\dot{Q}$ ratio (Figure 8.7). The alveolar dead space is too small to be measured with confidence in healthy supine humans, but becomes appreciable under some circumstances:

Low cardiac output, regardless of the cause, results in pulmonary hypotension and failure of perfusion of the uppermost parts of the lungs (Zone 1, see page 105). During anaesthesia with controlled ventilation, sudden changes in end-expiratory CO_2 therefore usually indicate changing alveolar dead space secondary to abrupt variations in cardiac output (page 171).

Pulmonary embolism is considered separately in Chapter 29. Apart from its effect on cardiac output, pulmonary embolism is a direct cause of alveolar dead space that may reach massive proportions.

Posture. Changes in position have a significant effect on the distribution of pulmonary blood flow (page 124). Fortunately, during normal breathing there are similar changes in the distribution of ventilation so that $\dot{V}/\dot{Q}$ mismatch is uncommon and there are no significant changes in alveolar dead space. However, if a patient is ventilated artificially in the lateral position, ventilation is distributed in favour of the upper lung (Table 8.1), particularly in the presence of an open chest (page 499),[4] and under these conditions, part of the ventilation of the upper lung will constitute alveolar dead space.

PHYSIOLOGICAL DEAD SPACE

Physiological dead space is the sum of all parts of the tidal volume that do not participate in gaseous exchange. Nowadays it is universally defined by the Bohr mixing equation with substitution of arterial P_{CO_2} for alveolar P_{CO_2} as described below.

Physiological dead space remains a fairly constant fraction of the tidal volume over a wide range of tidal volumes. It is, therefore, generally more useful to use the Vd/Vt ratio: the alveolar ventilation will then be $(1 - Vd/Vt) \times$ the respiratory minute volume. Thus if the physiological dead space is 30% of the tidal volume (i.e. $Vd/Vt = 0.3$), then the alveolar ventilation will be 70% of the minute volume. This approach is radically different from the assumption of a constant 'dead space' which is subtracted from the tidal volume, the difference then being multiplied by the respiratory frequency to indicate the alveolar ventilation.

THE BOHR EQUATION

Bohr introduced his equation in 1891[34] when the dead space was considered simply as gas exhaled from the conducting airways (i.e. anatomical dead space only). It may be simply derived as follows. During expiration, all the CO_2 eliminated is contained in the alveolar gas. Therefore:

Volume of CO_2 eliminated in the alveolar gas =
  volume of CO_2 eliminated in the mixed expired gas

that is to say:

Alveolar CO_2 concentration $\times$ alveolar ventilation =
  mixed-expired CO_2 concentration $\times$ minute volume

or, for a single breath:

Alveolar CO_2 concentration $\times$ (tidal volume $-$
dead space) = mixed-expired CO_2 concentration
  $\times$ tidal volume

There are four terms in this equation. There is no serious difficulty in measuring two of them, the tidal volume and the mixed-expired CO_2 concentration. This leaves the alveolar CO_2 concentration and the dead space. Therefore the alveolar CO_2 concentration may be derived if the dead space is known or, alternatively, the dead space may be derived if the alveolar CO_2 concentration is known.

The use of this equation has been expanded to measure various components of the dead space by varying the interpretation of the term 'alveolar'. In the equations above, the word 'alveolar' may be taken to mean end-expiratory gas, and therefore this use of the Bohr equation indicates the anatomical dead space. If the 'ideal' alveolar CO_2 concentration were used, then the equation would indicate the physiological dead space comprising the sum of the anatomical and alveolar dead spaces (Figure 8.9). 'Ideal' alveolar gas cannot be sampled but arterial P_{CO_2} may be substituted for alveolar P_{CO_2} in the Bohr equation, and the value so derived is now widely accepted as the definition of the physiological dead space:

$$\frac{V_D}{V_T} = \frac{(Pa_{CO_2} - P\bar{E}_{CO_2})}{Pa_{CO_2}}$$

In the healthy conscious resting subject, there is no significant difference between P_{CO_2} of end-expiratory gas and arterial blood. The former may therefore be used as a substitute for the latter, since the anatomical and physiological dead spaces should be the same (the normal alveolar dead space being too small to measure). However, the use of the end-expiratory P_{CO_2} in the Bohr equation may cause difficulties in certain situations. In exercise, in acute hyperventilation, or if there is maldistribution of inspired gas with sequential emptying, the alveolar P_{CO_2} rises, often steeply, during expiration of the alveolar gas, and the end-tidal P_{CO_2} will depend on the duration of expiration. The dead space so derived will not necessarily correspond to any of the compartments of the dead space shown in Figure 8.9.

FACTORS INFLUENCING THE PHYSIOLOGICAL DEAD SPACE

This section summarises factors that affect physiological dead space in normal subjects, but reasons for the changes have been considered above in the sections on the anatomical and alveolar dead space.

Age and sex. There is a tendency for V_D and also the V_D/V_T ratio to increase with age, as a result of changes in the anatomical component. The volume of V_D in men is around 50 ml greater than in women, but the former group has larger tidal volumes and there is little difference between sexes in the V_D/V_T ratios.

Body size. As described above it is evident that anatomical dead space and therefore V_D, in common with other pulmonary volumes, will be larger in larger people. Physiological dead space correlates with either weight or height, for example, V_D (in millilitres) approximates to the weight of the subject in pounds (1 pound = 0.45 kg),[35] or increases by 17 ml for every 10 cm increase in height.[36]

Posture. The V_D/V_T ratio decreases from a mean value of 34% in the upright position to 30% in the supine position.[37] This is largely explained by the change in anatomical dead space described above.

Pathology. Changes in dead space are important features of many causes of lung dysfunction such as pulmonary embolism, smoking, anaesthesia, artificial ventilation etc. These topics are discussed in Part 3 of this book.

EFFECTS OF AN INCREASED PHYSIOLOGICAL DEAD SPACE

Regardless of whether an increase in physiological dead space is in the anatomical or the alveolar component, alveolar ventilation is reduced unless there is a compensatory increase in minute volume. Reduction of alveolar ventilation due to an increase in physiological dead space produces changes in the 'ideal' alveolar gas tensions that are identical to those produced when alveolar ventilation is decreased by reduction in respiratory minute volume (see Figure 10.9).

It is usually possible to counteract the effects of an increase in physiological dead space by a corresponding increase in the respiratory minute volume. If, for example, the minute volume is $10 \, l.min^{-1}$ and the Vd/Vt ratio 30%, the alveolar ventilation will be $7 \, l.min^{-1}$. If the patient were then subjected to pulmonary embolism resulting in an increase of the Vd/Vt RATIO TO 50%, THE MINUTE VOLUME WOULD NEED TO BE INCREASED TO 14 LM IN $^{-1}$ to maintain an alveolar ventilation of $7 \, l.min^{-1}$. However, should the Vd/Vt increase to 80%, the minute volume would need to be increased to $35 \, l.min^{-1}$. Ventilatory capacity may be a limiting factor with massive increases in dead space, and this is a rare cause of ventilatory failure (Chapter 27).

VENOUS ADMIXTURE OR SHUNT

Admixture of arterial blood with poorly oxygenated or mixed venous blood is an important cause of arterial hypoxaemia.

NOMENCLATURE OF VENOUS ADMIXTURE

Venous admixture refers to the degree of admixture of mixed venous blood with pulmonary end-capillary blood that would be required to produce the observed difference between the arterial and the pulmonary end-capillary Po_2 (usually taken to equal ideal alveolar Po_2), the principles of the calculation being shown in Figure 8.10. Note that the venous admixture is not the *actual* amount of venous blood that mingles with the arterial blood, but the *calculated* amount that would be required to produce the observed value for the arterial Po_2. Calculated venous admixture and the actual volume of blood mixing differ because of two factors. First, the Thebesian and bronchial venous drainage does

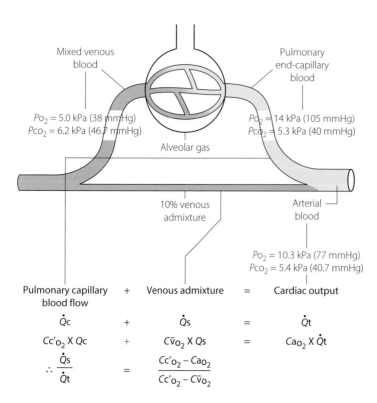

Fig. 8.10 A schematic representation of venous admixture. It makes the assumption that all the arterial blood has come either from alveoli with normal $\dot{V}/\dot{Q}$ ratios or from a shunt carrying only mixed venous blood. This is never true, but it forms a convenient method of quantifying venous admixture from whatever cause. The shunt equation is similar to the Bohr equation and is based on the axiomatic relationship that the total amount of oxygen in 1 minute's flow of arterial blood equals the sum of the amount of oxygen in 1 minute's flow through both the pulmonary capillaries and the shunt. Amount of oxygen in 1 minute's flow of blood equals the product of blood flow rate and the oxygen content of the blood. $\dot{Q}t$, total cardiac output; $\dot{Q}c$, pulmonary capillary blood flow; $\dot{Q}s$, blood flow through shunt; Cao_2, oxygen content of arterial blood; $Cc'o_2$, oxygen content of pulmonary end-capillary blood; $C\bar{v}o_2$, oxygen content of mixed venous blood.

not necessarily have the same Po_2 as mixed venous blood. Secondly, venous admixture includes the contribution to the arterial blood from alveoli having a $\dot{V}/\dot{Q}$ ratio of more than zero but less than the normal value (Figure 8.6), when again, Po_2 will differ from that of mixed venous blood. *Venous admixture* is thus a convenient index but defines neither the precise volume nor the anatomical pathway of the shunt. Nevertheless, it is often loosely termed 'shunt'.

Anatomical (extra-pulmonary) shunt refers to the amount of venous blood that mixes with the pulmonary end-capillary blood on the arterial side of the circulation. The term embraces bronchial and Thebesian venous blood flow and also admixture of mixed venous blood caused by atelectasis, bronchial obstruction, congenital heart disease with right-to-left shunting, etc. Clearly different components may have different oxygen contents, which will not necessarily equal the mixed venous oxygen content. Anatomical shunt excludes blood draining any alveoli with a $\dot{V}/\dot{Q}$ ratio of more than zero.

Virtual shunt refers to shunt values derived from calculations in which the arterial to mixed-venous oxygen difference is assumed rather than actually measured (see below).

Pathological shunt is sometimes used to describe the forms of anatomical shunt that do not occur in the normal subject.

Physiological shunt. This term is, unfortunately, used in two senses. In the first sense it is used to describe the degree of venous admixture that occurs in a normal healthy subject. Differences between the actual measured venous admixture and the normal value for the 'physiological shunt' thus indicate the amount of venous admixture that results from the disease process. In its alternative sense, physiological shunt is synonymous with venous admixture as derived from the mixing equation (Figure 8.10). The term is probably best avoided.

FORMS OF VENOUS ADMIXTURE

The contribution of $\dot{V}/\dot{Q}$ mismatch to venous admixture is discussed in detail below. Other important sources of venous admixture, both normal and pathological, include:

Venae cordis minimae (Thebesian veins). Some small veins of the left heart drain directly into the chambers of the left heart and so mix with the pulmonary venous blood. The oxygen content of this blood is probably very low, and therefore the flow (believed to be about 0.3% of cardiac output[38]) causes an appreciable fall in the mixed arterial oxygen tension.

Bronchial veins. Figure 7.1 shows that part of the venous drainage of the bronchial circulation passes by way of the deep true bronchial veins to reach the pulmonary veins. It is uncertain how large this component is in the healthy subject but it is probably less than 1% of cardiac output. In bronchial disease and coarctation of the aorta, the flow through this channel may be greatly increased, and in bronchiectasis and emphysema may be as large as 10% of cardiac output. In these circumstances it becomes a major cause of arterial desaturation.

Congenital heart disease. Right-to-left shunting in congenital heart disease is the cause of the worst examples of venous admixture. When there are abnormal communications between right and left heart, shunting will usually be from left to right unless the pressures in the right heart are raised above those of the left heart. This occurs in conditions involving obstruction to the right ventricular outflow tract (e.g. Fallot's tetralogy) or in prolonged left-to-right shunt when the increased pulmonary blood flow causes pulmonary hypertension and eventually a reversal of the shunt (Eisenmenger's syndrome).

Pulmonary pathology often results in increased venous admixture, thus causing hypoxaemia. Venous drainage from lung tumours constitutes a pathological shunt, but more commonly venous admixture results from pulmonary blood flow past non-ventilated alveoli in conditions such as lobar and bronchopneumonia, pulmonary collapse and acute lung injury. The amount of venous admixture that occurs with lung disease is variable, depending on the balance between hypoxic pulmonary vasoconstriction (page 108) and pathological vasodilation of the pulmonary vessels by inflammatory mediators.

EFFECT OF VENOUS ADMIXTURE ON ARTERIAL Pco_2 AND Po_2

Qualitatively, it will be clear that venous admixture reduces the overall efficiency of gas exchange and results in arterial blood gas tensions that are closer to those of mixed venous blood than would otherwise be the case. Quantitatively, the effect is simple provided that we consider the *contents* of gases in blood. In the case of the anatomical shunt in Figure 8.10, conservation of mass (oxygen) is the basis of the equations, which simply state that the amount of oxygen flowing in the arterial system equals the sum of the amount of oxygen leaving the pulmonary capillaries and the amount of oxygen flowing through the shunt. For each term in this equation the amount of oxygen flowing may be expressed as the product of the blood flow rate and the oxygen content of blood flowing in the vessel (the symbols are explained in Figure 8.10 and Appendix D). Figure 8.10 shows how the equation may be cleared and solved for the ratio of the venous admixture to the cardiac output. The final equation has a form that is rather similar to that of the Bohr equation for the physiological dead space.

In terms of *content*, the shunt equation is very simple to solve for the effect of venous admixture on arterial oxygen content. If, for example, pulmonary end-capillary oxygen content is $20\,ml.dl^{-1}$ and mixed venous blood oxygen content is $10\,ml.dl^{-1}$ then a 50% venous admixture will result in an arterial oxygen content of $15\,ml.dl^{-1}$, a 25% venous admixture will result in an arterial oxygen content of $17.5\,ml.dl^{-1}$, and so on. It is then necessary to convert arterial oxygen content to Po_2 by reference to the haemoglobin dissociation curve (see page 191). Since arterial Po_2 is usually on the flat part of the haemoglobin dissociation curve, small changes in content tend to have a very large effect on Po_2, though this effect diminishes at lower arterial Po_2 when the dissociation curve becomes steeper.

The effect of venous admixture on arterial CO_2 *content* is roughly similar in magnitude to that of oxygen content. However, due to the steepness of the CO_2 dissociation curve near the arterial point (see Figure 10.2), the effect on arterial Pco_2 is very small and far less than the change in arterial Po_2 (Table 8.2).

Two conclusions may be drawn:

- Arterial Po_2 is the most useful blood gas measurement for the detection of venous admixture.
- Venous admixture reduces the arterial Po_2 markedly, but has relatively little effect on arterial Pco_2 or on the content of either CO_2 or O_2 unless the venous admixture is large.

Elevations of arterial Pco_2 are seldom caused by venous admixture and it is customary to ignore the effect of moderate shunts on Pco_2. In the clinical situation, it is more usual for venous admixture to lower the Pco_2 indirectly, because the decreased Po_2 commonly causes hyperventilation, which more

Table 8.2 Effect of 5% venous admixture on the difference between arterial and pulmonary end-capillary blood levels of carbon dioxide and oxygen

	PULMONARY END-CAPILLARY BLOOD	ARTERIAL BLOOD
CO_2 content $(ml.dl^{-1})$	49.7	50.0
Pco_2 (kPa)	5.29	5.33
(mmHg)	39.7	40.0
O_2 content $(ml.dl^{-1})$	19.9	19.6
O_2 saturation (%)	97.8	96.8
Po_2 (kPa)	14.0	12.0
(mmHg)	105	90

It has been assumed that the arterial/venous oxygen content difference is $4.5\,ml.dl^{-1}$ and that the haemoglobin concentration is $14.9\,g.dl^{-1}$.

than compensates for the very slight elevation of Pco_2 that would otherwise result from the venous admixture (see Figure 27.1).

EFFECT OF CARDIAC OUTPUT ON SHUNT

Cardiac output influences venous admixture, and its consequences, in two opposing ways. First, a reduction of cardiac output leads to a decrease in mixed venous oxygen content, with the result that a given shunt causes a greater reduction in arterial Po_2 *provided the shunt fraction is unaltered*, a relationship that is illustrated in Figure 11.5. Secondly, it has been observed that, in a range of pathological and physiological circumstances, a reduction in cardiac output causes an approximately proportional reduction in the shunt fraction.[39,40] One possible explanation for the reduced shunt fraction is activation of hypoxic pulmonary vasoconstriction as a result of the reduction in Po_2 of the mixed venous blood flowing through the shunt (page 108). It is remarkable that these two effects tend to have approximately equal and opposite effects on arterial Po_2. Thus with a decreased cardiac output there is usually a reduced shunt of a more desaturated mixed venous blood, with the result that the arterial Po_2 is scarcely changed.

THE ISO-SHUNT DIAGRAM

If we assume normal values for arterial Pco_2, haemoglobin and arterial/mixed venous oxygen content

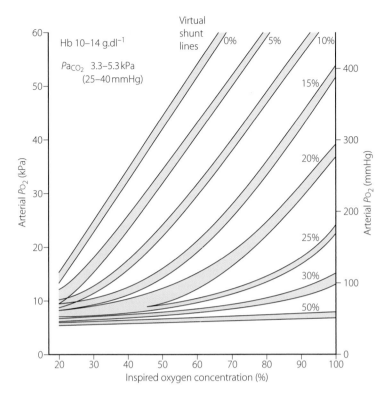

Fig. 8.11 Iso-shunt diagram. On coordinates of inspired oxygen concentration (abscissa) and arterial Po_2 (ordinate), iso-shunt bands have been drawn to include all values of Hb and arterial Pco_2 shown above. Arterial to mixed-venous oxygen content difference is assumed to be $5\,ml.dl^{-1}$, and normal barometric pressure is assumed. (After reference 41 by permission of the Editor of the British Journal of Anaesthesia and Oxford University Press.)

difference, the arterial Po_2 is determined mainly by the inspired oxygen concentration and venous admixture considered in the context of the three-compartment model (Figure 8.8). The relationship between inspired oxygen concentration and arterial Po_2 is a matter for constant attention in clinical situations, and it has been found useful to prepare a graph of the relationship at different levels of venous admixture (Figure 8.11). The arterial/mixed venous oxygen content difference is often unknown in the clinical situation and therefore the diagram has been prepared for an assumed content difference of 5 ml oxygen per 100 ml of blood. Iso-shunt bands have then been drawn on a plot of arterial Po_2 against inspired oxygen concentration. Since calculation of the venous admixture requires knowledge of the actual arterial/mixed venous oxygen content difference, the iso-shunt lines in Figure 8.11 refer to the *virtual shunt*, which is defined above.

In practice, the iso-shunt diagram is useful for adjusting the inspired oxygen concentration to obtain a required level of arterial Po_2. Under stable pathological conditions, changing the inspired oxygen concentration results in changes in arterial Po_2 that are reasonably well predicted by the iso-shunt diagram.[42] In critical care environments, the iso-shunt graph may therefore be used to determine the optimal inspired oxygen concentration to prevent hypoxaemia while avoiding the administration of an unnecessarily high concentration of oxygen.[41] For example, if a patient is found to have an arterial Po_2 of 30 kPa (225 mm Hg) while breathing 90% oxygen, he has a virtual shunt of 20%, and if it is required to attain an arterial Po_2 of 10 kPa (75 mmHg), this should be achieved by reducing the inspired oxygen concentration to 45%.

With inspired oxygen concentrations in excess of 40%, perfusion of alveoli with low (but not zero) $\dot{V}/\dot{Q}$ ratios has relatively little effect on arterial Po_2. However, with inspired oxygen concentrations in the range 21–35% increased scatter of $\dot{V}/\dot{Q}$ ratios has an appreciable effect on arterial Po_2 for reasons that are explained below. Therefore in these circumstances, the standard iso-shunt diagram is not

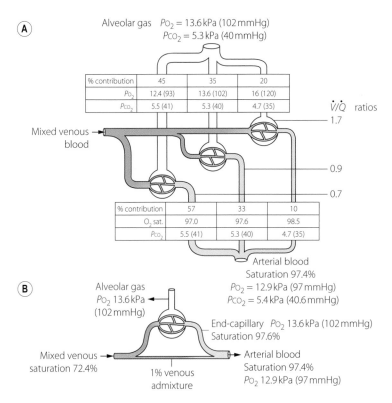

Fig. 8.12 Alveolar to arterial Po_2 difference caused by scatter of $\dot{V}/\dot{Q}$ ratios and its representation by an equivalent degree of venous admixture. (A) Scatter of $\dot{V}/\dot{Q}$ ratios corresponding roughly to the three zones of the lung in the normal upright subject. Mixed alveolar gas Po_2 is calculated with allowance for the volume contribution of gas from the three zones. Arterial saturation is similarly determined and the Po_2 derived. There is an alveolar/arterial Po_2 difference of 0.7 kPa (5 mmHg). (B) A theoretical situation that would account for the same alveolar to arterial Po_2 difference, caused solely by venous admixture. This is a useful method of quantifying the functional effect of scattered $\dot{V}/\dot{Q}$ ratios but should be carefully distinguished from the actual situation.

applicable, since arterial Po_2 is less than predicted as the inspired oxygen concentration is reduced towards 21%, and a modified iso-shunt diagram is required as described below.

THE EFFECT OF SCATTER OF $\dot{V}/\dot{Q}$ RATIOS ON ARTERIAL Po_2

It is usually extremely difficult to say whether reduction of arterial Po_2 is due to true shunt (areas of zero $\dot{V}/\dot{Q}$ ratio), or increased scatter of $\dot{V}/\dot{Q}$ ratios with an appreciable contribution to arterial blood from alveoli with very low (but not zero) $\dot{V}/\dot{Q}$ ratios. In the clinical field, it is quite usual to ignore scatter of $\dot{V}/\dot{Q}$ ratios (which are difficult to quantify) and treat blood-gas results *as if* the alveolar/arterial Po_2 difference was caused entirely by true shunt. In the example shown in Figure 8.12, it is quite impossible to distinguish between scatter of $\dot{V}/\dot{Q}$ ratios and a shunt on the basis of a single measurement of arterial Po_2. However, the two conditions are quite different in the effect of increased inspired oxygen

concentrations on the alveolar/arterial Po_2 difference and therefore the apparent shunt.

Figure 8.11 shows that, for a true shunt, with increasing inspired oxygen concentration, the effect on arterial Po_2 increases to reach a plateau value of 2–3 kPa (15–22 mmHg) for each 1% of shunt. This is more precisely shown in terms of alveolar/arterial Po_2 difference, plotted as a function of alveolar Po_2 in Figure 11.4.

It is not intuitively obvious why an increased spread of $\dot{V}/\dot{Q}$ ratios should increase the alveolar/arterial Po_2 difference. There are essentially two reasons. First, there tends to be more blood from the alveoli with low $\dot{V}/\dot{Q}$ ratio. For example, in Figure 8.12, 57% of the arterial blood comes from the alveoli with low $\dot{V}/\dot{Q}$ ratio and low Po_2, while only 10% is contributed by the alveoli with high $\dot{V}/\dot{Q}$ ratio and high Po_2. Therefore, the latter cannot compensate for the former, when arterial oxygen levels are determined with due allowance for volume contribution. The second reason is illustrated in Figure 8.13. Alveoli with high $\dot{V}/\dot{Q}$ ratios are on a flatter part of the haemoglobin dissociation curve than are alveoli

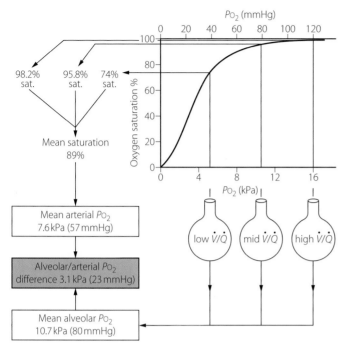

Fig. 8.13 Alveolar/arterial P_{O_2} difference caused by scatter of $\dot{V}/\dot{Q}$ ratios resulting in oxygen tensions along the upper inflexion of the oxygen dissociation curve. The diagram shows the effect of three groups of alveoli with P_{O_2} values of 5.3, 10.7 and 16.0 kPa (40, 80 and 120 mmHg). Ignoring the effect of the different volumes of gas and blood contributed by the three groups, the mean alveolar P_{O_2} is 10.7 kPa. However, due to the shape of the dissociation curve, the saturations of the blood leaving the three groups are not proportional to their P_{O_2}. The mean arterial saturation is, in fact, 89% and the P_{O_2} therefore is 7.6 kPa. The alveolar/arterial P_{O_2} difference is thus 3.1 kPa. The actual difference would be somewhat greater since gas with a high P_{O_2} would make a relatively greater contribution to the alveolar gas, and blood with a low P_{O_2} would make a relatively greater contribution to the arterial blood. In this example, a calculated venous admixture of 27% would be required to account for the scatter of $\dot{V}/\dot{Q}$ ratios in terms of the measured alveolar/arterial P_{O_2} difference, at an alveolar P_{O_2} of 10.7 kPa.

with low $\dot{V}/\dot{Q}$ ratios. Therefore, the adverse effect on oxygen *content* is greater for alveoli with a low $\dot{V}/\dot{Q}$ and therefore low P_{O_2} than is the beneficial effect of alveoli with a high $\dot{V}/\dot{Q}$ and therefore high P_{O_2}. Therefore, the greater the spread of $\dot{V}/\dot{Q}$ ratios, the larger the alveolar/arterial P_{O_2} difference.

Modification of the iso-shunt diagram to include $\dot{V}/\dot{Q}$ scatter. The iso-shunt diagram described above does not take into account $\dot{V}/\dot{Q}$ scatter so has bands too wide for practical use below an inspired oxygen concentration of approximately 40% (Figure 8.11). This problem has been overcome by the development of a two-compartment model including both true shunt and $\dot{V}/\dot{Q}$ scatter components,[43] which for the latter factor assumes a bimodal distribution of $\dot{V}/\dot{Q}$ scatter and uses five grades of $\dot{V}/\dot{Q}$ mismatch 'severity'. Figure 8.14 shows the effect of $\dot{V}/\dot{Q}$ mismatch on the 0% iso-shunt line (blue lines), clearly displaying the variation in arterial P_{O_2} with $\dot{V}/\dot{Q}$ scatter at lower inspired oxygen concentrations. Further examples are shown in Figure 8.14 of the effect of $\dot{V}/\dot{Q}$ scatter on the inspired to arterial oxygen gradients. This model is clearly an over-simplification of the situation in lung disease (see Figure 8.7). Nevertheless, the second grade of $\dot{V}/\dot{Q}$ mismatch, when combined with a range of shunt values, was found to provide a close simulation of the relationship between arterial

P_{O_2} and inspired oxygen concentration for a wide variety of patients with moderate respiratory dysfunction requiring inspired oxygen concentration in the range 25–35%.[43,44]

PRINCIPLES OF ASSESSMENT OF DISTRIBUTION OF VENTILATION AND PULMONARY BLOOD FLOW

REGIONAL DISTRIBUTION OF VENTILATION AND PERFUSION

Radioactive tracers. Regional distribution of ventilation and perfusion may both be conveniently studied with a gamma camera. Ventilation is assessed following inhalation of a suitable radioactive gas that is not too soluble in blood. Both ^{133}Xe and ^{81}Kr are suitable for this purpose, the latter usually being used because its short half-life (13 s) reduces uptake by the pulmonary circulation. For assessment of regional perfusion, a relatively insoluble gas such as ^{133}Xe or ^{99}Tc may be dissolved in saline and administered intravenously, and its distribution within the lung again recorded with a gamma camera. The technique defines both ventilation and perfusion in zones of the lung that can

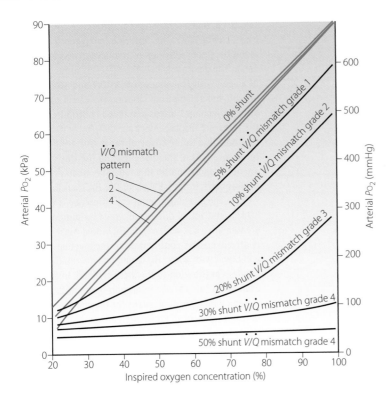

Fig. 8.14 Iso-shunt lines modified to incorporate the effect on arterial P_{O_2} of increasing degrees of $\dot{V}/\dot{Q}$ mismatch.[43] Blue lines show the effects of differing degrees of $\dot{V}/\dot{Q}$ mismatch in the absence of a true shunt. At lower inspired oxygen the arterial P_{O_2} is progressively decreased below normal for the reasons shown in Figures 8.12 and 8.13. The other iso-shunt lines shown are examples of progressively more severe degrees of combined shunt and $\dot{V}/\dot{Q}$ mismatch.

be related to anatomical subdivisions by comparing anteroposterior and lateral scans.

Scanning techniques. A variety of scanners are now used, mostly for research purposes, to assess regional ventilation and perfusion including:

- Positron emission tomography.[8] For this technique radioactive isotopes are inhaled or injected intravenously, for example $^{13}N_2$, and the radioisotopic concentration in a three dimensional field measured during normal breathing. Resolutions of less than $1\,cm^3$ of lung tissue are now possible.

- Magnetic resonance imaging (MRI).[9] Low proton density in lung tissue due to the presence of air makes MRI scanning of the lungs challenging. However, technological advances in MRI scanning have led to more functionally relevant scans.[10,45] By using non-radioactive tracer gases, such as ^3He that has been magnetically 'hyperpolarised', MRI scans can be greatly enhanced in a similar way to the use of contrast for traditional x-ray radiographs. Hyperpolarised ^3He used in this way interacts with the paramagnetic oxygen molecules (page 208) in the lungs, causing oxygen-dependent decay of the

hyperpolarisation, and this phenomenon can be used to generate scans showing regional P_{O_2} in the lung.[9]

- Single-photon-emission computed tomography (SPECT).[7] This technique also uses inhaled or intravenous radioactive tracers. Though of low resolution compared with the other scans, it does have the advantage of being able to image more than one process simultaneously, for example lung ventilation and perfusion.

MEASUREMENT OF VENTILATION AND PERFUSION AS A FUNCTION OF $\dot{V}/\dot{Q}$ RATIO

The information of the type displayed in Figures 8.6 and 8.7 is obtained by the MIGET,[23,25] which employs six tracer gases with different blood solubility ranging from very soluble (acetone) to very insoluble (sulphur hexafluoride). Saline is equilibrated with these gases and infused intravenously at a constant rate. Once steady state is achieved levels of the tracer gases in the arterial blood are then measured by gas chromatography, and levels in the mixed venous blood are derived by use of the Fick principle.

It is then possible to calculate the retention of each tracer in the blood passing through the lung and the elimination of each in the expired gas. Retention and elimination are related to the solubility coefficient of each tracer in blood and therefore it is possible to compute a distribution curve for pulmonary blood flow and alveolar ventilation respectively in relation to the spectrum of $\dot{V}/\dot{Q}$ ratios (Figure 8.6).

The technique is technically demanding and laborious. It has not become widely used, but studies using the technique from a small number of laboratories have made major contributions to our understanding of gas exchange in a variety of circumstances.

MEASUREMENT OF VENOUS ADMIXTURE

Venous admixture, according to the Riley three-compartment model (Figure 8.8), is calculated by solution of the equation shown in Figure 8.10. When the alveolar P_{O_2} is less than about 30 kPa (225 mmHg), scatter of $\dot{V}/\dot{Q}$ ratios contributes appreciably to the total calculated venous admixture (Figure 8.14). When the subject breathes 100% oxygen, the component due to scatter of $\dot{V}/\dot{Q}$ ratios is minimal. Nevertheless, the calculated quantity still does not indicate the precise value of shunted blood because some of the shunt consists of blood of which the oxygen content is unknown (e.g. from bronchial veins and venae cordis minimae). The calculated venous admixture is thus at best an index rather than a precise measurement of contamination of arterial blood with venous blood.

To solve the equation shown in Figure 8.10, there are three quantities required:

1. *Arterial oxygen content.* Arterial P_{O_2} or oxygen saturation may be measured on blood drawn from any convenient systemic artery. If arterial P_{O_2} is measured, this must first be converted to oxygen saturation (page 191 et seq.), before the oxygen content can be calculated (page 202).
2. *Mixed venous oxygen content.* Mixed venous blood must be sampled from the right ventricle or pulmonary artery. Blood from inferior and superior venae cavae and coronary sinus, each with quite different O_2 contents, remain separate in the right atrium. Oxygen content may then be calculated from measured P_{O_2} as for the arterial sample. An assumed value for arterial/mixed venous blood oxygen content difference is often made if it is not feasible to sample mixed venous blood.
3. *Pulmonary end-capillary oxygen content.* This cannot be measured directly, and is assumed equal to the alveolar P_{O_2} (page 149). If Figure 8.8 is studied in conjunction with Figure 8.10, it will be seen that the 'alveolar' P_{O_2} required is the 'ideal' alveolar P_{O_2} and not the end-expiratory P_{O_2}, which may be contaminated with alveolar dead space gas. The 'ideal' alveolar P_{O_2} is derived by solution of one of the alveolar air equations (see below), and again converted to oxygen content.

THE ALVEOLAR AIR EQUATION

The difference between inspired and alveolar gas concentrations is equal to the ratio of the output (or uptake) of the gas to the alveolar ventilation according to the universal alveolar air equation:

$$\begin{array}{l} \text{Alveolar} \\ \text{concentration} \\ \text{of gas } X \end{array} = \begin{array}{l} \text{inspired concentration of gas } X \\ \pm \dfrac{\text{output (or uptake) of gas } X}{\text{alveolar ventilation}} \end{array}$$

This equation uses fractional concentrations and does not correct for any difference between inspired and expired minute volumes (see below). The sign on the right-hand side is + for output of a gas (e.g. carbon dioxide) and − for uptake (e.g. oxygen).

For the derivation of P_{O_2} in 'ideal' alveolar gas the universal air equation was first modified with some precision by Riley et al. in 1946.[46] The equation exists in several forms that appear very different but give the same result.

Derivation of the ideal alveolar P_{O_2} is based on the following assumptions.

● Quite large degrees of venous admixture or $\dot{V}/\dot{Q}$ scatter cause relatively little difference between the P_{CO_2} of ideal alveolar gas (or pulmonary end-capillary blood) and arterial blood (Table 8.2). Therefore ideal alveolar P_{CO_2} is approximately equal to arterial P_{CO_2}.
● The respiratory exchange ratio of ideal alveolar gas (in relation to inspired gas) equals the respiratory exchange ratio of mixed expired gas (again in relation to inspired gas).

From these assumptions it is possible to derive an equation that indicates the ideal alveolar P_{O_2} in terms of arterial P_{CO_2} and inspired gas P_{O_2}. As a very rough approximation, the oxygen and carbon dioxide in the alveolar gas replace the oxygen in the inspired gas. Therefore, very approximately:

$$\text{Alveolar } Po_2 \approx \text{inspired } Po_2 - \text{arterial } Pco_2$$

This equation is not sufficiently accurate for use, except in the special case when 100% oxygen is breathed. In other situations, three corrections are required to overcome errors due to the following factors:

1. Usually, less carbon dioxide is produced than oxygen is consumed (effect of the respiratory exchange ratio, RQ).
2. The respiratory exchange ratio produces a secondary effect due to the fact that the expired volume does not equal the inspired volume.
3. The inspired and expired gas volumes may also differ because of inert gas exchange.

The simplest practicable form of the equation makes correction for the principal effect of the respiratory exchange ratio (1), but not the small supplementary error due to the difference between the inspired and expired gas volumes (2):

$$\text{Alveolar } Po_2 \approx \text{inspired } Po_2 - \text{arterial } Pco_2 / RQ$$

This form is suitable for rapid bedside calculations of alveolar Po_2, when great accuracy is not required.

One stage more complicated is an equation that allows for differences in the volume of inspired and expired gas due to the respiratory exchange ratio, but still does not allow for differences due to the exchange of inert gases. This equation exists in various forms, all algebraically identical:[46]

$$\text{Alveolar } Po_2 = PI_{O_2} - \frac{Pa_{CO_2}}{RQ}(1 - FI_{O_2}(1 - RQ))$$

This equation is suitable for use whenever the subject has been breathing the inspired gas mixture long enough for the inert gas to be in equilibrium. It is unsuitable for use when the inspired oxygen concentration has recently been changed, when the ambient pressure has recently been changed (e.g. during hyperbaric oxygen therapy) or when the inert gas concentration has recently been changed (e.g. soon after the start or finish of a period of inhaling nitrous oxide).

Perhaps the most satisfactory form of the alveolar air equation is that which was advanced by Filley, MacIntosh & Wright in 1954.[47] This equation makes

no assumption that inert gases are in equilibrium and allows for the difference between inspired and expired gas from whatever cause. It also proves to be very simple in use and does not require the calculation of the respiratory exchange ratio, though does require sampling of mixed-expired gas:

$$\text{Alveolar } Po_2 = PI_{O_2} - Pa_{CO_2}\left(\frac{PI_{O_2} - P\bar{E}_{O_2}}{P\bar{E}_{CO_2}}\right)$$

If the alveolar Po_2 is calculated separately according to the last two equations, the difference (if any) will be that due to inert gas exchange.

When using these equations in practice it is important to take into account water vapour, as alveolar gas will be saturated with water at body temperature, such that:

$$PI_{O_2} = FI_{O_2} \times (PB - PH_2O)$$

Where FI_{O_2} is the fractional inspired oxygen concentration, PB is barometric pressure, and PH_2O is saturated vapour pressure of water at 37°C (6.3 kPa, 47 mmHg).

DISTINCTION BETWEEN SHUNT AND THE EFFECT OF $\dot{V}/\dot{Q}$ SCATTER

Shunt and scatter of $\dot{V}/\dot{Q}$ ratios will each produce an alveolar/arterial Po_2 difference from which a value for venous admixture may be calculated. It is usually impossible to say to what extent the calculated venous admixture is due to a true shunt or to perfusion of alveoli with low $\dot{V}/\dot{Q}$ ratio. Three methods are available for distinction between the two conditions.

If the inspired oxygen concentration is altered, the effect on the arterial Po_2 will depend upon the nature of the disorder. If oxygenation is impaired by a shunt, the arterial Po_2 WILL INCREASE AS SHOWN IN THE ISO-SHUNT DIAGRAM (FIGURE 8.11). IF, HOWEVER, THE DISORDER IS DUE TO SCATTER OF $\dot{V}/\dot{Q}$ RATIOS, THE ARTERIAL Po_2 will approach the normal value for the inspired oxygen concentration as the inspired oxygen concentration is increased (Figure 8.14). $\dot{V}/\dot{Q}$ scatter has virtually no effect when the subject breathes 100% oxygen. This difference between shunt and $\dot{V}/\dot{Q}$ scatter forms the basis of a non-invasive method for investigating the mechanism of impaired gas exchange in the clinical setting.[48,49] Oxygen saturation is measured at several different inspired

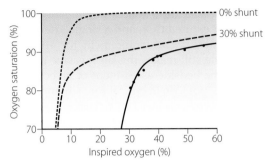

Fig. 8.15 Non-invasive evaluation of impaired gas exchange during one lung anaesthesia and thoracotomy. Oxygen saturation has been measured at nine different inspired oxygen concentrations (circles) and a curve fitted to the points (solid line). Mathematical modelling (broken lines) shows that shunt displaces the curve downwards (0% and 30% shunt shown) whilst $\dot{V}/\dot{Q}$ mismatch displaces the curve to the right. A computer algorithm, using an assumed value for arterio-venous oxygen difference, can compute the virtual shunt and the shift due to $\dot{V}/\dot{Q}$ mismatch from the actual curve obtained from the patient, in this case 30% shunt *and* marked $\dot{V}/\dot{Q}$ mismatch in the patient during one-lung ventilation (page 498). (After reference 48 with permission of the authors and the Editor of Anaesthesia.)

oxygen concentrations and an Sp_{O_2} versus $P_{I_{O_2}}$ curve drawn. Mathematical modelling, again using an assumed value for arterio-venous oxygen difference, and studies during one lung anaesthesia have shown that shunt depresses the curve downwards whilst increasing $\dot{V}/\dot{Q}$ mismatch moves the curve to the right (Figure 8.15).[48]

The multiple inert gas elimination technique for analysis of distribution of blood flow in relation to $\dot{V}/\dot{Q}$ ratio is the best method for distinction between shunt and areas of low $\dot{V}/\dot{Q}$ ratio (see above).

MEASUREMENT OF DEAD SPACE

Anatomical dead space is most conveniently measured by the technique illustrated in Figure 8.16, originally developed for use with a nitrogen analyser by Fowler.[28] The CO_2 concentration at the lips is measured continuously with a rapid gas analyser, and then displayed against the volume actually expired. The 'alveolar plateau' of CO_2 concentration is not flat but slopes gently. Anatomical dead space is easily derived from the graph as shown in Figure 8.16 or by a variety of mathematical methods.[50]

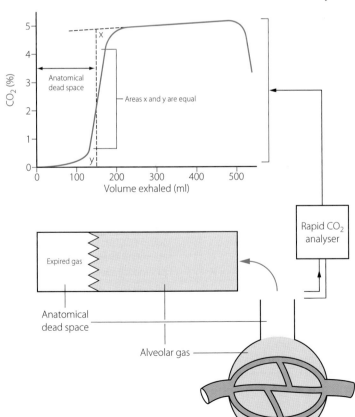

Fig. 8.16 Measurement of anatomical dead space using CO_2 as the tracer gas. If the gas passing the patient's lips is continuously analysed for CO_2 concentration, there is a sudden rise to the alveolar plateau level, after the expiration of gas from the anatomical dead space. If the instantaneous CO_2 concentration is plotted against the volume exhaled (allowing for delay in the CO_2 analyser), a graph similar to that shown is obtained. A vertical line is constructed so that the two areas *x* and *y* are equal. This line will indicate the volume of the anatomical dead space. Note that the abscissa records *volume* rather than *time* as seen with capnography performed in clinical situations.

Physiological dead space. Mixed expired air is collected over a period of two or three minutes, during which time an arterial blood sample is collected, and the P_{CO_2} of blood and gas are then determined. Provided that the inspired gas is free from carbon dioxide, physiological dead space is indicated by the following form of the Bohr equation:

$$\text{Physiological dead space} = \text{tidal volume} \left(\frac{Pa_{CO_2} - P\bar{E}_{CO_2}}{Pa_{CO_2}} \right) - \text{apparatus dead space}$$

Alveolar dead space is measured as the difference between the physiological and anatomical dead space, determined separately but at the same time. When only the physiological dead space is measured, it is often possible to attribute a large increase in physiological dead space to an increase in the alveolar component, since there are few circumstances in which the anatomical dead space is greatly enlarged. Methods are now available for the estimation of anatomical, physiological and therefore alveolar dead spaces from a single breath recording of expired CO_2, and a single arterial P_{CO_2} measurement.[51,52] The requirement for an arterial blood sample still makes this an invasive measurement, but the bedside assessment of alveolar dead space is now possible in critical care situations.[52]

The arterial/end-expiratory P_{CO_2} difference is a convenient and relatively simple method of assessing the magnitude of the alveolar dead space. In Figure 8.9, end-expiratory gas is shown to consist of a mixture of ideal alveolar gas and alveolar dead space gas. If the patient has an appreciable alveolar dead space, the end-expiratory P_{CO_2} will be less than the arterial P_{CO_2}, which is assumed equal to the ideal alveolar P_{CO_2}.

If, for example, ideal alveolar gas has a P_{CO_2} of 5.3 kPa (40 mmHg) and the end-expiratory P_{CO_2} is found to be 2.65 kPa (20 mmHg), it follows that the end expiratory gas consists of equal parts of ideal alveolar gas and alveolar dead space gas. Thus if the tidal volume is 500 ml, and the anatomical dead space 100 ml, then alveolar dead space and ideal alveolar gas components would be 200 ml each.

References

1. Svanberg L. Influence of posture on lung volumes, ventilation and circulation in normals. *Scand J Clin Lab Invest.* 1957;9(supp 25).
2. Rehder K, Sessler AD. Function of each lung in spontaneously breathing man anesthetized with thiopentalmeperidine. *Anesthesiology.* 1973;38:320–327.
3. Rehder K, Hatch DJ, Sessler AD, Fowler WS. The function of each lung of anesthetized and paralyzed man during mechanical ventilation. *Anesthesiology.* 1972;37:16–26.
4. Nunn JF. The distribution of inspired gas during thoracic surgery. *Ann R Coll Surg Eng.* 1961;28:223–237.
*5. Galvin I, Drummond GB, Nirmalan M. Distribution of blood flow and ventilation in the lung: gravity is not the only factor. *Br J Anaesth.* 2007;98:420–428.
6. Hopkins SR, Henderson AC, Levin DL, et al. Vertical gradients in regional lung density and perfusion in the supine human lung: the Slinky effect. *J Appl Physiol.* 2007;103:240–248.
7. Petersson J, Sánchez-Crespo A, Larsson SA, Mure M. Physiological imaging of the lung: single-photon-emission computed tomography (SPECT). *J Appl Physiol.* 2007;102:468–476.
8. Harris RS, Schuster DP. Visualising lung function with positron emission tomography. *J Appl Physiol.* 2007;102:448–458.
9. Hopkins SR, Levin DL, Emami K, et al. Advances in magnetic resonance imaging of lung physiology. *J Appl Physiol.* 2007;102:1244–1254.
*10. Kauczor HU, Chen XJ, van Beek EJR, Schreiber WG. Pulmonary ventilation imaged by magnetic resonance: at the doorstep of clinical application. *Eur Respir J.* 2001;17:1008–1023.
11. Kaneko K, Milic-Emili ME, Dolovich MB, Dawson A, Bates DV. Regional distribution of ventilation and perfusion as a function of body position. *J Appl Physiol.* 1966;21:767–777.
12. Hughes JMB, Glazier JB, Maloney JE, West JB. Effect of lung volume on the distribution of pulmonary blood flow in man. *Respir Physiol.* 1968;4:58–72.
13. Brudin LH, Rhodes CG, Valind SO, Jones T, Hughes JB. Interrelationship between regional blood flow, blood volume, and ventilation in supine humans. *J Appl Physiol.* 1994;76: 1205–1210.
14. Brudin LH, Rhodes CG, Valind SO, Jones T, Jonson B, Hughes JB. Relationship between regional ventilation and vascular and extravascular volume in supine humans. *J Appl Physiol.* 1994;76:1195–1204.

15. Hughes M, West JB. Gravity is the major factor determining the distribution of blood flow in the human lung. *J Appl Physiol.* 2008;104:1531–1533.

16. Glenny R. Gravity is not the major factor determining the distribution of blood flow in the healthy human lung. *J Appl Physiol.* 2008;104:1533–1536.

17. Jones AT, Hansell DM, Evans TW. Pulmonary perfusion in supine and prone positions: an electron-beam computed tomography study. *J Appl Physiol.* 2001;90:1342–1348.

18. Prisk GK, Yamada K, Henderson AC, et al. Pulmonary perfusion in the prone and supine postures in the normal human lung. *J Appl Physiol.* 2007;103:883–894.

19. Hakim TS, Lisbona R, Dean GW. Gravity-independent inequality in pulmonary blood flow in humans. *J Appl Physiol.* 1987;63:1114–1121.

*20. Hlastala MP, Glenny RW. Vascular structure determines pulmonary blood flow distribution. *News Physiol Sci.* 1999;14:182–186.

21. Burrowes KS, Hunter PJ, Tawhai MH. Anatomically based finite element models of the human pulmonary arterial and venous trees including supernumerary vessels. *J Appl Physiol.* 2005;99:731–738.

22. Hlastala MP. Ventilation/perfusion: from the bench to the patient. *Cardiologia.* 1996;41:405–415.

23. Roca J, Wagner PD. Principles and information content of the multiple inert gas elimination technique. *Thorax.* 1993;49:815–824.

24. Wagner PD, Laravuso RB, Uhl RR, West JB. Continuous distributions of ventilation-perfusion ratios in normal subjects breathing air and 100% O_2. *J Clin Invest.* 1974;54:54–68.

25. West JB. *Ventilation: blood flow and gas exchange.* Oxford: Blackwell Scientific; 1990.

26. Fenn WO, Rahn H, Otis AB. A theoretical analysis of the composition of alveolar air at altitude. *Am J Physiol.* 1946;146:637–653.

27. Riley RL, Cournard A. 'Ideal' alveolar air and the analysis of ventilation perfusion relationships in the lung. *J Appl Physiol.* 1949;1:825–849.

28. Fowler WS. Lung function studies. II. The respiratory dead space. *Am J Physiol.* 1948;154:405–416.

29. Numa AH, Newth CJL. Anatomic dead space in infants and children. *J Appl Physiol.* 1996;80:1485–1489.

30. Nunn JF, Campbell EJM, Peckett BW. Anatomical subdivisions of the volume of respiratory dead space and effect of position of the jaw. *J Appl Physiol.* 1959;14:174–176.

31. Lifshay A, Fast CW. Glazier JB. Effects of changes in respiratory pattern on physiological dead space. *J Appl Physiol.* 1971;31:478–483.

32. Nunn JF, Hill DW. Respiratory dead space and arterial to end-tidal CO_2 tension difference in anesthetized man. *J Appl Physiol.* 1960;15:383–389.

33. Casati A, Fanelli G, Torri G. Physiological dead space/tidal volume ratio during face mask, laryngeal mask, and cuffed oropharyngeal airway spontaneous ventilation. *J Clin Anesth.* 1998;10:652–655.

34. Bohr C. Über die Lungenathmung. *Skand Arch Physiol.* 1891;2:236.

35. Radford EP. Ventilation standards for use in artificial respiration. *J Appl Physiol.* 1955;7:451–463.

36. Harris EA, Hunter ME, Seelye ER, Vedder M, Whitlock RML. Prediction of the physiological dead-space in resting normal subjects. *Clin Sci.* 1973;45:375–386.

37. Craig DB, Wahba WM, Don HF, Couture JG, Becklake MR. 'Closing volume' and its relationship to gas exchange in seated and

supine positions. *J Appl Physiol.* 1971;31:717–721.

38. Ravin MG, Epstein RM, Malm JR. Contribution of thebesian veins to the physiologic shunt in anesthetized man. *J Appl Physiol.* 1965;20:1148–1152.

39. Dantzker DR, Lynch JP, Weg JG. Depression of cardiac output is a mechanism of shunt reduction in the therapy of acute respiratory failure. *Chest.* 1980;77:636–647.

40. Lynch JP, Mhyre JG, Dantzker DR. Influence of cardiac output on intrapulmonary shunt. *J Appl Physiol.* 1979;46:315–321.

41. Benator SR, Hewlett AM, Nunn JF. The use of iso-shunt lines for control of oxygen therapy. *Br J Anaesth.* 1973;45:711–718.

42. Lawler PGP, Nunn JF. A reassessment of the validity of the iso-shunt graph. *Br J Anaesth.* 1984;56:1325–1335.

43. Petros AJ, Doré CJ, Nunn JF. Modification of the iso-shunt lines for low inspired oxygen concentrations. *Br J Anaesth.* 1994;72:515–522.

44. Drummond GB, Wright DJ. Oxygen therapy after abdominal surgery. *Br J Anaesth.* 1977;49:789–797.

*45. Mills GH, Wild JM, Eberle B, Van Beek EJR. Functional magnetic resonance imaging of the lung. *Br J Anaesth.* 2003;91:16–30.

46. Riley RL, Lilienthal JL, Proemmel DD, Franke RE. On the determination of the physiologically effective pressures of oxygen and carbon dioxide in alveolar air. *Am J Physiol.* 1946;147:191–198.

47. Filley GF, MacIntosh DJ, Wright GW. Carbon monoxide uptake and pulmonary diffusing capacity in normal subject at rest and during exercise. *J Clin Invest.* 1954;33:530–539.

*48. de Gray L, Rush EM, Jones JG. A noninvasive method for evaluating the effect of thoracotomy on shunt and ventilation perfusion inequality. *Anaesthesia*. 1997;52:630–635.

49. Kjaergaard S, Rees S, Malczynski J, et al. Non-invasive estimation of shunt and ventilation-perfusion mismatch. *Intensive Care Med*. 2003;29:727–734.

50. Tang Y, Turner MJ, Baker AB. Systematic errors and susceptibility to noise of four methods for calculating anatomical dead space from the CO_2 expirogram. *Br J Anaesth*. 2007;98:828–834.

*51. Åström E, Niklason L, Drefeldt B, Bajc M, Jonson B. Partitioning of dead space – a method and reference values in the awake human. *Eur Respir J*. 2000;16:659–664.

52. Arnold JH. Measurement of alveolar deadspace: Are we there yet? *Crit Care Med*. 2001;29:1287–1288.

Chapter 9

Diffusion of respiratory gases

KEY POINTS

- For gas to transfer between the alveolus and the haemoglobin in the red blood cell it must diffuse across the alveolar and capillary walls, through the plasma and across the red cell membrane.

- The reaction rate for oxygen with haemoglobin also affects the rate at which red blood cells become saturated with oxygen on passing through the pulmonary capillary.

- Transfer of oxygen and carbon dioxide is very rapid, and impairment of this transfer is rarely a cause of impaired gas exchange.

- Carbon monoxide, because of its high affinity for haemoglobin, is used to assess the diffusing capacity of the lungs.

The previous chapters have described in detail how alveolar gases and pulmonary capillary blood are delivered to their respective sides of the alveolar wall. This chapter deals with the final step of lung function by discussing the transfer of respiratory gases between the alveolus and blood.

Nomenclature in this field is confusing. In Europe, measurement of the passage of gases between the alveoli and pulmonary capillaries is referred to as lung 'transfer factor' (e.g. $T_{L_{CO}}$ represents lung transfer factor for carbon monoxide). However, the older term 'diffusing capacity' (e.g. $D_{L_{CO}}$ for lung diffusing capacity for carbon monoxide) which has been used for many years in the USA is now the recommended term[1] despite the fact that some of the barrier to oxygen transfer is unrelated to diffusion (see below).

FUNDAMENTALS OF THE DIFFUSION PROCESS

Diffusion of a gas is a process by which a net transfer of molecules takes place from a zone in which the gas exerts a high partial pressure to a zone in which it exerts a lower partial pressure. The mechanism of transfer is the random movement of molecules and the term excludes both active biological transport and transfer by mass movement of gas in response to a *total* pressure difference (i.e. gas flow as occurs during tidal ventilation). The partial pressure (or tension) of a gas in a gas mixture is the pressure which it would exert if it occupied the space alone (equal to total pressure multiplied by fractional concentration). Gas molecules pass in each direction but at a rate proportional to the partial pressure of the gas in the zone from which they are leaving. The net transfer of the gas is the difference in the number of molecules passing in each direction, and is thus proportional to the difference in partial pressure between the two zones. Typical examples of diffusion are shown in Figure 9.1.

In each of the examples shown in Figure 9.1, there is a finite resistance to the transfer of the gas molecules. In Figure 9.1A, the resistance is concentrated at the restriction in the neck of the bottle. Clearly, the narrower the neck, the slower will be the process of equilibration with the outside air. In Figure 9.1B, the site of the resistance to diffusion is less circumscribed but includes gas diffusion within the alveolus, the alveolar/capillary membrane, the diffusion path through the plasma, and the delay in combination of oxygen with the reduced haemoglobin in the red blood cell (RBC). In Figure 9.1C,

DOI: 10.1016/B978-0-7020-2996-7.00009-X

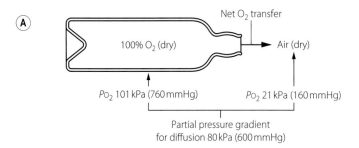

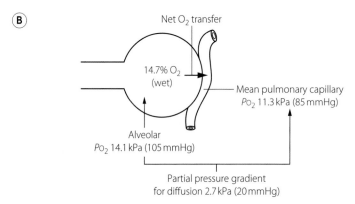

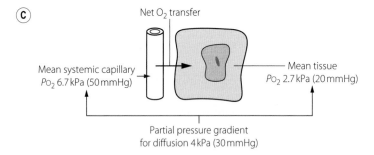

Fig. 9.1 Three examples of diffusion of oxygen. In each case there is a net transfer of oxygen from left to right in accord with the partial pressure gradient. (A) Oxygen passes from one gaseous phase to another. (B) Oxygen passes from a gaseous phase to a liquid phase. (C) Oxygen passes from one liquid to another.

the resistance commences with the delay in the release of oxygen by haemoglobin, and includes all the interfaces between the RBC membrane and the site of oxygen consumption in the mitochondria. There may then be an additional component in the rate at which oxygen enters into chemical reactions.

In the living body oxygen is constantly being consumed, while carbon dioxide is being produced, so equilibrium cannot be attained as in the case of the open bottle of oxygen in Figure 9.1A. Instead, a dynamic equilibrium is attained with diffusion down a gradient between the alveolus and the mitochondria for oxygen and the reverse for carbon dioxide. The maintenance of these partial pressure gradients is, in fact, a characteristic of life.

In the case of gases that are not metabolised to any great extent, such as nitrogen and most inhalational anaesthetic agents, there is always a tendency towards a static equilibrium at which all tissue partial pressures become equal to the partial pressure of the particular gas in the inspired air. This occurs with nitrogen and would also be attained with an inhalational anaesthetic agent if it were administered for a very long time.

QUANTIFICATION OF RESISTANCE TO DIFFUSION

The propensity of a gas to diffuse as a result of a given pressure gradient is known as its diffusing capacity according to the equation:

$$\text{Diffusing capacity} = \frac{\text{Net rate of gas transfer}}{\text{Partial pressure gradient}}$$

The usual biological unit of diffusing capacity is $ml.min^{-1}.mmHg^{-1}$ or, in SI units, $ml.min^{-1}.kPa^{-1}$.

Small molecules diffuse more easily than large molecules. Graham's law states that the rate of diffusion of a gas is inversely proportional to the square root of its density. In addition, gases also diffuse more readily at higher temperatures. Apart from these factors, inherent in the gas, the resistance to diffusion is related directly to the length of the diffusion path and inversely to the area of interface that is available for diffusion.

DIFFUSION OF GASES IN SOLUTION

The partial pressure of a gas in solution in a liquid is defined as being equal to the partial pressure of the same gas in a gas mixture that is in equilibrium with the liquid. When a gas is diffusing into or through an aqueous phase, the solubility of the gas in water becomes an important factor, and the diffusing capacity under these circumstances is considered to be directly proportional to the solubility. Nitrous oxide would thus be expected to have about 20 times the diffusing capacity of oxygen in crossing a gas–water interface. High solubility does not confer an increased 'agility' of the gas in its negotiation of an aqueous barrier, but simply means that, for a given partial pressure, more molecules of the gas are present in the liquid.

Partial pressure versus concentration gradients. Nongaseous substances in solution diffuse in response to concentration gradients. This is also true for gas mixtures at the same total pressure, when the partial pressure of any component gas is directly proportional to its concentration. This is not the case when a gas in solution in one liquid diffuses into a different liquid in which it has a different solubility coefficient. When gases are in solution, the partial pressure they exert is directly proportional to their concentration in the solvent but inversely to the solubility of the gas in the solvent. Thus, if water and oil have the same concentration of nitrous oxide dissolved in each, the partial pressure of nitrous oxide in the oil will be only one-third of the partial pressure in the water since the oil/water solubility ratio is about 3:1. If the two liquids are shaken up together, there will be a net transfer of nitrous oxide from the water to the oil until the tension in each phase is the same. At that time the concentration of nitrous oxide in the oil will be about three times the concentration in the water. There is thus a net transfer of nitrous oxide against the concentration

gradient, but always with the partial pressure gradient. It is therefore useful to consider partial pressure rather than concentrations in relation to movement of gases and vapours from one compartment of the body to another. The same units of pressure may be used in gas, aqueous and lipid phases.

DIFFUSION OF OXYGEN IN THE LUNGS

It is now widely accepted that oxygen passes from the alveoli into the pulmonary capillary blood by a passive process of diffusion according to physical laws, though for a while it was believed that oxygen was actively secreted into the blood (page 242). It is believed that diffusion equilibrium is very nearly achieved for oxygen during the normal pulmonary capillary transit time in the resting subject. Therefore, in these circumstances, the uptake of oxygen is limited by pulmonary blood flow and not by diffusing capacity. However, when exercising, while breathing gas mixtures deficient in oxygen or at reduced barometric pressure, the diffusing capacity becomes important and may limit oxygen uptake.

COMPONENTS OF THE ALVEOLAR/ CAPILLARY DIFFUSION PATHWAY

The gas space within the alveolus. At functional residual capacity, the diameter of the average human alveolus is of the order of $200\,\mu m$ (page 20), and it is likely that mixing of normal alveolar gas is almost instantaneous over the small distance from the centre to the periphery. Precise calculations are impossible on account of the complex geometry of the alveolus, but the overall efficiency of gas exchange within the lungs suggests that mixing must be complete within less than 10 ms. Therefore, in practice it is usual to consider alveolar gas of normal composition as uniformly mixed.

This generalisation does not seem to hold when subjects inhale gases of widely different molecular weights. This was first demonstrated in normal subjects inhaling mixtures of sulphur hexafluoride (SF_6) and helium when the SF_6 concentration was found to be higher (relative to helium) earlier in the breath.[2] According to Graham's law SF_6 (molecular weight 146), would diffuse six times less readily than helium (molecular weight 4) and would therefore tend to remain concentrated at the core of the alveolus. A similar problem is seen with inhaled anaesthetic agents, for example a large proportion of the end expiratory/arterial partial pressure gradient for the anaesthetic isoflurane (molecular weight 184.5) cannot be explained by alveolar dead space or shunt and may be due to failure to achieve uniformity within the alveolus.[3] Nevertheless, it seems unlikely that non-uniformity within a single alveolus is an important factor limiting diffusing capacity under normal conditions with gases such as oxygen, nitrogen and carbon dioxide, which have molecular weights that are not greatly different.

Alveolar lining fluid. Alveoli contain a thin layer of surfactant rich fluid (page 218) through which respiratory gases must diffuse.[4] The depth of this fluid layer, and therefore its impediment to diffusion, is very variable. There are 'pools' of fluid in alveolar corners (see Figure 2.8) and in the depressions between where the capillaries bulge into the alveolus, with only a very thin layer on the surface of the capillary bulges, thus providing the minimal diffusion barrier in the most vital area.

Tissue barrier. Electron microscopy reveals details of the actual path between alveolar gas and pulmonary capillary blood, shown in Figure 2.7. Each alveolus is lined with epithelium which, with its basement membrane, is about $0.2\,\mu m$ thick, except where epithelial cell nuclei bulge into the alveolar lumen. Beyond the basement membrane is the interstitial space, which is very thin where it overlies the capillaries, particularly on the active side; elsewhere it is thicker and contains collagen and elastic fibres. The pulmonary capillaries are lined with endothelium, also with its own basement membrane, which is approximately the same thickness as the alveolar epithelium, except where it is expanded to enclose the endothelial cell nuclei. The total thickness of the active part of the tissue barrier is thus about $0.5\,\mu m$, containing two pairs of lipid bilayers separated by the interstitial space.

Plasma layer. Human pulmonary capillaries are estimated to have a mean diameter of $7\,\mu m$, similar to the diameter of a RBC, part of which is therefore forced into contact with the endothelial cell surface (see Figure 2.7). The diffusion path through plasma may therefore be very short indeed, but only a small proportion of the RBC surface will be in such close proximity with the endothelium, much of the RBC passing through the middle of the capillary, up to $3.5\,\mu m$ from the endothelial cell. Furthermore, since the diameter of the capillary is about 14 times the thickness of the tissue barrier, it is clear that the diffusion path within the capillary is likely to be much longer than the path through the alveolar/capillary membrane. A complex pattern of diffusion gradients is therefore established within the plasma depending on the oxygen tension in the alveolus and the number of RBCs present.[5] This is discussed in more detail below with respect to carbon monoxide.

Diffusion into and within the RBC.[6] Confining haemoglobin within the RBC reduces the oxygen diffusing capacity by 40% in comparison with free haemoglobin solution.[7] There are three possible explanations for this observation. First, there is evidence that the rapid uptake of O_2 and CO by RBCs causes depletion of gas in the plasma layer immediately surrounding the RBC.[8] Referred to as the 'unstirred layer', this phenomenon is most likely to occur at low packed cell volume (PCV) when adjacent RBCs in the pulmonary capillary have more plasma between them.[9] Secondly, oxygen must diffuse across the RBC membrane, though this is not normally believed to be a significant diffusion barrier. Thirdly, once in the cell, oxygen must diffuse through a varying amount of intracellular fluid before combining with haemoglobin, a process that is aided by mass movement of the haemoglobin molecules caused by the deformation of the RBC as it passes through the capillary bed, in effect 'mixing' the oxygen with the haemoglobin.

RBCs change shape as they pass through capillaries (both pulmonary and systemic) and this plays an important role in the uptake and release of oxygen.[6] The dependence of diffusing capacity on RBC shape changes may result from reducing the unstirred layer by 'mixing' the plasma around the RBC, from changes in the cell membrane surface area to RBC volume ratio or from assisting the mass movement of haemoglobin within the cell. This has led to further studies in which the deformability of RBCs is reduced (using chlorpromazine) or increased (using sodium salicylate), which have demonstrated that diffusing capacity is increased with greater RBC deformability.[9] Of more clinical significance is the effect of plasma cholesterol on RBC function.[10] Elevated cholesterol concentration in the plasma causes increased cholesterol in the RBC membrane, a change that is known to make the membrane thicker and less deformable, both of which lead to reduced efficiency of diffusion across the membrane. Oxygen uptake by RBCs in the lung, and its release in the tissues, are both believed to be significantly impaired by hypercholesterolaemia, particularly in tissues with high oxygen extraction ratios such as the heart.

Uptake of oxygen by haemoglobin. The greater part of the oxygen that is taken up in the lungs enters into chemical combination with haemoglobin. This chemical reaction takes a finite time and forms an appreciable part of the total resistance to the transfer of oxygen.[11] This important discovery resulted in an extensive reappraisal of the whole concept of diffusing capacity. In particular, it became clear that measurements of 'diffusing capacity' did not necessarily give an indication of the degree of permeability of the alveolar/capillary membrane.

QUANTIFICATION OF THE DIFFUSING CAPACITY FOR OXYGEN

The diffusing capacity of oxygen is simply the oxygen uptake divided by the partial pressure gradient from alveolar gas to pulmonary capillary blood where the relevant tension is the mean pulmonary capillary P_{O_2}:

Oxygen diffusing capacity

$$= \frac{\text{Oxygen uptake}}{\text{Alveolar } P_{O_2} - \text{mean pulmonary capillary } P_{O_2}}$$

The alveolar P_{O_2} can be derived with some degree of accuracy (page 140) but there are very serious problems in estimating the mean pulmonary capillary P_{O_2}.

The mean pulmonary capillary P_{O_2}. It is clearly impossible to make a direct measurement of the mean P_{O_2} of the pulmonary capillary blood, and therefore attempts have been made to derive this quantity indirectly from the presumed changes of P_{O_2} that occur as blood passes through the pulmonary capillaries.

The earliest analysis of the problem was made by Bohr in 1909.[12] He made the assumption that, at any point along the pulmonary capillary, the rate of diffusion of oxygen was proportional to the P_{O_2} difference between the alveolar gas and the pulmonary capillary blood at that point. Using this approach, and *assuming a value for the alveolar/pulmonary end-capillary P_{O_2} gradient*, it seemed possible to construct a graph of capillary P_{O_2}, plotted against the time the blood had been in the pulmonary capillary. A typical curve drawn on this basis is shown as the broken line in Figure 9.2A. Once the curve has been drawn, it is relatively easy to derive the mean pulmonary capillary P_{O_2}, which then permits calculation of the oxygen diffusing capacity. The validity of the assumption of the alveolar/pulmonary end-capillary P_{O_2} gradient is considered below.

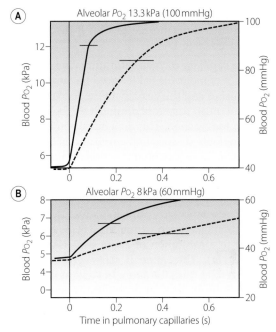

Fig. 9.2 Each graph shows the rise in blood P_{O_2} as blood passes along the pulmonary capillaries. The horizontal line at the top of the graph indicates the alveolar P_{O_2} that the blood P_{O_2} is approaching. In (A) the subject is breathing air, while in (B) the subject is breathing about 14% oxygen. The broken curve shows the rise in P_{O_2} calculated according to the Bohr procedure on an assumed value for the alveolar/end-capillary P_{O_2} gradient. The continuous curve shows the values obtained by forward integration.[13] Horizontal bars indicate mean pulmonary capillary P_{O_2} calculated from each curve.

Unfortunately this approach, known as the Bohr integration procedure, was shown to be invalid when it was found that the fundamental assumption was untrue. The rate of transfer of oxygen is not proportional to the alveolar/capillary P_{O_2} gradient at any point along the capillary. It would no doubt be true if the transfer of oxygen were a purely physical process but the rate of transfer is actually limited by the chemical combination of oxygen with haemoglobin, which is sufficiently slow to comprise a major part of the total resistance to transfer of oxygen.

Studies in vitro of the rate of combination of oxygen with haemoglobin have shown that this is not directly proportional to the P_{O_2} gradient, for two distinct reasons:

1. The combination of the fourth molecule of oxygen with the haemoglobin molecule $(Hb_4(O_2)_3 + O_2 \rightleftharpoons Hb_4(O_2)_4)$ has a much higher

velocity constant than that of the combination of the other three molecules. This is discussed further on page 190.

2. As the capillary oxygen saturation rises, the number of molecules of reduced haemoglobin diminishes and the velocity of the forward reaction must therefore diminish by the law of mass action. This depends upon the haemoglobin dissociation curve and is therefore not a simple exponential function of the actual Po_2 of the blood.

When these two factors are combined it is found that the resistance to 'diffusion' due to chemical combination of oxygen within the RBC is fairly constant up to a saturation of about 80% ($Po_2 = 6\,kPa$ or 45 mmHg). Thereafter, it falls very rapidly to become zero at full saturation. In view of these findings the Bohr integration procedure was elaborated to allow for changes in the rate of combination of haemoglobin with oxygen.[13] Assuming traditional values for the alveolar/end-capillary Po_2 difference, the resulting curve lies well to the left of the original Bohr curve as shown by the continuous curve in Figure 9.2A. This indicated a mean pulmonary capillary Po_2 greater than had previously been believed, and therefore an oxygen diffusing capacity that was substantially greater than the accepted value. The situation is actually more complicated still, as quick-frozen sections of lung show that the colour of haemoglobin begins to alter to the red colour of oxyhaemoglobin within the pulmonary arterioles before the blood has even entered the pulmonary capillaries. Furthermore, pulmonary capillaries do not cross a single alveolus but may pass over three or more.

Both the classic and the modified Bohr integration procedures for calculation of mean capillary Po_2 depended critically on the precise value of the pulmonary end-capillary Po_2. The constructed curve (Figure 9.2A) and therefore the derived mean capillary Po_2 were considerably influenced by very small variations in the value that was assumed. The 'ideal' alveolar/arterial Po_2 difference could be measured, but the problem was to separate this into its two components, the 'ideal' alveolar/pulmonary end-capillary Po_2 difference (due to diffusion block) and the pulmonary end-capillary/arterial Po_2 difference (due to venous admixture). Figure 8.8 will make this clear. Ingenious attempts were made to resolve the alveolar/arterial Po_2 gradient into its two components,[14] but these failed to produce results that were compatible with observed diffusing capacity, mainly because of the lack of appreciation of the part played by the reaction times of oxygen with haemoglobin.

Forward integration.[15] This involved a new and entirely opposite approach based on the new understanding of the kinetics of the combination of oxygen with haemoglobin (see above) and the pattern of blood flow through the pulmonary capillaries. Starting at the arterial end of the pulmonary capillaries, the Po_2 of the capillary blood is calculated progressively along the capillary until an estimate is obtained of the remaining alveolar/capillary Po_2 gradient at the end of the capillary. This procedure of forward integration was thus the reverse of the classic approach which, starting from the alveolar/end capillary Po_2 gradient, worked backwards to see what was happening along the capillary.

Forward integrations gave important results suggesting that alveolar/end capillary Po_2 gradients were very much smaller than had previously been thought. For example when breathing air, the gradient was always less than 0.0001 kPa, and only when exercising and breathing low inspired oxygen concentrations did the gradient become significant.

CAPILLARY TRANSIT TIME[16]

Capillary transit time is a most important factor determining both the pulmonary end-capillary Po_2 and the diffusing capacity. It will be seen from Figure 9.2A that, if the capillary transit time is reduced below 0.25 s, there will be an appreciable gradient between the alveolar and end-capillary Po_2. Because the diffusion gradient from alveolar gas to mean pulmonary capillary blood will be increased, the oxygen diffusing capacity must be decreased.

The mean pulmonary capillary transit time equals the pulmonary capillary blood volume divided by the pulmonary blood flow (approximately equal to cardiac output). This gives a normal time of the order of 0.8 s with a subject at rest. However, because of difficulties measuring pulmonary capillary blood volume and many other methodological problems, there appears to be a wide range of values on either side of the mean with estimates varying from 0.1 s to 3 s. It is therefore likely that, in a similar fashion to ventilation and perfusion, there is a wide range of normal capillary transit times affected by many factors such as posture, lung volume, cardiac output etc. Blood from capillaries with the shortest time will yield desaturated blood and this will not be compensated by blood from capillaries with longer than average transit times, for the reason shown in Figure 8.13.

DIFFUSION OF CARBON DIOXIDE IN THE LUNGS

Carbon dioxide has a much higher water solubility than oxygen and, although its vapour density is greater, it may be calculated to penetrate an aqueous membrane about 20 times as rapidly as oxygen (Table 9.1). Therefore it was formerly believed that diffusion problems could not exist for carbon dioxide because the patient would have succumbed from hypoxia before hypercapnia could attain measurable proportions. All of this ignored the fact that chemical reactions of the respiratory gases were sufficiently slow to affect the measured 'diffusing capacity', and in fact were generally the limiting factor in gas transfer. The carriage of carbon dioxide in the blood is discussed in Chapter 10, but for the moment it is sufficient to note the essential reactions in the release of chemically combined carbon dioxide:

1. Release of some carbon dioxide from carbamino carriage.
2. Conversion of bicarbonate ions to carbonic acid followed by dehydration to release molecular carbon dioxide.

The latter reaction involves the movement of bicarbonate ions across the RBC membrane, but its rate is probably limited by the dehydration of carbonic acid. This reaction would be very slow indeed if it were not catalysed by carbonic anhydrase, which is present in abundance in the RBC and also on the endothelium. The important limiting role of the rate of this reaction was elegantly shown in a study of the effect of inhibition of carbonic anhydrase on carbon dioxide transport. This resulted in a large increase in the arterial/alveolar P_{CO_2} gradient, corresponding to a gross decrease in the apparent 'diffusing capacity' of carbon dioxide.[17]

Equilibrium of carbon dioxide is probably very nearly complete within the normal pulmonary capillary transit time. However, even if it were not so, it would be of little significance since the mixed venous/alveolar P_{CO_2} difference is itself quite small (about 0.8 kPa or 6 mmHg). Therefore an end-capillary gradient as large as 20% of the initial difference would still be too small to be of any importance and, indeed, could hardly be measured by modern analytical methods.

Hypercapnia is, in fact, never caused by decreased 'diffusing capacity', except when carbonic anhydrase is completely inhibited by drugs such as acetazolamide (page 161). Pathological hypercapnia may always be explained by other causes, usually alveolar ventilation that is inadequate for the metabolic rate of the patient.

The assumption that there is no measurable difference between the P_{CO_2} of the alveolar gas and the pulmonary end-capillary blood is used when the alveolar P_{CO_2} is assumed equal to the arterial P_{CO_2} for the purpose of derivation of the 'ideal' alveolar P_{O_2} (page 139). The assumption is also made that there is no measurable difference between end-capillary and arterial P_{CO_2}. We have seen in the previous chapter (Table 8.2) that this is not strictly true and a large shunt of 50% will cause an arterial/end-capillary P_{CO_2} gradient of about 0.4 kPa.

DIFFUSION OF CARBON MONOXIDE IN THE LUNGS

Diffusing capacity is usually measured for carbon monoxide, for the very practical reason that affinity of carbon monoxide for haemoglobin is so high that the partial pressure of the gas in the pulmonary capillary blood remains effectively zero. The formula for calculation of this quantity then simplifies to the following:

Diffusing capacity for carbon monoxide

$$= \frac{\text{Carbon monoxide uptake}}{\text{Alveolar } P_{CO}}$$

(compare with corresponding equation for oxygen, page 149).

There are no insuperable difficulties in the measurement of either of the remaining quantities on the

Table 9.1 The influence of physical properties on the diffusion of gases through a gas–liquid interface

GAS	DENSITY RELATIVE TO OXYGEN	WATER SOLUBILITY RELATIVE TO OXYGEN	DIFFUSING CAPACITY RELATIVE TO OXYGEN
Oxygen	1.00	1.00	1.00
Carbon dioxide	1.37	24.0	20.5
Nitrogen	0.88	0.515	0.55
Carbon monoxide	0.88	0.75	0.80
Nitrous oxide	1.37	16.3	14.0
Helium	0.125	0.37	1.05
Nitric oxide	0.94	1.70	1.71

right-hand side of the equation, and the methods are outlined at the end of the chapter. Traditional units for CO diffusing capacity are ml.min^{-1}.mmHg^{-1}, though in SI units the volume of CO is usually described in molar terms, i.e. mmol.min^{-1}.kPa^{-1}.

Measurement of the carbon monoxide diffusing capacity is firmly established as a valuable routine pulmonary function test, which may show changes in a range of conditions in which other pulmonary function tests yield normal values. It provides an index that shows that something is wrong, and changes in the index provide a useful indication of progress of the disease. It is also used as an epidemiological tool for assessing lung function in seemingly healthy subjects.[18] However, it is much more difficult to explain a reduced diffusing capacity for carbon monoxide in terms of the underlying pathophysiology (see below).

THE DIFFUSION PATH FOR CARBON MONOXIDE

Diffusion of carbon monoxide within the alveolus, through the alveolar/capillary membrane and through the plasma into the RBC is governed by the same factors that apply to oxygen and these have been outlined above. The quantitative difference is due to the different vapour density and water solubility of the two gases (Table 9.1). These factors indicate that the rate of diffusion of oxygen up to the point of entry into the RBC is 1.25 times the corresponding rate for carbon monoxide.

Diffusion of CO in plasma. The frequent use of carbon monoxide for measurement of lung diffusing capacity has focused attention on the diffusion pathway for CO, which, in spite of the slight differences in the physical properties of CO and oxygen, are likely to be very similar in vivo. Clearly, direct measurement of diffusion gradients in a pulmonary capillary is not possible, so attempts to elucidate the diffusion pattern of gases in capillary plasma are based on mathematical models. The most recent analysis assumed that there is a gradient of CO concentration within the capillary, with minimal CO in the centre, and used a 'finite element analysis' to show that diffusion paths for CO are likely to be non-linear.[5] Figure 9.3 shows a theoretical drawing of the CO flux in the capillary at both high and low haematocrit, showing clearly that except in severe anaemia CO uptake is achieved long before diffusion to the centre of the capillary is able to take place. In spite of these detailed

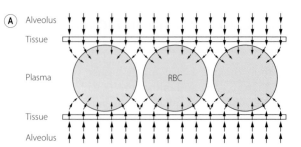

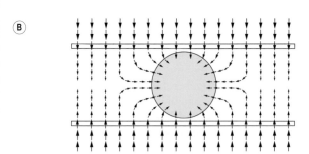

Fig. 9.3 Mathematical model of diffusion paths for CO between the alveolus and the red blood cell (RBC). The size and direction of the arrows indicates the magnitude and direction of the CO flux respectively. The RBC is assumed to be an infinite 'sink' for CO. (A) Normal. Packed cell volume 66%, under which conditions CO is absorbed by the RBC mainly at the periphery of the capillary. (B) Severe anaemia. Packed cell volume 12%. Diffusion occurs into the centre of the plasma and follows a non-linear path into the RBC. The thickness of the tissue barrier relative to capillary diameter is drawn to scale, showing the relatively small contribution that the alveolar capillary membrane makes to the diffusion barrier in total. (After reference 5.)

models, agreement with observed CO diffusion remains poor under most situations.[5]

UPTAKE OF CARBON MONOXIDE BY HAEMOGLOBIN[19]

The affinity of haemoglobin for carbon monoxide is about 250 times as great as for oxygen. Nevertheless, it does not follow that the *rate* of combination of carbon monoxide with haemoglobin is faster than the *rate* of combination of oxygen with haemoglobin: it is, in fact, rather slower. The reaction is slower still when oxygen must first be displaced from haemoglobin according to the equation:

$$CO + HbO_2 \rightarrow O_2 + HbCO$$

Therefore the reaction rate of carbon monoxide with haemoglobin is reduced when the oxygen saturation of the haemoglobin is high. The inhalation of different concentrations of oxygen thus causes changes in the reaction rate of carbon monoxide with the haemoglobin of a patient, an observation that has been utilised to study different components of the resistance to diffusion of carbon monoxide in humans.

QUANTIFICATION OF THE COMPONENTS OF THE RESISTANCE TO DIFFUSION OF CARBON MONOXIDE

When two resistances are arranged in series, the total resistance of the pair is equal to the sum of the two individual resistances. Diffusing capacity is analogous to conductance, which is the reciprocal of resistance. Therefore, the reciprocal of the diffusing capacity of the total system equals the sum of the reciprocals of the diffusing capacities of the two components.

$$\frac{1}{\text{total diffusing capacity for CO}} = \frac{1}{\text{diffusing capacity of CO for the alveolar/capillary membrane}} + \frac{1}{\text{'diffusing capacity' of CO in the blood}}$$

In theory, diffusing capacity of carbon monoxide in the blood includes diffusion across the plasma, red cell membrane, diffusion within the red cell, and the chemical combination of CO with haemoglobin. However in vivo, as in the case of oxygen, the reaction rate of CO with haemoglobin is a significant factor. This 'diffusing capacity' for blood is equal to the product of the pulmonary capillary blood volume (Vc) and the rate of reaction of carbon monoxide with haemoglobin (θ_{CO}), a parameter which varies with the oxygen saturation of the haemoglobin. The equation may now be rewritten:

$$\frac{1}{\text{total diffusing capacity for CO}} = \frac{1}{\text{diffusing capacity of CO for the alveolar/capillary membrane}} + \frac{1}{\text{pulmonary capillary blood volume reaction rate of CO with blood}}$$

The usual symbols for representation of this equation are as follows:

$$\frac{1}{D_{L_{CO}}} = \frac{1}{Dm_{CO}} + \frac{1}{Vc \times \theta_{CO}}$$

The term Dm is often described simply as membrane diffusing capacity. Dm_{CO} equals $0.8\ Dm_{O_2}$ under similar conditions (see Table 9.1).

The total diffusing capacity for carbon monoxide is a routine clinical measurement and is described at the end of this chapter: θ_{CO} may be determined, at different values of oxygen saturation, by studies in vitro. This leaves two unknowns – the diffusing capacity through the alveolar/capillary membrane and the pulmonary capillary blood volume. By repeating the measurement of total diffusing capacity at different arterial oxygen saturations (obtained by inhaling different concentrations of oxygen) it is possible to obtain two simultaneous equations with two unknowns which may then be solved to obtain values for Dm_{CO} and pulmonary capillary blood volume. Measurement of pulmonary capillary blood volume by this technique yields normal values between 60–110ml (depending on subject height),[20] which agrees well with a morphometric estimate of about 100ml.

FACTORS AFFECTING 'DIFFUSING CAPACITY'

The basic principles of pulmonary diffusion described so far indicate that there are three major mechanisms by which diffusing capacity may alter: changes in the effective surface area of the gas exchange membrane, a change in the physical properties of the membrane, or changes related to the uptake of gases by the RBC. Each of these mechanisms will be discussed individually, and then other factors that affect diffusion capacity by either multiple or unknown mechanisms will be described.

Most of the factors outlined in this section will apply equally to oxygen and CO diffusion, though the majority have been studied using CO for the reasons described in the previous section.

FACTORS INFLUENCING DIFFUSING CAPACITY BY CHANGES IN MEMBRANE SURFACE AREA

Total lung volume, and therefore the number of alveoli available for gas exchange, will clearly affect diffusing capacity. However, only those alveoli that are adequately ventilated and perfused will contribute to gas exchange, and the scatter of ventilation/perfusion therefore has an important influence on the diffusing capacity.

Body size. Stature influences diffusing capacity directly due to the relationship between height and lung volume. Normal values for total diffusing capacity may be calculated from the formulae:[20]

Males:

$$D_{L_{CO}} = 10.9 \times \text{height (m)} - 0.067 \times \text{age (years)} - 5.89$$

Females:

$$D_{L_{CO}} = 7.1 \times \text{height (m)} - 0.054 \times \text{age (years)} - 0.89$$

A healthy 30-year-old male 1.78 m tall would therefore have a CO diffusing capacity of 11.5 mmol. min^{-1}.kPa^{-1} (34.4 ml.min.$^{-1}$mmHg^{-1}).

Lung volume. Diffusing capacity is directly related to lung volume and so maximal at total lung capacity.[21] Different techniques for the measurement of diffusing capacity use different lung volumes, so it is now standard practice to simultaneously measure 'alveolar volume' (lung volume at which diffusing capacity was measured) by inert gas dilution, usually with helium or methane. Diffusing capacity can then be measured as diffusing capacity per litre alveolar volume, referred to as the diffusion constant (K_{CO}), with units of mmol.min^{-1}.kPa^{-1}.l^{-1} (ml.min.$^{-1}$mmHg^{-1}.l^{-1}).

Ventilation/perfusion mismatch results in a physiological dysfunction that presents many of the features of a reduction in diffusing capacity. If, for example, most of the ventilation is distributed to the left lung and most of the pulmonary blood flow to the right lung, then the effective interface must be reduced. Minor degrees of maldistribution greatly complicate the interpretation of a reduced diffusing capacity. Both maldistribution and impaired diffusing capacity have a similar effect on the alveolar/arterial P_{O_2} gradient in relation to inspired oxygen concentration (Figure 8.14), and a distinction cannot be made by simple means.

Posture. Diffusing capacity is substantially increased when the subject is supine rather than standing or sitting, in spite of the fact that lung volume is reduced.[20] This change is probably explained by the increase in pulmonary blood volume, and the more uniform distribution of perfusion of the lungs in the supine position.

Pathology. The total area of the alveolar/capillary membrane may be reduced by any disease process or surgery that removes a substantial number of alveoli. For example emphysema reduces the diffusing capacity mainly by destruction of alveolar septa such that $D_{L_{CO}}$ correlates with the anatomical degree of emphysematous changes in the lung.[22]

FACTORS INFLUENCING THE MEMBRANE DIFFUSION BARRIER

'Alveolar/capillary block' is a term used in the past to describe a syndrome characterised by reduced lung volume, reasonably normal ventilatory capacity, hyperventilation and normal arterial P_{O_2} at rest, but with desaturation on exercise. These patients had reduced diffusing capacity that was believed to be due to an impediment at the alveolar/capillary membrane itself, which might either be thickened or have its permeability to gas transfer reduced by some chemical abnormality. Evidence for such a mechanism was never found, and it now seems likely that most of the patients thought to have alveolar/capillary block actually had hypoxaemia as a result of disturbances in distribution of ventilation and/or perfusion.

It will be clear that the oxygen diffusing capacity may be influenced by many factors that are really nothing at all to do with diffusion per se. In fact, there is considerable doubt as to whether a true defect of alveolar/capillary membrane diffusion is ever the limiting factor in transfer of oxygen from the inspired gas to the arterial blood.

Chronic heart failure and pulmonary oedema remain the only likely causes of a membrane diffusion barrier. This may occur either via pulmonary capillary congestion increasing the length of the diffusion pathway for oxygen through plasma, by interstitial oedema increasing the thickness of the membrane, or by raised capillary pressure damaging the endothelial and epithelial cells leading to proliferation of type II alveolar cells and thickening of the membrane. The membrane component of diffusing capacity (D_m) is reduced in heart failure, and the reduction correlates with symptom severity, whilst capillary volume increases only in severe heart failure.[23] It is therefore possible that with heart failure of a suitable severity over a prolonged period a form of 'alveolar/capillary block' can occur.

FACTORS RELATED TO UPTAKE OF GASES BY HAEMOGLOBIN

Haemoglobin concentration affects diffusing capacity by influencing the rate and amount of oxygen or CO uptake by blood flowing through the pulmonary capillary. Measurements of diffusing capacity are therefore usually mathematically corrected to account for abnormalities in the patient's haemoglobin concentration.[20]

Decreased capillary transit time. In the section above, it has been explained how a reduction in capillary transit time may reduce the diffusing capacity. The mean transit time is reduced when cardiac output is raised and this may increase diffusing capacity substantially, for example during exercise (see below).

OTHER DETERMINANTS OF DIFFUSING CAPACITY

Age. Even when corrected for changes in lung volume, $D_{L_{CO}}$ declines in a linear fashion with increasing age (see above).[21]

Sex. Women have a reduced total pulmonary diffusing capacity in comparison with men. This difference is almost totally explained by differences in stature and haemoglobin concentration.[18] $D_{L_{CO}}$ in women varies throughout the menstrual cycle reaching a peak prior to menstruation, and seems to result from changes in θ, the reaction rate of CO with blood. The finding may however represent a technical problem with measuring $D_{L_{CO}}$ in that the low value during menstruation could result from a high *endogenous* production of carboxyhaemoglobin during the catabolism of haem compounds.[24]

Exercise. During exercise diffusing capacity may be double the value obtained at rest, as a result of increased cardiac output causing a reduction in capillary transit time and pulmonary capillary recruitment in non-dependent lung zones (page 103). Because of this large effect of cardiac output on the measurement of diffusing capacity, some groups advocate using simultaneous non-invasive measures of cardiac output to aid interpretation of the diffusing capacity result.[25] Paradoxically, hypoxaemia from diffusion limitation during exercise is more common among elite, trained athletes than the average individual.[16] Physiological changes in exercise are discussed in Chapter 15.

Racial origin. In a study in the US of over 4000 healthy individuals, $D_{L_{CO}}$ was significantly lower in black subjects compared with white.[18] The reasons for this are not clear.

Smoking history affects diffusing capacity even when most of the other determinants listed in this section are taken into account. $D_{L_{CO}}$ is reduced in proportion to the number of cigarettes per day currently smoked, and the total lifetime number of cigarettes ever smoked.[18] The causes of this decline in lung function with smoking are discussed in Chapter 21.

DIFFUSION OF GASES IN THE TISSUES

OXYGEN[26,27]

Oxygen leaves the systemic capillaries by the reverse of the process by which it entered the pulmonary capillaries. Chemical release from haemoglobin is followed by diffusion through the capillary wall and thence through the tissues to its site of utilisation in the mitochondria.

Krogh, in 1919, was the first to describe the factors that influence the diffusion of oxygen through tissues,[28] and his ideas developed into the first mathematical model to quantify the transfer of oxygen from the capillaries into the tissues (Figure 9.4).[29] In Krogh's model, an individual capillary is assumed to be surrounded by a cylindrical area of tissue that derives its oxygen from the single capillary under consideration. There is a non-linear gradient in P_{O_2} along the length of the capillary, referred to as the axial or longitudinal gradient, from a maximum at the arteriolar end of the capillary to a minimum at the venule. This curve is an inverted form of the oxy-haemoglobin dissociation curve (see Figure 11.9) between oxygen saturation values of 100% and 75%. At each point along the capillary there is a further non-linear radial P_{O_2} gradient where the oxygen diffuses across the capillary wall and surrounding tissues to its site of use in the mitochondria of the cells in the tissue cylinder. Using this model, a theoretical value for the P_{O_2} at any point in the tissue cylinder can be calculated using the Krogh–Erlang equation.[29] Although Krogh's model did not include axial diffusion within the tissues, this is also believed to occur.[29] With axial gradients along the capillary and in the tissue, and radial gradients throughout, P_{O_2} is always minimal at the outer edge of the tissue cylinder at the venous end of the capillary, a region referred to as the 'lethal corner'. The concept of the Krogh cylinder makes no pretence to histological

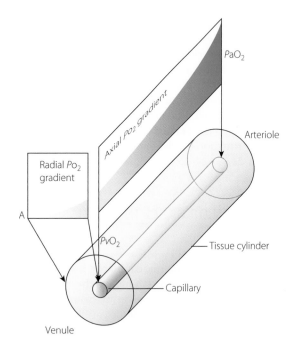

Fig. 9.4 Schematic representation of the Krogh model of tissue oxygenation. See text for details. Point A is the 'lethal corner', or tissue region where Po_2 will always be the lowest, i.e. at the point furthest away from the venular end of the capillary.

accuracy but it does illustrate the difficulty of talking about the 'mean tissue Po_2', which is not an entity like the arterial or mixed venous Po_2.

The Krogh model has numerous unrealistic assumptions,[29] for example that capillaries are all straight, parallel, of constant length and radius, with no connections between them. Values obtained for tissue Po_2 from the Krogh–Erlang equation are therefore only theoretical, and measurement of tissue Po_2 on a small enough scale to confirm Krogh's cylinder model remains impossible. Even so, studies of tissue Po_2 have provided some support for Krogh's model. For example, heterogeneity of tissue Po_2 is considerable, with measurements in the kidney cortex showing Po_2 values ranging from 0.7 to 11.3 kPa (5.3–85 mmHg).[27] Studies of Po_2 along the length of individual pial capillaries has demonstrated a non-linear decline in Po_2 along the capillary that closely matches the Krogh model.[30]

Diffusion paths are much longer in tissues than in the lung. In well-vascularised tissue, such as brain, each capillary serves a zone of radius about 20 μm, but the corresponding distance is about 200 μm in skeletal muscle and greater still in fat

and cartilage, though in muscle tissue, myoglobin accelerates the rate of transfer of oxygen within the cell.

It is also impracticable to talk about mean tissue Po_2 since this varies from one organ to another and must also depend on perfusion in relation to metabolic activity. Furthermore, within a tissue there must be some cells occupying more favourable sites towards the arterial ends of capillaries, while others must accept oxygen from the venous ends of the capillaries, where the Po_2 is lower. This is well demonstrated in the liver where the centrilobular cells must exist at a lower Po_2 than those at the periphery of the lobule. Even within a single cell, there can be no uniformity of Po_2. Not only are there 'low spots' around the mitochondria, but those mitochondria in regions of the cell nearest to the capillary presumably enjoy a higher Po_2 than those lying further away.

CARBON DIOXIDE

Little is known about the magnitude of carbon dioxide gradients between the mitochondria and the tissue capillaries. It is, however, thought that the tissue/venous Pco_2 gradient can be increased by two methods. The first is by inhibition of carbonic anhydrase, which impairs the uptake of carbon dioxide by the blood. The second is by hyperoxygenation of the arterial blood caused by breathing 100% oxygen at high pressures. If the Po_2 of the arterial blood exceeds about 300 kPa (2250 mmHg), the dissolved oxygen will be sufficient for the usual tissue requirements. Therefore there will be no significant amount of reduced haemoglobin, which is more effective than oxyhaemoglobin for carbamino carriage of carbon dioxide. The effect of this on tissue Pco_2 is likely to be too small to be clinically significant, and the alternative method of carbon dioxide carriage as bicarbonate seems to be adequate.

PRINCIPLES OF MEASUREMENT OF CARBON MONOXIDE DIFFUSING CAPACITY[20]

All the methods are based on the general equation:

$$D_{CO} = \frac{\dot{V}_{CO}}{P_{A_{CO}} - P\bar{c}_{CO}}$$

In each case it is usual to assume that the mean partial pressure of carbon monoxide in the pulmonary capillary blood ($P\bar{c}_{co}$) is effectively zero. It is, therefore, only necessary to measure the carbon monoxide uptake ($\dot{V}_{co}$), and the alveolar carbon monoxide tension ($P_{A_{CO}}$). The diffusing capacity so measured (D_{CO}) is the total diffusing capacity including that of the alveolar capillary membrane, plasma and the component due to the reaction time of carbon monoxide with haemoglobin.

THE STEADY STATE METHOD

The subject breathes a gas mixture containing about 0.3% carbon monoxide for about a minute. After this time, expired gas is collected when the alveolar P_{CO} is steady but the mixed venous P_{CO} has not yet reached a level high enough to require consideration in the calculation.

Carbon monoxide uptake ($\dot{V}_{CO}$) is measured in exactly the same way as oxygen consumption by the open method (page 211): the amount of carbon monoxide expired (expired minute volume × mixed expired CO concentration) is subtracted from the amount of carbon monoxide inspired (inspired minute volume × inspired CO concentration). The alveolar P_{CO} is calculated from the Filley version of the alveolar air equation (page 140) using carbon monoxide in place of oxygen.

The steady state method requires no special respiratory manoeuvre and is therefore particularly suitable for use in children.[20]

THE SINGLE–BREATH METHOD[1]

This method is the most frequently used in clinical practice and has a long history of progressive refinement. There are many variations on the exact method used, which yield broadly similar results,[31]

but the multitude of techniques and factors affecting the results have led to attempts to standardise the method between centres.[1]

The patient is first required to exhale maximally. He then draws in a vital-capacity breath of a gas mixture containing about 0.3% carbon monoxide and about 10% helium. The breath is held for 10s and a gas sample is then taken after the exhalation of the first 0.75 litre, which is sufficient to wash out the patient's dead space. The breath-holding time is sufficient to overcome maldistribution of the inspired gas.

It is assumed that no significant amount of helium has passed into the blood and, therefore, the ratio of the concentration of helium in the inspired gas to the concentration in the end-expiratory gas, multiplied by the volume of gas drawn into the alveoli during the maximal inspiration, will indicate the total alveolar volume during the period of breath holding. The alveolar P_{CO} at the commencement of breath holding is equal to the same ratio multiplied by the P_{CO} of the inspired gas mixture. The end-expiratory P_{CO} is measured directly.

From these data, together with the time of breath holding, it is possible to calculate the carbon monoxide uptake and the mean alveolar P_{CO}. Lung diffusing capacity for carbon monoxide can then be calculated and normalised for lung volume using the alveolar volume measured at the same time with helium.

THE REBREATHING METHOD

Somewhat similar to the single-breath method is the rebreathing method by which gas mixture containing about 0.3% carbon monoxide and 10% helium is rebreathed rapidly from a bag. The bag and the patient's lungs are considered as a single system, with gas exchange occurring in very much the same way as during breath holding. The calculation proceeds in a similar way to that for the single-breath method.

References

1. MacIntyre N, Crapo RO, Viegi G, et al. Standardisation of the single-breath determination of carbon monoxide uptake in the lung. *Eur Respir J.* 2005;26:720–735.
2. Georg G, Lassen NA, Mellemgaard K, Vinther A. Diffusion in the gas phase of the lungs in normal and emphysematous subjects. *Clin Sci.* 1965;29:525–532.
3. Landon MJ, Matson AM, Royston BD, Hewlett AM, White DC, Nunn JF. Components of the inspiratory-arterial isoflurane partial pressure difference. *Br J Anaesth.* 1993;70:605–611.
4. Weibel ER, Federspiel WJ, Fryder-Doffey F, et al. Morphometric model for pulmonary diffusing capacity I. Membrane diffusing capacity. *Respir Physiol.* 1993;93:125–149.
5. Hsia CCW, Chuong CJC, Johnson RL. Critique of conceptual basis of diffusing capacity estimates: a finite element analysis. *J Appl Physiol.* 1995;79:1039–1047.
6. Sarelius I. Invited editorial on 'Effect of RBC shape and deformability on pulmonary O_2 diffusing capacity and resistance to flow in rabbit lungs'. *J Appl Physiol.* 1995;78:763–764.

7. Geiser J, Betticher DC. Gas transfer in isolated lungs perfused with red cell suspension or haemoglobin solution. *Respir Physiol*. 1989;77:31–40.

8. Yamaguchi K, Nguyen-Phu D, Scheid P, Piiper J. Kinetics of O_2 uptake and release by human erythrocyte studied by a stopped-flow technique. *J Appl Physiol*. 1985;58:1215–1224.

9. Betticher DC, Reinhart WH, Geiser J. Effect of RBC shape and deformability on pulmonary O_2 diffusing capacity and resistance to flow in rabbit lungs. *J Appl Physiol*. 1995;78:778–783.

*10. Buchwald H, O'Dea TJ, Menchaca HJ, Michalek VN, Rohde TD. Effect of plasma cholesterol on red blood cell oxygen transport. *Clin Exp Pharmacol Physiol*. 2000;27:951–955.

11. Staub NC, Bishop JM, Forster RE. Velocity of O_2 uptake by human red blood cells. *J Appl Physiol*. 1961;16:511–516.

12. Bohr C. Über die spezifische Tätigkeit der Lungen bei der respiratorischen Gasaufnahme. *Skand Arch Physiol*. 1909;22:221.

13. Staub NC, Bishop JM, Forster RE. Importance of diffusion and chemical reaction rates in O_2 uptake in the lung. *J Appl Physiol*. 1962;17:21–27.

14. Riley RL, Lilienthal JL, Proemmel DD, Franke RE. On the determination of the physiologically effective pressures of oxygen and carbon dioxide in alveolar air. *Am J Physiol*. 1946;147:191–198.

15. Staub NC. Alveolar-arterial oxygen tension gradient due to diffusion. *J Appl Physiol*. 1963;18:673–680.

16. Wagner PD. Vascular transit times in the lung. *J Appl Physiol*. 1995;79:380–381.

17. Cain SM, Otis AB. Carbon dioxide transport in anaesthetised dogs during inhibition of carbonic anhydrase. *J Appl Physiol*. 1961;16:1023–1028.

18. Neas LM, Schwartz J. The determinants of pulmonary diffusing capacity in a national sample of US adults. *Am J Respir Crit Care Med*. 1996;153:656–664.

19. Reeves RB, Park HK. CO uptake kinetics of red cells and CO diffusing capacity. *Respir Physiol*. 1992;88:1–21.

20. Cotes JE, Chinn DJ, Miller MR. *Lung function. Physiology, measurement and application in medicine*. Oxford: Blackwell Publishing; 2006.

21. Stam H, Hrachovina V, Stijnen T, Versprille A. Diffusing capacity dependent on lung volume and age in normal subjects. *J Appl Physiol*. 1994;76:2356–2363.

22. Cotton DJ, Sparkar GR, Graham BL. Diffusing capacity in the clinical assessment of chronic airflow limitation. *Med Clin North Am*. 1996;80:549–564.

23. Puri S, Baker BL, Dutka DP, Oakley CM, Hughes JMB, Cleland JGF. Reduced alveolar-capillary membrane diffusing capacity in chronic heart failure. *Circulation*. 1995;91:2769–2774.

24. Sansores RH, Abboud RT, Kennell C, Haynes N. The effect of menstruation on the pulmonary carbon monoxide diffusing capacity. *Am J Respir Crit Care Med*. 1995;152:381–384.

25. Hsia CCW. Recruitment of lung diffusing capacity. Update of concept and application. *Chest*. 2002;122:1774–1783.

*26. Tsai AG, Johnson PC, Intaglietta M. Oxygen gradients in the microcirculation. *Physiol Rev*. 2003;83:933–963.

27. Lübbers DW, Baumgärtl H. Heterogeneities and profiles of oxygen pressure in brain and kidney as examples of the pO_2 distribution in living tissue. *Kidney Int*. 1997;51:372–380.

28. Krogh A. The rate of diffusion of gases through animal tissues, with some remarks on the coefficient of invasion. *J Physiol (Lond)*. 1919;52:391–408.

29. Kreuzer F. Oxygen supply to the tissues: the Krogh model and its assumptions. *Experientia*. 1982;38:1415–1426.

30. Ivanov KP, Sokolova IB, Vovenko EP. Oxygen transport in the rat brain cortex at normobaric hyperoxia. *Eur J Appl Physiol*. 1999;80:582–587.

31. Beck KC, Offord KP, Scanlon PD. Comparison of four methods for calculating diffusing capacity by the single breath method. *Chest*. 1994;105:594–600.

Chapter 10

Carbon dioxide

KEY POINTS

- Most of the carbon dioxide carried in blood is in the form of bicarbonate, production and breakdown of which is catalysed by the enzyme carbonic anhydrase.
- Formation of bicarbonate is enhanced by the buffering of hydrogen ions by haemoglobin, and by active removal of bicarbonate ions from the red blood cell by Band 3 protein.
- Smaller amounts of carbon dioxide are carried in solution in plasma, as carbonic acid, or as carbamino compounds formed with plasma proteins and haemoglobin.
- There is normally a small gradient between arterial and alveolar $P\text{co}_2$ caused by scatter of ventilation-perfusion ratios.

Carbon dioxide is the end-product of aerobic metabolism and is produced almost entirely in the mitochondria where the $P\text{co}_2$ is highest. From its point of origin, there are a series of partial pressure gradients as carbon dioxide passes through the cytoplasm and the extracellular fluid into the blood. In the lungs, the $P\text{co}_2$ of the blood entering the pulmonary capillaries is normally higher than the alveolar $P\text{co}_2$, and therefore carbon dioxide diffuses from the blood into the alveolar gas, where a dynamic equilibrium is established. The equilibrium concentration equals the ratio between carbon dioxide output and alveolar ventilation (page 139). Blood leaving the alveoli has, for practical purposes, the same $P\text{co}_2$ as alveolar gas, and arterial blood $P\text{co}_2$ is usually very close to 'ideal' alveolar $P\text{co}_2$.

Abnormal levels of arterial $P\text{co}_2$ occur in a number of pathological states and have many important physiological effects throughout the body, some as a result of changes in pH, and these are discussed in Chapter 23. Fundamental to all problems relating to $P\text{co}_2$ is the mechanism by which carbon dioxide is carried in the blood.[1]

CARRIAGE OF CARBON DIOXIDE IN BLOOD

IN PHYSICAL SOLUTION

Carbon dioxide is moderately soluble in water. According to Henry's law of solubility:

$$P\text{co}_2 \times \text{solubility coefficient} = \text{CO}_2 \text{ concentration in solution} \quad (1)$$

The solubility coefficient of carbon dioxide (α) is expressed in units of $\text{mmol.l}^{-1}\text{kPa}^{-1}$ (or $\text{mmol.l}^{-1}.\text{mmHg}^{-1}$). The value depends on temperature, and examples are listed in Table 10.1. The contribution of dissolved carbon dioxide to the total carriage of the gas in blood is shown in Table 10.2.

AS CARBONIC ACID

In solution, carbon dioxide hydrates to form carbonic acid:

$$\text{CO}_2 + \text{H}_2\text{O} \rightleftharpoons \text{H}_2\text{CO}_3 \quad (2)$$

The equilibrium of this reaction is far to the left under physiological conditions. Published work shows some disagreement on the value of the

Table 10.1 Values for solubility of carbon dioxide in plasma and pK′ at different temperatures

| TEMPERATURE (°C) | SOLUBILITY OF CO$_2$ IN PLASMA | | pK′ | | |
	mmol.l^{-1}.kPa^{-1}	mmol.l^{-1}mmHg^{-1}	at pH 7.6	at pH 7.4	at pH 7.2
40	0.216	0.0288	6.07	6.08	6.09
39	0.221	0.0294	6.07	6.08	6.09
38	0.226	0.0301	6.08	6.09	6.10
37	0.231	0.0308	6.08	6.09	6.10
36	0.236	0.0315	6.09	6.10	6.11
35	0.242	0.0322	6.10	6.11	6.12
25	0.310	0.0413	6.15	6.16	6.17
15	0.416	0.0554	6.20	6.21	6.23

Data from references 2 and 3.

Table 10.2 Normal values for carbon dioxide carriage in blood

	ARTERIAL BLOOD (Hb sat. 95%)	MIXED VENOUS BLOOD (Hb sat. 75%)	ARTERIAL/VENOUS DIFFERENCE
Whole blood			
pH	7.40	7.37	−0.033
P_{CO_2} (kPa)	5.3	6.1	+0.8
(mmHg)	40.0	46.0	+6.0
Total CO$_2$ (mmol.l^{-1})	21.5	23.3	+1.8
(ml.dl^{-1})	48.0	52.0	+4.0
Plasma (mmol.l^{-1})			
Dissolved CO$_2$	1.2	1.4	+0.2
Carbonic acid	0.0017	0.0020	+0.0003
Bicarbonate ion	24.4	26.2	+1.8
Carbamino CO$_2$	Negligible	Negligible	Negligible
Total	25.6	27.6	+2.0
Red blood cell fraction of 1 litre of blood			
Dissolved CO$_2$	0.44	0.51	+0.07
Bicarbonate ion	5.88	5.92	+0.04
Carbamino CO$_2$	1.10	1.70	+0.60
Plasma fraction of 1 litre of blood			
Dissolved CO$_2$	0.66	0.76	+0.10
Bicarbonate ion	13.42	14.41	+0.99
Total in 1 litre of blood (mmol.l^{-1})	21.50	23.30	+1.80

equilibrium constant, but it seems likely that less than 1% of the molecules of carbon dioxide are in the form of carbonic acid. There is a very misleading medical convention by which both forms of carbon dioxide in equation (2) are sometimes shown as carbonic acid. Thus the term H$_2$CO$_3$ may, in some situations, mean the total concentrations of dissolved CO$_2$ and H$_2$CO$_3$; to avoid confusion it is preferable to use αP_{CO_2} as in equation (7) below. This does not apply to equations (4) and (5) below, where H_2CO_3 has its correct meaning.

Carbonic anhydrase.[4,5] The reaction of carbon dioxide with water (equation 2) is non-ionic and slow, requiring a period of minutes for equilibrium to be attained. This would be far too slow for the time available for gas exchange in pulmonary and systemic capillaries if the reaction were not catalysed in both directions by the enzyme carbonic anhydrase (CA). In addition to its role in the respiratory transport of carbon dioxide, CA plays a fundamental role in many body tissues, for example the generation of hydrogen and bicarbonate ions in secretory organs including the stomach and kidney, and the intracellular transfer of carbon dioxide within both skeletal and cardiac muscle. In mammals there are now 16 isozymes of CA identified, of which two are involved in blood carbon dioxide transport.

Red blood cells (RBCs) contain large amounts of CA II, one of the fastest enzymes known, whilst CA IV is a membrane bound isozyme present in pulmonary capillaries. There is no CA activity in plasma. Carbonic anhydrase is a zinc-containing enzyme of low molecular weight, and there is now extensive knowledge of the molecular mechanisms of CA.[5,6] First, the zinc atom hydrolyses water to a reactive $Zn–OH^-$ species, whilst a nearby histidine residue acts as a 'proton shuttle', removing the H^+ from the metal-ion centre and transferring it to any buffer molecules near the enzyme. Carbon dioxide then combines with the $Zn–OH^-$ species and the HCO_3^- formed rapidly dissociates from the zinc atom. The maximal rate of catalysis is determined by the buffering power in the vicinity of the enzyme, as the speed of the enzyme reactions are so fast that its kinetics are determined mostly by the ability of the surrounding buffers to provide/remove H^+ ions to/from the enzyme.

Carbonic anhydrase is inhibited by a large number of compounds, including some drugs such as thiazide diuretics and various heterocyclic sulphonamides, of which acetazolamide is the most important. Acetazolamide is non-specific for the different CA isozymes and so inhibits CA in all organs at a dose of $5–20\,mg.kg^{-1}$ and has no other pharmacological effects of importance. Acetazolamide has been used extensively in the study of carbonic anhydrase and has revealed the surprising fact that it is not essential to life. The quantity and efficiency of RBC CA is such that more than 98% of activity must be blocked before there is any discernible change in carbon dioxide transport, though when total inhibition is achieved, P_{CO_2} gradients between tissues and alveolar gas are increased, pulmonary ventilation is increased and alveolar P_{CO_2} is decreased.

AS BICARBONATE ION

The largest fraction of carbon dioxide in the blood is in the form of bicarbonate ion, which is formed by ionisation of carbonic acid thus:

$$H_2CO_3 \rightleftharpoons H^+ + HCO_3^- \rightleftharpoons 2H^+ + CO_3^{2-} \qquad (3)$$

The second dissociation occurs only at high pH (above 9) and is not a factor in the carriage of carbon dioxide by the blood. The first dissociation is, however, of the greatest importance within the physiological range. The pK_1' is about 6.1 and carbonic acid is about 96% dissociated under physiological conditions.

According to the law of mass action:

$$\frac{[H^+] \times [HCO_3^-]}{[H_2CO_3]} = K_1' \qquad (4)$$

where K_1' is the equilibrium constant of the first dissociation. The subscript 1 indicates that it is the first dissociation, and the prime indicates that we are dealing with concentrations rather than the more correct thermodynamic activities.

Rearrangement of equation (4) gives the following:

$$[H^+] = K_1' \frac{[H_2CO_3]}{[HCO_3^-]} \qquad (5)$$

The left-hand side is the hydrogen ion concentration, and this equation is the non-logarithmic form of the Henderson–Hasselbalch equation.[7] The concentration of carbonic acid cannot be measured and the equation may be modified by replacing this term with the total concentration of dissolved CO_2 and H_2CO_3, most conveniently quantified as αP_{CO_2} as described above. The equation now takes the form:

$$[H^+] = K_1' \frac{\alpha P_{CO_2}}{[HCO_3^-]} \qquad (6)$$

The new constant K' is the *apparent* first dissociation constant of carbonic acid, and includes a factor that allows for the substitution of total dissolved carbon dioxide concentration for carbonic acid.

The equation is now in a useful form and permits the direct relation of plasma hydrogen ion concentration, P_{CO_2} and bicarbonate concentration, all quantities that can be measured. The value of K' cannot be derived theoretically and is determined experimentally by simultaneous measurements of the three variables. Under normal physiological conditions, if $[H^+]$ is in $nmol.l^{-1}$, P_{CO_2} in kPa, and $[HCO_3^-]$ in $mmol.l^{-1}$, the value of the combined parameter $(\alpha K')$ is about 180. If P_{CO_2} is in mmHg, the value of the parameter is 24.

Most people prefer to use the pH scale and so follow the approach described by Hasselbalch in 1916 and take logarithms of the reciprocal of each term in equation (6) with the following familiar result:[8]

$$pH = pK' + \log\frac{[HCO_3^-]}{\alpha P_{CO_2}} = pK' + \log\frac{[CO_2] - \alpha P_{CO_2}}{\alpha P_{CO_2}}$$

$$(7)$$

where pK' has an experimentally derived value of the order of 6.1, but varies with temperature and pH (see Table 10.1). '$[CO_2]$' refers to the total concentration of carbon dioxide in all forms (dissolved CO_2, H_2CO_3 and bicarbonate) in plasma and not in whole blood.

CARBAMINO CARRIAGE

Amino groups in the uncharged $R–NH_2$ form have the ability to combine directly with carbon dioxide to form a carbamic acid. At body pH, the carbamic acid then dissociates almost completely to carbamate:

$$\begin{array}{ccc} H & H & H \\ | & | & | \\ R-N-H + CO_2 \rightleftharpoons R-N-C-OH \rightleftharpoons R-N-C-O^- + H^+ \\ & \parallel & \parallel \\ & O & O \end{array}$$

In a protein, the amino groups involved in the peptide linkages between amino acid residues cannot combine with carbon dioxide. The potential for carbamino carriage is therefore restricted to the one terminal amino group in each protein chain and to the side chain amino groups that are found in lysine and arginine. Since both hydrogen ions and carbon dioxide compete to react with uncharged amino groups, the ability to combine with carbon dioxide is markedly pH dependent. The terminal α-amino groups are the most effective at physiological pH, and one binding site per protein monomer is more than sufficient to account for the quantity of carbon dioxide carried as carbamino compounds.

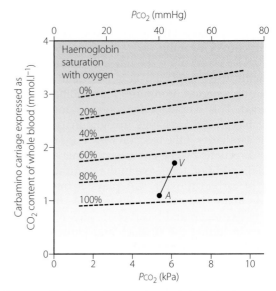

Fig. 10.1 The broken lines on the graph indicate the carbamino carriage of carbon dioxide at different levels of oxygen saturation of haemoglobin. It will be seen that oxygen saturation has a far greater influence on carbamino carriage than the actual P_{CO_2} (abscissa). Points A and V represent the saturation and P_{CO_2} of arterial and venous blood respectively. Note that the arterial/venous difference in carbamino carriage is large in relation to the actual amounts of carbamino carriage.

Carbamino carriage and haemoglobin. Only very small quantities of carbon dioxide are carried in carbamino compounds with plasma proteins. Almost all is carried by haemoglobin, and reduced haemoglobin is about 3.5 times as effective as oxyhaemoglobin (Figure 10.1), this being a major component of the Haldane effect (see below). Carbon dioxide binds to α-amino groups at the ends of both the α- and β-chains of haemoglobin. Earlier studies of CO_2-haemoglobin reactions using free haemoglobin solution overestimated the magnitude of carbamino binding with haemoglobin, as later work showed that 2,3-diphosphoglycerate (2,3-DPG) present in vivo antagonises the binding of CO_2 with haemoglobin. This antagonism results from direct competition between CO_2 and 2,3-DPG for the end-terminal valine of the β-chain of haemoglobin, an effect that is not observed on the α-chains.

The Haldane effect. This is the difference in the quantity of carbon dioxide carried, at constant P_{CO_2}, in oxygenated and deoxygenated blood (Figure 10.2). Although the amount of carbon dioxide carried in the blood by carbamino carriage is small, the *difference* between the amount carried in venous and

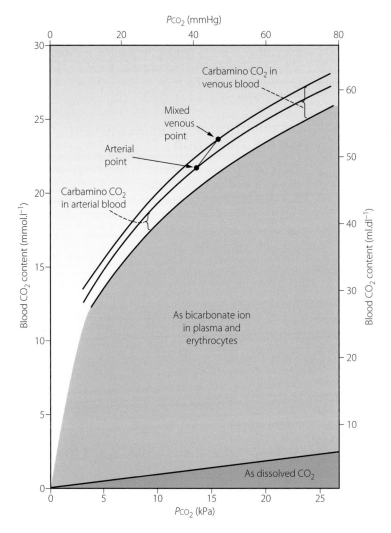

Fig. 10.2 Components of the CO_2 dissociation curve for whole blood. Dissolved CO_2 and bicarbonate ion vary with $P\text{co}_2$ but are little affected by the state of oxygenation of the haemoglobin. (Increased basic properties of reduced haemoglobin cause a slight increase in formation of bicarbonate ion.) Carbamino carriage of CO_2 is strongly influenced by the state of oxygenation of haemoglobin but hardly at all by $P\text{co}_2$.

arterial blood is about a third of the total arterial/venous difference (Table 10.2). This therefore accounts for the major part of the Haldane effect, the remainder being due to the increased buffering capacity of reduced haemoglobin, which is discussed below. When the Haldane effect was described by Christiansen, Douglas & Haldane in 1914, they believed that the whole effect was due to altered buffering capacity:[9] carbamino carriage was not demonstrated until much later (1934).[10]

Formation of carbamino compounds does not require the dissolved carbon dioxide to be hydrated and so is independent of carbonic anhydrase. The reaction is very rapid and would be of particular importance in a subject who had received a carbonic anhydrase inhibitor.

EFFECT OF BUFFERING POWER OF PROTEINS ON CARBON DIOXIDE CARRIAGE

Amino and carboxyl groups concerned in peptide linkages have no buffering power. Neither have most side chain groups (e.g. in lysine and glutamic acid) because their pK values are far removed from the physiological range of pH. In contrast is the imidazole group of the amino acid histidine, which is almost the only amino acid to be an effective buffer in the normal range of pH. Imidazole groups constitute the major part of the considerable buffering power of haemoglobin, each tetramer containing 38 histidine residues. The buffering power of plasma proteins is less and is directly proportional to their histidine content.

H
C
N N⁻
| |
HC=C   + H⁺ ⇌
    |
   CH₂
    |
NH₂—C—COOH
     |
     H

Basic form of histidine

H
C
N NH
| |
HC=C
    |
   CH₂
    |
NH₂—C—COOH
     |
     H

Acidic form of histidine

The four haem groups of a molecule of haemoglobin are attached to the corresponding four amino acid chains at one of the histidine residues on each chain (page 188), and the dissociation constant of the imidazole groups of these four histidine residues is strongly influenced by the state of oxygenation of the haem. Reduction causes the corresponding imidazole group to become more basic. The converse is also true: in the acidic form of the imidazole group of the histidine, the strength of the oxygen bond is weakened. Each reaction is of great physiological interest and both effects were noticed many decades before their mechanisms were elucidated.

1. The reduction of haemoglobin causes it to become more basic. This results in increased carriage of carbon dioxide as bicarbonate, since hydrogen ions are removed, permitting increased dissociation of carbonic acid (first dissociation of equation 3). This accounts for part of the Haldane effect, the other and greater part being due to increased carbamino carriage (see above).

2. Conversion to the basic form of histidine causes increased affinity of the corresponding haem group for oxygen. This is, in part, the cause of the Bohr effect (page 192).

Total deoxygenation of the haemoglobin in blood would raise the pH by about 0.03 if the P_{CO_2} were held constant at 5.3 kPa (40 mmHg), and this would correspond roughly to the addition of 3 mmol of base to 1 litre of blood. The normal degree of desaturation in the course of the change from arterial to venous blood is about 25%, corresponding to a pH increase of about 0.007 if P_{CO_2} remains constant. In

fact, P_{CO_2} rises by about 0.8 kPa (6 mmHg), which would cause a decrease of pH of 0.040 if the oxygen saturation were to remain the same. The combination of an increase of P_{CO_2} of 0.8 kPa and a decrease of saturation of 25% thus results in a fall of pH of 0.033 (Table 10.2).

DISTRIBUTION OF CARBON DIOXIDE WITHIN THE BLOOD

Table 10.2 shows the forms in which carbon dioxide is carried in normal arterial and mixed venous blood. Although the amount carried in solution is small, most of the carbon dioxide enters and leaves the blood as CO_2 itself (Figure 10.3). Within the

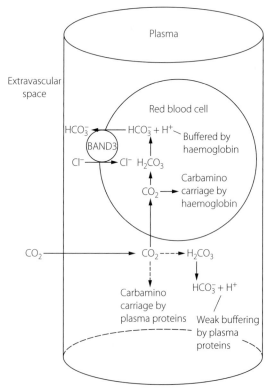

Fig. 10.3 How carbon dioxide enters the blood in molecular form. Within the plasma, there is only negligible carbamino carriage by plasma proteins and a slow rate of hydration to carbonic acid due to the absence of carbonic anhydrase. The greater part of CO_2 diffuses into the red blood cell where conditions for carbamino carriage (by haemoglobin) are more favourable. In addition, more rapid formation of carbonic acid is facilitated by carbonic anhydrase, the removal of hydrogen ions by haemoglobin buffering and the transfer of bicarbonate out of the red blood cell in exchange for chloride by the Band 3 ion-exchange protein (Hamburger shift).

plasma there is little chemical combination of carbon dioxide, for three reasons. First, there is no carbonic anhydrase in plasma and therefore carbonic acid is formed only very slowly. Secondly, there is little buffering power in plasma to promote the dissociation of carbonic acid. Thirdly, the formation of carbamino compounds by plasma proteins is not great, and must be almost identical for arterial and venous blood.

Carbon dioxide can, however, diffuse freely into the RBC, where two courses are open. First, increasing intracellular $P\text{co}_2$ will increase carbamino carriage of CO_2 by haemoglobin, an effect greatly enhanced by the fall in oxygen saturation which is likely to be occurring at the same time (Figure 10.1). The second course is hydration and dissociation of CO_2 to produce hydrogen and bicarbonate ions, facilitated by the presence of carbonic anhydrase in the RBC. However, accumulation of intracellular hydrogen and bicarbonate ions will quickly tip the equilibrium of the reaction against further dissociation of carbonic acid, a situation that is avoided in the RBC by two mechanisms:

Haemoglobin buffering. Hydrogen ions produced by carbonic anhydrase are quickly buffered by the imidazole groups on the histidine residues of the haemoglobin, as described above. Once again, the concomitant fall in haemoglobin saturation enhances this effect by increasing the buffering capacity of the haemoglobin.

Hamburger shift. Hydration of CO_2 and buffering of the hydrogen ions results in the formation of considerable quantities of bicarbonate ion within the RBC. These excess bicarbonate ions are actively transported out of the cell into the plasma in exchange for chloride ions to maintain electrical neutrality across the RBC membrane. This ionic exchange was first suggested by Hamburger in 1918,[11] and believed to be a passive process. It is now known to be facilitated by a complex membrane bound protein that has been extensively studied and named Band 3 after its position on a gel electrophoresis plate.[12,13,14] Band 3 exchanges bicarbonate and chloride ions by a 'ping-pong' mechanism in which one ion first moves out of the RBC before the other ion moves inwards, in contrast to most other ion pumps, which simultaneously exchange the two ions. Band 3 protein is also intimately related to other proteins in the RBC (Figure 10.4):[13,14]

- RBC cytoskeleton. The cytoplasmic domain of band 3 acts as an anchoring site for many of the proteins involved in the maintenance of cell shape and membrane stability such as ankyrin and spectrin. A genetically engineered deficiency of band 3 in animals results in small, fragile, spherical RBCs,[12] and in humans an inherited defect of band 3 is responsible for hereditary spherocytosis in which RBCs become spheroidal in shape and fragile.[15,16]

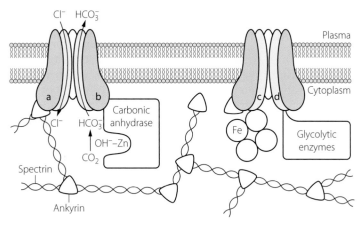

Fig. 10.4 Proteins associated with band 3 in the red blood cell membrane. Band 3 has twelve trans-membrane domains forming the bicarbonate/chloride exchange ion channel, and four globular cytoplasmic domains (a–d), each of which is associated with different groups of intra-cellular proteins. (a) Ankyrin and spectrin, to maintain and possibly alter red cell shape; (b) Carbonic anhydrase, with which band 3 acts as a metabolon to directly export bicarbonate ions from the red cell; (c) Haemoglobin, with which band 3 may act as a metabolon to export nitric oxide; (d) Glycolytic enzymes – the functional significance of this association is unknown.

RBC shape and deformability are now known to be important in oxygen transport in the capillaries (page 148) and it is possible that band 3 is involved in bringing about these shape changes.

- Carbonic anhydrase. Band 3 is also closely associated with carbonic anhydrase, and the protein complex formed is believed to act as a metabolon, a term describing the channelling of a substrate directly between proteins that catalyse sequential reactions in a metabolic pathway.[13] In this case the substrate is bicarbonate, which after its formation by CA is transferred directly to band 3, which rapidly exports it from the cell.
- Haemoglobin. Band 3 is also associated with haemoglobin, with which it is believed to form another metabolon system exporting nitric oxide derived nitrosothiols, possibly to regulate capillary blood flow and oxygen release from haemoglobin (page 195).
- Glycolytic enzymes. Some of the enzymes involved in glycolysis (page 198), including glyceraldehyde-3-phosphate dehydrogenase, phosphofructokinase and aldolase, are bound to band 3; the functional significance of this is unknown.

In the pulmonary capillary, where Pco_2 is low, the series of events described above goes into reverse and the CO_2 released from the RBC diffuses into the alveolus and is excreted.

DISSOCIATION CURVES OF CARBON DIOXIDE

Figure 10.2 shows the classic form of the dissociation curve of carbon dioxide relating blood content to tension. For decades there has been great interest in curves that relate any pair of the following: (1) plasma bicarbonate concentration; (2) Pco_2; (3) pH. These three quantities are related by the Henderson–Hasselbalch equation (equation 7) and therefore the third variable can always be derived from the other two. The most famous is the Siggaard-Andersen plot, which relates Pco_2 on a logarithmic scale to pH (Figure 10.5). These graphs can be used to explore the effects of changes in respiratory and metabolic acid-base balance, but care must be taken in using these in vitro data in intact subjects. For example, if the Pco_2 of an entire patient is altered, the pH changes are not

the same as those of a blood sample of which the Pco_2 is altered in vitro. This is because the blood of a patient is in continuity with the extracellular fluid (of very low buffering capacity) and also with intracellular fluid (of high buffering capacity). Bicarbonate ions pass rapidly and freely across the various interfaces. As a result, the in vivo change in pH is normally greater than the in vitro change in the patient's blood when subjected to the same change in Pco_2.

FACTORS INFLUENCING THE CARBON DIOXIDE TENSION IN THE STEADY STATE

In common with other catabolites, the level of carbon dioxide in the body fluids depends on the balance between production and elimination. There is a continuous gradient of Pco_2 from the mitochondria to the expired air and thence to ambient air. The Pco_2 in all cells is not identical, but is lowest in tissues with the lowest metabolic activity and the highest perfusion (e.g. skin) and highest in tissues with the highest metabolic activity for their perfusion (e.g. the myocardium). Therefore the Pco_2 of venous blood differs substantially from one tissue to another.

In the pulmonary capillaries, carbon dioxide passes into the alveolar gas and this causes the alveolar Pco_2 to rise steadily during expiration. During inspiration, the inspired gas dilutes the alveolar gas and the Pco_2 falls by about 0.4 kPa, imparting a sawtooth curve to the alveolar Pco_2 when it is plotted against time (Figure 10.6).

Blood leaving the pulmonary capillaries has a Pco_2 that is very close to that of the alveolar gas and, therefore, varies with time in the same manner as the alveolar Pco_2. These oscillations in arterial Pco_2 with respiratory rate may be involved in respiratory control, particularly during exercise and at altitude.[18] There is also a regional variation, with Pco_2 inversely related to the ventilation/perfusion ratio of different parts of the lung (Figure 8.12). The mixed arterial Pco_2 is the integrated mean of blood from different parts of the lung, and a sample drawn over several seconds will average out the cyclical variations.

It is more convenient to consider partial pressure than content, because carbon dioxide always moves in accord with partial pressure gradients even if they are in the opposite direction to concentration gradients. Also, the concept of partial pressure may

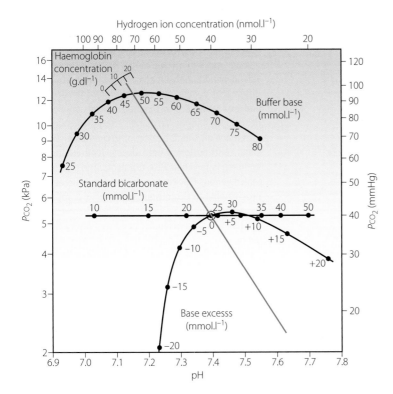

Fig. 10.5 The Siggaard-Andersen nomogram. The blue line shows the normal in vitro relationship between pH and log P_{CO_2}, and is derived by varying the P_{CO_2} of a blood sample and measuring its pH. The slope is that of a line joining the normal arterial point (shown by a small circle) and the relevant point on the haemoglobin scale. Intersections of this line indicate three other indices of metabolic acid–base state: buffer base, standard bicarbonate and base excess. If both pH and P_{CO_2} are measured in vivo a single point may be plotted on the graph and a line parallel to the in vitro one is drawn that passes through this point. All three acid–base indices can then be read from the nomogram. This process is now routinely performed mathematically by blood-gas analysers. (Reprinted from reference 17 by permission of Taylor & Francis AS).

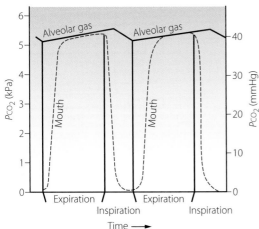

Fig. 10.6 Changes in alveolar and mouth P_{CO_2} during the respiratory cycle. The alveolar P_{CO_2} is shown by a continuous curve, and the mouth P_{CO_2} by the broken curve. The mouth P_{CO_2} falls at the commencement of inspiration but does not rise during expiration until the anatomical dead space gas is washed out. The alveolar P_{CO_2} rises during expiration and also during the early part of inspiration until fresh gas penetrates the alveoli after the anatomical dead space is washed out. The alveolar P_{CO_2} then falls until expiration commences. This imparts a sawtooth curve to the alveolar P_{CO_2}.

be applied with equal significance to gas and liquid phases, content having a rather different connotation in the two phases. Furthermore, the effects of carbon dioxide (e.g. upon respiration) are a function of partial pressure rather than content. Finally, it is easier to measure blood P_{CO_2} than CO_2 content. Normal values for partial pressure and content are shown in Figure 10.7.

Each factor that influences the P_{CO_2} has already been mentioned in this book and in this chapter they will be drawn together, illustrating their relationship to one another. It is convenient first to summarise the factors influencing the alveolar P_{CO_2}, and then to consider the factors that influence the relationship between the alveolar and the arterial P_{CO_2} (Figure 10.8).

THE ALVEOLAR P_{CO_2} ($P_{A_{CO_2}}$)

Carbon dioxide is constantly being added to the alveolar gas from the pulmonary arterial blood,

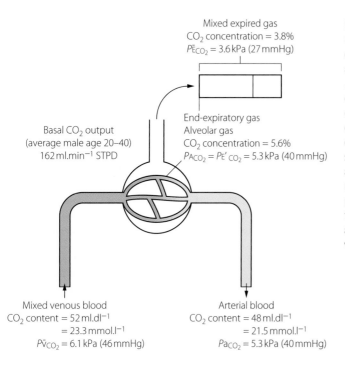

Mixed expired gas
CO_2 concentration = 3.8%
$P\bar{E}CO_2$ = 3.6 kPa (27 mmHg)

End-expiratory gas
Alveolar gas
CO_2 concentration = 5.6%
$PACO_2 = PE'CO_2$ = 5.3 kPa (40 mmHg)

Basal CO_2 output
(average male age 20–40)
162 ml.min⁻¹ STPD

Mixed venous blood
CO_2 content = 52 ml.dl⁻¹
= 23.3 mmol.l⁻¹
$P\bar{v}CO_2$ = 6.1 kPa (46 mmHg)

Arterial blood
CO_2 content = 48 ml.dl⁻¹
= 21.5 mmol.l⁻¹
$PaCO_2$ = 5.3 kPa (40 mmHg)

Fig. 10.7 Normal values of CO_2 levels. These normal values are rounded off and ignore the small difference in PCO_2 between end-expiratory gas, alveolar gas and arterial blood. Actual values of PCO_2 depend mainly on alveolar ventilation but the differences depend on maldistribution; the alveolar/end-expiratory PCO_2 difference depends on alveolar dead space and the very small arterial/alveolar PCO_2 difference on shunt. Scatter of $\dot{V}/\dot{Q}$ ratios makes a small contribution to both alveolar/end-expiratory and arterial/alveolar PCO_2 gradients. The arterial/mixed venous CO_2 content difference is directly proportional to CO_2 output and inversely proportional to cardiac output. Secondary symbols: A, alveolar; a, arterial; $\bar{E}$, mixed expired; E', end-expiratory; $\bar{v}$, mixed venous.

and removed from it by the alveolar ventilation. Therefore, ignoring inspired carbon dioxide, it follows that:

$$\text{Alveolar } CO_2 \text{ concentration} = \frac{\text{Carbon dioxide output}}{\text{Alveolar ventilation}}$$

This axiomatic relationship is the basis for prediction of the alveolar concentration of any gas that enters or leaves the body. With inclusion of the inspired concentration, it may be written as a form of alveolar air equation (page 139), for which the version for carbon dioxide is as follows:

$$\text{Alveolar } PCO_2 = \frac{\text{dry}}{\text{barometric}}_{\text{pressure}} \left(\begin{array}{l} \text{mean inspired } CO_2 \\ \text{concentration} \\ + \frac{CO_2 \text{ output}}{\text{alveolar ventilation}} \end{array} \right)$$

This equation includes all the more important factors influencing PCO_2 (Figure 10.8), and examples of the hyperbolic relationship between PCO_2 and alveolar ventilation are shown in Figure 10.9. Individual factors will now be considered.

The dry barometric pressure is not a factor of much importance in the determination of alveolar PCO_2, and normal variations of barometric pressure at sea level are unlikely to influence the PCO_2 by more

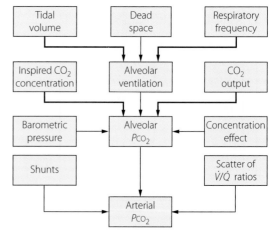

Fig. 10.8 Summary of factors that influence PCO_2; the more important ones are indicated with the thicker arrows. In the steady state, the CO_2 output of a resting subject usually lies within the range 150–200 ml.min⁻¹ and the alveolar PCO_2 is largely governed by the alveolar ventilation, provided that the inspired CO_2 concentration is zero. See text for explanation of the concentration effect.

than 0.3 kPa (2 mmHg). At high altitude, the hypoxic drive to ventilation lowers the PCO_2 (Chapter 17).

The mean inspired CO_2 concentration. The effect of inspired carbon dioxide on the alveolar PCO_2 is

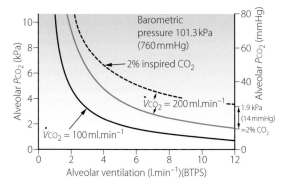

Fig. 10.9 The effect of CO_2 output, alveolar ventilation and inspired CO_2 concentration on alveolar Pco_2. The lowest continuous curve shows the relationship between ventilation and alveolar Pco_2 for a CO_2 output of 100 ml.min^{-1} (STPD). The blue curve shows the normal relationship when the CO_2 output is 200 ml.min^{-1}. The broken curve represents the relationship when the CO_2 output is 200 ml.min^{-1} and there is an inspired CO_2 concentration of 2%. Two per cent CO_2 is equivalent to about 1.9 kPa (14 mmHg) and each point on the broken curve is 1.9 kPa above the upper of the two continuous curves.

additive. If, for example, a patient breathes gas containing 4.2% carbon dioxide (Pco_2 = 4.0 kPa or 30 mmHg), the alveolar Pco_2 will be raised 4.0 kPa above the level that it would be if there were no carbon dioxide in the inspired gas, *and other factors, including ventilation, remained the same.*

Carbon dioxide output. It is carbon dioxide output and not production that directly influences the alveolar Pco_2. Output equals production in a steady state, but they may be quite different during unsteady states. During acute hypoventilation, much of the carbon dioxide production is diverted into the body stores, so that the output may temporarily fall to very low figures until the alveolar carbon dioxide concentration has risen to its new level. Conversely, acute hyperventilation results in a transient increase in carbon dioxide output. A sudden fall in cardiac output decreases the carbon dioxide output until the carbon dioxide concentration in the mixed venous blood rises. The unsteady state is considered in more detail later in this chapter.

Alveolar ventilation for present purposes means the product of the respiratory frequency and the difference between the tidal volume and the physiological dead space (page 128). It can change over very wide limits and is the most important factor influencing alveolar Pco_2. Factors governing ventilation are considered in Chapter 5, and dead space in Chapter 8.

The concentration effect. Apart from the factors shown in the equation above and in Figure 10.9, the alveolar Pco_2 may be temporarily influenced by net transfer of soluble inert gases across the alveolar/capillary membrane. Rapid uptake of an inert gas increases the concentration (and partial pressure) of carbon dioxide (and oxygen) in the alveolar gas. This occurs, for example, at the beginning of an anaesthetic when large quantities of nitrous oxide are passing from the alveolar gas into the body stores, and a much smaller quantity of nitrogen is passing from the body into the alveolar gas. The converse occurs during elimination of the inert gas and results in transient reduction of alveolar Pco_2 and Po_2.

THE END–EXPIRATORY Pco_2 (PE'_{CO_2})

In the normal, healthy, conscious subject, the end-expiratory gas consists almost entirely of alveolar gas. If, however, appreciable parts of the lung are ventilated but not perfused, they will contribute a significant quantity of CO_2-free gas from the alveolar dead space to the end-expiratory gas (see Figure 8.9). As a result, the end-expiratory Pco_2 will have a lower Pco_2 than that of the alveoli which are perfused. Gas cannot be sampled selectively from the perfused alveoli. However, since arterial Pco_2 usually approximates closely to Pco_2 of the perfused alveoli (see below), it is possible to compare arterial and end-expiratory Pco_2 to demonstrate the existence of an appreciable proportion of underperfused alveoli. Studies during anaesthesia have, for example, shown an arterial/end-tidal Pco_2 gradient between 0.7 and 1.3 kPa (5–10 mmHg).[19,20]

THE ALVEOLAR/ARTERIAL Pco_2 GRADIENT

For reasons that have been discussed in Chapter 9, we may discount the possibility of any significant gradient between the Pco_2 of alveolar gas and that of pulmonary end-capillary blood (page 151). Arterial Pco_2 may, however, be slightly greater than the mean alveolar Pco_2 because of shunting or scatter of ventilation/perfusion ratios. Factors governing the magnitude of the gradient were considered in Chapter 8, where it was shown that a shunt of 10% will cause an alveolar/arterial Pco_2 gradient of only about 0.1 kPa (0.7 mmHg) (Figure 8.10). Because the normal degree of ventilation/perfusion ratio scatter causes a gradient of the same order, neither has much significance for carbon dioxide (in contrast to oxygen), and there is an established convention by which the arterial and 'ideal' alveolar P_{CO_2} values are taken to be identical. It is only in exceptional patients with, for example, a shunt in excess of 30% that the gradient is likely to exceed 0.3 kPa (2 mmHg).

THE ARTERIAL P_{CO_2} (P_{ACO_2})

Pooled results for the normal arterial P_{CO_2} reported by various authors show a mean of 5.1 kPa (38.3 mmHg) with 95% confidence limits of ±1.0 kPa (7.5 mmHg). This means that 5% of normal subjects will lie outside these limits and it is therefore preferable to call it the reference range rather than the normal range. There is no evidence that P_{CO_2} is influenced by age in the healthy subject.

CARBON DIOXIDE STORES AND THE UNSTEADY STATE

The quantity of carbon dioxide and bicarbonate ion in the body is very large – about 120 litres, which is almost 100 times greater than the volume of oxygen. Therefore, when ventilation is altered out of accord with metabolic activity, carbon dioxide levels change only slowly and new equilibrium levels are only attained after about 20–30 minutes. In contrast, corresponding changes in oxygen levels are very rapid.

Figure 10.10 shows a three-compartment hydraulic model in which depth of water represents P_{CO_2} and the volume in the various compartments corresponds to volume of carbon dioxide. The metabolic production of carbon dioxide is represented by the variable flow of water from the supply tank. The outflow corresponds to alveolar ventilation, and the controller watching the P_{CO_2} represents the central chemoreceptors. The rapid compartment represents circulating blood, brain, kidneys and other well-perfused tissues. The medium compartment represents skeletal muscle (resting) and other tissues with a moderate blood flow. The slow compartment includes bone, fat and other tissues with a large capacity for carbon dioxide. Each compartment has its own time constant (see Appendix E), and the long time constants of the medium and slow compartments buffer changes in the rapid compartment.

Hyperventilation is represented by a wide opening of the outflow valve with subsequent exponential decline in the levels in all three compartments, the rapid compartment falling most quickly. The rate of decrease of P_{CO_2} is governed primarily by ventilation and the capacity of the stores. Hypoventilation is fundamentally different. The rate of increase of P_{CO_2} is now limited by the metabolic production of carbon dioxide, which is the *only* factor directly increasing the quantity of carbon dioxide in the body compartments. Therefore, the time course of the increase of P_{CO_2} following step decrease of ventilation is not the mirror image of the time course of decrease of P_{CO_2} when ventilation is increased. The rate of rise is much slower than the rate of fall, which is fortunate for patients in asphyxial situations.

When *all* metabolically produced carbon dioxide is retained, the rate of rise of arterial P_{CO_2} is of the order of 0.4–0.8 kPa.min^{-1} (3–6 mmHg.min^{-1}).

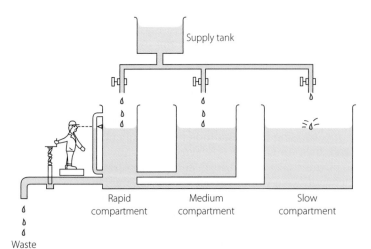

Fig. 10.10 A hydrostatic analogy of the elimination of carbon dioxide. See text for full description.

This is the resultant of the rate of production of carbon dioxide and the capacity of the body stores for carbon dioxide. During hypoventilation, the rate of increase in P_{CO_2} will be less than this and Figure 10.11 shows typical curves for P_{CO_2} increase and decrease following step changes in ventilation of anaesthetised patients. The time course of rise of P_{CO_2} after step reduction of ventilation is faster when the previous level of ventilation has been of short duration.[21]

The difference in the rate of change of P_{CO_2} and P_{O_2} after a step change in ventilation (see Figure 11.19) has two important implications for monitoring and measurement. First, changes in P_{O_2} (or oxygen saturation) will often provide an earlier warning of acute hypoventilation than will the capnogram, provided that the alveolar P_{O_2} is not much above the normal range. However, *in the steady state* P_{CO_2} gives the best indication of the adequacy of ventilation, because oxygenation is so heavily influenced by intra-pulmonary shunting and the inspired oxygen concentration. Secondly, step changes in ventilation are followed by temporary changes in the respiratory exchange ratio because, in the unsteady state, carbon dioxide output changes more than oxygen uptake. However, if the ventilation is held constant at its new level, the respiratory exchange ratio must eventually return to the value determined by the metabolic process of the body.

Cardiac output and CO₂ transport. In the normal subject, fluctuations in cardiac output have little effect on arterial, alveolar or end-expiratory P_{CO_2} because of the efficiency of the chemical control of breathing. However, with a constant level of artificial ventilation, for example during anaesthesia or cardiopulmonary resuscitation, the situation is quite different. In the extreme circumstance of a total cessation of cardiac output, then alveolar and end-expiratory P_{CO_2} will fall dramatically as the delivery of blood containing carbon dioxide to the lung also ceases. In a similar fashion, a sudden reduction in cardiac output during anaesthesia causes an abrupt reduction in end-expiratory P_{CO_2}.[22] This almost certainly results from increased alveolar dead space caused by an increase in the number of non-perfused but ventilated alveoli (Zone 1, page 105). If low cardiac output is sustained for more than a few minutes, blood P_{CO_2} will rise and the expired P_{CO_2} returns towards normal as the blood passing through the still-perfused lung regions releases more carbon dioxide into the expired gas. Apart from being a useful early warning of cardiovascular catastrophe during anaesthesia, the measurement of expired carbon dioxide has also been advocated during cardiopulmonary resuscitation both as a method of monitoring the efficacy of chest compressions and as an indicator of the return of spontaneous cardiac output.[23]

APNOEA

When a patient becomes apnoeic while breathing air, alveolar gas reaches equilibrium with mixed

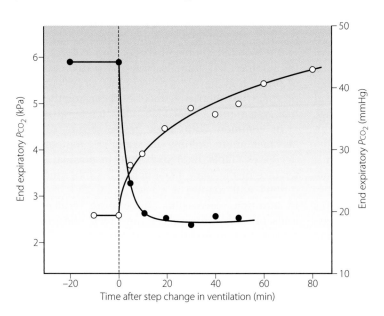

Fig. 10.11 Time course of changes in end-expiratory P_{CO_2} following step changes in ventilation. The solid circles indicate the changes in end-expiratory P_{CO_2} that follow a change in ventilation from 3.3 to 14 l.min⁻¹. The open circles show the change following a reduction in ventilation from 14 to 3.3 l.min⁻¹ in the same patient. During the fall in P_{CO_2}, half the total change is completed in about 3 minutes; during the rise in P_{CO_2}, half-change takes approximately 16 minutes.

venous blood within a few minutes. Assuming normal starting conditions and ignoring changes in the composition of the recirculated mixed venous blood, this would entail a rise of alveolar P_{CO_2} from 5.3 to 6.1 kPa (40 to 46 mmHg) and a fall of P_{O_2} from 14 to 5.3 kPa (105 to 40 mmHg). These changes correspond to the uptake of 230 ml of oxygen but the output of only 21 ml of carbon dioxide. Carbon dioxide appears to reach equilibrium within about 10 seconds,[24] while oxygen would take about a minute, being limited by the ability of the cardiac output and the arterial/mixed venous oxygen content difference to remove some two thirds of the oxygen in the alveolar gas (normally about 450 ml).

These calculations assume that alveolar gas is not replenished from outside the patient. What actually happens to the arterial blood gases in apnoea depends upon the patency of the airway and the composition of the ambient gas if the airway is patent.

With airway occlusion. As described above, there is rapid attainment of equilibrium between alveolar and mixed venous P_{CO_2}. Thereafter, arterial, alveolar and mixed venous P_{CO_2} values remain close, and, with recirculation of the blood, increase together at the rate of about 0.4–0.8 kPa.min^{-1} (3–6 mmHg. min^{-1}), more than 90% of the metabolically produced carbon dioxide passing into the body stores. Alveolar P_{O_2} decreases close to the mixed venous P_{O_2} within about a minute, and then decreases further as recirculation continues. The lung volume falls by the difference between the oxygen uptake and the carbon dioxide output. Initially the rate would be $230 - 21 = 209$ ml.min^{-1}. The change in alveolar P_{O_2} may be calculated, and gross hypoxia supervenes after about 90 seconds if apnoea with airway occlusion follows air breathing at functional residual capacity.

With patent airway and air as ambient gas. The initial changes are as described above. However, instead of the lung volume falling by the net gas exchange rate (initially 209 ml.min^{-1}), this volume of ambient gas is drawn in by mass movement down the trachea. If the ambient gas is air, the oxygen in it will be removed but the nitrogen will accumulate and rise above its normal concentration until gross hypoxia supervenes after about 2 minutes. This is likely to occur when the accumulated nitrogen has reached 90% since the alveolar carbon dioxide concentration will then have reached about 8%. Carbon dioxide elimination cannot occur as there is mass-movement of air down the trachea, preventing loss of carbon dioxide by either convection or diffusion.

With patent airway and oxygen as the ambient gas. Oxygen is continuously removed from the alveolar gas as described above, but is replaced by oxygen drawn in by mass-movement. No nitrogen is added to the alveolar gas, and the alveolar P_{O_2} only falls as fast as the P_{CO_2} rises (about 0.4–0.8 kPa.min^{-1} or 3–6 mmHg.min^{-1}). Therefore the patient will not become seriously hypoxic for several minutes. If the patient has been breathing 100% oxygen prior to the respiratory arrest, the starting alveolar P_{O_2}, would be of the order of 88 kPa (660 mmHg) and therefore the patient could theoretically survive about 100 minutes of apnoea *provided that his airway remained clear and he remained connected to a supply of 100% oxygen.* This does, in fact, happen and has been demonstrated in both animals and man, and is referred to as apnoeic mass-movement oxygenation or diffusion respiration. The phenomenon enjoyed a brief vogue in anaesthetic practice as a means of maintaining oxygenation during apnoea, particularly for airway surgery or bronchoscopy (page 492), and remains a widely used method for oxygenation of the non-ventilated lung during one-lung ventilation (page 502).

CARBON DIOXIDE CARRIAGE DURING HYPOTHERMIA

Understanding the carriage of CO_2 during hypothermia is of importance both to clinicians involved in the care of hypothermic patients and to the comparative physiologist studying differences between warm-blooded (homeothermic) and cold-blooded (poikilothermic) animals. These two diverse areas of physiology have over recent years converged to produce two alternative theories regarding the optimal system for CO_2 carriage at low temperature.

In common with most gases, carbon dioxide becomes more soluble in water as temperature decreases (Table 10.1) such that, in plasma, maintenance of the same P_{CO_2} under hypothermic conditions will require a greater total CO_2 content. In addition, decreasing temperature reduces the ionisation of water into H^+ and OH^- ions, so pH increases by approximately 0.016 per degree Celsius fall in temperature.[25] If CO_2 production and excretion remain constant, hypothermia would therefore be expected to result in alkalotic conditions in both the intra- and extracellular spaces. Different animals are believed to respond to these changes in two ways, as follows.

The pH-stat hypothesis,[26] as the name suggests, involves the animal responding to hypothermia by maintaining the same blood pH regardless of its body temperature. This is achieved by hypoventilation, which increases the $P\text{CO}_2$ to maintain pH at close to 7.4, and is seen in hibernating mammals. Indeed it is thought possible that the high $P\text{CO}_2$, and the resulting intracellular acidosis, may contribute to the hypothermic 'sleep' state.

The alpha-stat hypothesis is more complex.[25,27] In this situation, the pH of the animal is allowed to change in keeping with the physical chemistry laws described above. As temperature falls, the blood pH, again measured at the animal's body temperature, increases. Studies of protein function and acid–base disturbances have revealed the importance of the α-imidazole moiety of histidine in buffering changes in pH, and that the state of dissociation of these α-imidazole groups is crucial to protein function. The pK of α-imidazole is unique among amino acids in that it changes with temperature to a similar degree as the dissociation of water.[27] Thus as temperature decreases, blood and tissue pH rise but the dissociative state of α-imidazole, and thus protein function, remains close to normal. Most poikilothermic animals use an alpha-stat system and can function well through a broad range of temperatures. Even hibernators, with their pH stat regulation, maintain an alpha-stat type control of some vital tissues such as heart and brain.[28]

There is controversy about whether the blood gases of humans undergoing cardiac surgery during hypothermia should be managed by the alpha-stat or pH-stat techniques.[26,29] In the former case, arterial blood drawn from the cold patient is warmed to 37°C before measurement of $P\text{CO}_2$ and the cardiopulmonary bypass adjusted to achieve normal values. For pH-stat control, $P\text{CO}_2$ is again measured at 37°C but mathematically corrected to the patient's temperature, and then CO_2 administered to the patient to achieve a pH of 7.4. Increased arterial $P\text{CO}_2$ during pH-stat will in theory improve cerebral perfusion, and possibly thereby improve cerebral function.[29] However, there remains little evidence that the two forms of blood gas management result in differences in patient well-being during or after hypothermic surgery except at very low temperatures, when pH-stat may be superior.[30]

OUTLINE OF METHODS OF MEASUREMENT OF CARBON DIOXIDE

FRACTIONAL CONCENTRATION IN GAS MIXTURES[31]

Infrared analysis. This is the most widely used method for rapid breath-to-breath analysis and is also convenient for analysis of discrete gas samples. Most diatomic gases absorb infra-red radiation, and errors may arise due to overlap of absorption bands and collision broadening. Infrared analysers are available with a response time of less than $300\,\mu s$ and will follow the respiratory cycle provided the respiratory frequency is not too high. Breathe-through cells (placed near the patient's airway) have a better frequency response than systems which draw gas from the airway for analysis in a distant machine, as mixing of the inspired and expired gases occurs along the sampling tube. Capnography is described in more detail below.

Mass spectrometry. This powerful technique is established as an alternative method for the rapid analysis of carbon dioxide. The cost is much greater than for infrared analysis, but response times tend to be shorter and there is usually provision for analysis of up to four gases at the same time. In spite of this, mass spectrometry for measurement of respiratory gases remains essentially a research tool.

BLOOD CO$_2$ PARTIAL PRESSURE

The $P\text{CO}_2$-sensitive electrode. This technique was first described by Severinghaus & Bradley in 1958,[32] and allows the $P\text{CO}_2$ of any gas or liquid to be determined directly. The $P\text{CO}_2$ of a film of bicarbonate solution is allowed to come into equilibrium with the $P\text{CO}_2$ of a sample on the other side of a membrane permeable to carbon dioxide but not to hydrogen ions. The pH of the bicarbonate solution is constantly monitored by a glass electrode and the log of the $P\text{CO}_2$ is inversely proportional to the recorded pH. Analysis may now be satisfactorily performed by untrained staff on a do-it-yourself basis with results available within 2 minutes.

Handling of blood samples.[33,34] It is important that samples be preserved from contact with air, including bubbles and froth in the syringe, to which they may lose carbon dioxide, and either lose or gain oxygen depending on the relative $P\text{O}_2$ of the sample and the air. Dilution with excessive volumes of heparin or 'dead space' fluids from indwelling arterial cannulae should be avoided. At very high Po_2 values, oxygen can diffuse across the wall of plastic syringes and glass syringes may therefore be preferable.[34] Analysis should be undertaken quickly, as the Pco_2 of blood in vitro rises by about 0.013 kPa per min (0.1 mmHg per min) at 37°C, whilst Po_2 declines at 0.07–0.3 kPa (0.5–2.3 mmHg) per minute depending on the Po_2. If rapid analysis is not possible (within 10 minutes), the specimen should be stored on ice, which reduces this carbon dioxide production and oxygen consumption by about 90%. Modern blood gas analysers invariably work at 37°C, so for patients with abnormal body temperatures a correction factor should be applied. Nomograms allow correction for both pre-analytic metabolism and patient temperature.[35]

Continuous measurement of arterial Pco_2 using indwelling arterial catheters is rapidly becoming a realistic clinical technique.[36] The method uses a 'photochemical optode', which consists of a small optical fibre (140 μm diameter) along which light of a specific wavelength is passed to impinge on a dye incorporated into the tip of the fibre, which lies within the patient's artery. The dye may either absorb the light or fluoresce (give off light of a different wavelength) in a pH sensitive fashion, and these changes are transmitted back to the analyser via the same or a second optical fibre. For analysis of Pa_{CO_2}, the pH sensitive optode is again enclosed within a CO_2 permeable membrane with a bicarbonate buffer, as for the Pco_2-sensitive electrode but on a very small scale. The current generation of intra-arterial sensors are reasonably accurate with a precision of 0.4–0.8 kPa (3–6 mmHg).

Transcutaneous Pco_2. This technique is an indirect measurement of arterial Pco_2. A CO_2-sensitive electrode is heated to about 44°C to maximise blood flow to the skin but this temperature is, however, close to the temperature that causes burns. Transcutaneous Pco_2 should be within about 0.5 kPa (3.8 mmHg) of the simultaneous arterial value, but it is necessary to apply a large correction factor for the difference in temperature between body and electrode.[37]

CAPNOGRAPHY[31,38]

Capnograms consist of plots of CO_2 concentration in airway gas against either time or expired volume. Despite the curves being of similar shape

(Figures 8.16 and 10.12) they contain quite different information; for example, time capnography has both inspiratory and expiratory phases whilst CO_2 against volume plots only involve expiration. Plots of CO_2 and expired volume allow calculation of anatomical dead space (see Figure 8.16), physiological dead space and tidal volume, but this form of capnography is not commonly used clinically. Current generations of capnometer allow the CO_2 concentration to be displayed as either volume %, kPa or mmHg. Infrared analysers measure the partial pressure of CO_2, while mass spectrometers measure fractional concentration. Conversions between fractional concentration and partial pressure will be affected by the atmospheric pressure, for example by the altitude at which the capnometer is being used. Current technical specifications for capnometers therefore require that the equipment must automatically compensate for barometric pressure when converting the measured units into the displayed units.[31]

In the past there has been confusion over the nomenclature of a normal time capnogram, but the most widely accepted terms are shown in Figure 10.12A. There is an inspiratory phase (0), and expiration is divided into three phases: phase I represents CO_2-free gas from the apparatus and anatomical dead space; phase II a rapidly changing mixture of alveolar and dead space gas; phase III the alveolar plateau, the peak of which represents end-expiratory Pco_2 $\left(PE'_{CO_2} \right)$. The alpha and beta angles allow quantification of abnormalities of the capnogram. Much information may be obtained from a time capnogram:

1. The inspiratory carbon dioxide concentration.
2. Respiratory rate
3. The demonstration of the capnogram is a reliable indication of the correct placement of a tracheal tube.
4. PE'_{CO_2} is related to arterial Pco_2 (see below)
5. Sudden decrease in PE'_{CO_2} at a fixed level of ventilation is a valuable indication of a sudden reduction in cardiac output (page 171) or a pulmonary embolus (Chapter 29).
6. Cardiac arrest during artificial ventilation will cause PE'_{CO_2} to fall to zero.

There are three principal abnormalities of a capnogram,[31] which may occur separately or together and are shown in Figure 10.12B. Line A, with an increased alpha angle and phase III slope, results from increased ventilation perfusion mismatch.

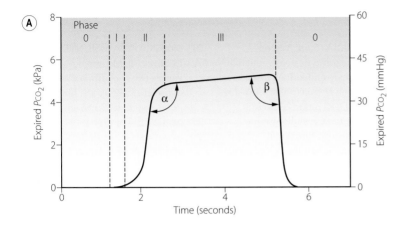

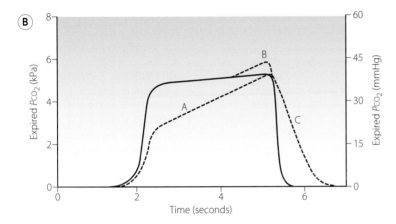

Fig. 10.12 Time capnography.
(A) Normal trace showing the phases of the respiratory cycle and the angles used to quantify the shape of the capnogram. See text for details. (B) Dashed lines show abnormalities of the trace, which may occur separately or together. A, varying alveolar time constants (page 123) such as asthma; B, phase IV terminal upswing seen in pregnancy or obesity; C, rebreathing of expired gases.

Almost any lung pathology may result in a sloping phase III, and a common clinical cause is acute asthma: line A is typical of a patient with bronchospasm. The gradient of phase III on a capnogram has been proposed as a non effort-dependent test of the severity of acute asthma.[39] Line B, sometimes referred to as phase IV, is occasionally seen in pregnancy or severe obesity,[38] but more commonly results from a leak between the sampling tube and analyser in an artificially ventilated patient.[31] Line C and an increase in the beta angle occur with rebreathing from either excessive apparatus dead space or a malfunctioning anaesthetic breathing system.

Technical considerations should always be borne in mind when considering abnormalities of a capnogram. The response time of the analyser, excessive lengths of sampling tube and inadequate sampling rates will all tend to 'blunt' the normal capnogram trace. This is a particular problem when the tidal volume is low, for example in children or tachypnoeic patients.

Arterial to end-expiratory Pco_2 gradient. has already been mentioned above (page 170) and occurs to some extent in almost all subjects, but particularly in elderly patients, smokers, those with lung disease or during anaesthesia.[40] The magnitude of the difference is greatest in patients with significant alveolar dead space (page 130) who can be identified from the slope of phase III. Attempts to reduce the gradient by forced or prolonged expiration have generally been unsuccessful.[19] Use of PE'_{CO_2} as a monitor of absolute arterial Pco_2 is therefore unhelpful, but the assessment remains useful for following changes within a subject.

References

1. Geers C, Gros G. Carbon dioxide transport and carbonic anhydrase in blood and muscle. *Physiol Rev*. 2000;80:681–715.

2. Severinghaus JW, Stupfel M, Bradley AF. Accuracy of blood pH and Pco_2 determinations. *J Appl Physiol*. 1956;9:189–196.

3. Severinghaus JW, Stupfel M, Bradley AF. Variations in serum carbonic acid pK' with pH and temperature. *J Appl Physiol*. 1956;9:197–200.

4. Henry RP. Multiple roles of carbonic anhydrase in cellular transport and metabolism. *Annu Rev Physiol*. 1996;58:523–538.

*5. Esbaugh AJ, Tufts BL. The structure and function of carbonic anhydrase isozymes in the respiratory system of vertebrates. *Respir Physiol Neurobiol*. 2006;154:185–198.

6. Chegwidden WR, Carter ND, Edwards YH, eds. *The Carbonic Anhydrases. New Horizons*. Basel: Birkhäuser Verlag; 2000.

7. Henderson LJ. Das Gleichgewicht zwischen Basen und Säuren im tierischen Organismus. *Ergebn Physiol*. 1909;8:254.

8. Hasselbalch KA. Die Berechnung der Wasserstoffzahl des Blutes usw. *Biochem Z*. 1916;78:112–144.

9. Christiansen J, Douglas CG, Haldane JS. The adsorption and dissociation of carbon dioxide by human blood. *J Physiol*. 1914;48:244–271.

10. Ferguson JKW, Roughton FJW. The direct chemical estimation of carbamino compounds of CO_2 with haemoglobin. *J Physiol*. 1934;83:68–86.

11. Hamburger HJ. Anionenwanderungen in serum und Blut unter dem Einfluss von CO_2. Säure und Alkali. *Biochem Z*. 1918;86:309.

*12. Jay DG. Role of band 3 in homeostasis and cell shape. *Cell*. 1996;86:853–854.

13. Tanner MJA. Band 3 anion exchanger and its involvement in erythrocyte and kidney disorders. *Curr Opin Hematol*. 2002;9:133–139.

14. Zhang D, Kiyatkin A, Bolin JT, Low PS. Crystallographic structure and functional interpretation of the cytoplasmic domain of erythrocyte membrane band 3. *Blood*. 2000;96:2925–2933.

15. Williamson RC, Toye AM, Glycophorin A. Band 3 aid. *Blood Cells Mol Diseases*. 2008;41:35–43.

16. Perrotta S, Gallagher PG, Mohandas N. Hereditary spherocytosis. *Lancet*. 2008;372:1411–1426.

17. Siggaard-Andersen O. The pH, log Pco_2 blood acid-base nomogram revisited. *Scand J Clin Lab Invest*. 1962;14:598–604.

18. Collier DJ, Nickol AH, Milledge JS, et al. Alveolar Pco_2 oscillations and ventilation at sea level and at high altitude. *J Appl Physiol*. 2008;104:404–415.

19. Tavernier B, Rey D, Thevenin D, Triboulet J-P, Scherpereel P. Can prolonged expiration manoeuvres improve the prediction of arterial Pco_2 from end-tidal Pco_2. *Br J Anaesth*. 1997;78:536–540.

20. Nunn JF, Hill DW. Respiratory dead space and arterial to end tidal CO_2 tension difference in anesthetized man. *J Appl Physiol*. 1960;15:383–389.

21. Ivanov SD, Nunn JF. Influence of the duration of hyperventilation on rise time of Pco_2 after step reduction of ventilation. *Respir Physiol*. 1968;5:243–249.

22. Shibutani K, Muraoka M, Shirasaki S, Kubal K, Sanchala VT, Gupte P. Do changes in end-tidal Pco_2 quantitatively reflect changes in cardiac output. *Anesth Analg*. 1994;79:829–833.

23. Sanders AB. Capnometry in emergency medicine. *Ann Emerg Med*. 1989;18:1287–1290.

24. Stock MC, Downs JB, McDonald JS, Silver MJ, McSweeney TD, Fairley DS. The carbon dioxide rate of rise in awake apneic humans. *J Clin Anesth*. 1988;1:96–99.

25. Nattie EE. The alpha-stat hypothesis in respiratory control and acid–base balance. *J Appl Physiol*. 1990;69:1201–1207.

26. Burrows FA. Con: pH-stat management of blood gases is preferable to alpha-stat in patients undergoing brain cooling for cardiac surgery. *J Cardiothorac Vasc Anesth*. 1995;9:219–221.

27. Reeves RB. An imidazole alpha-stat hypothesis for vertebrate acid-base regulation: tissue carbon dioxide content and body temperature in bullfrogs. *Respir Physiol*. 1972;14:219–236.

28. Swain JA, McDonald TJ, Robbins RC, Balaban RS. Relationship of cerebral and myocardial intracellular pH to blood pH during hypothermia. *Am J Physiol*. 1991;260:H1640–H1644.

29. Kern FH, Greeley WJ. Pro: pH-stat management of blood gases is not preferable to alpha-stat in patients undergoing brain cooling for cardiac surgery. *J Cardiothorac Vasc Anesth*. 1995;9:215–218.

30. Laussen PC. Optimal blood gas management during deep hypothermic paediatric cardiac surgery: alpha-stat is easier, but pH-stat may be preferable. *Paediatr Anaesth*. 2002;12:199–204.

*31. Gravenstein JS, Jaffe MB, Paulus DA. *Capnography: Clinical Aspects*. Cambridge: Cambridge University Press; 2004.

32. Severinghaus JW, Bradley AF. Electrodes for blood Po_2 and Pco_2 determination. *J Appl Physiol*. 1958;13:515–520.

33. Szaflarski NL. Preanalytic error associated with blood gas/pH measurement. *Crit Care Nurse*. 1996;16:89–100.

34. d'Ortho MP, Delclaux C, Zerah F, Herigault R, Adnot S, Harf A. Use of glass capillaries avoids the time changes in high blood Po_2 observed with plastic syringes. *Chest*. 2001;120:1651–1654.

35. Kelman GR, Nunn JF. Nomograms for correction of blood Po_2, Pco_2, pH and base excess for time and temperature. *J Appl Physiol*. 1966;21: 1484–1490.

36. Ganter M, Zollinger A. Continuous intravascular blood gas monitoring: development, current techniques, and clinical use of a commercial device. *Br J Anaesth*. 2003;91:397–407.

37. Severinghaus JW. A combined transcutaneous Po_2–Pco_2 electrode with electrochemical HCO_3^- stabilization. *J Appl Physiol*. 1981;51:1027–1032.

38. Bhavani-Shankar K, Kumar AY, Moseley HSL, Ahyee-Hallsworth R. Terminology and the current limitations of time capnography: a brief review. *J Clin Monit*. 1995;11:175–182.

39. Yaron M, Padyk P, Hutsinpiller M, Cairns CB. Utility of the expiratory capnogram in the assessment of bronchospasm. *Ann Emerg Med*. 1996;28:403–407.

40. Wahba RWM, Tessler MJ. Misleading end-tidal CO_2 tensions. *Can J Anaesth*. 1996;43: 862–866.

Chapter 11

Oxygen

KEY POINTS

- Oxygen moves down a partial pressure gradient between the inspired gas and its point of use in the mitochondria, where the oxygen partial pressure may be only 0.13 kPa (1 mmHg).
- Significant barriers to oxygen transfer are between inspired and alveolar gas, between alveolar and arterial oxygen partial pressures, and on diffusion from the capillary to the mitochondria.
- Each 100 ml of arterial blood carries 0.3 ml of oxygen in physical solution and around 20 ml of oxygen bound to haemoglobin, which reduces to around 15 ml.dl^{-1} in venous blood.
- Oxygen carriage by haemoglobin is influenced by carbon dioxide, pH, temperature and red blood cell 2,3-diphosphoglycerate; the molecular mechanism of haemoglobin is now well elucidated.
- Glucose and other substrates are used to produce energy in the form of adenosine triphosphate (ATP), each glucose molecule yielding 38 molecules of ATP in the presence of oxygen, compared with only 2 in anaerobic conditions.
- Oxygen delivery is the total amount of oxygen leaving the heart per minute and is around 1000 ml.min^{-1}, compared with oxygen consumption of around 250 ml.min^{-1}.

The appearance of oxygen in the atmosphere of the Earth has played a crucial role in the development of life (see Chapter 1). The whole of the animal kingdom is totally dependent on oxygen, not only for function but also for survival. This is notwithstanding the fact that oxygen is extremely toxic in the absence of elaborate defence mechanisms at a cellular level (see Chapter 26). Before considering the role of oxygen within the cell, it is necessary to bring together many strands from previous chapters and outline the transport of oxygen all the way from the atmosphere to the mitochondria.

THE OXYGEN CASCADE

The Po_2 of dry air at sea level is 21.2 kPa (159 mmHg). Oxygen moves down a partial pressure gradient from air, through the respiratory tract, the alveolar gas, the arterial blood, the systemic capillaries, the tissues and the cell. It finally reaches its lowest level in the mitochondria where it is consumed (Figure 11.1). At this point, the Po_2 is probably within the range 0.5–3 kPa (3.8–22.5 mmHg), varying from one tissue to another, from one cell to another, and from one region of a cell to another.

The steps by which the Po_2 decreases from air to the mitochondria are known as the oxygen cascade and are of great practical importance. Any one step in the cascade may be increased under pathological circumstances and this may result in hypoxia. The steps will now be considered *seriatim*.

DILUTION OF INSPIRED OXYGEN BY WATER VAPOUR

The normally quoted value for the concentration of atmospheric oxygen (20.94% or 0.2094 fractional concentration) indicates the concentration of oxygen in *dry* gas. As gas is inhaled through the respiratory tract, it becomes humidified at body temperature and the added water vapour dilutes the oxygen and so reduces the Po_2 below its level in the ambient

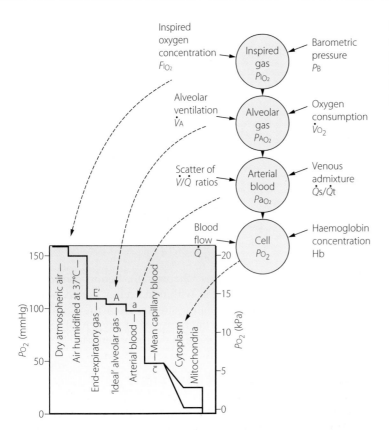

Fig. 11.1 On the left is shown the oxygen cascade with Po_2 falling from the level in the ambient air down to the level in mitochondria. On the right is a summary of the factors influencing oxygenation at different levels in the cascade.

air. When dry gas at normal barometric pressure becomes fully saturated with water vapour at 37°C, 100 volumes of the dry gas take up about 6 volumes of water vapour, giving a total gas volume of 106 units but containing the same number of molecules of oxygen. The Po_2 is thus reduced by the fraction 6/106. It follows from Boyle's law that Po_2 after humidification is indicated by the following expression:

$$\begin{array}{c}\text{fractional} \\ \text{concentration} \\ \text{of oxygen in} \\ \text{the dry gas phase}\end{array} \times \left(\begin{array}{cc}\text{barometric} & \text{saturated water} \\ \text{pressure} & \text{vapour pressure}\end{array}\right)$$

(the quantity in parentheses is known as the dry barometric pressure). Therefore the effective Po_2 of inspired air at a body temperature of 37°C is:

$$0.2094 \times (101.3 - 6.3) = 0.2094 \times 95$$
$$= 19.9 \text{kPa}$$

or, in mmHg:

$$0.2094 \times (760 - 47) = 0.2094 \times 713$$
$$= 149 \text{mmHg}$$

PRIMARY FACTORS INFLUENCING ALVEOLAR OXYGEN TENSION

Dry barometric pressure. If other factors remain constant, the alveolar Po_2 will be directly proportional to the dry barometric pressure. Thus with increasing altitude, alveolar Po_2 falls progressively to become zero at 19 kilometres where the actual barometric pressure equals the saturated vapour pressure of water at body temperature (see Table 17.1). The effect of increased pressure is complex (see Chapter 18), for example, a pressure of 10 atmospheres (absolute) increases the alveolar Po_2 by a factor of about 15 if other factors remain constant (see Table 18.1).

Inspired oxygen concentration. The alveolar Po_2 will be raised or lowered by an amount equal to

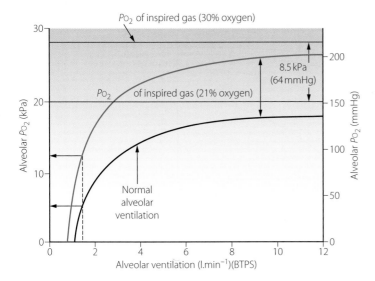

Fig. 11.2 The effect on alveolar Po_2 of increasing the inspired oxygen concentration from 21% (black curve) to 30% (blue curve). In this example, the alveolar Po_2 is reduced to a dangerously low level when breathing air at an alveolar minute ventilation of 1.5 l.min^{-1}. In this situation, oxygen enrichment of the inspired gas to 30% is sufficient to raise the alveolar Po_2 almost to within the normal range. Oxygen consumption is assumed to be 200 ml.min^{-1} (STPD).

the change in the inspired gas Po_2, provided that other factors remain constant. Because the concentration of oxygen in the inspired gas should always be under control, it is a most important therapeutic tool that may be used to counteract a number of different factors that may impair oxygenation.

Figure 11.2 shows the effect of an increase in the inspired oxygen concentration from 21% to 30% on the relationship between alveolar Po_2 and alveolar ventilation. For any alveolar ventilation, the improvement of alveolar Po_2 will be 8.5 kPa (64 mmHg). This will be of great importance if, for example, hypoventilation while breathing air has reduced the alveolar Po_2 to 4 kPa (30 mmHg), a value that presents a significant threat to life. Oxygen enrichment of inspired gas to 30% will then increase the alveolar Po_2 to 12.5 kPa (94 mmHg), which is almost within the normal range. However, at this level of hypoventilation, arterial Pco_2 would be about 13 kPa (98 mmHg) and might well have risen further on withdrawal of the hypoxic drive to ventilation. In fact, 30% is the maximum concentration of oxygen in the inspired gas that should be required to correct the alveolar Po_2 of a patient breathing air, who has become hypoxaemic purely as a result of hypoventilation. This problem is discussed further in Chapter 27 (pages 399 et seq).

An entirely different problem is hypoxaemia due to venous admixture. This results in an increased alveolar/arterial Po_2 difference, which, within limits, can be offset by increasing the alveolar Po_2. Quantitative aspects are quite different from the problem of hypoventilation and are considered later in this chapter.

Oxygen consumption. In the past there has been an unfortunate tendency to consider that all patients consume 250 ml of oxygen per minute under all circumstances. Oxygen consumption must, of course, be raised by exercise but is often well above basal in a patient supposedly 'at rest'. This may be due to restlessness, pain, increased work of breathing, shivering or fever. These factors may well coexist with failure of other factors controlling the arterial Po_2. Thus, for example, a patient may be caught by the pincers of a falling ventilatory capacity and a rising ventilatory requirement (see Figure 27.4).

Figure 11.3 shows the effect of different values for oxygen consumption on the relationship between alveolar ventilation and alveolar Po_2 for a patient breathing air and clearly shows the potential for an increase in oxygen consumption to cause hypoxia. Altered oxygen consumption is very common in patients, being substantially increased with sepsis, thyrotoxicosis or convulsions, the first of which may lead to difficulties with weaning patients from artificial ventilation (page 474). Oxygen consumption is reduced with general anaesthesia, hypothyroidism or hypothermia, the last of which causes a marked reduction in oxygen consumption with values of about 50% of normal at 31°C.

Alveolar ventilation. The alveolar air equation (page 139) implies a hyperbolic relationship between alveolar Po_2 and alveolar ventilation. This relationship, which is considered in Appendix E, is clinically very

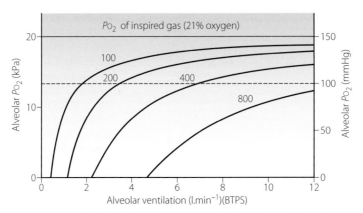

Fig. 11.3 The relationship between alveolar ventilation and alveolar P_{O_2} for different values of oxygen consumption for a patient breathing air at normal barometric pressure. The figures on the curves indicate the oxygen consumption in ml.min^{-1} (STPD). A value of 100 ml.min^{-1} is typical of a hypothermic patient at 30°C; 200 ml.min^{-1} a normal subject at rest or during anaesthesia; higher values result from exercise or fever. Note that the alveolar ventilation required to maintain any particular alveolar P_{O_2} is directly proportional to the oxygen consumption. (In calculations of this type it is important to make the correction required by the fact that oxygen consumption and alveolar ventilation values are commonly expressed at different temperatures and pressures – see Appendix C.)

important. As ventilation is increased, the alveolar P_{O_2} rises asymptomatically towards (but never reaches) the P_{O_2} of the inspired gas (Figure 11.2). It will be seen from the shape of the curves that changes in ventilation above the normal level have comparatively little effect on alveolar P_{O_2}. In contrast, changes in ventilation below the normal level may have a very marked effect. At very low levels of ventilation, the alveolar ventilation becomes critical and small changes may precipitate severe hypoxia. Note that there is a finite alveolar ventilation at which alveolar P_{O_2} becomes zero.

SECONDARY FACTORS INFLUENCING ALVEOLAR OXYGEN TENSION

Cardiac output. In the short term, cardiac output can influence the alveolar P_{O_2}. For example, if other factors remain constant, a sudden reduction in cardiac output will temporarily increase the alveolar P_{O_2}, because less blood passes through the lungs to remove oxygen from the alveolar gas. However, the reduced cardiac output also causes increased oxygen extraction in the tissues supplied by the systemic circulation, and before long the mixed venous oxygen level decreases. When that has happened, the removal of oxygen from the alveolar gas returns to its original level as the reduction in blood flow rate is compensated by the greater amount of oxygen that is taken up per unit volume of blood

flowing through the lungs. Thus, in the long term, cardiac output does not directly influence the alveolar P_{O_2}, and therefore it does not appear in the alveolar air equation.

The 'concentration', third gas or Fink effect. The diagrams and equations above have ignored a factor that influences alveolar P_{O_2} during exchanges of large quantities of soluble gases such as nitrous oxide. This effect was mentioned briefly in connection with carbon dioxide on page 169 but its effect on oxygen is probably more important. During the early part of the administration of nitrous oxide, large quantities of the more soluble gas replace smaller quantities of the less soluble nitrogen previously dissolved in body fluids. There is thus a net transfer of 'inert' gas from the alveoli into the body, causing a temporary increase in the alveolar concentration of both oxygen and carbon dioxide, which will thus temporarily exert a higher partial pressure than would otherwise be expected. Conversely, during recovery from nitrous oxide anaesthesia, large quantities of nitrous oxide leave the body to be replaced with smaller quantities of nitrogen. There is thus a net outpouring of 'inert' gas from the body into the alveoli, causing dilution of oxygen and carbon dioxide, both of which will temporarily exert a lower partial pressure than would otherwise be expected. There may then be temporary hypoxia, the direct reduction of alveolar P_{O_2} sometimes being exacerbated by ventilatory depression due to decreased alveolar P_{CO_2}.

Fortunately such effects last only a few minutes and hypoxia can easily be avoided by small increases in the inspired oxygen concentration when nitrous oxide administration is stopped.

THE ALVEOLAR/ARTERIAL Po_2 DIFFERENCE

The next step in the oxygen cascade is of great clinical relevance. In the healthy young adult breathing air, the alveolar/arterial Po_2 difference does not exceed 2 kPa (15 mmHg) but it may rise to above 5 kPa (37.5 mmHg) in aged but healthy subjects. These values may be exceeded in a patient with any lung disease that causes shunting or mismatching of ventilation to perfusion. An increased alveolar/arterial Po_2 difference is the commonest cause of arterial hypoxaemia in clinical practice and it is therefore a very important step in the oxygen cascade.

Unlike the alveolar Po_2, the alveolar/arterial Po_2 difference cannot be predicted from other more easily measured quantities. There is no simple means of knowing the magnitude of the alveolar/arterial Po_2 difference in a particular patient other than by measurement of the arterial blood gas tensions and calculation of alveolar Po_2. Therefore, it is particularly important to understand the factors that influence the difference, and the principles of restoration of arterial Po_2 by increasing the inspired oxygen concentration when hypoxia is due to an increased alveolar/arterial Po_2 difference.

FACTORS INFLUENCING THE MAGNITUDE OF THE ALVEOLAR/ARTERIAL Po_2 DIFFERENCE

In Chapter 8 it was explained how the alveolar/arterial Po_2 difference results from venous admixture (or physiological shunt) which consists of two components: (1) shunted venous blood that mixes with the oxygenated blood leaving the pulmonary capillaries; (2) a component due to scatter of ventilation/perfusion ratios in different parts of the lungs. Any component due to impaired diffusion across the alveolar/capillary membrane is likely to be very small and in most circumstances can probably be ignored.

Figure 8.10 shows the derivation of the following axiomatic relationship for the first component, shunted venous blood:

$$\frac{\dot{Q}s}{\dot{Q}t} = \frac{Cc'_{O_2} - Ca_{O_2}}{Cc'_{O_2} - C\bar{v}_{O_2}}$$

Two points should be noted.

1. The equation gives a slightly false impression of precision because it assumes that all the shunted blood has the same oxygen content as mixed venous blood. This is not the case, Thebesian and bronchial venous blood being obvious exceptions (Figure 7.1).

2. Oxygen content of pulmonary end-capillary blood (Cc'_{O_2}) is, in practice, calculated on the basis of the end-capillary oxygen tension (Pc'_{O_2}) being equal to the 'ideal' alveolar Po_2 which is derived by means of the alveolar air equation (see page 139).

The equation may be cleared and solved for the pulmonary end-capillary/arterial oxygen content difference as follows:

$$Cc'_{O_2} - Ca_{O_2} = \frac{\dfrac{\dot{Q}s}{\dot{Q}t}(Ca_{O_2} - C\bar{v}_{O_2})}{1 - \dfrac{\dot{Q}s}{\dot{Q}t}} \qquad (1)$$

(scaling factors are required to correct for the inconsistency of the units which are customarily used for the quantities in this equation).

$Ca_{O_2} - C\dot{v}_{O_2}$ is the arterial/mixed venous oxygen content difference and is a function of the oxygen consumption and the cardiac output thus

$$\dot{Q}t(Ca_{O_2} - C\bar{v}_{O_2}) = \dot{V}o_2 \qquad (2)$$

Substituting for $Ca_{O_2} - C\dot{v}_{O_2}$ in equation (1), we have:

$$Cc'_{O_2} - Ca_{O_2} = \frac{\dot{V}o_2 \dfrac{\dot{Q}s}{\dot{Q}t}}{\dot{Q}t\left(1 - \dfrac{\dot{Q}s}{\dot{Q}t}\right)} \qquad (3)$$

This equation shows the content difference in terms of oxygen consumption ($\dot{V}o_2$), the venous admixture ($\dot{Q}s/\dot{Q}t$) and the cardiac output ($\dot{Q}t$).

The final stage in the calculation is to convert the end-capillary/arterial oxygen *content* difference to the *partial pressure* difference. The oxygen content of blood is the sum of the oxygen in physical solution and that which is combined with haemoglobin:

Oxygen content of blood $= \alpha Po_2 + (So_2 \times [Hb] \times 1.39)$

Table 11.1 Oxygen content of human blood $(ml.dl^{-1})$ as a function of Po_2 and other variables		
HAEMOGLOBIN CONCENTRATION $(g.dl^{-1})$		
10	14	18
Normal Po_2 at pH 7.4, 37°C, base excess zero:		
6.7 kPa (50 mmHg)	11.99	16.72	21.45
13.3 kPa (100 mmHg)	13.85	19.27	24.69
26.7 kPa (200 mmHg)	14.41	19.94	25.47
Respiratory acidosis Po_2 at pH 7.2, 37°C, base excess zero:		
6.7 kPa (50 mmHg)	10.45	14.57	18.69
13.3 kPa (100 mmHg)	13.62	18.94	24.27
26.7 kPa (200 mmHg)	14.37	19.87	25.38
Hypothermia Po_2 at pH 7.4, 34°C, base excess zero:		
6.7 kPa (50 mmHg)	12.81	17.87	22.93
13.3 kPa (100 mmHg)	13.96	19.43	24.89
26.7 kPa (200 mmHg)	14.44	19.98	25.51

Data are from reference 1.

where: α is the solubility coefficient of oxygen in blood (not plasma); So_2 is the haemoglobin saturation, and varies with Po_2 according to the oxygen dissociation curve, which itself is influenced by temperature, pH and base excess (Bohr effect); [Hb] is the haemoglobin concentration $(g.dl^{-1})$; 1.39 is the volume of oxygen (ml) that has been found to combine with 1 g of haemoglobin (page 189). Carriage of oxygen in the blood is discussed in detail on pages 187 et seq.

Derivation of the oxygen content from the Po_2 is laborious if due account is taken of pH, base excess, temperature and haemoglobin concentration. Derivation of Po_2 from content is even more laborious, as an iterative approach is required. Tables of partial pressure/content relationships therefore need to be used, and Table 11.1 is an extract from one such table to show the format and general influence of the several variables.[1]

The principal factors influencing the magnitude of the alveolar/arterial Po_2 difference caused by venous admixture may be summarised as follows.

The magnitude of the venous admixture increases the alveolar/arterial Po_2 difference with direct proportionality for small shunts, although this is lost with larger shunts (Figure 11.4). The resultant effect on arterial Po_2 is shown in Figure 8.11. Different forms of venous admixture are considered on pages 133 et seq.

$\dot{V}/\dot{Q}$ scatter. It was explained in Chapter 8 that scatter in ventilation/perfusion ratios produces an alveolar/arterial Po_2 difference for the following reasons:

1. More blood flows through the underventilated overperfused alveoli, and the mixed arterial blood is therefore heavily weighted in the direction of the poorly-oxygenated blood from areas of low $\dot{V}/\dot{Q}$ ratio. The smaller amount of blood flowing through areas of high $\dot{V}/\dot{Q}$ ratio cannot compensate for this (see Figure 8.12).
2. Due to the bend in the dissociation curve around a Po_2 of 8 kPa the fall in saturation of blood from areas of low $\dot{V}/\dot{Q}$ ratio tends to be greater than the rise in saturation of blood from areas of correspondingly high $\dot{V}/\dot{Q}$ (see Figure 8.13).

These two reasons in combination explain why blood from alveoli with a high $\dot{V}/\dot{Q}$ ratio cannot compensate for blood from alveoli with a low $\dot{V}/\dot{Q}$ ratio.

The actual alveolar Po_2 has a profound but complex and non-linear effect on the alveolar/arterial Po_2 gradient (see Figure 11.4). The alveolar/arterial oxygen *content* difference for a given shunt is uninfluenced by the alveolar Po_2 (equation 3), and the effect on the *partial pressure* difference arises entirely in conversion from content to partial pressure: it is thus a function of the slope of the dissociation curve at the Po_2 of the alveolar gas. For example, a loss of 1 ml per 100 ml of oxygen from blood with a Po_2 of 93 kPa (700 mmHg) causes a fall of Po_2 of about 43 kPa (325 mmHg), most of the oxygen being lost from physical solution. However, if the initial Po_2 were 13 kPa (100 mmHg), a loss of 1 ml per 100 ml would cause a fall of Po_2 of only 4.6 kPa (35 mmHg), most of the oxygen being lost from combination with haemoglobin. If the initial Po_2 is only 6.7 kPa (50 mmHg), a loss of 1 ml per 100 ml would cause a very small change in Po_2 of the order of 0.7 kPa (5 mmHg), drawn almost entirely from combination with haemoglobin at a point where the dissociation curve is steep.

The quantitative considerations outlined in the previous paragraph have most important clinical implications. Figure 11.4 clearly shows that, for the same degree of shunt, the alveolar/arterial Po_2 difference will be greatest when the alveolar Po_2

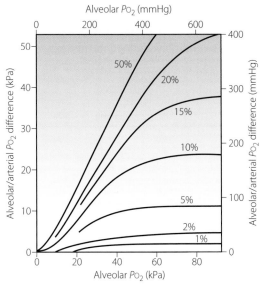

Fig. 11.4 Influence of shunt on alveolar/arterial P_{O_2} difference at different levels of alveolar P_{O_2}. Figures in the graph indicate shunt as percentage of total pulmonary blood flow. For small shunts, the difference (at constant alveolar P_{O_2}) is roughly proportional to the magnitude of the shunt. For a given shunt, the alveolar/arterial P_{O_2} difference increases with alveolar P_{O_2} in a non-linear manner governed by the oxygen dissociation curve. At high alveolar P_{O_2}, a plateau of alveolar/arterial P_{O_2} difference is reached, but the alveolar P_{O_2} at which the plateau is reached is higher with larger shunts. Note that, with a 50% shunt, an increase in alveolar P_{O_2} produces an almost equal increase in alveolar/arterial P_{O_2} difference. Therefore, the arterial P_{O_2} is virtually independent of changes in alveolar P_{O_2}, if other factors remain constant. Constants incorporated into the diagram: arterial/venous oxygen content difference, 5 ml.dl^{-1}; Hb concentration 14 g.dl^{-1}; temperature of blood, 37°C; pH of blood, 7.40; base excess, zero.

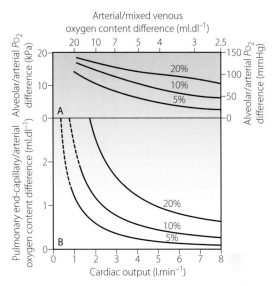

Fig. 11.5 Influence of cardiac output on the alveolar/arterial P_{O_2} difference in the presence of shunts (values indicated for each curve). In this example it is assumed that the patient has an oxygen consumption of 200 ml.min^{-1} and an alveolar P_{O_2} of 24 kPa (180 mmHg). Changes in cardiac output produce an inverse change in the pulmonary end-capillary/arterial oxygen content difference (graph B). When converted to partial pressure differences, the inverse relationship is distorted by the effect of the oxygen dissociation curve in a manner that is applicable only to the particular alveolar P_{O_2} of the patient (graph A). (Alveolar P_{O_2} is assumed to equal pulmonary end-capillary P_{O_2}.)

is highest. If the alveolar P_{O_2} is reduced (e.g. by underventilation), the alveolar/arterial P_{O_2} gradient will also be diminished if other factors remain the same. The arterial P_{O_2} thus falls less than the alveolar P_{O_2}. This is fortunate and may be considered as one of the many benefits deriving from the shape of the oxyhaemoglobin dissociation curve. With a 50% venous admixture, changes in the alveolar P_{O_2} are almost exactly equal to the resultant changes in the alveolar/arterial P_{O_2} difference (Figure 11.4). Therefore the arterial P_{O_2} is almost independent of changes in alveolar P_{O_2} and administration of oxygen will do little to relieve hypoxia (see Figure 8.11).

Cardiac output changes have extremely complex effects on the alveolar/arterial P_{O_2} difference. The

Fick relationship (equation 2, page 183) tells us that a reduced cardiac output per se must increase the arterial/mixed venous oxygen content difference if the oxygen consumption remains the same. This means that the shunted blood will be more desaturated, and will therefore cause a greater decrease in the arterial oxygen level than would less desaturated blood flowing through a shunt of the same magnitude. Equation (3) shows an inverse relationship between the cardiac output and the alveolar/arterial oxygen content difference if the venous admixture is constant (Figure 11.5B). However, when the content difference is converted to partial pressure difference, the relationship to cardiac output is no longer truly inverse, but assumes a complex non-linear form in consequence of the shape of the oxyhaemoglobin dissociation curve. An example of the relationship between cardiac output and alveolar/arterial P_{O_2} difference is shown in Figure 11.5A but this applies only to the conditions specified, with an alveolar P_{O_2} of 24 kPa (180 mmHg).

Unfortunately the influence of cardiac output is even more complicated because it has been observed that a reduction in cardiac output is almost always associated with a reduction in the shunt fraction. Conversely an increase in cardiac output usually results in an increased shunt fraction. This approximately counteracts the effect on mixed venous desaturation, so that arterial Po_2 tends to be relatively little influenced by changes in cardiac output (see Chapter 8, page 134). Nevertheless, it must be remembered that, even if the arterial Po_2 is unchanged, the oxygen delivery (flux) will be reduced in proportion to the change in cardiac output.

Temperature, pH and base excess of the patient's blood influence the oxyhaemoglobin dissociation curve (page 192). In addition, temperature affects the solubility coefficient of oxygen in blood. Thus all three factors influence the relationship between partial pressure and content (see Table 11.1), and therefore the effect of venous admixture on the alveolar/arterial Po_2 difference, although the effect is not usually important except in extreme deviations from normal.

Haemoglobin concentration influences the partition of oxygen between physical solution and chemical combination. Although the haemoglobin concentration does not influence the pulmonary end-capillary/arterial oxygen *content* difference (equation 3), it does alter the *partial pressure* difference. An increased haemoglobin concentration causes a small decrease in the alveolar/arterial Po_2 difference. Table 11.2 shows an example with a cardiac output of $5 l.min^{-1}$, oxygen consumption of $200 ml.min^{-1}$ and a venous admixture of 20%. This would result in a pulmonary end-capillary/arterial oxygen content difference of 0.5 ml per 100 ml. Assuming an alveolar Po_2 of 24 kPa (180 mmHg), the alveolar/arterial Po_2 difference is influenced by haemoglobin concentration as shown in Table 11.2. (Different figures would be obtained by selection of a different value for alveolar Po_2.)

Alveolar ventilation. The overall effect of changes in alveolar ventilation on the arterial Po_2 presents an interesting problem and serves to illustrate the integration of the separate aspects of the factors discussed above. An increase in the alveolar ventilation may be expected to have the following results.

1. The alveolar Po_2 must be raised provided the barometric pressure, inspired oxygen concentration and oxygen consumption remain the same (Figure 11.2).

Table 11.2 Effect of different haemoglobin concentrations on the arterial Po_2 under venous admixture conditions defined in the text

HAEMOGLOBIN CONCENTRATION	ALVEOLAR/ARTERIAL Po_2 DIFFERENCE		ARTERIAL Po_2	
g.dl^{-1}	kPa	mmHg	kPa	mmHg
8	15.0	113	9.0	67
10	14.5	109	9.5	71
12	14.0	105	10.0	75
14	13.5	101	10.5	79
16	13.0	98	11.0	82

2. The alveolar/arterial Po_2 difference is increased for the following reasons:
   - The increase in the alveolar Po_2 will increase the alveolar/arterial Po_2 difference by the same proportion if other factors remain the same (see Figure 11.4).
   - Under many conditions it has been demonstrated that a fall of Pco_2 (resulting from an increase in alveolar ventilation) reduces the cardiac output, with the consequent changes that have been outlined above.
   - The change in arterial pH resulting from the reduction in Pco_2 causes a small, unimportant increase in alveolar/arterial Po_2 difference.

Thus an increase in alveolar ventilation may be expected to increase both the alveolar Po_2 and the alveolar/arterial Po_2 difference. The resultant change in arterial Po_2 will depend upon the relative magnitude of the two changes. Figure 11.6 shows the changes in arterial Po_2 caused by variations of alveolar ventilation at an inspired oxygen concentration of 30% in the presence of varying degrees of venous admixture, assuming that cardiac output is influenced by Pco_2 as described in the legend. Up to an alveolar ventilation of $1.5 l.min^{-1}$, an increase in ventilation will always raise the arterial Po_2. Beyond that, in the example cited, further increases in alveolar ventilation will increase the arterial Po_2 only if the venous admixture is less than 3 per cent. For larger values of venous admixture, the increase in the alveolar/arterial Po_2 difference exceeds the increase in the alveolar Po_2 and the arterial Po_2 is thus decreased.

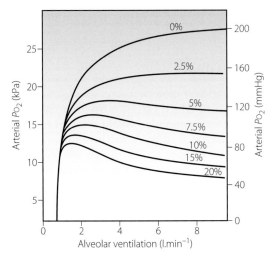

Fig. 11.6 The effect of alveolar ventilation on arterial Po_2 is the algebraic sum of the effect upon the alveolar Po_2 (Figure 11.2) and the consequent change in alveolar/arterial Po_2 difference (Figure 11.4). When the increase in the latter exceeds the increase in the former, the arterial Po_2 will be diminished. The figures in the diagram indicate the percentage venous admixture. The curve corresponding to 0% venous admixture will indicate alveolar Po_2. Constants incorporated in the design of this figure: inspired O_2 concentration, 30%; O_2 consumption, 200 ml.min^{-1}; respiratory exchange ratio, 0.8. It has been assumed that the cardiac output is influenced by the Pco_2 according to the equation $\dot{Q} = 0.039 \times Pco_2 + 2.23$ (mmHg). (After reference 2 by permission of the Editor of British Journal of Anaesthesia and Oxford University Press.)

COMPENSATION FOR INCREASED ALVEOLAR/ARTERIAL Po_2 DIFFERENCE BY RAISING THE INSPIRED OXYGEN CONCENTRATION

Many patients with severe respiratory dysfunction are hypoxaemic while breathing air. The main objective of treatment is clearly to remove the cause of the hypoxaemia but, when this is not immediately possible, it is often possible to relieve the hypoxaemia by increasing the inspired oxygen concentration. The principles for doing so depend upon the cause of the hypoxaemia. As a broad classification, hypoxaemia may be due to hypoventilation or to venous admixture or to a combination of the two. When hypoxaemia is primarily due to hypoventilation, and when it is not appropriate or possible to restore normal alveolar ventilation, the arterial Po_2 can usually be restored by elevation of the inspired

oxygen within the range 21–30% as explained above (page 181 and Figure 11.2) and also in Chapter 27.

Quantitatively, the situation is entirely different when hypoxaemia is primarily due to venous admixture. It is then only possible to restore the arterial Po_2 by oxygen enrichment of the inspired gas when the venous admixture does not exceed the equivalent of a shunt of 30% of the cardiac output, and at this level may require up to 100% inspired oxygen (page 135). The quantitative aspects of the relationship are best considered in relation to the iso-shunt diagram (see Figure 8.11).

THE CARRIAGE OF OXYGEN IN THE BLOOD

The preceding section has considered in detail the factors that influence the Po_2 of the arterial blood. It is now necessary to consider how oxygen is carried in the blood and, in particular, the relationship between the Po_2 and the quantity of oxygen that is carried. The latter is crucially important to the delivery of oxygen and is no less important than the partial pressure at which it becomes available to the tissue.

Oxygen is carried in the blood in two forms. Much the greater part is in reversible chemical combination with haemoglobin, while a smaller part is in physical solution in plasma and intracellular fluid. The ability to carry large quantities of oxygen in the blood is of great importance to the organism. Without haemoglobin the amount carried would be so small that the cardiac output would need to be increased by a factor of about 20 to give an adequate delivery of oxygen. Under such a handicap, animals could not have developed to their present extent. The biological significance of the haemoglobin-like compounds is thus immense. It is interesting that the tetrapyrrole ring, which contains iron in haemoglobin is also a constituent of chlorophyll (which has magnesium in place of iron) and the cytochromes responsible for cellular oxygen metabolism. This chemical structure is thus concerned with production, transport and utilisation of oxygen.

PHYSICAL SOLUTION OF OXYGEN IN BLOOD[3]

Oxygen is carried in physical solution in both red blood cells (RBCs) and plasma. There does not appear to have been any recent determination of the solubility coefficient, and we tend to rely on earlier studies indicating that the amount carried in normal blood in solution at 37°C is about 0.0232 $ml.dl^{-1}.kPa^{-1}$ or $0.00314\,ml.dl^{-1}.mmHg^{-1}$. At normal arterial Po_2, the oxygen in physical solution is thus about $0.25–0.3\,ml.dl^{-1}$, or rather more than 1% of the total oxygen carried in all forms. However, when breathing 100% oxygen, the level rises to about $2\,ml.dl^{-1}$. Breathing 100% oxygen at 3 atmospheres pressure absolute (303 kPa), the amount of oxygen in physical solution rises to about $6\,ml.dl^{-1}$, which is sufficient for the normal resting arterio-venous extraction. The amount of oxygen in physical solution rises with decreasing temperature for the same Po_2.

HAEMOGLOBIN[4]

The haemoglobin molecule consists of four protein chains, each of which carries a haem group (Figure 11.7A), the total molecular weight being 64 458. In the commonest type of adult human haemoglobin (HbA) there are two types of chain, two of each occurring in each molecule. The two α-chains each have 141 amino acid residues, with the haem attached to a histidine residue occupying position 87. The two

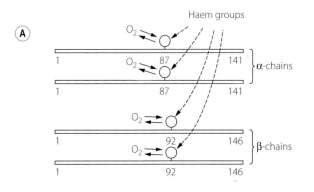

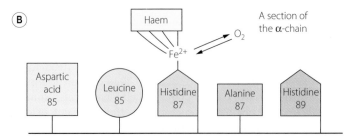

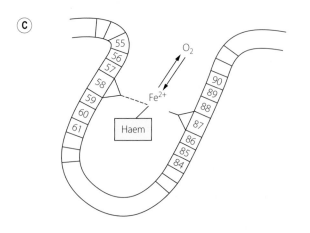

Fig. 11.7 The haemoglobin molecule consists of four amino acid chains, each carrying a haem group. (A) There are two pairs of identical chains: α-chains each with 141 amino acid residues and β-chains each with 146 amino acid residues. (B) The attachment of the haem group to the α-chain. (C) The crevice that contains the haem group.

β-chains each have 146 amino acid residues, with the haem attached to a histidine residue occupying position 92. Figure 11.7B shows details of the point of attachment of the haem in the α-chain.

MOLECULAR MECHANISMS OF OXYGEN BINDING[4,5]

The four chains of the haemoglobin molecule lie in a ball, like a crumpled necklace. However, the form is not random and the actual shape (the quaternary structure) is of critical importance and governs the reaction with oxygen. The shape is maintained by loose (electrostatic) bonds between specific amino acids on different chains and also between some amino acids on the same chain. One consequence of these bonds is that the haem groups lie in crevices formed by electrostatic bonds between the haem groups and histidine residues, other than those to which they are attached by normal valency linkages. For example, Figure 11.7C shows a section of an alpha chain with the haem group attached to the iron atom, which is bound to the histidine residue in position 87. However, the haem group is also attached by an electrostatic bond to the histidine residue in position 58 and also by non-polar bonds to many other amino acids. This forms a loop and places the haem group in a crevice, the shape of which controls the ease of access for oxygen molecules.

In deoxyhaemoglobin, the electrostatic bonds within and between the protein chains are strong, holding the haemoglobin molecule in a tense (T) conformation, in which the molecule has a relatively low affinity for oxygen. In oxyhaemoglobin the electrostatic bonds are weaker, and the haemoglobin adopts its relaxed (R) state, in which the crevices containing the haem groups can open and bind oxygen, and the molecule's affinity for oxygen becomes 500 times greater than in the T state. Binding of oxygen to just one of the four protein chains induces a conformational change in the whole haemoglobin molecule, which increases the affinity of the other protein chains for oxygen. This 'cooperativity' between oxygen binding sites is fundamental to the physiological role of haemoglobin, and affects the kinetics of the reaction between haemoglobin and oxygen, which are described below. The conformational state (R or T) of the haemoglobin molecule is also altered by other factors that influence the strength of the electrostatic bonds; such factors include carbon dioxide, pH and temperature.

The Bohr effect describes the alteration in haemoglobin oxygen affinity that arises from changes in hydrogen ion or carbon dioxide concentrations, and is generally considered in terms of its influence upon the dissociation curve (see Figure 11.10 below). Changes in pH affect the numerous electrostatic bonds that maintain the quaternary structure of haemoglobin, and so stabilises the molecule in the T conformation, reducing its affinity for oxygen. Similarly, carbon dioxide binds to the *N*-terminal amino acid residues of the α-chain to form carbaminohaemoglobin (page 162), and this small alteration in the function of the protein chains stabilises the T conformation and facilitates release of the oxygen molecule from haemoglobin.

Conversely, the Haldane effect describes the smaller amount of carbon dioxide that can be carried in oxygenated blood compared with deoxygenated blood (page 162). Crystallographic studies have shown that in deoxyhaemoglobin the histidine in position 146 of the β-chain is loosely bonded to the aspartine residue at position 94, and that when haemoglobin binds oxygen and changes to the R conformation the histidine 146 moves 10 Å further away from the aspartine, which is sufficient distance to change its p*K* value.[6] Once again, this small change in one area of the β-chains has widespread effects on electrostatic bonds throughout the molecule, changing the quaternary structure of the entire molecule and altering its ability to buffer hydrogen ions and form carbamino compounds with carbon dioxide.

Oxygen-binding capacity of haemoglobin (B$_{O_2}$) or Hüfner constant. Following the determination of the molecular weight of haemoglobin, the theoretical value for B_{O_2} of 1.39 ml.g^{-1} was easily derived (4 moles of oxygen of 22 414 ml STPD each bind to 1 mole of haemoglobin with molecular mass 64 458 g) and passed into general use. However, it gradually became clear that this value was not obtained when direct measurements of haemoglobin concentration and oxygen capacity were compared. Gregory in 1974 proposed the value of 1.306 ml g^{-1} for human adult blood,[7] and just a few years later two studies[8,9] reported values of 1.36 and 1.368 ml.g^{-1}. The difference between the theoretical and in vivo values results from the presence of dyshaemoglobins,[3,10] which includes any form of haemoglobin that lacks oxygen binding capacity, the most common being methaemoglobin (metHb) and carboxyhaemoglobin (COHb). If the dyshaemoglobins are taken into account, then the theoretical value for Hüfner's constant may be used and the oxygen binding capacity for the blood sample (Bo_2) calculated as:

$$Bo_2 = 1.39 \times (tHb - (metHb + COHb))$$

where tHb = total haemoglobin present in the sample.

Current blood gas analysers routinely measure all four forms of haemoglobin that make up the majority of tHb in blood i.e. oxyhaemoglobin (O_2Hb), deoxyhaemoglobin (HHb), metHb and COHb. If the first two of these have been measured, then the dyshaemoglobins can be excluded completely and the calculation of Bo_2 becomes even simpler:

$$Bo_2 = 1.39 \times (HHb + O_2Hb)$$

KINETICS OF THE REACTION OF OXYGEN WITH HAEMOGLOBIN

Adair first proposed in 1925 that the binding of oxygen to haemoglobin proceeds in four separate stages:[11]

$$Hb + 4O_2 \overset{K_1}{\rightleftharpoons} HbO_2 + 3O_2 \overset{K_2}{\rightleftharpoons} Hb(O_2)_2 + 2O_2$$
$$\overset{K_3}{\rightleftharpoons} Hb(O_2)_3 + O_2 \overset{K_4}{\rightleftharpoons} Hb(O_2)_4$$

For each of the four reactions there are two velocity constants with small k indicating the reverse reaction (towards deoxyhaemoglobin) and small k prime (k') indicating the forward reaction. Large K is used to represent the ratio of the forward and reverse reactions, thus for example $K_1 = k'_1/k_1$. In this way, the dissociation between deoxy- and oxyhaemoglobin may be represented by the four velocity constants K_1–K_4.

The Adair equation described assumes that the α- and β-chains of haemoglobin behave identically in their chemical reactions with oxygen, which is unlikely in vivo. When α- and β-chains are taken into account there are many different reaction routes that may be followed between deoxy- and oxy-haemoglobin, in theory giving rise to 16 different reversible reactions (Figure 11.8).[12] However, the multiple separate forward and reverse reactions can again be combined to give a single value for K, which does not differ significantly from those obtained using the simpler Adair equation.

In both cases, the separate velocity constants have been measured[12] and values for K_1–K_4 are shown in Figure 11.8. It can be seen that the last reaction has a forward velocity that is many times higher than that of the other reactions. During the oxygenation of the final 25% of deoxyhaemoglobin, the last reaction will predominate and the high velocity constant counteracts the effect of the ever-diminishing number of oxygen binding sites that would otherwise slow the reaction rate by the law of mass action. The magnitude of the forward reaction for K_4 also explains why the dissociation of oxyhaemoglobin is somewhat slower than its formation.

The velocity constant of the combination of carbon monoxide with haemoglobin is of the same order, but the rate of dissociation of carboxyhaemoglobin is extremely slow by comparison.

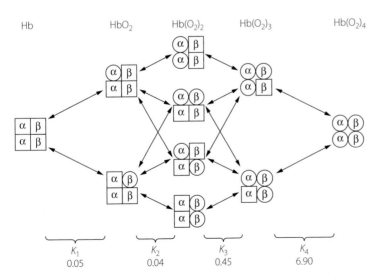

Fig. 11.8 Oxygenation of tetrameric haemoglobin. If chemical interactions with oxygen differ between α- and β-chains then the transition from deoxyhaemoglobin to fully oxygenated haemoglobin can take a variety of routes as shown. Arrows indicate the 16 possible separate dissociation equilibria, which must be combined to derive the four Adair constants K_1–K_4, the values of which are indicated. It can be clearly seen that the final stage of oxygenation is considerably faster than the previous three.[12]

THE OXYHAEMOGLOBIN DISSOCIATION CURVE

As a result of the complex kinetics of the chemical reaction between oxygen and haemoglobin, the relationship between Po_2 and percentage saturation of haemoglobin is non-linear, and the precise form of the non-linearity is of fundamental biological importance. It is shown, under standard conditions, in graphical form for adult and fetal haemoglobin and also for myoglobin and carboxyhaemoglobin in Figure 11.9.

Equations to represent the dissociation curve. An 'S' shaped oxyhaemoglobin dissociation curve was first described by Bohr in 1904 (page 241 and Figure 13.11). Adair[11] and Kelman[13] subsequently developed equations that would reproduce the observed oxygen dissociation curve, using a variety of coefficients. Kelman's equation, which uses seven coefficients, generates a curve indistinguishable from the true curve above a Po_2 of about 1 kPa (7.5 mmHg) and this has remained the standard. Calculation of Po_2 from saturation requires an iterative approach, but saturation may be conveniently determined from Po_2 by computer, a calculation that is automatically carried out by most blood gas analysers in clinical

use. The following simplified version of the Kelman equation is convenient to use and yields similar results at Po_2 values above 4 kPa (30 mmHg):[14]

$$So_2 = \frac{100(Po_2^3 + 2.667 \times Po_2)}{Po_2^3 + 2.667 \times Po_2 + 55.47}$$

(Po_2 values here are in kilopascals; So_2 is percentage)

This equation takes no account of the position of the dissociation curve as described in the next section, so must be used with caution in clinical situations.

FACTORS CAUSING DISPLACEMENT OF THE DISSOCIATION CURVE

Several physiological and pathological changes to blood chemistry cause the normal dissociation curve to be displaced in either direction along its x axis. A convenient approach to quantifying a shift of the dissociation curve is to indicate the Po_2 required for 50% saturation and, under the standard conditions shown in Figure 11.9, this is 3.5 kPa (26.3 mmHg). Referred to as the P_{50} this is the usual method of reporting shift of the dissociation curve.

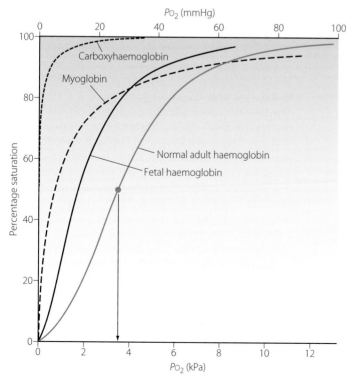

Fig. 11.9 Dissociation curves of normal adult and fetal haemoglobins. Curves for myoglobin and carboxyhaemoglobin are shown for comparison. The arrow shows the P_{50} for this curve which is the oxygen tension at which the Hb saturation is 50%. Note: (1) Fetal haemoglobin is adapted to operate at a lower Po_2 than adult blood. (2) Myoglobin approaches full saturation at Po_2 levels normally found in voluntary muscle (2–4 kPa, 15–30 mmHg); the bulk of its oxygen can only be released at very low Po_2 during exercise. (3) Carboxyhaemoglobin can be dissociated only by the maintenance of very low levels of Pco.

The Bohr effect, as a result of changes in blood pH, is shown in Figure 11.10. Shifts may be defined as the ratio of the P_{O_2} that produces a particular saturation under standard conditions, to the P_{O_2} which produces the same saturation with a particular shift of the curve. Standard conditions include pH 7.4, temperature 37°C and zero base excess. In Figure 11.10, a saturation of 80% is produced by P_{O_2} 6 kPa (45 mmHg) at pH 7.4 (standard). At pH 7.0 the P_{O_2} required for 80% saturation is 9.4 kPa (70.5 mmHg). The ratio is 0.64 and this applies to all saturations at pH 7.0.

The Bohr effect has an influence on oxygen carriage under normal physiological conditions. As blood moves along a capillary, either pulmonary or systemic, the transfer of CO_2 alters the pH of the blood and therefore the dissociation curve is shifted. Though the effect may seem to be small, for example the arteriovenous pH difference is only around 0.033, the effect on oxygen saturation at the venous point, where the dissociation curve is steep, will be significant. It has been suggested that 25% of oxygen release and uptake by haemoglobin as it traverses systemic and pulmonary capillaries respectively is due to the Bohr effect.

Temperature has a large influence on the dissociation curve with a left shift in hypothermia and *vice versa.*

Base excess is a parameter derived from blood pH and P_{CO_2} to quantify the metabolic (as opposed to respiratory) component of an observed change in blood pH. Compared with pH itself, alterations in base excess have only a small effect on the position of the dissociation curve but must be taken into account for accurate results.

Quantifying displacement of the haemoglobin dissociation curve. Estimation of haemoglobin saturation from P_{O_2} using the modified Kelman equation has been shown above. However, this equation assumes a normal P_{50}, so will yield erroneous results in all but the most 'normal' physiological circumstances. In clinical practice, the type of patient who requires blood gas measurement invariably also has abnormalities of pH, temperature and base excess. Automated calculation of saturation from P_{O_2} by blood gas analysers routinely takes these factors into account, using a variety of equations to correct for dissociation curve displacement of which one example is:[15]

Corrected P_{O_2} =
$$P_{O_2} \times 10^{[0.48(pH-7.4)-0.024(T-37)-0.0013 \times \text{Base Excess}]}$$

where P_{O_2} is in kPa and temperature (T) in °C. The corrected P_{O_2} may then be entered into any version of the haemoglobin dissociation curve equation as shown above (page 191).

Clinical significance of displacement of the haemoglobin dissociation curve. The important effect is on tissue P_{O_2}, and the consequences of a shift in the dissociation curve are not intuitively obvious. It is essential to think quantitatively. For example, a shift to the right (caused by low pH or high temperature) impairs oxygenation in the lungs but aids release of oxygen in the tissues. Do these effects in combination increase or decrease tissue P_{O_2}? An illustrative example is set out in Figure 11.10. The arterial P_{O_2} is assumed to be 13.3 kPa (100 mmHg) and there is a decrease in arterial saturation with a reduction of pH. At normal arterial P_{O_2} the effect on arterial saturation is relatively small, but at the venous point the position is quite different, and the examples in Figure 11.10 show the venous oxygen tensions to be very markedly affected. Assuming that the arterial/venous oxygen saturation difference is constant at 25% it will be seen that at low pH the venous P_{O_2} is raised to 6.9 kPa (52 mmHg), while at high pH the venous P_{O_2} is reduced to 3.5 kPa (26 mmHg). This is

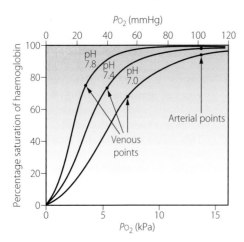

Fig. 11.10 The Bohr effect and its effect upon oxygen partial pressure. The centre curve is the normal curve under standard conditions; the other two curves show the displacement caused by differing blood pH as indicated, other factors remaining constant. The venous points have been determined on the basis of a fixed arterial/mixed venous oxygen saturation difference of 25%. They are thus 25% saturation less than the corresponding arterial saturation, which is equivalent to a P_{O_2} of 13.3 kPa (100 mmHg) in each case. Under the conditions shown, alkalosis lowers venous P_{O_2} and acidosis raises venous P_{O_2}. Temperature, 37°C; base excess, zero.

important as the tissue Po_2 equates more closely to the venous Po_2 than to the arterial Po_2 (page 155). Thus, in the example shown, the shift to the right is beneficial for tissue oxygenation.

It is a general rule that a shift to the right (increased P_{50}) will benefit venous Po_2, provided that the arterial Po_2 is not critically reduced. Below an arterial Po_2 of about 5 kPa (38 mmHg), the arterial point is on the steep part of the dissociation curve, and the deficiency in oxygenation of the arterial blood would outweigh the improved off-loading of oxygen in the tissues. Thus, with severe arterial hypoxaemia, the venous Po_2 would tend to be reduced by a shift to the right and a *leftward* shift would then be advantageous. It is therefore of great interest that a spontaneous leftward shift occurs at extreme altitude when arterial Po_2 is critically reduced (see below).

2,3–DIPHOSPHOGLYCERATE

For many years it has been known that the presence of certain organic phosphates in the RBC has a pronounced effect on the P_{50}. The most important of these compounds is 2,3-diphosphoglycerate (DPG),[16] one molecule of which becomes bound by electrostatic bonds between the two β-chains, stabilising the T conformation of haemoglobin,[4] reducing its oxygen affinity, and so displacing the dissociation curve to the right. The percentage of haemoglobin molecules containing a DPG molecule governs the overall P_{50} of a blood sample within the range 2–4.5 kPa (15–34 mmHg).

DPG is formed in the Rapoport–Luebering shunt off the glycolytic pathway, and its level is determined by the balance between synthesis and degradation (Figure 11.11). Activity of DPG mutase is enhanced and DPG phosphatase diminished at high pH, which thus increases the level of DPG.

The relationship between DPG levels and P_{50} suggested that DPG levels would have a most important bearing on clinical practice. Much research effort was devoted to this topic, which mostly failed to substantiate the theoretical importance of DPG for oxygen delivery. In fact, the likely effects of changes in P_{50} mediated by DPG seem to be of marginal significance in comparison with changes in arterial Po_2, acid–base balance and tissue perfusion.[17]

DPG levels with blood storage and transfusion remains the only area where red cell DPG levels may have significant effects in clinical practice. Storage of blood for transfusion at below 6°C reduces glycolysis to less than 5% of normal rates, and so reduces DPG production by a similar amount. Thus, after one to two weeks of storage, red cell DPG levels are effectively zero. Blood preservation solutions have evolved through the years to include the addition of dextrose to encourage glycolytic activity, citrate to buffer the resulting lactic acid and adenine or phosphate to help maintain ATP levels. Thus storage of blood with citrate-phosphate-dextrose (CPD) reduces the rate of DPG depletion when compared with older preservation solutions,[18] but levels still become negligible within two weeks.

Once transfused, the red blood cells are quickly warmed and provided with all required metabolites, and the limiting factor for return to normal DPG levels will be reactivation of DPG mutase (Figure 11.11). In vivo studies in healthy volunteers indicate that red cell DPG levels in transfused red cells are approximately 50% of normal 7 hours after transfusion, and pretransfusion levels are not achieved until 48 hours (Figure 11.12).[19] This ingenious study involved the administration of 35 day old CPD-Adenine preserved type O blood to type A volunteers, and then in repeated venous samples red cells were separated according to their blood

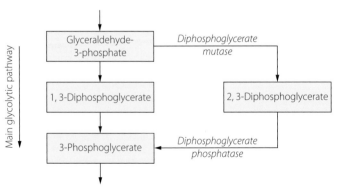

Fig. 11.11 Rapoport-Luebering shunt for synthesis of 2,3-diphosphoglycerate.

group before measuring DPG levels. In this way, DPG levels of both the recipients' own cells and the transfused cells could be monitored separately (Figure 11.12).

The clinical significance of the slow return to normal DPG levels is uncertain, and in most cases likely to be minimal, as the proportion of the patient's haemoglobin that consists of transfused blood will usually be small. However, rapid transfusion of large volumes of DPG depleted blood does result in a reduced P_{50}, which will in theory impair tissue oxygenation (page 192). However, in humans, little evidence has been found of tissue hypoxia under these circumstances, with no changes in cardiac output or oxygen consumption following transfusion with DPG depleted blood.[20] Changes in the P_{50} of a patient do not usually exceed 0.5 kPa (3.8 mmHg), and it is possible that changes in the haemoglobin dissociation curve are compensated for by changes in blood flow at a capillary level.[21]

Other causes of altered DPG levels. Anaemia results in a raised DPG level, with P_{50} of the order of 0.5 kPa (3.8 mmHg) higher than control levels.[22] The problem of oxygen delivery in anaemia is considered in Chapter 25.

Altitude causes an increased red cell concentration of DPG. However, there is a progressive respiratory alkalosis with increasing altitude, which has an opposite and much more pronounced effect on displacement of the dissociation curve. There is now a firm consensus that there is a *leftward* displacement of the haemoglobin dissociation curve at high altitude (see Chapter 17).

NORMAL ARTERIAL P_{O_2}

In contrast to the arterial P_{CO_2}, the arterial P_{O_2} shows a progressive decrease with age. Using the pooled results from 12 studies of healthy subjects, one review suggested the following relationship in subjects breathing air:[23]

Arterial P_{O_2} = 13.6 − 0.044 × age in years (kPa)
or   = 102 − 0.33 × age in years (mmHg)

About this regression line there are 95% confidence limits of ± 1.33 kPa (10 mmHg) (Table 11.3) so 5% of normal patients will lie outside these limits and it is therefore preferable to refer to this as the reference range rather than the normal range.

NITRIC OXIDE AND HAEMOGLOBIN[24,25,26]

The enormous interest over recent years in both endogenous and exogenous nitric oxide (NO) has inevitably led to intensive research into its interaction with haemoglobin. It has been known for some time that NO binds to haemoglobin very rapidly, and this observation is fundamental to its therapeutic use when inhaled NO exerts its effects in the pulmonary vasculature but is inactivated by binding to haemoglobin before it reaches the systemic circulation (page 111). There are two quite separate chemical reactions between NO and the haemoglobin molecule:[27]

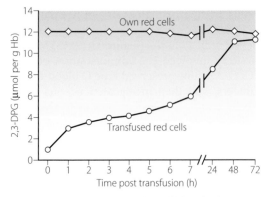

Fig. 11.12 Restoration of red cell 2,3-diphosphoglycerate (DPG) levels following blood transfusion. The Type O transfused red cells were stored for 35 days in CPD-A preservative solution before being given to type A volunteers. Red cells were subsequently separated into the transfused cells and the volunteer's own cells before analysis. The clinical implications of this slow return to normal DPG levels are unclear; see text for details. (After reference 19 with permission of the authors and the publishers of British Journal of Haematology.)

Table 11.3 Normal values for arterial P_{O_2}

AGE (YEARS)	MEAN (95% CONFIDENCE INTERVALS)	
	kPa	mmHg
20–29	12.5 (11.2–13.8)	94 (84–104)
30–39	12.1 (10.7–13.4)	90 (80–100)
40–49	11.6 (10.3–13.0)	87 (77–97)
50–59	11.2 (9.9–12.5)	84 (74–94)
60–69	10.7 (9.4–12.1)	81 (71–91)
70–79	10.3 (9.0–11.6)	77 (67–87)
80–89	9.9 (8.5–11.2)	74 (64–84)

Figures derived from reference 23.

1. NO binds to the haem moiety of each haemoglobin chain, but the resulting reaction differs with the state of oxygenation. For deoxyhaemoglobin, in the T conformation, a fairly stable Hb–NO complex is rapidly formed, which has little vasodilator activity, whilst for oxyhaemoglobin, in the R conformation, the oxygen is displaced by NO and in doing so the iron atom is oxidised to methaemoglobin and a nitrate ion produced:

$$Hb[Fe^{2+}] + NO \rightarrow Hb[Fe^{2+}]NO$$
$$\text{or} \quad Hb[Fe^{2+}]O_2 + NO \rightarrow Hb[Fe^{3+}] + NO_3^-$$

These reactions are so rapid that there is doubt that endogenous NO itself can exert any effects within blood (e.g. on platelets) before being bound by haemoglobin, and must therefore act via an intermediate substance.

2. Nitric oxide is also known to form stable compounds with sulphydryl groups termed S-nitrosothiols, with the general formula R-S-NO, where the R group may be glutathione or sulphur containing amino acid residues within proteins.[26,28] Nitrosothiols retain biological activity as vasodilators[29] and can survive for longer than free NO within the blood vessels. NO forms a nitrosothiol group with the cysteine residue at position 93 on the β-chains, producing S-nitrosohaemoglobin (SNO-Hb). As a result of conformational changes in haemoglobin the reaction is faster with R-state oxyhaemoglobin and under alkaline conditions.[27]

Thus in vivo NO in arterial blood is predominantly in the form of SNO-Hb, whilst in venous blood haem bound HbNO predominates.[27] It has been proposed that as haemoglobin passes through the pulmonary capillary, changes in oxygenation, Pco_2 and pH drive the change from the deoxygenated T conformation to the oxygenated R conformation, and this change in quaternary structure of haemoglobin causes the intramolecular transfer of NO from the haem to cysteine bound positions. In the peripheral capillaries, the opposite sequence of events occurs, which encourages release of NO from the RSNO group, where it may again bind to the haem group, or be released from the RBC to act as a local vasodilator, effectively improving flow to vessels with the greatest demand for oxygen.[30] Export of NO activity from the RBC is believed to occur via a complex mechanism. Deoxygenated T conformation haemoglobin binds to one of the cytoplasmic domains of the RBC transmembrane Band 3 protein (Figure 10.4),[31] which may act as a metabolon (page 166) and directly transfer the NO, via a series of nitrosothiol reactions, to the outside of the cell membrane where it can exert its vasodilator activity. The biological implications of this series of events are yet to be determined. The suggestion that haemoglobin is acting as a nitric oxide carrier to regulate capillary blood flow and oxygen release from the RBC represents a fundamental advance in our understanding of the delivery of oxygen to tissues.[25,32] One role postulated for these interactions between haemoglobin and NO is to modulate the vascular response to changes in oxygen availability,[33] for example during haemorrhage when NO activity from RBCs may be involved in overcoming the catecholamine mediated vasoconstriction in vital organs.[32]

ABNORMAL FORMS OF HAEMOGLOBIN

There are a large number of alternative amino acid sequences in the haemoglobin molecule. Most animal species have their own peculiar haemoglobins while, in humans, γ- and δ-chains occur in addition to the α- and β-monomers already described. γ- and δ-chains occur normally in combination with α-chains. The combination of two γ-chains with two α-chains constitutes fetal haemoglobin (HbF), which has a dissociation curve well to the left of adult haemoglobin (Figure 11.9). The combination of two δ-chains with two α-chains constitutes A$_2$ haemoglobin (HbA$_2$), which forms 2% of the total haemoglobin in normal adults. Other variations in the amino acid chains can be considered abnormal, and, although over 600 have been reported and named, only one third of these have any clinical effects.[34] Some abnormal haemoglobins (such as San Diego and Chesapeake) have a high P_{50} but it is more common for the P_{50} to be lower than normal (such as Sickle and Kansas). In the long term, a reduced P_{50} results in excessive production of RBCs (erythrocytosis), presumed to result from cellular hypoxia in the kidney leading to erythropoietin production.[35] However, many abnormal haemoglobins also have deranged quaternary protein structure and so are unstable, a situation that leads to haemoglobin chains becoming free within the RBC cytoplasm and membrane causing cell lysis.[35] These patients therefore have a higher than normal rate of RBC production but are generally anaemic because of even greater degrees of RBC destruction.

This combination of abnormalities results in severe long-term problems with body iron metabolism.

Sickle cell disease[36] is caused by the presence of HbS in which valine replaces glutamic acid in position 6 on the β-chains. This apparently trivial substitution is sufficient to cause critical loss of solubility of reduced haemoglobin, resulting in polymerisation of HbS within the RBC causing red cells to take on the characteristic 'sickle' shape and be more prone to haemolysis. It is a hereditary condition and in the homozygous state is a grave abnormality, with sickling occurring at an arterial Po_2 of less than 5.5 kPa (40 mmHg), which is close to the normal venous Po_2. Thus any condition that increases the arterio-venous oxygen difference, such as infection, risks precipitating a sickle 'crisis'. Sickle cells cause damage in two ways. First, the sickled cells are crescent shaped and rigid, so can more easily occlude small blood vessels, usually venules. Secondly, haemolysis releases free haemoglobin into the circulation which binds NO released from the vascular endothelium causing vasoconstriction, further impairing the ability of the sickle cells to pass through the microcirculation. In the long term these effects cause widespread microvascular damage, including pulmonary hypertension.[37]

Patients with sickle cell disease have varying degrees of compensatory production of HbF, and the amount of HbF found in RBCs is inversely related to the severity of clinical symptoms of sickle cell disease. Thus most therapies in recent years have focussed on increasing HbF synthesis by the bone marrow with cytotoxic drugs such as hydroxyurea.[38] Heterozygous carriers of the disease only sickle below an arterial Po_2 of 2.7 kPa (20 mmHg) and so are usually asymptomatic.

Thalassaemia is another hereditary disorder of haemoglobin. It consists of a suppression of formation of HbA, again with a compensatory production of HbF, which persists throughout life instead of falling to low levels after birth. The functional disorder thus includes a shift of the dissociation curve to the left (Figure 11.9).

Methaemoglobin is haemoglobin in which the iron has been oxidised and assumes the trivalent ferric form. One way in which methaemoglobin forms is when oxyhaemoglobin acts as a nitric oxide scavenger, a process that occurs physiologically to limit the biological activity of endogenous NO, or pharmacologically during treatment with inhaled NO. Other drugs may cause methaemoglobinaemia, most notably some local anaesthetics[39] (prilocaine, benzocaine)

but also nitrites and dapsone.[40] Methaemoglobin is unable to combine with oxygen but is slowly reconverted to haemoglobin in the normal subject by the action of four different systems:

1. NADH-methaemoglobin reductase system of enzymes, which is present in RBCs and uses NADH generated by glycolysis to reduce methaemoglobin. This system is by far the most important in normal subjects, accounting for over two thirds of methaemoglobin reducing activity, and is deficient in familial methaemoglobinaemia.

2. Ascorbic acid may also bring about the reduction of methaemoglobin by a direct chemical effect, though the rate of this reaction is slow.

3. Glutathione-based reductive enzymes have a small amount of methaemoglobin reductase activity.

4. NADPH-dehydrogenase enzyme in RBCs can reduce methaemoglobin using NADPH generated from the pentose phosphate pathway. Under physiological conditions, this system has almost no effect and is regarded as the 'reserve' methaemoglobin reductase.

Elevated methaemoglobin levels of whatever cause may be treated by the administration of either ascorbic acid or methylene blue.[39] The latter is extremely effective and brings about methaemoglobin reduction by activation of NADPH-dehydrogenase.

ABNORMAL LIGANDS

The iron in haemoglobin is able to combine with other inorganic molecules apart from oxygen. Compounds so formed are, in general, more stable than oxyhaemoglobin and therefore block the combination of haemoglobin with oxygen. The most important of these abnormal compounds is COHb, but ligands may also be formed with nitric oxide (see above), cyanide, sulphur, ammonia and a number of other substances. In addition to the loss of oxygen-carrying power, there is also often a shift of the dissociation curve to the left.

Carboxyhaemoglobin. Carbon monoxide is well known to displace oxygen from combination with haemoglobin, its affinity being approximately 300 times greater than the affinity for oxygen. Thus in a subject with 20% of their haemoglobin bound to carbon monoxide, blood oxygen content will be reduced by a similar amount (the small contribution from dissolved oxygen will be unchanged). However, the presence of carboxyhaemoglobin also causes a leftward shift of the dissociation curve of the remaining oxyhaemoglobin, partly mediated by a reduction in DPG levels. Tissue oxygenation is therefore impaired to an even greater extent than simply reducing the amount of haemoglobin available for oxygen carriage. This situation contrasts with that of anaemia, where P_{50} is increased so the reduced oxygen carrying capacity is partially alleviated by an improved unloading of oxygen in the tissues (page 192).

BLOOD SUBSTITUTES[41]

There are obvious advantages in the provision of an artificial oxygen-carrying solution that would avoid the infectious and antigenic complications seen with transfusion of another individual's red cells. The search for a blood substitute has followed two quite different parallel paths.

Perfluorocarbons.[42] Oxygen is highly soluble in these hydrophobic compounds, which with an 8–10 carbon chain are above the critical molecular size to act as anaesthetics. Perfluorooctyl bromide (Perflubron) is a 60% emulsion, which will carry about 50 ml of oxygen per 100 ml on equilibration with 100% oxygen at normal atmospheric pressure. Since oxygen is in physical solution in fluorocarbons, its 'dissociation curve' is a straight line, with the quantity of dissolved oxygen being directly proportional to Po_2. Because of the requirement to maintain adequate blood constituents apart from red cells (e.g. platelets, clotting factors, blood chemistry and oncotic pressure) the proportion of blood that may be replaced by Perflubron is small, so that even when breathing 100% oxygen the additional oxygen carrying capacity is limited. Even so, clinical uses for intravenous Perflubron have been identified, for example its administration may delay the need for blood transfusion.[43]

Flow resistance is considerably less than that of blood, and as it is virtually unaffected by shear rate, the rheological properties are particularly favourable at low flow rates. Fluorocarbons may therefore be useful in partial obstruction of the circulation, for example in myocardial infarction and during percutaneous transluminal coronary angioplasty.[44] Successful use of perflubron in the lungs for liquid or partial liquid ventilation is now widely reported in premature babies (page 255), children and adults (page 458).

Perfluorocarbons are cleared from the circulation into the reticuloendothelial system where they reside for varying lengths of time before being excreted unchanged from the lungs.

Haemoglobin-based oxygen carriers.[45,46] Early attempts at using RBC haemolysates resulted in acute renal failure due to the stroma from the RBC rather than the free haemoglobin. Development of stroma free haemoglobin solutions failed to solve the problem because although relatively stable in vitro, the haemoglobin tetramer dissociates in the body into dimers, which are excreted in the urine within a few hours. Other problems include the absence of DPG resulting in a low P_{50}, and a high colloid oncotic pressure limiting the amount that can be used. The short half life and high oncotic pressure can be improved by either polymerisation or cross-linking of haemoglobin molecules. The P_{50} of the solution can be improved by using recombinant human haemoglobin rather than animal haemoglobin, and by choosing a specific variant of human haemoglobin (Presbyterian Hb) which has a naturally higher P_{50}.[47] Unfortunately, despite these advances, haemoglobin based oxygen carriers all have significant drawbacks in clinical use, mostly due to the haemoglobin scavenging NO and so causing vasoconstriction, release of inflammatory mediators and inhibition of platelet function. These effects are not theoretical: a meta-analysis of studies shows haemoglobin based blood substitutes cause an increased number of deaths and myocardial infarctions compared with controls.[46]

These limitations of free haemoglobin molecules have led to attempts to encapsulate haemoglobin within liposomes or artificial cell membranes.[45] Haemoglobin can be incorporated into a lipid vesicle, sometimes even including reducing agents and oxygen-affinity modifiers to produce a more functional oxygen carrying unit. Animal studies show these solutions have the potential to deliver useful quantities of oxygen to hypoxic tissues.[48]

The latest attempt at producing a haemoglobin-based oxygen carrier without relying on blood donation uses stem cell technology.[49] With the application of suitable growth factors human stem cells can be developed in vitro to produce mature RBCs with all the physiological characteristics of a normal RBC.

THE ROLE OF OXYGEN IN THE CELL

Dissolved molecular oxygen (dioxygen) enters into many metabolic processes in the mammalian body. Quantitatively much the most important is the cytochrome c oxidase system, which is responsible for about 90% of the total oxygen consumption of the body. However, cytochrome c oxidase is only one of more than 200 oxidases, which may be classified as follows.

Electron transfer oxidases. As a group, these oxidases involve the reduction of oxygen to superoxide anion, hydrogen peroxide or water, the last being the fully reduced state (see Chapter 26, Figure 26.2). The most familiar of this group of enzymes is cytochrome c oxidase. It is located in the mitochondria and is concerned in the production of the high energy phosphate bond in adenosine triphosphate (ATP), which is the main source of biological energy. This process is described in greater detail below.

Oxygen transferases (dioxygenases). This group of oxygenases incorporate oxygen into substrates without the formation of any reduced oxygen product. Familiar examples are cyclo-oxygenase and lipoxygenase, which are concerned in the first stage of conversion of arachidonic acid into prostaglandins and leukotrienes (see Chapter 12).

Mixed function oxidases. These oxidases result in oxidation of both a substrate and a co-substrate, which is most commonly NADPH. The best known examples are the cytochrome P-450 hydroxylases, which play an important role in detoxification.

ENERGY PRODUCTION

Most of the energy deployed in the mammalian body is derived from the oxidation of food fuels, of which the most important is glucose:

$$C_6H_{12}O_6 + 6O_2 \rightarrow 6CO_2 + 6H_2O + energy$$

The equation accurately describes the combustion of glucose in vitro, but is only a crude, overall representation of the oxidation of glucose in the body. The direct reaction would not produce energy in a form in which it could be utilised by the body so biological oxidation proceeds by a large number of stages with phased production of energy. This energy is not immediately released but is stored mainly by means of the reaction of adenosine diphosphate (ADP) with inorganic phosphate ion to form ATP. The third phosphate group in ATP is held by a high energy bond that releases its energy when ATP is split back into ADP and inorganic phosphate ion during any of the myriad of biological reactions requiring energy input. ADP is thus recycled indefinitely, with ATP acting as a short-term store of energy, available in a form that may be used directly for work such as muscle contraction, ion pumping, protein synthesis and secretion.

There is no large store of ATP in the body and it must be synthesised continuously as it is being used. The ATP/ADP ratio is an indication of the level of energy that is currently carried in the ADP/ATP system, and the ratio is normally related to the state of oxidation of the cell. The ADP/ATP system is not the only short-term energy store in the body but it is the most important.

Complete oxidation of glucose requires a three-stage process, the first of which, glycolysis, is independent of oxygen supply.

GLYCOLYSIS AND ANAEROBIC ENERGY PRODUCTION

Figure 11.13 shows detail of the glycolytic (Embden–Meyerhof) pathway for the conversion of glucose to lactic acid. Glycolysis occurs entirely within the cytoplasm, and under normal conditions proceeds only as far as pyruvic acid, which then enters the citric acid cycle (see below). In RBCs, where there is an absence of the respiratory enzymes located in the mitochondria, or in other cells when cellular P_{O_2} falls below its critical level, lactic acid is produced. Figure 11.13 shows that, over all, four molecules of ATP are produced, but two of these are consumed in the priming stages prior to the formation of fructose-1,6-diphosphate. The conversion of glyceraldehyde-3-phosphate to 3-phosphoglyceric acid produces a hydrogen ion, which becomes bound to extramitochondrial nicotinamide adenine dinucleotide (NAD). This hydrogen cannot enter the mitochondria for further oxidative metabolism so is taken up lower down the pathway by the reduction of pyruvic acid to lactic acid.

This series of changes is therefore associated with the net formation of only two molecules of ATP from one of glucose:

$$Glucose + 2Pi + 2ADP \rightarrow$$
$$2Lactic\ acid + 2ATP + 2H_2O$$

(Pi = inorganic phosphate)

However, considerable chemical energy remains in the lactic acid which, in the presence of oxygen, can be reconverted to pyruvic acid and then oxidised in the citric acid cycle, producing a further 36 molecules of ATP. Alternatively, lactic acid may be converted into liver glycogen to await more favourable conditions for oxidation.

In spite of their inefficiency for ATP production, anaerobic metabolism is of great biological importance and was universal before the atmospheric P_{O_2}

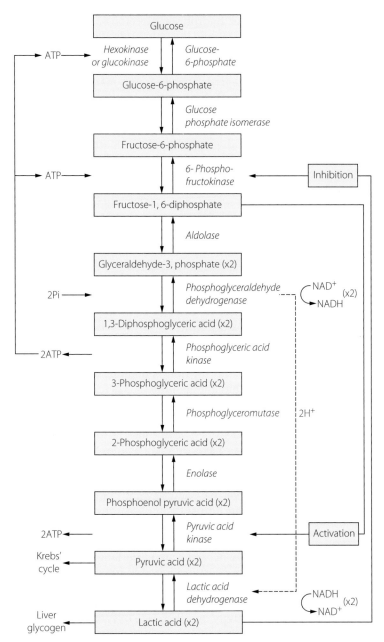

Fig. 11.13 The glycolytic (Embden–Meyerhof) pathway for anaerobic metabolism of glucose. From glyceraldehyde-3-phosphate downwards, two molecules of each intermediate are formed from one of glucose. Note the consumption of two molecules of ATP in the first three steps. These must be set against the total production of four molecules of ATP, leaving a net gain of only two molecules of ATP from each molecule of glucose. All the acids are largely ionised at tissue pH.

was sufficiently high for aerobic pathways (Chapter 1). Anaerobic metabolism is still the rule in anaerobic bacteria and also in the mammalian body when energy requirements outstrip oxygen supply as, for example, during severe exercise or during hypoxia.

AEROBIC ENERGY PRODUCTION

The aerobic pathway permits the release of far greater quantities of energy from the same amount of substrate and is therefore used whenever possible. Under aerobic conditions, most reactions of the glycolytic pathway remain unchanged, with two very important exceptions. The conversion of glyceraldehyde-3-phosphate to 3-phosphoglyceric acid occurs in the mitochondrion, when the two NADH molecules formed may enter oxidative phosphorylation (see below) rather than producing lactic acid. Similarly, pyruvate does not continue along the pathway to lactic acid but diffuses

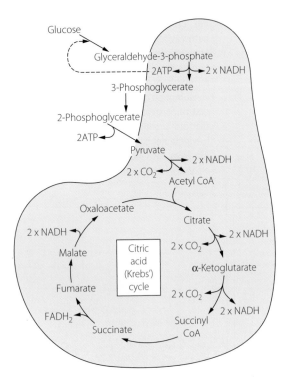

Fig. 11.14 Oxidative metabolic pathway of glucose by the citric acid cycle. The shaded area represents the mitochondrion and indicates the reactions that can take place only within them. Substances shown straddling the shaded area are capable of diffusion across the mitochondrial membrane. Many stages of the glycolytic pathway (Figure 11.13) have been omitted for clarity. Note that one molecule of glucose will produce two molecules of all the other intermediate substances. Only 2 molecules of ATP are produced, along with 12 molecules of $NADPH_2$, each of which enters oxidative phosphorylation within the mitochondria producing 3 molecules of ATP (Figure 11.15).

into the mitochondria and enters the next stage of oxidative metabolism.

The citric acid (Krebs') cycle occurs within the mitochondria as shown in Figure 11.14. It consists of a series of reactions to reduce the length of the carbon chain of the molecules before adding a new 2-carbon chain (acetyl CoA) derived from glycolysis. During these reactions, six molecules of carbon dioxide are produced (for each molecule of glucose) along with a further 8 molecules of NADH and one molecule of $FADH_2$. Therefore in total, each glucose molecule yields 12 hydrogen ions bound to either NAD or FAD carrier molecules.

The scheme shown in Figure 11.14 also accounts for the consumption of oxygen in the metabolism

of fat. After hydrolysis, glycerol is converted into pyruvic acid while the fatty acids shed a series of 2-carbon molecules in the form of acetyl CoA. Pyruvic acid and acetyl CoA enter the citric acid cycle and are then degraded in the same manner as though they had been derived from glucose. Amino acids are dealt with in similar manner after deamination.

Oxidative phosphorylation is the final stage of energy production and again occurs in the mitochondria. The hydrogen ions from NADH or $FADH_2$ are passed along a chain of hydrogen carriers to combine with oxygen at cytochrome a_3, which is the end of the chain. Figure 11.15 shows the transport of hydrogen along the chain, which consists of structural entities just visible under the electron microscope and arranged in rows along the cristae of the mitochondria. Three molecules of ATP are formed at various stages of the chain during the transfer of each hydrogen ion. The process is not associated directly with the production of carbon dioxide, which is formed only in the citric acid cycle.

Cytochromes have a structure similar to haemoglobin with an iron containing haem complex bound within a large protein. Their activity is controlled by the availability of oxygen and hydrogen molecules, the local concentration of ADP and by some unidentified cytosolic factors.[50] Different cytochromes have different values for P_{50} and so may act as oxygen sensors in several areas of the body (page 71). There is evidence for an interaction between NO and several cytochromes, with NO forming nitrosyl complexes in a similar fashion to its reaction with haemoglobin (page 194).[30] It is postulated that NO, or NO derived nitrosyl compounds, may play an important role in controlling oxygen consumption at a mitochondrial level. High levels of endogenous NO, for example during sepsis, may produce sufficient inhibition of cytochrome activity and therefore oxygen consumption to contribute to the impaired tissue function seen in vital organs such as the heart.[30] The reduction of oxygen to water by cytochrome a_3 is inhibited by cyanide.

Significance of aerobic metabolism. Glycolysis under aerobic conditions and the citric acid cycle yields a total of 12 hydrogen molecules for each glucose molecule used. In turn, each hydrogen molecule enters oxidative phosphorylation to yield 3 ATP molecules. These, along with the two produced during glycolysis result in a total production of 38 ATP molecules.

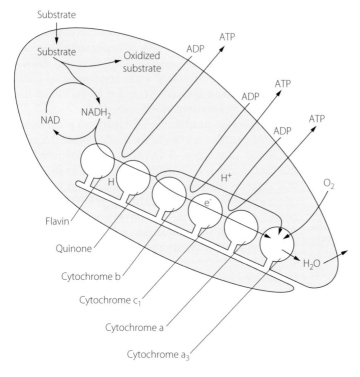

Substrate

Substrate

Oxidized
substrate

ATP

ADP

ATP

ADP

ATP

ADP

NADH$_2$

NAD

H

H$^+$

e$^-$

O$_2$

H$_2$O

Flavin

Quinone

Cytochrome b

Cytochrome c$_1$

Cytochrome a

Cytochrome a$_3$

Fig. 11.15 Diagrammatic representation of oxidative phosphorylation within the mitochondrion. Intramitochondrial NADH$_2$ produced from glycolysis and the citric acid cycle provides hydrogen to the first of a chain of hydrogen carriers that are attached to the cristae of the mitochondria. When the hydrogen reaches the cytochromes, ionisation occurs; the proton passes into the lumen of the mitochondrion while the electron is passed along the cytochromes where it converts ferric iron to the ferrous form. The final stage is at cytochrome a$_3$ where the proton and the electron combine with oxygen to form water. Three molecules of ADP are converted to ATP at the stages shown in the diagram. ADP and ATP can cross the mitochondrial membrane freely while there are separate pools of intra- and extra-mitochondrial NAD that cannot interchange.

In simplified form, the contrasting pathways can be shown as follows:

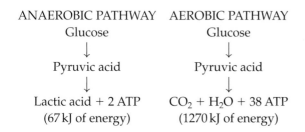

ANAEROBIC PATHWAY	AEROBIC PATHWAY
Glucose	Glucose
↓	↓
Pyruvic acid	Pyruvic acid
↓	↓
Lactic acid + 2 ATP	CO_2 + H_2O + 38 ATP
(67 kJ of energy)	(1270 kJ of energy)

In vitro combustion of glucose liberates 2820 kJ. mol^{-1} as heat. Thus, under conditions of oxidative metabolism, 45% of the total energy is made available for biological work, which compares favourably with most machines.

Use of anaerobic pathways must therefore either consume very much larger quantities of glucose or, alternatively, yield less ATP. In high energy consuming organs such as brain, kidney and liver it is not, in fact, possible to transfer the increased quantities of glucose and therefore these organs suffer ATP depletion under hypoxic conditions. In contrast, voluntary muscle is able to function satisfactorily on anaerobic metabolism during short periods of time and this is normal in the diving mammals.

The critical oxygen tension for aerobic metabolism. When the mitochondrial P_{O_2} is reduced, oxidative phosphorylation continues normally down to a level of about 0.3 kPa (2 mmHg). Below this level, oxygen consumption falls and the various members of the electron transport chain tend to revert to the reduced state. NADH/NAD$^+$ and lactate/pyruvate ratios rise and the ATP/ADP ratio falls. The critical P_{O_2} varies between different organs and different species but, as an approximation, a mitochondrial P_{O_2} of about 0.13 kPa (1 mmHg) may be taken as the level below which there is serious impairment of oxidative phosphorylation and a switch to anaerobic metabolism. This level is, of course, far below the critical arterial P_{O_2}, because there normally exists a large gradient of P_{O_2} between arterial blood and the site of utilisation of oxygen in the mitochondria, as part of the oxygen cascade (Figure 11.1). Tissue hypoxia is discussed further on page 367. The critical P_{O_2} for oxidative phosphorylation is also known as the Pasteur point and has applications beyond the pathophysiology of hypoxia in man. In particular, it has a powerful bearing on putrefaction, many forms of which are anaerobic metabolism resulting from a fall of P_{O_2} below the Pasteur point in, for example, polluted rivers.

TISSUE P_{O_2}

It is almost impossible to quantify tissue P_{O_2}. It is evident that there are differences between different organs, with the tissue P_{O_2} influenced not only by arterial P_{O_2} but also by the ratio of tissue oxygen consumption to perfusion. However, even greater difficulties arise from the regional variations in tissue P_{O_2} in different parts of the same organ, which are again presumably caused by regional variations in tissue perfusion and oxygen consumption. Nor is this the whole story. As described on page 155, movement of oxygen from capillaries into the tissue is by simple diffusion, with complex radial and longitudinal gradients in P_{O_2} around individual capillaries (see Figure 9.4). For a single cell, the capillary P_{O_2} will be that of the nearest section of capillary and so anywhere between the local arterial and venous values, and the final tissue P_{O_2} will also depend on the distance between the capillary and the cell, which may be up to $200\mu m$. These factors explain why the largest drop in P_{O_2} of the oxygen cascade is the final stage between capillary and mitochondrial P_{O_2} (Figure 11.1). In spite of this sometimes long diffusion path, and low value for mitochondrial P_{O_2}, oxygen supply is extremely efficient, and it is believed to be the supply of metabolic substrates (fatty acids and glucose) that normally limit cellular energy production.[51] Tissue P_{O_2} is thus an unsatisfactory quantitative index of the state of oxygenation of an organ, and indirect assessments must be made (page 210).

TRANSPORT OF OXYGEN FROM THE LUNGS TO THE CELL

THE CONCEPT OF OXYGEN DELIVERY

The most important function of the respiratory and circulatory systems is the supply of oxygen to the cells of the body in adequate quantity and at a satisfactory partial pressure. The quantity of oxygen made available to the body in one minute is known as oxygen delivery ($\dot{D}_{O_2}$) or oxygen flux, and is equal to cardiac output × arterial oxygen content.

At rest, the numerical values are approximately:

5000 ml blood per min × 20 ml O_2 per 100 ml blood
    (cardiac output)   (arterial oxygen content)
               = 1000 ml O_2 per min
               (oxygen delivery)

Of this $1000\,ml.min^{-1}$, approximately $250\,ml.min^{-1}$ are used by the conscious resting subject. The circulating blood thus loses 25% of its oxygen and the mixed venous blood is approximately 70% saturated (i.e. $95 - 25$). The 70% of unextracted oxygen forms an important reserve that may be drawn upon under the stress of such conditions as exercise, to which additional extraction forms one of the integrated adaptations (see Figure 15.3).

Oxygen consumption must clearly depend upon delivery but the relationship is non-linear. Modest reduction of oxygen delivery is well tolerated by the body, which is, within limits, able to draw on the reserve of unextracted venous oxygen without reduction of oxygen consumption. However, below a critical value for delivery, consumption is decreased and the subject shows signs of hypoxia. The important quantitative aspects of the relationship between oxygen consumption and delivery are considered below.

QUANTIFICATION OF OXYGEN DELIVERY

The arterial oxygen content consists predominantly of oxygen in combination with haemoglobin, and this fraction is given by the following expression:

$$Ca_{O_2} = Sa_{O_2} \times [Hb] \times 1.39$$

where Ca_{O_2} is the arterial oxygen content, Sa_{O2} is the arterial oxygen saturation (as a fraction) and [Hb] is the haemoglobin concentration of the blood; 1.39 is the volume of oxygen (ml) which has been found to combine with 1 g of haemoglobin (excluding dyshaemoglobins: see page 189).

To the combined oxygen must be added the oxygen in physical solution which will be of the order of $0.3\,ml.dl^{-1}$, and the expression for total arterial oxygen concentration may now be expanded thus:

$$
\begin{array}{cccccc}
Ca_{O_2} & = & (Sa_{O_2} & \times & [Hb] & \times & 1.39) & + & 0.3 \\
ml.dl^{-1} & & \%/100 & & g.dl^{-1} & & ml.g^{-1} & & ml.dl^{-1} \\
\end{array}
$$

e.g. $19 \quad = \quad (0.97 \quad \times \quad 14 \quad \times \quad 1.39) \quad + \quad 0.3$

$$(4)$$

Since oxygen delivery is the product of cardiac output and arterial oxygen content:

$$
\begin{array}{ccccc}
\dot{D}_{O_2} & = & \dot{Q} & \times & Ca_{O_2} \\
ml.min^{-1} & & l.min^{-1} & & ml.dl^{-1} \\
\end{array}
$$

e.g. $1000 \quad = \quad 5.25 \quad \times \quad 19 \quad\quad (5)$

$\dot{Q}$ is cardiac output (right-hand side is multiplied by a scaling factor of 10).

By combining equations (4) and (5) the full expression for oxygen delivery is as follows:

$$\dot{D}_{O_2} = \dot{Q} \times \{(Sa_{O_2} \times [Hb] \times 1.39) + 0.3\}$$

$$\text{ml.min}^{-1} \quad \text{l.min}^{-1} \quad \%/100 \quad \text{g.dl}^{-1} \quad \text{ml.g}^{-1} \quad \text{ml.dl}^{-1}$$

$$\text{e.g.} \quad 1000 = 5.25 \times \{(0.97 \times 14 \times 1.39) + 0.3\}$$

$$(6)$$

(right-hand side is multiplied by a scaling factor of 10).

For comparison between subjects, values for oxygen delivery must be related to body size, which is done by relating the value to body surface area. Oxygen delivery divided by surface area is known as oxygen delivery index and has units of $\text{ml.min}^{-1}.\text{m}^{-2}$.

INTERACTION OF THE VARIABLE FACTORS GOVERNING OXYGEN DELIVERY

Equation (6) contains, on the right hand side, three variable factors that govern oxygen delivery.

1. Cardiac output (or, for a particular organ, the regional blood flow). Failure of this factor has been termed 'stagnant anoxia'.
2. Arterial oxygen saturation. Failure of this (for whatever reason) has been termed 'anoxic anoxia'.
3. Haemoglobin concentration. Reduced haemoglobin as a cause of tissue hypoxia, has been termed 'anaemic anoxia'.

The classification of 'anoxia' into stagnant, anoxic and anaemic was proposed by Barcroft in 1920[52] and has stood the test of time. The three types of 'anoxia' may be conveniently displayed on a Venn diagram (Figure 11.16), which shows the possibility of combinations of any two types of anoxia or all three together. For example, the combination of anaemia and low cardiac output, which occurs in untreated haemorrhage, would be indicated by the overlapping area of the stagnant and anaemic circles (indicated by ×). If the patient also suffered from lung injury, he might then move into the central area, indicating the addition of anoxic anoxia. On a more cheerful note, compensations are more usual. Patients with anaemia normally have a high cardiac output; subjects resident at altitude have polycythaemia, and so on.

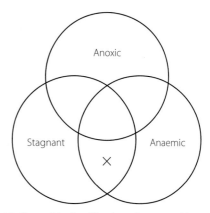

Fig. 11.16 Barcroft's classification of causes of hypoxia displayed on a Venn diagram to illustrate the possibility of combinations of more than one type of hypoxia. The lowest overlap, marked with a cross, shows coexistent anaemia and low cardiac output. The central area illustrates a combination of all three types of hypoxia (e.g. a patient with sepsis resulting in anaemia, circulatory failure and lung injury).

THE RELATIONSHIP BETWEEN OXYGEN DELIVERY AND CONSUMPTION

The relationship between $\dot{D}_{O_2}$ and oxygen consumption ($\dot{V}_{O_2}$) is best illustrated on the coordinates shown in Figure 11.17. The abscissa shows oxygen delivery as defined above, while consumption is shown on the ordinate. The fan of lines originating from the zero point indicate different values for oxygen extraction ($\dot{V}_{O_2}/\dot{D}_{O_2}$) expressed as a percentage. Because the mixed venous oxygen saturation is the arterial saturation less the extraction, it is a simple matter to indicate the mixed venous saturation, which corresponds to a particular value for extraction. The black dot indicates a typical normal resting point, with $\dot{D}_{O_2}$ of 1000 ml.min^{-1}, $\dot{V}_{O_2}$ of 250 ml.min^{-1} and extraction 25%.

When oxygen delivery is moderately reduced, for whatever reason, oxygen consumption tends to be maintained at its normal value by increasing oxygen extraction and therefore decreasing mixed venous saturation. There should be no evidence of additional anaerobic metabolism, such as increased lactate production. This is termed 'supply-independent oxygenation', a condition that applies provided that delivery remains above a critical value. This is shown by the horizontal line in Figure 11.18. Below the critical level of oxygen delivery, oxygen consumption decreases as a linear function of delivery. This is termed 'supply-dependent oxygenation'

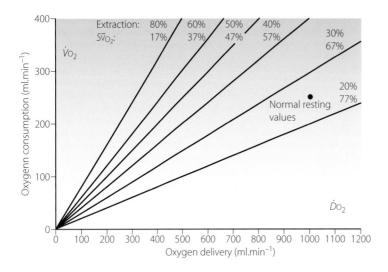

Fig. 11.17 Grid relating oxygen delivery and consumption to extraction and mixed venous oxygen saturation, on the assumption of 97% saturation for arterial blood. The spot marks the normal resting values.

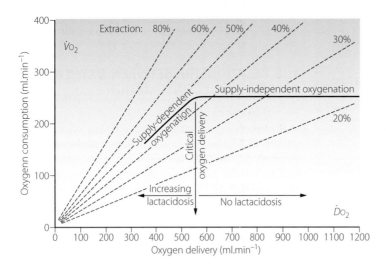

Fig. 11.18 This diagram is based on the grid shown in Figure 11.17. For an otherwise healthy subject, the thick horizontal line shows the extent to which oxygen delivery can be reduced without reducing oxygen consumption and causing signs of cellular hypoxia (supply-independent oxygenation). Below the postulated critical delivery, oxygen consumption becomes supply-dependent and there are signs of hypoxia. There is uncertainty of the exact values for critical delivery in otherwise healthy subjects.

and is usually accompanied by evidence of hypoxia, such as increased blood lactate and organ failure.

Pathological supply dependency of oxygen consumption has been a source of controversy for many years.[53] In critically ill patients, the transition between supply-dependent and supply-independent oxygen consumption (critical oxygen delivery, see Figure 11.18) was thought to move to the right, such that increasing oxygen delivery continued to increase oxygen consumption even at levels greater than those seen in normal healthy subjects.[54] Early work in critical care units claimed better survival in patients in whom oxygen delivery, and therefore consumption,

was increased above normal values.[53,55] Sadly, larger randomised studies failed to confirm the benefits of this aggressive management of oxygen delivery.[56] Furthermore, a value for the critical oxygen delivery in ill patients remained elusive,[57] mostly due to the considerable difficulties in assessing the relationship between oxygen consumption and delivery in this group. It is therefore possible that the value for critical oxygen delivery is unchanged in critically ill patients, and that pathological supply dependency may not exist at all, with much of the earlier data resulting from methodological problems and mathematical coupling of the variables being measured. Outcome benefits to patients from deliberately increasing $\dot{D}o_2$ seem to be minimal or non-existent,[56,58] and current advice is to concentrate more closely on achieving normal values for cardiac output, haemoglobin and blood volume, rather than pursuing supra-normal targets.

OXYGEN STORES

In spite of its great biological importance, oxygen is a very difficult gas to store in a biological system. There is no satisfactory method of physical storage in the body. Haemoglobin is the most efficient chemical carrier, but more than 0.5 kg is required to carry 1 g of oxygen. The concentration of haemoglobin in blood far exceeds the concentration of any other protein in any body fluid. Even so, the quantity of oxygen in the blood is barely sufficient for three minutes' metabolism in the resting state. It is a fact of great clinical importance that the body oxygen stores are so small and, if replenishment ceases, they are normally insufficient to sustain life for more than a few minutes. The principal stores are shown in Table 11.4.

While breathing air, not only are the total oxygen stores very small but also, to make matters worse, only part of the stores can be released without an unacceptable reduction in Po_2. Half of the oxygen in blood is still retained when the Po_2 is reduced to 3.5 kPa (26 mmHg). Myoglobin is even more reluctant to part with its oxygen and very little can be released above a Po_2 of 2.7 kPa (20 mmHg).

Breathing oxygen causes a substantial increase in total oxygen stores. Most of the additional oxygen is accommodated in the alveolar gas from which 80% may be withdrawn without causing the Po_2 to fall below the normal value. With 2400 ml of easily available oxygen after breathing oxygen, there is no difficulty in breath holding for several minutes without becoming hypoxic.

The small size of the oxygen stores means that changes in factors affecting the alveolar or arterial Po_2 will produce their full effects very quickly after the change. This is in contrast to carbon dioxide where the size of the stores buffers the body against rapid changes (page 170). Figure 11.19 compares the time course of changes in Po_2 and Pco_2 produced by the same changes in ventilation. Figure 10.11 showed how the time course of changes of Pco_2 is different for falling and rising Pco_2.

Table 11.4 Principal stores of body oxygen

	WHILE BREATHING AIR (ml)	WHILE BREATHING 100% OXYGEN (ml)
In the lungs (FRC)	450	3000
In the blood	850	950
Dissolved in tissue fluids	50	?100
Combined with myoglobin	?200	?200
Total	1550	4250

FRC, functional residual capacity.

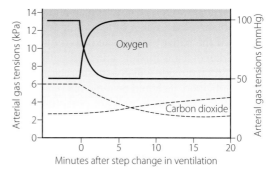

Fig. 11.19 The upper pair of curves indicate the rate of change of arterial Po_2 following a step change in ventilation. Half of the total change occurs in about 30 seconds. The rising curve could be produced by an increase of alveolar ventilation from 2 to 4 l.min^{-1} while breathing air (see Figure 11.2). The falling curve could result from the corresponding reduction of alveolar ventilation from 4 to 2 l.min^{-1}. The lower pair of broken curves indicate the time course of changes in Pco_2, which are much slower than for oxygen (these changes are shown in greater detail in Figure 10.11).

Factors that reduce the Po_2 always act rapidly, but two examples of changes that produce anoxia illustrate different degrees of 'rapid'.

Circulatory arrest. When the circulation is arrested, hypoxia supervenes as soon as the oxygen in the tissues and stagnant capillaries has been exhausted. In the case of the brain, with its high rate of oxygen consumption, there is only about 10 seconds before consciousness is lost. Circulatory arrest also differs from other forms of hypoxia in the failure of clearance of products of anaerobic metabolism (e.g. lactic acid) which should not occur in arterial hypoxaemia.

Apnoea. The rate of onset of anoxia depends on the initial alveolar Po_2, the lung volume and the rate of oxygen consumption. It is, for example, more rapid while swimming underwater than while breath holding at rest in the laboratory. Generally speaking, after breathing air, 90 seconds of apnoea results in a substantial fall of Po_2 to a level that threatens loss of consciousness. If a patient has previously inhaled a few breaths of oxygen, the arterial Po_2 should remain above 13.3 kPa (100 mmHg) for at least 3 minutes of apnoea, and this is the basis of the usual method of protection against hypoxia during any deliberate interference with ventilation, as for example during tracheal intubation.

In view of the rapid changes shown in Figure 11.19, it follows that, for a patient breathing air, a pulse oximeter will probably give an earlier indication of underventilation than will a carbon dioxide analyser. However, if the patient is protected from hypoxia by the inhalation of a gas mixture enriched with oxygen, then the carbon dioxide will give the earlier indication of hypoventilation. It should be remembered that oxygen levels change quickly and are potentially much more dangerous. Carbon dioxide levels change only slowly (in response to a change in ventilation) and are usually less dangerous.

CONTROL OF THE INSPIRED OXYGEN CONCENTRATION[59]

Much of this chapter has been concerned with the theoretical basis for selection of the optimal inspired oxygen concentration for a particular pathophysiological state. In clinical practice the administration of oxygen to ill patients has become almost ubiquitous, both in the hospital and community settings. Recently published guidelines[59] have sought to challenge this 'oxygen culture'[60] by recommending that oxygen therapy should, wherever possible, by guided by the patient's oxygen saturation. Also, where oxygen is being used to treat tissue hypoxia treatment should also encompass correcting anaemia and low cardiac output states. Numerous systems exist for increasing the inspired oxygen concentration, and an understanding of these is crucial for effective therapy.

FIXED PERFORMANCE SYSTEMS

These allow the delivery of a known concentration of oxygen, independent of the patient's respiratory system – that is, the oxygen concentration delivered is unaffected by respiratory rate, tidal volume and inspiratory flow rate. Methods may be divided into low flow (closed) or high flow (open) delivery systems.

Closed delivery systems. A crucial factor in oxygen therapy is the nature of the seal between the patient's airway and the external breathing apparatus. Airtight seals may be obtained with cuffed tracheal or tracheostomy tubes or, at low airway pressures, with a tight fitting facemask or laryngeal mask airway. These devices should give complete control over the composition of the inspired gas. Any closed delivery system requires the use of a breathing system that provides suitable separation of inspired and expired gases to prevent rebreathing, and does not present significant resistance to breathing.

Open delivery systems. Most disposable oxygen masks do not attempt to provide an airtight fit. An alternative solution to the problem of the airtight seal is to provide a high flow of gas, which can vent to atmosphere between the mask and the face, thus preventing the inflow of air. The required flow of air/oxygen mixture needs to be in excess of the peak inspiratory flow rate. For normal resting ventilation this is approximately $30 \, l.min^{-1}$ but in patients with respiratory distress may be considerably greater.

Oxygen may be passed through the jet of a Venturi to entrain air. Venturi based devices are a convenient and highly economical method of preparing high flows of oxygen mixtures in the range 25–40% concentration. For example, $3 \, l.min^{-1}$ of oxygen passed through the jet of a Venturi with an entrainment ratio of 8:1 will deliver $27 \, l.min^{-1}$ of 30% oxygen. Higher oxygen concentrations require a lower entrainment ratio and therefore a higher oxygen flow in order to maintain an adequate total delivered flow rate. Commercially available Venturi masks now have a variety of colour coded Venturi attachments that indicate the required oxygen flow rate, the inspired oxygen concentration achieved and the total gas flow rate. With an adequate flow rate of the air/oxygen mixture, the Venturi mask need not fit the face with an airtight seal. The high flow rate escapes round the cheeks as well as through the holes in the mask, and room air is effectively excluded. Numerous studies have indicated that the Venturi mask gives excellent control over the inspired oxygen concentration that is mostly unaffected by variations in the ventilation of the patient except at high oxygen concentrations.[61] There is no doubt that this is the most satisfactory method of controlling the inspired oxygen concentration of a patient who is breathing spontaneously without tracheal intubation.

Control of the patient's gaseous environment. The popularity of oxygen tents declined because of their large volume and high rate of leakage, which made it difficult to attain and maintain a high oxygen concentration unless the volume was reduced and a high gas flow rate used. In addition, the fire hazard cannot be ignored. These problems are minimised when the patient is an infant, and oxygen control within an incubator is a satisfactory method of administering a precise oxygen concentration.

VARIABLE PERFORMANCE DEVICES[61]

Simple disposable oxygen masks and nasal catheters aim to blow oxygen at or into the air passages. The oxygen is mixed with inspired air to give an inspired oxygen concentration that is a complex function of the geometry of the device, the oxygen flow rate, the patient's ventilation and whether the patient is breathing through his mouth or nose. The effective inspired oxygen concentration is impossible to predict and may vary between very wide limits. These devices cannot be used for oxygen therapy when the exact inspired oxygen concentration is critical (e.g. ventilatory failure), but are useful in less critical situations such as recovery from routine anaesthesia. With simple oxygen masks a small inspiratory reservoir will store fresh gas during expiration for use during inspiration, which will tend to increase the inspired oxygen concentration but, again, in a somewhat unpredictable fashion.

With a device such as a nasal catheter or prongs, the lower the ventilation, the greater will be the fractional contribution of the fixed flow of oxygen to the inspired gas mixture. There is thus an approximate compensation for hypoventilation, with greater oxygen concentrations being delivered at lower levels of ventilation. Arterial P_{O_2} may then be maintained in spite of a progressively falling ventilation. However, this will do nothing to prevent the rise in P_{CO_2}, which may reach a dangerous level without the appearance of cyanosis to warn that all is not well.[62]

CYANOSIS

Cyanosis describes a blue discoloration of a subject's skin and mucous membranes, and is almost universally caused by arterial hypoxaemia. Though now regarded as a sign of rather advanced hypoxia, there must have been countless occasions in which the appearance of cyanosis has given warning of hypoventilation, pulmonary shunting, stagnant circulation or decreased oxygen concentration of inspired gas. Indeed, it is interesting to speculate on the additional hazards to life if gross arterial hypoxaemia could occur without overt changes in the colour of the blood.

CENTRAL AND PERIPHERAL CYANOSIS

If shed arterial blood is seen to be purple, this is a reliable indication of arterial desaturation. However, when skin or mucous membrane is inspected, most of the blood which colours the tissue is lying in veins (i.e. sub-papillary venous plexuses) and its oxygen content is related to the arterial oxygen content as follows:

$$\begin{matrix} \text{venous oxygen} \\ \text{content} \end{matrix} = \begin{matrix} \text{arterial oxygen} \\ \text{content} \end{matrix} - \begin{matrix} \text{arterial/venous} \\ \text{oxygen content} \\ \text{difference} \end{matrix}$$

The last term may be expanded in terms of the tissue metabolism and perfusion:

$$\begin{matrix} \text{venous} \\ \text{oxygen} \\ \text{content} \end{matrix} = \begin{matrix} \text{arterial} \\ \text{oxygen} \\ \text{content} \end{matrix} - \frac{\text{tissue oxygen consumption}}{\text{tissue blood flow}}$$

In normal circumstances, the oxygen consumption by the skin is low in relation to its circulation, so the second term on the right hand side of the second equation is generally small. Therefore, the cutaneous venous oxygen content is close to that of the arterial blood and inspection of the skin usually gives a reasonable indication of arterial oxygen content. However, when circulation is reduced in relation to skin oxygen consumption, cyanosis may occur in the presence of normal arterial oxygen levels. This occurs typically in patients with low cardiac output or in cold weather. Vigorous coughing, particularly when lying flat, or placing a patient in the Trendelenburg position causes the skin capillaries of the upper body to become engorged with venous blood, once again causing the appearance of cyanosis with normal arterial oxygen content.

SENSITIVITY OF CYANOSIS AS AN INDICATION OF HYPOXAEMIA

Two factors may affect the ability to detect cyanosis. Anaemia will inevitably make cyanosis less likely to occur, and it is now generally accepted that cyanosis can be detected when *arterial* blood contains greater than $1.5 \, g.dl^{-1}$ of reduced haemoglobin,[63] or at an arterial oxygen saturation of 85–90%, although there is much variation. Such levels would probably correspond to a 'capillary' reduced haemoglobin concentration of about $3 \, g.dl^{-1}$. The source of illumination can also affect the perceived colour of a patient's skin.[64] Some fluorescent tubes tend to make the patient look pinker and others impart a bluer tinge to the patient. The former gives false negatives (no cyanosis in the presence of hypoxaemia), while the latter gives false positives (cyanosis in the absence of hypoxaemia). However, the total number of false results is approximately the same with all tubes and provided all areas of the same hospital are illuminated with the same type of tube this effect is unlikely to adversely affect the assessment of a patient's colour.

Thus the appearance of cyanosis is considerably influenced by the circulation, patient position, haemoglobin concentration and lighting conditions. Even when all these are optimal, cyanosis is by no means a precise indication of the arterial oxygen level and it should be regarded as a warning sign rather than a measurement. Cyanosis is detected in about half of patients who have an arterial saturation of 93%, and about 95% of patients with a saturation of 89%.[64] In other words, cyanosis is not seen in 5% of patients at or below a saturation of 89% (arterial $Po_2 \approx 7.5 \, kPa$ or $56 \, mmHg$). It is quite clear that absence of cyanosis does not necessarily mean normal arterial oxygen levels.

Non-hypoxic cyanosis has several causes, all of which are rare, but worth considering in a patient who appears cyanosed but displays no other evidence of hypoxia. Sulph-haemoglobin, and more importantly methaemoglobin (at concentrations of $1.5 \, g.dl^{-1}$) cause a blue-grey appearance, and chronic use of drugs or remedies that include gold or silver have been reported to cause 'pseudo-cyanosis'.[65]

PRINCIPLES OF MEASUREMENT OF OXYGEN LEVELS

OXYGEN CONCENTRATION IN GAS SAMPLES

Para-magnetic analysers rely on the fact that oxygen will influence an electrically generated magnetic field in direct proportion to its concentration in a mixture of gases. A particularly attractive feature of the method for physiological use is the complete lack of interference by other gases likely to be present as significant paramagnetic properties are unique to oxygen. Early paramagnetic analysers were cumbersome, delicate and had slow response times, but technological progress has led to the availability of inexpensive, accurate and robust analysers that are now found in a whole range of anaesthetic and intensive care equipment. Measurement of breath-to-breath changes in oxygen concentrations of respired gases requires an instrument with a response time of less than about $300 \, ms$ and current paramagnetic analysers are easily capable of this.

Fuel cells have similarities to the polarographic electrode described below. An oxygen permeable membrane covers a cell made up of a gold cathode and lead anode separated by potassium hydroxide, which generates a current in proportion to the oxygen concentration. The response time is many seconds, so these analysers are not suitable for measuring inspired and expired oxygen concentrations. No electrical input is needed, the fuel cell acting like a battery generating its own power from the absorption of oxygen. However, the cell therefore also has a limited lifespan, depending on the total amount of oxygen to which it is exposed over time, but in normal clinical use, fuel cells last several months.

BLOOD Po_2

Previous chemical based analyses have now been completely replaced by a single method:

Polarography. This method, first described by Clark in 1956,[66] is based on a cell formed by a silver anode and a platinum cathode, both in contact with an electrolyte in dilute solution. If a potential difference of about $700 \, mV$ is applied to the cell, a current is passed that is directly proportional to the Po_2 of the electrolyte in the region of the cathode. In use, the electrolyte is separated from the sample by a thin membrane that is permeable to oxygen. The electrolyte rapidly attains the same Po_2 as the sample and the current passed by the cell is proportional to the Po_2 of the sample, which may be gas, blood or other liquids. Gas mixtures are normally used for regular calibration, and an important source of error is the difference in reading between blood and gas of the same Po_2. Estimates of the ratio vary between 1.0 and 1.17 but it may change unexpectedly due to changes in the position of the membrane. This source of error has been greatly reduced in modern micro-electrodes which consume much less oxygen at the cathode. The error may be detected and prevented by calibration with tonometer-equilibrated blood, which is simple to perform. Frequent measurement of Po_2 in blood samples leads to protein deposition on the membrane, which over time forms a diffusion barrier between the sample and the electrolyte. Regular cleaning with a proteolytic solution is therefore required.

Polarographic electrodes may now be made small enough to facilitate continuous intra-arterial monitoring of Po_2, and a photochemical Po_2 sensor has also been developed.[67] Along with pH and Pco_2 sensors (page 174) the intra-arterial catheter remains less than 0.5 mm in diameter.

Errors in measuring oxygen levels. Errors arising from the handling of samples for blood gas analysis are considered on page 174. Temperature has a marked effect on Po_2 measurement. If blood Po_2 is measured at a lower temperature than the patient's, the measured Po_2 will be less than the Po_2 of the blood while it was in the patient. It is usual to maintain the measuring apparatus at 37°C, and, if the patient's body temperature differs from this by more than 1°C, then a significant error will result. Automated blood gas machines correct for this automatically, provided the patient's temperature is entered.

Transcutaneous Po_2.[68] Cutaneous venous or capillary blood Po_2 may, under ideal conditions, be close to the arterial Po_2, but a modest reduction in skin perfusion will cause a substantial fall in Po_2 since the oxygen is consumed at the flat part of the dissociation curve, where small changes in content correspond to large changes in Po_2. As for transcutaneous Pco_2 (page 174), heating of skin to 44°C minimises differences between arterial and capillary/skin Po_2, which can be measured by a directly applied polarographic electrode.

OXYGEN SATURATION[10]

Blood oxygen saturation is measured photometrically. Near infra-red absorption spectra for different forms of haemoglobin[69] are shown in Figure 11.20. Methods are based on the fact that the absorption of monochromatic light of certain wavelengths is the same (isobestic) for reduced and oxygenated haemoglobin (800 nm). At other wavelengths there is a marked difference between the absorption of transmitted or reflected light by the two forms of haemoglobin. Use of a greater number of different wavelengths also allows the detection and quantification of other commonly present haemoglobins. For example current generations of co-oximeter measure absorption at 128 different wavelengths and from the spectra obtained can calculate the quantities of O_2Hb, HHb, $COHb$ and $metHb$.

Oxygen saturation (So_2) may be derived from Po_2, a process which is performed automatically by some blood gas analysers (page 191). This is reasonably accurate above a Po_2 of about 7.3 kPa (55 mmHg) but is inaccurate at lower tensions because, on the steep

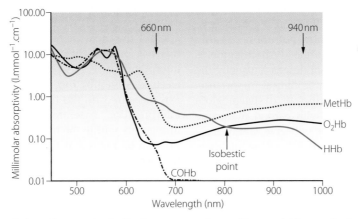

Fig. 11.20 Near infra-red absorption spectra for the four common types of haemoglobin seen *in vivo*. The isobestic point for oxyhaemoglobin (O_2Hb) and deoxyhaemoglobin (HHb) is shown. To measure oxygen saturation, pulse oximeters use two wavelengths at around 660 and 940 nm, where the absorptivities of O_2Hb and HHb differ significantly. If measurement of carboxyhaemoglobin and methaemoglobin is also required, a greater number of wavelengths must be used, and current generations of co-oximeter use over 100 different wavelengths. (Data from reference 69.)

part of the curve, the saturation changes by 3% for a Po_2 change of only 0.13 kPa (1 mmHg).

Pulse oximetry.[70] Saturation may be measured photometrically in vivo as well as in vitro. Light at two different wavelengths is either transmitted through a finger or an ear lobe or else is reflected from the skin, usually on the forehead. The usual wavelengths used are 660 nm, where there is a large difference between the oxy- and deoxyhaemoglobin spectra (Figure 11.20), and 940 nm, close to the isobestic point. With the original techniques, most of the blood that was visualised was venous or capillary rather than arterial, and the result therefore depended on there being a brisk cutaneous blood flow to minimise the arterial/venous oxygen difference. The older techniques have now been completely replaced by pulse oximeters, which relate the optical densities at the two wavelengths to the pulse wave detected by the same sensor. The signal between the pulse waves is subtracted from the signal at the height of the pulse wave, the difference being due to the inflowing arterial blood and so reflecting the saturation of the arterial blood.

In the same manner as for the measurement of Hüfner's constant (page 189), the presence of dyshaemoglobins (COHb and metHb) has caused controversy regarding the terminology used when discussing pulse oximetry.[10] Oxygen saturation, as originally defined by Christian Bohr, is the ratio of O_2Hb to active, oxygen binding, Hb (= O_2Hb + HHb), rather than the more commonly used definition of the ratio of O_2Hb to total Hb. The original definition is the more relevant as the COHb and metHb do not carry oxygen and do not affect pulse oximeter readings.[10] Pulse oximeter So_2 values are therefore a good assessment of pulmonary oxygenation, but not necessarily of oxygen carriage. Provided the dyshaemoglobins are only present in small quantities, as is usually the case, this distinction is of minor clinical importance. However, when larger quantities of dyshaemoglobins are present, particularly with carbon monoxide poisoning, the pulse oximeter will give falsely reassuring readings. For example, if 30% of the total haemoglobin present is bound to CO and Po_2 is normal, the pulse oximeter will read normal values despite the oxygen content of the blood being reduced by 30%. With metHb a more complex situation results because its absorption spectrum is more similar to O_2Hb and HHb than that of COHb (Figure 11.20) so it causes a slight reduction in So_2 readings up to about 20% metHb. At higher levels of metHb pulse oximeter readings tend to become fixed at about 85%.

There are many other sources of error with pulse oximetry. Currently available pulse oximeters continue to function even in the presence of arterial hypotension, although there may be a delayed indication of changes in So_2,[71] and readings become less accurate below a systolic blood pressure of 80 mmHg.[72] Anaemia tends to exaggerate desaturation readings: at a haemoglobin concentration of 8 g.dl^{-1} normal saturations were correctly recorded but there was a mean bias of -15% at a true So_2 of 53.6%.[73] Patients with dark skin were previously reported to have accurate readings with pulse oximetry, but some bias has been demonstrated at lower So_2 values (<80%).[74] If fingers or toes are used for pulse oximetry then nail polish should be removed. Different coloured polishes cause variable decreases in So_2 values, with red/purple colours having less effect and darker or green/blue colours causing an average of between 1.6 and 5.5% fall in So_2 values.[75,76] Acrylic nails have also been shown to cause minor inaccuracies in pulse oximeter readings with some, but not all, instruments.[77]

Calibration of pulse oximeters presents a problem. Optical filters may be used for routine calibration, but the gold standard is calibration against arterial blood Po_2 or saturation, which is seldom undertaken. When oxygenation is critical, there is no substitute for direct measurement of arterial Po_2.

TISSUE Po_2

Clearly the tissue Po_2 is of greater significance than the Po_2 at various intermediate stages higher in the oxygen cascade. It would therefore appear logical to attempt the measurement of Po_2 in the tissues, but this has proved difficult both in technique and in interpretation. For experimental procedures needle electrodes may be inserted directly into tissue, and Po_2 measured on the tip of a needle. Difficulties of interpretation arise from the fact that Po_2 varies immensely within the tissue, so even if a mean tissue Po_2 can be measured this may not represent Po_2 in the more relevant 'lethal corner' region (page 156).

Tissue surface electrodes. A miniaturised polarographic electrode may be placed on or attached to the surface of an organ to indicate the Po_2. Interpretation of the reading is subject to many of the same limitations as with the needle electrode. Nevertheless, tissue surface Po_2 may provide the surgeon with useful information regarding perfusion and viability in cases of organ ischaemia.

Near infra-red spectroscopy.[78] In tissues that are relatively translucent the biochemical state of tissue oxidation may be determined by the use of transmission spectroscopy in the near infra-red (700–1000 nm). The state of relative oxidation of haemoglobin and cytochrome a_3 may be determined within this wave band. At present it is feasible to study *transmission* spectroscopy over a path length up to about 9 cm, which is sufficient to permit monitoring of the brain of newborn infants. Use in adults requires *reflectance* spectroscopy and does allow assessment of oxygenation in, for example, an area of a few cubic centimetres of brain tissue. This is useful, for example, during surgery on the carotid arteries when changes in oxygenation in the area supplied by the artery concerned can be followed. However, the technique has failed to gain widespread acceptance because of interference from extracranial tissue, particularly scalp blood flow, and difficulties with calibrating the readings and defining any 'normal' values.

Indirect assessment of tissue oxygenation.[79] Such are the difficulties of measurements of tissue Po_2 that in clinical practice it is more usual simply to seek evidence of anaerobic tissue metabolism. In the absence of this, tissue perfusion and oxygenation can be assumed to be acceptable. Indirect methods that assess global (i.e. whole body) tissue perfusion include mixed venous oxygen saturation, measured either by sampling pulmonary arterial blood or using a fibreoptic catheter to measure oxygen saturation continuously in the pulmonary artery. Blood lactate levels also provide a global indication of tissue perfusion. However, acceptable global tissue oxygenation provides no reassurance about function either of regions in an individual organ or in an entire organ. Methods of assessing oxygenation in a specific tissue have focused on the gut because of ease of access and the observation that gut blood flow is often the first to be reduced when oxygen delivery is inadequate. Gastric intramucosal pH measurement allows an assessment to be made of cellular pH within the stomach mucosa, which has been shown to correlate with other assessments of tissue oxygenation and patient well-being during critical illness.

MEASUREMENT OF OXYGEN CONSUMPTION AND DELIVERY

OXYGEN CONSUMPTION

There are three main methods for the measurement of oxygen consumption:

1. Oxygen loss from (or replacement into) a closed breathing system.
2. Subtraction of the expired from the inspired volume of oxygen.
3. Multiplication of cardiac output by arterial/mixed venous oxygen content difference.

Oxygen loss from a closed breathing system. Probably the simplest method of measuring oxygen consumption is by observing the loss of volume from a closed-circuit spirometer, with expired carbon dioxide absorbed by soda lime. It is essential that the spirometer should initially contain an oxygen enriched mixture so that the inspired oxygen concentration does not fall to a level that is dangerous for the subject or patient. Alternatively, a known flow rate of oxygen may be added to maintain the volume of the spirometer and its oxygen concentration constant: under these conditions, the oxygen inflow rate must equal the oxygen consumption. The technique may be adapted to the conditions of artificial ventilation (Figure 11.21), but the technique, although accurate, is cumbersome.[80]

Subtraction of expired from inspired volume of oxygen. The essence of the technique is subtraction of the volume of oxygen breathed out (expired minute volume × mixed expired oxygen concentration) from the volume of oxygen breathed in (inspired minute volume × inspired oxygen concentration). The difference between the inspired and expired minute volumes is a very important factor in achieving accuracy with the method, particularly when a high concentration of oxygen is inhaled. Inspired and expired minute volumes differ as a result of the respiratory exchange ratio, and also any exchange of inert gas (e.g. nitrogen) that might occur. On the assumption that the patient is in equilibrium for nitrogen, and the mass of nitrogen inspired is the same as that expired, it follows that the ratio of inspired/expired minute volumes is inversely proportional to the respective ratios of nitrogen concentrations. Therefore:

$$\text{Inspired minute volume} = \text{expired minute volume} \times \frac{\text{Expired nitrogen concentration}}{\text{Inspired nitrogen concentration}}$$

This is the basis of the classical Douglas bag technique, in which expired gas is measured for volume, and analysed for oxygen and carbon dioxide concentrations. The expired nitrogen concentration is determined by subtraction and the inspired minute

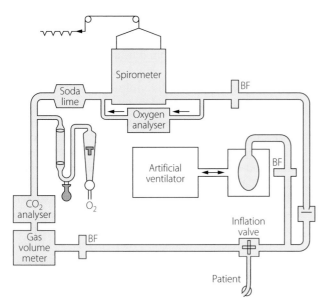

Fig. 11.21 A closed circuit spirometer system for measurement of oxygen consumption of a patient ventilated artificially by means of a box-bag system. When the system is in equilibrium, oxygen consumption is indicated by the oxygen added to the system, and carbon dioxide output is measured as the product of expired minute volume and mean carbon dioxide concentration in the expired gas. BF, bacterial filter. (Reproduced from reference 81 by permission of the Editor and publishers of Critical Care Medicine.)

volume derived. The approach has been automated by several manufacturers and their systems can be used satisfactorily during artificial ventilation.[81]

Multiplication of cardiac output by arterial/mixed venous oxygen content difference. This approach is the reverse of using the Fick principle for measurement of cardiac output (see page 113) and is commonly known as the reversed Fick technique:

$$\dot{V}_{O_2} = \dot{Q}\,(Ca_{O_2} - C\bar{v}_{O_2})$$

where $\dot{V}_{O_2}$ is the oxygen consumption, $\dot{Q}$ is the cardiac output, Ca_{O_2} is the arterial oxygen content and $C\bar{v}_{O_2}$ is the mixed venous oxygen content.

The technique is essentially invasive as the cardiac output must be measured by an independent method (usually thermodilution), and it is also necessary to sample arterial and mixed venous blood, the latter preferably from the pulmonary artery. Nevertheless it is convenient in the critical care situation where the necessary vascular lines may be in place.

The method has a larger random error than the gasometric techniques described above,[82] but also has a systematic error as it excludes the oxygen consumption of the lungs. Studies comparing the two methods in humans show wide variations between different patient groups. The necessity for invasive

monitoring prevents the study of normal awake subjects, but results from patients in intensive care (with presumed lung pathology) do not seem to differ from patients with normal lungs undergoing cardiac surgery. The contribution of the lungs to total oxygen consumption therefore remains to be fully elucidated, but studies so far indicate that the pulmonary contribution may be very variable depending on many physiological and pathological factors.[82,83,84]

OXYGEN DELIVERY

Oxygen delivery is measured as the product of cardiac output and arterial oxygen content. This excludes oxygen delivered for consumption within the lung. In the intensive care situation, cardiac output is now commonly measured by thermal dilution and simultaneously an arterial sample is drawn for measurement of oxygen content by any of the methods described above. If oxygen delivery is determined at the same time as oxygen consumption is measured by the reversed Fick technique, it should be remembered that two of the variables (cardiac output and arterial oxygen content) are common to both measurements. This linking of data is a potential source of error in inferring the consequences of changes in one product on the other (see page 204).[85]

References

1. Kelman GR, Nunn JF. *Computer Produced Physiological Tables*. London and Boston, Mass.: Butterworth; 1968.

2. Kelman GR, Nunn JF, Prys-Roberts C, Greenbaum R. The influence of cardiac output on arterial oxygenation. *Br J Anaesth*. 1967;39:450–458.

3. Moran RF, Clausen JL, Ehrmayer S, Feil M, Van Kessel AL, Eichhorn JH. *Oxygen content, hemoglobin oxygen "saturation," and related quantities in blood: terminology, measurement, and reporting*. Villanova PA: National Committee for Clinical Laboratory Standards publication C25-P; 1990.

4. Hsia CCW. Respiratory function of hemoglobin. *N Engl J Med*. 1998;338:239–247.

*5. Russo R, Benazzi L, Perrella M. The Bohr effect of hemoglobin intermediates and the role of salt bridges in the tertiary/quaternary transitions. *J Biol Chem*. 2001;276:13628–13634.

6. Ho C, Perussi JR. Proton nuclear magnetic resonance studies of haemoglobin. *Methods Enzymol*. 1994;232:97–139.

7. Gregory IC. The oxygen and carbon monoxide capacities of foetal and adult blood. *J Physiol*. 1974;236:625–634.

8. Zander R. The oxygen capacity of normal human blood. *Pflügers Archiv*. 1978;373(suppl 1):R43.

9. Dijkhuizen P, Buursma A, Fongers TME, Gerding AM, Oeseburg B, Zijlstra WG. The oxygen binding capacity of human haemoglobin: Hüfner's factor redetermined. *Pflügers Archiv*. 1977;369:223–231.

*10. Toffaletti J, Zijlstra WG. Misconceptions in reporting oxygen saturation. *Anesth Analg*. 2007;105:S5–S9.

11. Adair GS. The hemoglobin system. VI. The oxygen dissociation curve of hemoglobin. *J Biol Chem*. 1925;63:529–545.

12. Imai K. Adair fitting to oxygen equilibration curves of hemoglobin. *Methods Enzymol*. 1994;232:559–576.

13. Kelman GR. Digital computer subroutine for the conversion of oxygen tension into saturation. *J Appl Physiol*. 1966;21:1375–1376.

14. Severinghaus JW, Stafford M, Thunstrom AM. Estimation of skin metabolism and blood flow with tcPO$_2$ and tcPCO$_2$ electrodes by cuff occlusion of the circulation. *Acta Anaesthiol Scand Supp*. 1978;68:9–15.

15. Thomas LJ. Algorithms for selected blood acid-base and blood gas calculations. *J Appl Physiol*. 1972;33:154–158.

16. MacDonald R. Red cell 2, 3-diphosphoglycerate and oxygen affinity. *Anaesthesia*. 1977;32:544–553.

17. Morgan TJ, Koch D, Morris D, Clague A, Purdie DM. Reduced red cell 2,3-diphosphoglycerate concentrations in critical illness without decreased in vivo P50. *Anaesth Intensive Care*. 2001;29:479–483.

18. Shafer AW, Tague LL, Welch MH, Guenter CA. 2, 3-Diphosphoglycerate in red cells stored in acid-citrate-dextrose and citrate-phosphate-dextrose: Implications regarding delivery of oxygen. *J Lab Clin Med*. 1971;77:430–437.

19. Heaton A, Keegan T, Holme S. In vivo regeneration of red cell 2, 3-diphosphoglycerate following transfusion of DPG-depleted AS-1, AS-3 and CPDA-1 red cells. *Br J Haematol*. 1989;71:131–136.

20. Sheldon GF. Diphosphoglycerate in massive transfusion and erythrophoresis. *Crit Care Med*. 1979;7:407–411.

21. Bowen JC, Fleming WH. Increased oxyhaemoglobin affinity after transfusion of stored blood: evidence for circulatory compensation. *Ann Surg*. 1974;180:760–764.

22. Torrance J, Jacobs P, Restrepo A, Eschbach J, Lenfant C, Finch CA. Intraerythrocytic adaptation to anemia. *N Engl J Med*. 1970;283:165–169.

23. Marshall BE, Whyche MQ. Hypoxemia during and after anesthesia. *Anesthesiology*. 1972;37:178–209.

24. Hobbs AJ, Gladwin MT, Patel RP, Williams DLH, Butler AR. Haemoglobin: NO transporter, NO inactivator or none the above. *Trends Pharmacol Sci*. 2002;23:406–411.

25. Gross SS. Targeted delivery of nitric oxide. *Nature*. 2001;409:577–578.

*26. Gaston B, Singel D, Doctor A, Stamler JS. S-nitrosothiol signaling in respiratory biology. *Am J Respir Crit Care Med*. 2006;173:1186–1193.

27. Jia L, Bonaventura C, Bonaventura J, Stamler JS. S-nitrosohaemoglobin: a dynamic activity of blood involved in vascular control. *Nature*. 1996;380:221–226.

28. Hogg N. The biochemistry and physiology of S-nitrosothiols. *Annu Rev Pharmacol Toxicol*. 2002;42:585–600.

29. Stamler JS, Simon DL, Osborne JA, et al. S-Nitrosylation of proteins with nitric oxide: Synthesis and characterisation of biologically active compounds. *Proc Natl Acad Sci USA*. 1992;89:444–448.

30. Shen W, Hintze TH, Wolin MS. Nitric oxide: An important signaling mechanism between vascular endothelium and parenchymal cells in the regulation of oxygen consumption. *Circulation*. 1995;92:3505–3512.

31. Pawloski JR, Hess DT, Stamler JS. Export by red blood cells of nitric oxide bioactivity. *Nature*. 2001;409:622–626.

32. Atkins JL, Day BW, Handrigan MT, Zhang Z, Pamnani MB, Gorbunov NV. Brisk production of nitric oxide and associated formation of S-nitrosothiols in early hemorrhage. *J Appl Physiol.* 2006;100:1267–1277.

33. Cabrales P, Tsai AG, Intaglietta M. Nitric oxide regulation of microvascular oxygen exchange during hypoxia and hyperoxia. *J Appl Physiol.* 2006;100:1181–1187.

34. Huisman TH. The structure and function of normal and abnormal haemoglobins. *Baillière's Clin Haematol.* 1993;6:1–30.

35. Wajcman H, Galacteros F. Abnormal haemoglobins with high oxygen affinity and erythrocytosis. *Hematol Cell Ther.* 1996;38:305–312.

36. Gladwin MT, Vichinsky E. Pulmonary complications of sickle cell disease. *N Engl J Med.* 2008;359:2254–2265.

37. McLaughlin VV, Channick R. Sickle cell disease-associated pulmonary hypertension. A coat of many colors. *Am J Respir Crit Care Med.* 2007;175:1218–1219.

38. Platt OS. Hydroxyurea for the treatment of sickle cell anemia. *N Engl J Med.* 2008;358:1362–1369.

39. Guay J. Methemoglobinemia related to local anesthetics: A summary of 242 episodes. *Anesth Analg.* 2009;108:837–845.

40. Choi A, Sarang A. Drug-induced methaemoglobinaemia following elective coronary artery bypass grafting. *Anaesthesia.* 2007;62:737–740.

41. Goodnough LT, Shander A, Brecher ME. Transfusion medicine: looking to the future. *Lancet.* 2003;361:161–169.

42. Spiess BD. Perflurocarbon emulsions: One approach to intravenous artificial respiratory gas transport. *Int Anesthesiol Clin.* 1995;33:103–113.

43. Spahn DR, van Brempt R, Theilmeier G, et al. Perflubron emulsion delays blood transfusions in orthopaedic surgery. European Perflubron emulsion study group. *Anesthesiology.* 1999;91:1195–1208.

44. Tobias MD, Longnecker DE. Recombinant haemoglobin and other blood substitutes. *Baillières Clin Anaesth.* 1995;9:165–179.

*45. Chang TMS. Future generations of red blood cell substitutes. *J Intern Med.* 2003;253:527–535.

46. Natanson C, Kern SJ, Lurie P, Banks SM, Wolfe SM. Cell-free hemoglobin-based blood substitutes and risk of myocardial infarction and death. A meta-analysis. *JAMA.* 2008;299:2304–2312.

47. Looker D, Abbott-Brown D, Kozart P, et al. A human recombinant hemoglobin designed for use as a blood substitute. *Nature.* 1992;356:258–260.

48. Awasthi V, Yee S-H, Jerabek P, Goins B, Phillips WT. Cerebral oxygen delivery by liposome-encapsulated hemoglobin: a positron-emission tomographic evaluation in a rat model of hemorrhagic shock. *J Appl Physiol.* 2007;103:28–38.

49. Lu S-J, Feng Q, Park JS. Biologic properties and enucleation of red blood cells from human embryonic stem cells. *Blood.* 2008;112:4475–4484.

50. Korzeniewski B. Theoretical studies on the regulation of oxidative phosphorylation in intact tissues. *Biochim Biophys Acta.* 2001;1504:31–45.

51. Weibel ER, Taylor CR, Weber J-M, Vock R, Roberts TJ, Hoppeler H. Design of the oxygen substrate pathways. VII Different structural limits for oxygen and substrate supply to muscle mitochondria. *J Exp Biol.* 1996;199:1699–1709.

52. Barcroft J. Physiological effects of insufficient oxygen supply. *Nature.* 1920;106:125–129.

53. Hinds C, Watson D. Manipulating hemodynamics and oxygen transport in critically ill patients. *N Engl J Med.* 1995;333:1074–1075.

54. Pinsky MR. Beyond global oxygen supply-demand relations: in search of measures of dysoxia. *Intensive Care Med.* 1994;20:1–3.

55. Shoemaker WC, Bland RD, Apel PL. Therapy of critically ill postoperative patients based on outcome prediction and prospective clinical trials. *Surg Clin North Am.* 1985;65:811–833.

56. Gattinoni L, Brazzi L, Pelosi P, et al. A trial of goal-oriented hemodynamic therapy in critically ill patients. *N Engl J Med.* 1995;333:1025–1032.

57. Steltzer H, Hiesmayr M, Mayer N, Krafft P, Hammerle AF. The relationship between oxygen delivery and uptake in the critically ill: is there a critical or optimal therapeutic value? A meta-analysis. *Anaesthesia.* 1994;49:229–236.

58. Kem JW, Shoemaker WC. Meta-analysis of haemodynamic optimization in high-risk patients. *Crit Care Med.* 2002;30:1686–1672.

59. O'Driscoll BR, Howard LS, Davison AG. BTS guideline for emergency oxygen use in adult patients. *Thorax.* 2008;63(suppl VI):1–68.

60. Leach RM, Davidson AC. Use of emergency oxygen in adults. *BMJ.* 2009;338:366–367.

61. Wagstaff TAJ, Soni N. Performance of six types of oxygen delivery devices at varying respiratory rates. *Anaesthesia.* 2007;62:492–503.

62. Davies RJO, Hopkin JM. Nasal oxygen in exacerbations of ventilatory failure; an underappreciated risk. *BMJ.* 1989;299:43–44.

63. Goss GA, Hayes JA, Burdon JAW. Deoxyhaemoglobin in the

detection of central cyanosis. *Thorax.* 1988;43:212–213.

64. Kelman GR, Nunn JF. Clinical recognition of hypoxaemia under fluorescent lamps. *Lancet.* 1966;1:1400–1403.

65. Timmins AC, Morgan GAR. Argyria or cyanosis. *Anaesthesia.* 1988;43:755–756.

66. Clark LC. Monitor and control of tissue oxygen tensions. *Trans Am Soc Artif Inter Organs.* 1956;2:41–48.

67. Ganter M, Zollinger A. Continuous intravascular blood gas monitoring: development, current techniques, and clinical use of a commercial device. *Br J Anaesth.* 2003;91:397–407.

68. Severinghaus JW. A combined transcutaneous Po_2-Pco_2 electrode with electrochemical HCO_3^- stabilization. *J Appl Physiol.* 1981;51:1027–1032.

69. Zijlstra WG, Buursma A, Meeuwsen-van der Roest WP. Absorption spectra of human fetal and adult oxyhemoglobin, de-oxyhemoglobin, carboxyhemoglobin, and methemoglobin. *Clin Chem.* 1991;37:1633–1638.

70. Severinghaus JW, Kelleher JF. Recent developments in pulse oximetry. *Anesthesiology.* 1992;76:1018–1038.

71. Severinghaus JW, Spellman MJ. Pulse oximeter failure thresholds in hypotension and vasoconstriction. *Anesthesiology.* 1990;73:532–537.

72. Hinkelbein J, Genzwuerker HV, Fiedler F. Detection of a systolic pressure threshold for reliable readings in pulse oximetry. *Resuscitation.* 2005;64:315–319.

73. Severinghaus JW, Koh SO. Effect of anemia on pulse oximeter accuracy at low saturation. *J Clin Monit.* 1990;6:85–88.

74. Feiner JR, Severinghaus JW, Bickler PE. Dark skin decreases the accuracy of pulse oximeters at low oxygen saturation: the effects of oximeter probe. *Anesth Analg.* 2007;105:S18–S23.

75. Coté CJ, Goldstein A, Fuchsman WH, Hoaglin DC. The effect of nail polish on pulse oximetry. *Anesth Analg.* 1988;67:683–686.

76. Hinkelbein J, Genzwuerker HV, Sogl R, Fiedler F. Effect of nail polish on oxygen saturation determined by pulse oximetry in critically ill patients. *Resuscitation.* 2007;72:82–91.

77. Hinkelbein J, Koehler H, Genzwuerker HV, Fiedler F. Artificial acrylic finger nails may alter pulse oximetry measurement. *Resuscitation.* 2007;74:75–82.

78. Harris DNF. Near infra-red spectroscopy. *Anaesthesia.* 1995;50:1015–1016.

79. Vincent JL. Monitoring tissue perfusion. *Can J Anaesth.* 1996;43:R55–R57.

80. Nunn JF, Makita K, Royston B. Validation of oxygen consumption measurements during artificial ventilation. *J Appl Physiol.* 1989;67:2129–2134.

81. Makita K, Nunn JF, Royston B. Evaluation of metabolic measuring instruments for use in critically ill patients. *Crit Care Med.* 1990;18:638–644.

82. Smithies MN, Royston B, Makita K, Konieczko K, Nunn JF. Comparison of oxygen consumption measurements: indirect calorimetry versus the reversed Fick method. *Crit Care Med.* 1991;19:1401–1406.

83. Jolliet P, Thorens JB, Nicod L, Pichard C, Kyle U, Chevrolet JC. Relationship between pulmonary oxygen consumption, lung inflammation, and calculated venous admixture in patients with acute lung injury. *Intensive Care Med.* 1996;22:277–285.

84. Saito H, Minamiya Y, Kawai H, et al. Estimation of pulmonary oxygen consumption in the early postoperative period after thoracic surgery. *Anaesthesia.* 2007;62:648–653.

85. Walsh TS, Lee A. Mathematical coupling in medical research: lessons from studies of oxygen kinetics. *Br J Anaesth.* 1998;81:118–120.

Chapter 12

Non-respiratory functions of the lung

KEY POINTS

- The entire cardiac output passes through the pulmonary circulation, so the lungs act as a filter, preventing emboli from passing to the left side of the circulation.
- The lungs constitute a huge interface between the outside environment and the body, requiring the presence of multiple systems for defence against inhaled biological and chemical hazards.
- In the pulmonary circulation there is active uptake and metabolism of many endogenous compounds including amines, peptides and eicosanoids.

The lungs are primarily adapted for the purpose of gas exchange, and to achieve this with such efficiency almost the entire blood volume passes through the lungs during a single circulation. This characteristic makes the lungs ideally suited to undertake many other important functions. The location of the lungs within the circulatory system is ideal for its role as a filter to protect the systemic circulation, not only from particulate matter but also from a wide range of chemical substances that undergo removal or biotransformation in the pulmonary circulation. The pulmonary arterial tree is well adapted for the reception of emboli without resultant infarction, and the very large area of endothelium gives the lung a metabolic role out of proportion to its total mass. This large interface between the external atmosphere and the circulation is not without its own hazards, and the lung must protect the circulation from many potentially harmful inhaled substances.

FILTRATION

Sitting astride the whole output of the right ventricle, the lung is ideally situated to filter out particulate matter from the systemic venous return. Without such a filter, there would be a constant risk of particulate matter entering the arterial system, where the coronary and cerebral circulations are particularly vulnerable to damaging emboli.

Pulmonary capillaries have a diameter of about $7\,\mu m$, but this does not appear to be the effective pore size of the pulmonary circulation when considered as a filter. There is no clear agreement on the maximal diameter of particles that can traverse the pulmonary circulation. Animal studies have demonstrated the passage through perfused lungs of glass beads up to $500\,\mu m$.[1] It is well known that small quantities of gas and fat emboli may gain access to the systemic circulation in patients without intracardiac shunting. Emboli may bypass the alveoli via some of the pre-capillary anastomoses that are known to exist in the pulmonary circulation (page 99), though the functional role of these anastomoses remains uncertain. More extensive invasion of the systemic arteries may occur in the presence of an overt right-to-left intracardiac shunt, which is now known to be quite common. Post mortem studies show that over 25% of the population have a 'probe-patent' foramen ovale, usually in the form of a slit-like defect that acts as a valve, and which is therefore normally kept closed by the left atrial pressure being slightly greater than the right.[2] In 10% of normal subjects, a simple Valsalva manoeuvre or cough results in easily demonstrable

DOI: 10.1016/B978-0-7020-2996-7.00012-X

blood flow between the right and left atria.[3] Paradoxical embolism may therefore result from a relative increase in right atrial pressure caused by physiological events or pulmonary embolus (Chapter 29).

So far as the survival of the lung is concerned, the geometry of the pulmonary microcirculation is particularly well adapted to maintaining alveolar perfusion in the face of quite large degrees of embolisation. However, a significant degree of embolisation inevitably blocks the circulation to parts of the lung, disturbing the balance between ventilation and perfusion. This situation is considered in Chapter 29. Pulmonary microembolism with small clumps of fibrin and/or platelets will not have a direct effect on gas exchange until it is very extensive. Plugging of pulmonary capillaries by microemboli does, however, initiate neutrophil activation in the area, leading to an increase in endothelial permeability and alveolar oedema, and has been implicated in the aetiology of acute lung injury (Chapter 31).

Thrombi are cleared more rapidly from the lungs than from other organs. The lung possesses well-developed proteolytic systems not confined to the removal of fibrin. Pulmonary endothelium is known to be rich in plasmin activator, which converts plasminogen into plasmin, which in turn converts fibrin into fibrin degradation products. However, the lung is also rich in thromboplastin, which converts prothrombin to thrombin. To complicate the position further, the lung is a particularly rich source of heparin, and bovine lung is used in its commercial preparation. The lung can thus produce high concentrations of substances necessary to promote or delay blood clotting and also for fibrinolysis. Apart from the lung's ability to clear itself of thromboemboli, it may play a role in controlling the overall coagulability of the blood.

DEFENCE AGAINST INHALED SUBSTANCES

The skin, gastrointestinal tract and lungs form the major interfaces between the outside world and the carefully controlled internal body systems. Efficient gas exchange in the lung requires a physically very thin interface between air and blood, which leaves the lung vulnerable to invasion by many airborne hazards, both chemical and biological. These are almost entirely prevented from reaching the distal

airways by the airway lining fluid found throughout the tracheobronchial tree.

AIRWAY LINING FLUID

Within the airway lining fluid there are two distinct layers,[4,5] a periciliary or 'sol' layer which is of low viscosity containing water and solutes and in which the cilia are embedded, and a mucous or 'gel' layer above.

Mucous layer. Large airways are completely lined by a mucous layer, whilst in smaller, more distal, airways the mucus is found in 'islands', and a mucous layer is absent in small bronchioles and beyond. Mucus is composed mostly of glycoproteins called mucins,[6,7] which determine the visco-elastic and other properties of the mucus. Mucin is released by rapid (<150 ms) exocytosis from the mucus secreting goblet cells in response to a range of stimuli including direct chemical irritation, inflammatory cytokines[8] and neuronal stimulation, predominantly by cholinergic nerves.[9,10] Mucins have a core composed of glycoprotein subunits joined by disulphide bonds and their length may extend up to 6 μm. The core is 80% glycosylated with side chains attached via *O*-glycosidic bonds. Almost all terminate in sialic acid and possess micro-organism binding sites. Mucus plays a vital role in pathogen entrapment and removal, and also has a variety of antimicrobial actions (see below).

Ciliary function.[11,12] The mucous layer is propelled cephalad by the ciliated epithelial cells (Figure 12.1)

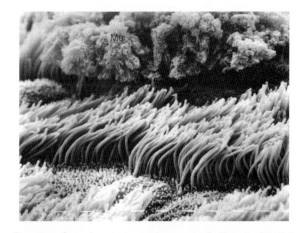

Fig. 12.1 Scanning electron micrograph of ciliated epithelial cells beneath the mucous (Mu) lining the larger airways. (Kindly reproduced by permission of Dr P. K. Jeffery, Imperial College School of Science, Technology and Medicine, London and the publishers of Respiratory Medicine.[13])

at an average rate of $4\,mm.min^{-1}$, to be removed by expectoration or swallowing on reaching the larynx and pharynx. The cilia beat mostly within the low-viscosity periciliary layer of airway lining fluid, with the cilia tips intermittently gripping the underside of the mucous layer, so propelling the mucous layer along the airway wall.

Cilial beat frequency is 12–14 beats per second and can be affected by pollutants, smoke, anaesthetic agents and infection. Two phases occur for each beat (Figure 12.2). First is the recovery stroke which occupies 75% of the time of each cycle and involves a slow bowing movement away from the resting position by a sideways action of the cilium. There then follows the effective stroke in which the cilium extends to its full height, gripping the mucous layer above with claws on its tip, before moving forward in a plane perpendicular to the cell below and returning to its resting position. Adjacent cilia somehow coordinate their strokes to produce waves of activity that move the mucous layer along, probably by a physical effect of cilia stimulating adjacent cilia during the sideways sweep of the recovery stroke.

Periciliary layer. For this propulsion system to work effectively, it is crucial that the depth of the periciliary fluid layer be closely controlled,[4,5] particularly considering the increasing amount of mucus that will occur each time two smaller airways converge into one larger airway. The depth of both layers of the airway lining fluid is controlled by changes in the volume of secretions and the speed of their reabsorption. If the periciliary layer reduces in depth, the gel layer will compensate for this by donating liquid to the periciliary layer to maintain the correct depth of fluid, an effect probably mediated by simple osmotic gradients between the two layers. The mucous layer may donate fluid to the periciliary layer until its volume is diminished by 70%. The reverse happens as the mucus converges on the larger airways, with the mucous layer absorbing excess periciliary water. The volume of periciliary fluid is therefore effectively determined by its salt concentration, which is in turn controlled by active ion transport on the surface of the epithelial cells. The ion channels responsible for active control are amiloride sensitive Na^+ and Cl^- channels, the latter better known as the cystic fibrosis transmembrane regulator (CFTR) protein. CFTR is likely to be partially active at rest but is stimulated when Na^+ channels are inhibited. The factors responsible for this critical system are unknown, though adenosine diphosphate release in response to cyclical airway movements may be involved.[14]

In patients with cystic fibrosis an inherited defect of CFTR leads to dysfunction in the regulation of airway lining fluid homeostasis, with severe consequences (Chapter 28).

Humidification. The airway lining fluid acts as a heat and moisture exchanger to humidify and warm inspired gas. During inspiration, relatively cool, dry air causes evaporation of surface water and cooling of the airway lining, then on expiration moisture condenses on the surface of the mucus and warming occurs. Thus only about one half of the heat and moisture needed to condition (fully warm and saturate) each breath is lost to the atmosphere. With quiet nasal breathing, air is conditioned before reaching the trachea, but as ventilation increases smaller airways are recruited until at minute volumes of over $50\,l.min^{-1}$ airways of $1\,mm$ diameter are involved in humidification.

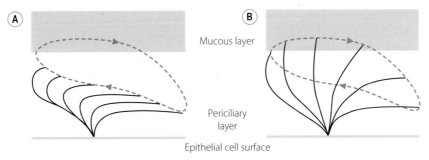

Fig. 12.2 Mechanism of action of a single cilium on the respiratory epithelium. (A) Recovery stroke in which the cilium bows backwards and sideways within the low-viscosity periciliary layer. (B) Effective stroke in which the cilium extends perpendicular to the epithelial cell into the mucous layer and propels it forwards. The blue line shows the trajectory of the cilium tip.

INHALED PARTICLES

Where in the respiratory tract inhaled particles are deposited depends on both their size and the breathing pattern during inhalation. Three mechanisms cause deposition:

1. Inertial impaction occurs with large particles (>3 μm). Large particles (>8 μm) rarely reach further than the pharynx before impaction, while smaller particles penetrate further into the respiratory tract. Inertial impaction is greatly influenced by the velocity of the particles, so a greater inspiratory flow rate and tidal volume will increase the penetration into the lungs of large particles.

2. Sedimentation occurs with particles of 1–3 μm, and occurs in the smaller airways or alveoli where slow gas velocity allows the particles to fall out of suspension and be deposited on lung tissue. Breathholding after inhalation of particles encourages sedimentation. Particles of this size pass easily into the alveoli and may either diffuse back out of the alveolus to be exhaled, or be deposited on the alveolar walls where they will be ingested by alveolar macrophages. After deposition, different dust types have variable persistence in the lung, some being rapidly cleared and others persisting within the pulmonary macrophage for many years. Differing particle types activate the macrophage to a varying extent, but may stimulate cytokine release causing lung inflammation that then proceeds to lung tissue repair, the deposition of collagen, and pulmonary fibrosis.

3. Diffusion, caused by Brownian motion of particles, occurs with particles below 1 μm in size. These particles should simply be inhaled and exhaled with minimal contact with the airway or alveolar walls.

Aiding all these mechanisms is the high humidity within the respiratory tract. Absorption of water by the particle during its journey along the airways will increase the particle's weight, and so encourage both inertial impaction and sedimentation to occur. Naturally this affects hygroscopic particles to a greater degree.

DEFENCE AGAINST INHALED PATHOGENS

As an interface with the outside environment the lung is exposed to a great many organisms carried by the ~20 000 litres of air breathed each day. Pulmonary defence mechanisms have evolved to protect the respiratory tract from invasion by micro-organisms. They can be subdivided into direct removal of the pathogen, chemical inactivation of the invading organism and, if these fail, immune defences.

Direct removal of pathogens. With normal nasal breathing, a majority of inhaled pathogens impact on the nasal mucosa, which is swept backwards by the ciliated nasal epithelium and swallowed. At higher inspiratory flow rates, for example when dyspnoeic, pathogens will penetrate deeper into the airways and be trapped by the sticky mucous layer of the airway lining fluid, before being removed.

Chemical inactivation of pathogens.[15] Airway lining fluid is more than a simple transport mechanism for impacted micro-organisms. Some smaller particles will penetrate far into the bronchial tree and take some time to be transported out of the respiratory tract. To prevent these organisms from causing damage during this time, the airway lining fluid contains multiple systems for directly killing pathogens. Surfactant, in addition to its role in reducing lung compliance (page 30), also acts as part of the innate defences in the lung.[16] Surfactant protein A is the most active surfactant protein in pulmonary defence, its actions including stimulating macrophage migration, the production of reactive oxygen species, and the synthesis of immunoglobulins and cytokines. Both surfactant protein A and D are directly bactericidal,[17] with activity against many common pulmonary pathogens. Lysozyme is also present in airway lining fluid. This enzyme, secreted by neutrophils, is capable of destroying microbial cell walls causing bacterial lysis, particularly for Gram-positive bacteria.

Finally, airway lining fluid contains a range of natural antimicrobial peptides referred to as defensins. These are small molecular weight (3–5 kD) peptides with a broad antimicrobial range, acting either directly on the bacterial cell wall or indirectly by stimulating respiratory epithelial cells to release chemokines to recruit inflammatory cells. α-defensins are present in the α-granules of neutrophils and have activity against a range of bacteria and the Herpes simplex virus. β-defensins originate from the epithelial cells and at least four human β-defensins (HBD) have been identified. HBD-1 is found in lung secretions in normal individuals while HBD-2 is found in secretions of cystic fibrosis patients as well as those with inflammatory lung disease. These small peptides contribute to inflammation and repair. Defective functioning of HBDs in the airway lining fluid is believed to be a major contributor to chronic airway infection in cystic fibrosis (Chapter 28).[18]

Protease/antiprotease system. Protease enzymes such as neutrophil elastase and metalloproteinases are normally released in the lung following activation of neutrophils or macrophages in response to pathogens or tobacco smoke. These enzymes are powerful antimicrobial molecules in the airway lining fluid, but if left unchecked, they will damage lung tissue. There are at least two mechanisms that protect the lung from damage by its own protease enzymes. First, the proteases are mostly confined to the mucous layer of the airway surface liquid, so avoiding close contact with underlying epithelial cells whilst being in close proximity to inhaled micro-organisms. Secondly, they are inactivated by conjugation with anti-protease enzymes present in the lung.[19] Anti-protease enzymes active in the lung include α_1-antitrypsin, α_2-macroglobulin and α_1-chymotrypsin. α_1-antitrypsin is manufactured in the liver and transported to the lung. It constitutes a major proportion of antiprotease activity in the alveoli and is the most active inhibitor of neutrophil elastase.

Inactivation of such powerful protease enzymes presents a significant biochemical challenge, and the way that α_1-antitrypsin achieves this has recently been elucidated.[19,20] The α_1-antitrypsin molecule exists in a semi-stable state, held together by a loop of amino acids that projects from the molecule with a pair of methionine-serine residues at its tip, which acts as a 'bait' for protease enzymes. When a protease binds the peptide loop, the α_1-antitrypsin structure becomes unstable and rapidly flips the bound protease onto the other side of the molecule, an action that has been likened to a mousetrap. Once flipped to the other side of the molecule the protease becomes bound so tightly within a β-sheet of the α_1-antitrypsin that it is effectively crushed, preventing the conformational changes required for its function.

In 1963 a group of patients were described whose plasma proteins were deficient in α_1-antitrypsin and who had developed emphysema.[21] The enzyme deficiency is inherited as an autosomal recessive gene, with 7.7% of people of European descent being carriers for one of the two common mutations of the α_1-antitrypsin gene.[19,22] Lower plasma levels of α_1-antitrypsin in homozygous patients result not from failed production of α_1-antitrypsin, but from failure to secrete the protein from hepatocytes. The retained α_1-antitrypsin protein polymerises within the cell and leads to hepatic damage.[20]

About 1:3000 of the population are believed to be homozygous for the more severe Z mutation of the α_1-antitrypsin gene, though many of these are believed to succumb to pulmonary and liver disease before the α_1-antitrypsin deficiency is ever found.[19,23] Homozygotes do form a higher proportion of patients with emphysema and estimates range from 3% to 26%. These patients tend to have basal emphysema, onset at a younger age and a severe form of the disease. It thus appears that α_1-antitrypsin deficiency is an aetiological factor in a small proportion of patients with emphysema (page 411). Smoking, which increases neutrophil protease production (page 321), is associated with more severe lung disease in patients with a deficiency of α_1-antitrypsin.[23] Disturbances of the less well understood protease-antiprotease systems, such as the matrix metalloproteases group of enzymes, are now also believed to be involved in pathogenesis of a variety of inflammatory lung diseases.[24]

Immune systems. Humoral immunity is provided in the lung by immunoglobulins found in the airway lining fluid. IgA is the major type present in the nasopharyngeal area and large bronchi. Its role seems to be to prevent the binding of bacteria to the nasal mucosa, and specific IgA has the ability to act as an opsonin and induce complement. Deeper in the respiratory tract IgG is present in larger amounts, becoming the most prevalent immunoglobulin in the alveoli.

Cellular immunity involves the immunologically active epithelial cells and macrophages that are present in normal airways. In response to a variety of stimuli bronchial epithelial cells initiate an inflammatory response, and are probably also responsible for terminating the response and initiating tissue repair.[25] This is done by secretion of numerous molecules:

- adhesion molecules (e.g. ICAM-1) to induce margination of inflammatory cells in nearby pulmonary capillaries
- chemokines (e.g. IL-8) to recruit inflammatory cells into the lung tissue
- cytokines (e.g. IL-1, IL-6, tumour necrosis factor) to amplify the inflammatory response by further stimulation of inflammatory cells
- growth factors (e.g. TGF-β, EGF) to stimulate the cells responsible for tissue repair such as fibroblasts
- extra-cellular matrix proteins (e.g. collagen, hyaluronan) to begin the tissue repair process.

Once initiated, this response causes large numbers of phagocytic cells to enter the lung tissue. The presence of immunoglobulins, complement and other opsonins enhances the phagocytic cells' recognition process. In severe infections, the reactive oxygen species used in the killing of micro-organisms by phagocytic cells may spill out of the lysosome and into the lung tissue, exacerbating the tissue injury.

In patients with asthma, the inflammatory cells responsible for airway inflammation are eosinophils and mast cells, while in those with chronic obstructive pulmonary disease and other forms of lung inflammation, neutrophils predominate.

CHEMICAL HAZARDS

Many factors will influence the fate of inhaled chemicals:[26]

Particle size, as with biological particles described above, will affect where in the lung deposition occurs.

Water solubility. Once incorporated into the lung tissue, water solubility affects the rate at which chemicals are cleared from the lung, with water soluble substances taking longer than lipid soluble ones to be absorbed into the blood for disposal elsewhere.

Concentration of inhaled chemicals is important as metabolic activity within the lung is easily saturated.

Metabolism of inhaled chemicals is poorly understood in the human lung, and, though it has been extensively investigated in animals, there are known to be large species differences.[26] Metabolic activity is found in all cell types of the respiratory mucosa, but in animals is particularly well developed in Clara cells and type II alveolar cells (page 23).[26,27] As in the liver, metabolism of toxic chemicals involves two stages:

1. Phase I metabolism, in which the toxic molecule is converted into a different compound, usually by oxidative reactions. This is achieved in the lung by the cytochrome P-450 mono-oxygenase, and to a much lesser extent, flavin based mono-oxygenase systems. The lung is one of the major extrahepatic sites of mixed function oxidation by the cytochrome P-450 systems, but, gram-for-gram, remains considerably less active than the liver.

2. Phase II metabolism involves conjugation of the resulting compounds to 'carrier' molecules, which render them less biologically active, more water soluble and therefore easier to excrete. In the lung, phase II metabolism is normally by conjugation with glucuronide or glutathione.[26]

Metabolic changes to inhaled chemicals may not be beneficial, especially with many synthetic organic compounds and several chemicals in cigarette smoke (page 317). Bioactivation by phase I metabolism converts some quite innocuous compounds into potent carcinogens, while slightly different metabolic conversions may do the reverse.[26,28] The balance between activating and inactivating pathways varies between species. What little data is available on human lungs indicates that we are fortunate in having a very favourable ratio, the inactivation of potential carcinogens being 100-fold greater than in rodents.[26] Presumably, without this evolutionary advantage, the history of cigarette smoking would have been considerably different.

PROCESSING OF ENDOGENOUS COMPOUNDS BY THE PULMONARY VASCULATURE[29]

Hormones may pass through the lung unchanged, others may be almost entirely removed from the blood during a single pass, and some may be activated during transit (Table 12.1).

Of the many types of cell in the lungs, it is the endothelium that is most active metabolically. The

Table 12.1 Summary of metabolic changes to hormones on passing through the pulmonary circulation

GROUP	EFFECT OF PASSING THROUGH PULMONARY CIRCULATION		
	ACTIVATED	NO CHANGE	INACTIVATED
Amines		Dopamine Adrenaline Histamine	5-hydroxy-tryptamine Noradrenaline
Peptides	Angiotensin I	Angiotensin II Oxytocin Vasopressin	Bradykinin Atrial natriuretic peptide Endothelins
Arachidonic acid derivatives	Arachidonic acid	PGI_2 (prosta-cyclin) PGA_2	PGD_2 PGE_2 $PGF_{2\alpha}$ Leukotrienes
Purine derivatives			Adenosine ATP, ADP, AMP

most important location is the pulmonary capillary but it must be stressed that endothelium from a range of vessels throughout the body have been shown to possess a similar repertoire of metabolic processes. The extensive metabolic actions of the pulmonary endothelium take place in spite of the paucity of organelles that are normally associated with metabolic activity, in particular mitochondria and smooth endoplasmic reticulum or microsomes. Nevertheless, the caveolae result in a major increase in the already extensive surface area of these cells (about $126\,m^2$),[30] which is particularly advantageous for membrane bound enzymes.

CATECHOLAMINES AND ACETYLCHOLINE

Noradrenaline (norepinephrine). There is a striking difference in the handling of noradrenaline and adrenaline. Although each catecholamine has a half-life of about 20 seconds in blood, some 30% of noradrenaline is removed in a single pass through the lungs,[31] while adrenaline (and isoprenaline and dopamine) are unaffected. Monoamine oxidase and catechol-*O*-methyl transferase within the endothelial cells will metabolise all amine derivatives with equal efficiency. The specificity of pulmonary endothelium for noradrenaline therefore lies with the cell membrane, which selectively takes up only noradrenaline and 5-hydroxytryptamine.[32] Extraneuronal uptake of noradrenaline is not confined to the endothelium of the lungs, but uptake by the pulmonary circulation (uptake 1) differs from extraneuronal uptake (uptake 2) in other tissues, which is less specific for noradrenaline.

5-Hydroxytryptamine (5-HT, serotonin) is removed very effectively by the lungs, up to 98% being removed in a single pass. There are considerable similarities to the processing of noradrenaline. 5-HT is taken up by the endothelium, mainly in the capillaries, and is then rapidly metabolised by monoamine oxidase. The half-life of 5-HT in blood is about 1–2 minutes and pulmonary clearance plays the major role in the prevention of its recirculation.

Histamine, dopamine and adrenaline (epinephrine) are not removed from blood on passing through the pulmonary circulation, in spite of the high concentrations of monoamine oxidase in lung tissue. Their removal from the circulation is limited by the lack of a transport mechanism across the blood/endothelium barrier.

Acetylcholine is rapidly hydrolysed in blood where it has a half-life of less than 2 seconds. This tends to overshadow any changes attributable to the lung, which nevertheless does contain acetylcholinesterases and pseudocholinesterases.

PEPTIDES

Angiotensin. It has long been known that angiotensin I, a decapeptide formed by the action of renin on a plasma α_2-globulin (angiotensinogen), was converted into the vasoactive octapeptide angiotensin II by incubation with plasma. Angiotensin-converting enzyme (ACE) is found free in the plasma, but is also bound to the surface of endothelium. This appears to be a general property of endothelium but ACE is present in abundance on the vascular surface of pulmonary endothelial cells, also lining the inside of the caveolae and extending onto the projections into the lumen. Some 80% of angiotensin I passing through the lungs is converted to angiotensin II in a single pass. Angiotensin converting enzyme is a zinc containing carboxypeptidase with two active sites, each located within a deep groove in the side of the protein.[33] Binding sites in the groove attach the substrate firmly to the protein and the zinc moiety then cleaves either a phenylalanine-histidine bond (angiotensin I) or a phenylalanine-arginine bond (bradykinin). Drugs that inhibit ACE (see below) do so by becoming buried deep within the protein groove, simply covering the active site.[33]

Bradykinin, a vasoactive nonapeptide, is also very effectively removed during passage through the lung and other vascular beds. The half-life in blood is about 17 seconds but less than 4 seconds in various vascular beds. Like angiotensin I, ACE is the enzyme responsible for metabolism of bradykinin.

By its effects on bradykinin and angiotensin, ACE plays a crucial role in controlling arterial blood pressure. Bradykinin, which promotes blood vessel dilation and a lowering of blood pressure, is inactivated. Conversely, angiotensin II production results in a host of events that increase blood pressure such as renal sodium retention, vasoconstriction and release of noradrenaline. Drugs that inhibit ACE are now widely used in the treatment of cardiovascular disease. However, this also decreases the degradation of bradykinin by ACE, although other enzymes are capable of metabolising bradykinin, so allowing ACE inhibitors to exert their hypotensive effects.

Angiotensin II itself passes through the lung unchanged, as do vasopressin and oxytocin.

Atrial natriuretic peptide (ANP) is largely removed by the lung in many animal species. Methodological problems caused by the secretion of ANP from both left and right atria in humans led to uncertainty about the ability of human lungs to metabolise ANP. Studies using radiolabelled ANP have now shown that in humans, ANP is not metabolised by the lung to any significant extent.[34]

Endothelins, a group of 21 amino acid peptides with diverse biological activity (page 110) have a plasma half-life of just a few minutes, being cleared by the kidney, liver and lungs. The pulmonary enzymes responsible are not clearly defined, but there are believed to be several different types in humans.[35]

ARACHIDONIC ACID DERIVATIVES

The lung is a major site of synthesis, metabolism, uptake and release of arachidonic acid metabolites. The group as a whole are 20-carbon carboxylic acids, generically known as eicosanoids. The initial stages of eicosanoid synthesis involve the conversion, by phospholipase A_2, of membrane phospholipids into arachidonic acid. Metabolism of arachidonic acid involves its oxygenation by two main pathways for which the enzymes are cyclo-oxygenase (COX) and

lipoxygenase (Figures 12.3 and 4.9 respectively). Oxygenation and cyclisation of arachidonic acid by COX produces the prostaglandin PGG_2 (the subscript 2 indicates two double bonds in the carbon chain). A non-specific peroxidase then converts PGG_2 to PGH_2, which is the parent compound for synthesis of the many important derivatives shown in Figure 12.3.

Eicosanoids are not stored preformed, but are synthesised as required by many cell types in the lung, including endothelium, airway smooth muscle, mast cells, epithelial cells and vascular muscle. Activation of phospholipase initiates the pathway, and results from a variety of stimuli such as inflammatory cytokines, complement activation, hormones, allergens or mechanical stimuli. The enzyme for the next step of the pathway, COX, exists in multiple isoforms, including COX-1, which is a constitutive enzyme present at low concentrations, and COX-2, which is induced by inflammatory cytokines. In the normal lung, the physiological role of these COX isoforms is uncertain, but in some patients with asthma, inhibition of COX-1 by aspirin induces bronchospasm, whilst inhibition of COX-2 does not (page 408).

$PGF_{2\alpha}$, PGD_2, PGG_2, PGH_2 and thromboxane are bronchial and tracheal constrictors, $PGF_{2\alpha}$ and PGD_2

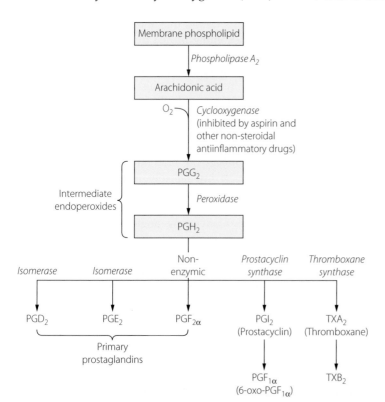

Fig. 12.3 The cyclo-oxygenase pathway for the production of arachidonic acid, and its subsequent conversion to form the prostaglandins and thromboxanes. See text for metabolism taking place in the lungs.

being much more potent in asthmatic patients compared with normal subjects. PGE_1 and PGE_2 are bronchodilators, particularly when administered by aerosol. Prostacyclin (PGI_2) has different effects in different species. In humans, it has no effect on airway calibre in doses that have profound cardiovascular effects. PGI_2 and PGE_1 are pulmonary vasodilators. PGH_2 and $PGF_{2\alpha}$ are pulmonary vasoconstrictors.

Various specific enzymes in the lung are responsible for extensive metabolism of PGE_2, PGE_1 and $PGF_{2\alpha}$, but PGA_2 and PGI_2 pass through the lung unchanged. As for catecholamine metabolism, specificity for pulmonary prostaglandin metabolism is in the uptake pathways rather than with the intracellular enzymes.[29]

Leukotrienes[36] are also eicosanoids derived from arachidonic acid but by the lipoxygenase pathway (see Figure 4.9). The leukotrienes LTC_4 and LTD_4 are mainly responsible for the bronchoconstrictor effects of what was formerly known as slow-reacting substance A or SRS-A. SRS-A also contains LTB_4, which is a less powerful bronchoconstrictor but increases vascular permeability. These compounds, which are synthesised by the mast cell, have an important role in asthma and the mechanism of their release is discussed in Chapter 28, whilst drugs that inhibit leukotrienes are described on page 53.

PURINE DERIVATIVES

Specific enzymes exist on the surface of pulmonary endothelial cells for the degradation of AMP, ADP and ATP to adenosine. Adenosine itself has potent effects on the circulation, but is also inactivated in the lungs by a rapid uptake mechanism into the endothelial cells, where it is either phosphorylated into AMP or deaminated to produce inosine and ultimately uric acid for excretion.

PHARMACOKINETICS AND THE LUNG

DRUG DELIVERY[37,38]

Inhalation of drugs to treat lung disease may be considered as topical administration of the drug to the respiratory tract, though systemic absorption of the drug is likely to be greater than other topical routes. Pulmonary administration of a drug that is intended to work systemically offers many advantages over other routes, such as very rapid delivery into the circulation and avoidance of first pass metabolism in the liver.

For delivery to the alveoli, particles around $3\,\mu m$ are the optimal size, as larger particles tend to deposit in the airways, and smaller particles tend to be inhaled and exhaled without being deposited in lung tissue (page 220). Targeted delivery of drugs to specific regions of the respiratory tract should be possible, by, for example, modifying the particle size, the timing of its addition to the breath or the breathing pattern during inhalation.[38,39] In future even more specific targeting of inhaled drugs may be possible, as demonstrated by a study in which magnetic iron oxide nanoparticles were added to aerosol solutions and a magnetic field used to modify where in the lung the aerosol was deposited.[40] In clinical practice, most delivery devices in clinical use produce aerosols containing a wide range of particle sizes, the most commonly used metered-dose inhaler used to treat asthma generating particles between $1-35\,\mu m$. Use of a spacer device before inhalation allows the largest particles to fall out of the aerosol before inhalation, and so reduces their impaction in the pharynx where they are responsible for some of the side effects of inhaled drugs.

DRUG ELIMINATION

The wide range of mechanisms present in the lung for the processing of endogenous and inhaled substances makes an effect on drug disposition almost inevitable.

Inhaled drugs will be subjected to the same metabolic activity in the airway and alveolar cells as other toxic chemicals described above. Mixed function oxidase and cytochrome P-450 systems are active in the lung and so are presumed to metabolise drugs in the same way as in hepatocytes. Steroids are known to be metabolised in lung airway tissue, as is isoprenaline.[29]

Pulmonary circulation.[29,41,42] Many drugs are removed from the circulation on passing through the lungs. However, in the majority of cases this occurs by retention of the drug in lung tissue rather than actual metabolism. This low activity of metabolic enzymes found in the lung occurs for two reasons. First, access to the metabolic enzymes in endothelial cells is closely controlled by highly specific uptake mechanisms that are vital to allow the highly selective metabolism of endogenous compounds. Secondly, it is possible that the oxidative systems responsible for drug metabolism elsewhere in the body are located mostly in the airways thus preventing blood borne drugs gaining access to them. Drugs that are basic (pKa >8) and lipophilic tend to be taken up in the pulmonary circulation while acidic drugs preferentially bind to plasma proteins.[29,42] Drug binding in the pulmonary circulation may act as a first pass filter for any drug administered intravenously.[41] This drug reservoir within the lung may then be released slowly, or even give rise to rapid changes in plasma drug levels when the binding sites either become saturated or when one drug is displaced by a different drug with greater affinity for the binding site.

Pulmonary toxicity of drugs. Accumulation of some drugs and other toxic substances in the lung may cause dangerous local toxicity.[43] Paraquat is an outstanding example: it is slowly taken up into alveolar epithelial cells where it promotes the production of reactive oxygen species (page 384), with resulting lung damage. Some drugs cause pulmonary toxicity by a similar mechanism, including nitrofurantoin and bleomycin, toxicity from the latter being strongly associated with exposure to high oxygen concentrations. Amiodarone, a highly effective and commonly used antiarrhythmic agent, is also associated with pulmonary toxicity which occurs in 6% of patients given the drug.[44] When toxicity occurs it may be severe and is fatal in up to 10% of cases. The cause is unknown, but formation of reactive oxygen species, immunological activation and direct cellular toxicity are all believed to contribute.[44]

THE ENDOCRINE LUNG

To qualify as a true endocrine organ, the lung must secrete a substance into the blood, which brings about a useful physiological response in a distant tissue. In spite of its wide-ranging metabolic activities already described, the endocrine functions of the lung remain ill-defined. Contenders include the following.

Inflammatory mediators. Histamine, endothelin and eicosanoids are released from the lung following immunological activation by inhaled allergens (Chapter 28). These mediators are undoubtedly responsible for cardiovascular and other physiological changes in the rest of the body, such as a rash, peripheral vasodilation and a reduction in blood pressure. However, it is doubtful if this can really be regarded as a desirable physiological effect.

Hypoxic endocrine responses.[45] Animal studies have demonstrated the presence of clusters of peptide and amine secreting cells in lung tissue. These cells degranulate in the presence of acute hypoxia, but the substances secreted and their effects are not known. The cells belong to the 'diffuse endocrine system' and are present in humans, but their role is extremely unclear.

Nitric oxide (NO) plays an important role in the regulation of airway smooth muscle (page 51) and pulmonary vascular resistance (page 107), and is well known for its effects on platelet function and the systemic vasculature elsewhere in the body. There is no evidence that pulmonary endothelium secretes NO into the blood in order to exert an effect elsewhere, mainly because of the rapid uptake of NO by haemoglobin (page 194). However, this does not rule out an indirect effect of pulmonary NO production in influencing peripheral blood flow, which may be controlled by the balance between different forms of NO–haemoglobin complexes (page 195).

References

1. Niden AH, Aviado DM. Effects of pulmonary embolism on the pulmonary circulation with special reference to arteriovenous shunts in the lung. *Circ Res*. 1956;4:67–73.

2. Kerut EK, Norfleet WT, Plotnick GD, Giles TD. Patent foramen ovale: A review of associated conditions and the impact of physiological size. *J Am Coll Cardiol*. 2001;38:613–623.

3. Fisher DC, Fisher EA, Budd JH, Rosen SE, Goldman ME. The incidence of patent foramen ovale in 1000 consecutive patients. *Chest*. 1995;107:1504–1509.

4. Widdicombe JH. Regulation of the depth and composition of airway surface liquid. *J Anat*. 2002;201:313–318.

5. Boucher RC. Regulation of airway surface liquid volume by human airway epithelia. *Pflugers Arch*. 2003;445:495–498.

6. Rose MC, Voynow JA. Respiratory tract mucin genes and mucin glycoproteins in health and disease. *Physiol Rev*. 2006;86:245–278.

7. Hattrup CL, Gendler SJ. Structure and function of the cell surface (tethered) mucins. *Annu Rev Physiol*. 2008;70:431–457.

8. Burgel P-R, Nadel JA. Epidermal growth factor receptor-mediated innate immune responses and their roles in airway diseases. *Eur Respir J*. 2008;32:1068–1081.

9. Rogers DF. Airway goblet cells: responsive and adaptable frontline defenders. *Eur Respir Journal*. 1994;7:1690–1706.

10. Rogers DF. Motor control of airway goblet cells and glands. *Respir Physiol*. 2000;125:129–144.

11. Houtmeyers E, Gosselink R, Gayan-Ramirez G, Decramer M. Regulation of mucociliary clearance in health and disease. *Eur Respir J*. 1999;13:1177–1188.

12. Salathe M. Regulation of mammalian ciliary beating. *Annu Rev Physiol*. 2007;69:401–422.

13. Jeffery PK. Microscopic structure of normal lung. In: Brewis RAL, Corrin B, Geddes DM, Gibson GJ, eds. *Respiratory Medicine*. London: WB Saunders Company Ltd; 1995:54–72.

14. Button B, Picher M, Boucher RC. Differential effects of cyclic and constant stress on ATP release and mucociliary transport by human airway epithelia. *J Physiol*. 2007;580:577–592.

15. Ganz T. Antimicrobial polypeptides in host defense of the respiratory tract. *J Clin Invest*. 2003;109:693–697.

16. Wright JR. Pulmonary surfactant: a front line of lung host defense. *J Clin Invest*. 2003;111:1453–1455.

17. Wu H, Kuzmenko A, Wan S, et al. Surfactant proteins A and D inhibit the growth of Gram-negative bacteria by increasing membrane permeability. *J Clin Invest*. 2003;111:1589–1602.

*18. Hiemstra PS. Antimicrobial peptides in the real world: implications for cystic fibrosis. *Eur Respir J*. 2007;29:617–618.

*19. Carrell RW, Lomas DA. Alpha$_1$-antitrypsin deficiency – a model for conformational diseases. *N Engl J Med*. 2002;346:45–53.

20. Lomas DA, Mahadeva R. α_1-antitrypsin polymerisation and the serpinopathies: pathobiology and prospects for therapy. *J Clin Invest*. 2002;110:1585–1590.

21. Laurell CB, Eriksson S. The electrophoretic α_1-globulin pattern of serum in α_1-antitrypsin deficiency. *Scand J Clin Lab Invest*. 1963;15:132–136.

22. Lomas DA. The selective advantage of α_1-antitrypsin deficiency. *Am J Respir Crit Care Med*. 2006;173:1072–1077.

23. Norman MR, Mowat AP, Hutchinson DCS. Molecular basis, clinical consequences and diagnosis of alpha-1 antitrypsin deficiency. *Ann Clin Biochem*. 1997;34:230–246.

*24. Greenlee KJ, Werb Z, Kheradmand F. Matrix metalloproteinases in lung: multiple, multifarious, and multifaceted. *Physiol Rev*. 2007;87:69–98.

25. Smyth RL. The airway epithelium in health and disease: "calm on the surface, paddling furiously underneath." *Thorax*. 2009;64:277–278.

26. Bond JA. Metabolism and elimination of inhaled drugs and airborne chemicals from the lungs. *Pharmacol Toxicol*. 1993;72(3):36–47.

27. Dahl AR, Gerde P. Uptake and metabolism of toxicants in the respiratory tract. *Environ Health Perspect*. 1994;102(supp 11):67–70.

28. Kikkawa Y. Diverse role of pulmonary cytochrome P-450 monooxygenase. *Lab Invest*. 1992;67:535–539.

29. Bahkle YS. Pharmacokinetic and metabolic properties of the lung. *Br J Anaesth*. 1990;65:79–93.

30. Weibel ER. How does lung structure affect gas exchange. *Chest*. 1983;83:657–665.

31. Sole MJ, Dobrac M, Schwartz L, Hussain MN, Vaughan-Neil EF. The extraction of circulating catecholamines by the lungs in normal man and in patients with pulmonary hypertension. *Circulation*. 1979;60:160–163.

32. Gillis CN, Pitt BR. The fate of circulating amines within the pulmonary circulation. *Annu Rev Physiol*. 1982;44:269–281.

33. Brew K. Structure of human ACE gives new insights into inhibitor binding and design. *Trends Pharmacol Sci*. 2003;24:391–394.

34. Iervasi G, Clerico A, Pilo A, et al. Atrial natriuretic peptide is not degraded by the lungs in humans. *J Clin Endocrinol Metab*. 1998;83:2898–2906.

35. Michael JR, Markewitz BA. Endothelins and the lung. *Am J Respir Crit Care Med*. 1996;154:555–581.

36. Peters-Golden M, Henderson WR. Leukotrienes. *N Engl J Med*. 2007;357:1841–1854.

*37. Groneberg DA, Witt C, Wagner U, Chung KF, Fischer A. Fundamentals of pulmonary drug delivery. *Respir Med*. 2003;97:382–387.

38. Bennett WD, Brown JS, Zeman KL, Hu S-C, Scheuch G, Sommerer K. Targeting delivery of aerosols to different lung regions. *J Aerosol Med*. 2002;15:179–188.

39. Usmani OS, Biddiscombe MF, Barnes PJ. Regional lung deposition and bronchodilator response as a function of β_2-agonist particle size. *Am J Respir Crit Care Med*. 2005;172:1497–1504.

*40. Coates AL. Guiding aerosol deposition in the lung. *N Engl J Med*. 2008;358:304–305.

41. Upton RN, Doolette DJ. Kinetic aspects of drug deposition in the lungs. *Clin Exp Pharmacol Physiol*. 1999;26:381–391.

*42. Boer F. Drug handling by the lungs. *Br J Anaesth*. 2003;91:50–60.

43. Foth H. Role of the lung in accumulation and metabolism of xenobiotic compounds – implications for chemically induced toxicity. *Crit Rev Toxicol*. 1995;25:165–205.

44. Reasor MJ, Kacew S. An evaluation of possible mechanisms underlying amiodarone-induced pulmonary toxicity. *Proc Soc Exp Biol Med*. 1996;212:297–305.

45. Gosney JR. The endocrine lung and its response to hypoxia. *Thorax*. 1994;49:S25–S26.

Chapter 13

The history of respiratory physiology

KEY POINTS

- That breathing was essential for life was clear to the ancient Egyptian civilisations 5000 years ago, but the reasons for this were unknown.
- Early explanations for the function of breathing involved the air drawn into the lungs fuelling combustion in the heart, and removing 'sooty and fuliginous spirits' from the body.
- In the Renaissance, advances in knowledge of anatomy led to the discovery of the pulmonary circulation and the observation that blood changed colour on passing through the lungs.
- Physiology in the 17th century involved more rigorous scientific experimentation, and led to several discoveries about the mechanics and function of breathing.
- Developments in fundamental sciences, particularly chemistry and physics, facilitated the elucidation of current knowledge of breathing and respiration.

The historical path along which we have gained our current knowledge of respiratory physiology is long and varied. There are periods when our understanding leapt forward in just a few years, interspersed by prolonged periods when progress was negligible, and even some periods when progress was reversed. That breathing is essential for life was clear from the beginnings of history, but the mechanism of breathing and the reasons for it remained elusive for many centuries. Progress usually occurred in parallel with understanding in other scientific disciplines, particularly chemistry, physics and anatomy. Innovative ideas on the physiology of breathing led, in more than one instance, to the premature

death of the physiologist, and the history of respiratory physiology includes some of the most famous controversies seen in medical science.

This chapter is of necessity only a brief overview of the subject, and ends around 100 years ago, when the explosion of scientific progress makes the subject too large for such a short account. Significant advances in respiratory physiology in the last 100 years are reported in the other chapters of this book, and the reader interested in the history of this period is referred to more authoritative accounts.[1,2,3] For more general information on the history of respiratory physiology numerous recent sources (by historical standards) are available.[4,5,6]

ANCIENT CIVILISATIONS

EGYPTIAN PHYSIOLOGY[7]

Ancient Egyptian civilisations existed from around 3100BC to 332BC when the Graeco-Roman period began. The most remarkable contribution made to history by ancient Egyptians is their writings, though knowledge of their language was mostly lost after 500AD. Approximately 1300 years later, 19th century scholars were able to use the Coptic language to assist in translating the ancient Egyptian writings. This has allowed an insight into medical knowledge from as early as 1820BC, the date of the earliest known medical writings in the Kahun papyrus.

Medical papyri. Many Egyptian papyri are concerned with medical topics, mostly descriptions of pragmatic 'recipes' for the treatment of a multitude of specific conditions.[7]

DOI: 10.1016/B978-0-7020-2996-7.00013-1

The longest and best known of the medical papyri is the Ebers Papyrus,[8,9] which dates from about 1534BC, and is accepted as being a compilation of various earlier works. The Ebers Papyrus is unique in containing a section on physiology, including comments on respiration. The overall purpose of respiration is described thus:

As to the air that penetrates into the nose. It enters into the heart and the lung. They are those which give air to the entire body.[9]

Further sections include detailed descriptions of specific numbers of *metu* conducting 'moisture and air' to many parts of the body. These *metu* seem to mostly relate to blood vessels but also probably included such structures as tendons, muscles and the ureters. At first, this primitive view of anatomy is surprising considering the embalming abilities of ancient Egyptians, though in practice, embalming was carried out using very small inconspicuous incisions that would have revealed very little internal anatomy. Two *metu* are described to each ear, through which '*the breath of life enters into the right ear and the breath of death enters into the left*',[9] illustrating the 'magical' aspect of medicine at the time.

ANCIENT GREECE

Greek writers were primarily philosophers, but they were also outstanding physicians, with one of their number, Hippocrates, forming a school that is now widely attributed with the foundation of modern medical conduct. Early Greek philosophers such as Anaximenes (570BC–?) clearly stated that 'pneuma' or air was essential to life,[6] but in contrast to this correct observation, Alcmaeon reportedly claimed that goats breathed through their ears and that some air passed from the nose directly to the brain.[4] Empedocles (495–435BC) disputed many of Alcmaeon's writings, suggesting instead that breathing occurred through the skin, and that blood flow from the heart was tidal in nature, ebbing and flowing to and from the heart. Empedocles successfully combined physiology and philosophy in his description of the 'innate heat' in the heart, which was closely related to the soul, and which was distributed throughout the body by the heart. This concept of heat generation within the heart gained acceptance throughout the ancient Greek period, and was to remain at the centre of respiratory physiological ideas for about 1000 years.

The writings of Plato, Aristotle and the Hippocratic school only rarely directed their attention to respiration, but their contribution to scientific method and thinking was enormous. Subsequent philosopher-physicians adopted a more scientific approach to investigating physiology. At this time, dissection became widely practised, sometimes in public, and on both animals and humans. Animal vivisection also undoubtedly took place, and there are even disputed reports of human vivisection of criminals.[4] Herophilus (circa 325BC) distinguished between arteries and veins, and, along with Aristotle, asserted that they contained air. Erasistratus (304–250BC), more widely renowned as the father of philosophy, was the first to apply scientific principles to explain breathing. His view was that air was taken into the lungs and passed to the heart along the pulmonary artery. In the heart, air was converted into a 'vital spirit' that was distributed to all parts of the body by the arteries, whilst the brain further converted the vital spirit into 'animal spirit' which travelled down the hollow nerves to activate muscles. Erasistratus seemed to understand that heart valves only allowed flow to occur in one direction, but failed to apply this knowledge to elucidate the transport of vital spirit or blood around the body. After Erasistratus, Greek interest moved away from medicine to philosophy and the physical sciences, and the progression of physiological knowledge halted for about 400 years.

ROMAN MEDICINE AND GALEN (129–199AD)

By the age of 28 years Claudius Galen was physician to the gladiators of Pergamun, and 12 years later became physician to the Roman emperor Marcus Aurelius. He wrote many works on anatomy and physiology, many of which still exist in modern form including two with much material on respiration *On the usefulness of the parts of the body* and *On the use of breathing*.[10,11] Galen's work provides the first direct evidence of experimentation and the application of clinical observations to explain physiology.

Galen's system of physiology and anatomy. In Galen's descriptions, food was processed in the gut before being used by the liver to produce blood, which passed to the right heart. Much of this blood flowed into the pulmonary artery to nourish the lung, whilst the remainder passed across invisible pores in the inter-ventricular septum, to be combined with 'pneuma' brought from the lung via the blood flow, realising that tidal blood flow to and from the lungs with each breath was *'in no way suitable for the blood'*.[10] He suggested the existence of capillaries 1500 years before they were discovered by stating:

> *'All over the body the arteries and veins communicate with one another by common openings and exchange blood and pneuma through certain invisible and extremely narrow passages'*.

2. Galen ligated both carotid arteries of a dog, an intervention that he observed caused the animal no detectable harm. He concluded that the brain could therefore derive pneuma directly from the nose, to make the animal spirit earlier described by the Greeks (termed 'psychic pneuma' by Galen).

3. During his time in the gladiator arena he observed that the level of neck injury sustained by gladiators affected their breathing,[6] so proving that respiration originated in the brain. He did many animal experiments to ascertain more precisely the spinal level at which the nerves responsible for respiration originated, and went on to describe the nerve roots and destination of the phrenic nerves.[11]

4. On the necessity for breathing via the mouth and nose Galen was unclear, writing in earlier works that pneuma could enter arteries via the pharynx, heart or skin as well as the lungs. An experiment to attempt to demonstrate this was carried out:

> *'Covering the mouth and nostrils of a boy with a large ox-bladder, or any such vessel, so that he was unable to draw breath at all outside it, we saw him breathing unhindered through a whole day'*.

Galen's conclusion from this study is contradictory: *'Hence it is clear that the arteries all through the animal draw in the outer air very little or not at all'*. Modern views of this experiment are that the ox-bladder was unlikely to be air tight, or that Galen's assistants must have removed the bladder to allow the boy to breathe easily when their master was not directly supervising the experiment.[11]

The functions of breathing. Apart from providing pneuma to the heart, Galen described other functions for breathing:

1. *Regulation of heat.* Galen's writings strengthened the analogy between the heart and a flame, and

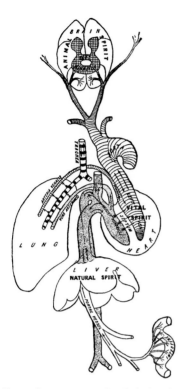

Fig. 13.1 Illustration reconstructing Galen's scheme of cardiovascular and respiratory physiology as described in the text. Galen did not use illustrations in his writings; this diagram is taken from reference 12.

pulmonary vein (Figure 13.1). In the left heart, the pneuma instilled the blood with vital spirit that was circulated to the body and brain as described by Erasistratus.

Anatomically Galen regarded the lungs as having three types of intertwining vessels, the pulmonary artery, pulmonary vein and the 'rough artery' (trachea). On respiratory mechanics, Galen regards the ribs as primarily providing protection for the intrathoracic organs, particularly the heart, but he also clearly describes the role of the intercostal muscles and diaphragm in effecting both inspiratory and expiratory movements. He understood the potential problems of diaphragmatic splinting, describing respiration as 'little and fast' in such conditions as pregnancy and 'water or phlegm in the liver'.

Experiments on respiration. Galen's experiments provided mixed results:

1. For the first time he proved that arteries contained no air, but only blood, by ligating an animal's artery in two places before opening the vessel under water. He wrote at length about

several pages of 'On the use of breathing' are concerned with the similarities between the two. For example, the observation that flames were extinguished when deprived of air or that an oil lamp burns out when its sustenance, the oil, is used up, were seen as analogous to humans seen *'perishing when deprived of air'* or who lacked sufficient nourishment. Galen was concerned about the contradictory requirements for the idea of the heart and lungs generating innate heat, realising that a fine balance must be drawn between *'fanning the source of the innate heat and from cooling in due proportion'*, citing examples such as fever, with increased breathing, when the balance was disturbed.

2. *Voice.* Galen described in detail the anatomy of the laryngeal cartilages and muscles, and wrote a whole treatise on the voice, clearly recognising the importance of the lungs. The rough artery (trachea) provided preliminary regulation of the voice, which was produced in the larynx and amplified off the roof of the mouth with the uvula acting as a plectrum. The purpose of having such a large volume of air in the lung was to allow continuous use of the voice.

3. *Removal of sooty and fuliginous spirits.* Waste products from the blood were discharged from the lung, and this was the function of expiration. Without doing so, the heart would have become stifled by its own 'smoky vapours', once again like a burning flame. Explanations by Galen as to how the body separated the fuliginous spirits from the pneuma have become uncertain with the passage of time, one explanation being that the fuliginous spirits were regurgitated through the incompetent mitral valve and passed back along the pulmonary vein to the lung.[6]

4. *Physical protection of the heart.* The spongy nature of lung tissue, and the position of the heart in the centre of the chest, led Galen to suggest that the lung served to cushion the heart from the effects of body movements.

Galen's legacy. Galen was the first physician to apply the Hippocratic method of scientific thinking to physiology, and he ingeniously combined the knowledge of his predecessors with his own thinking to produce an impressive treatise on the workings of the human body. Also, it is from the writings of Galen that we have obtained our knowledge of many of his predecessors: most of what is known of Erasistratus's views on physiology is derived from

Galens' comments on it. Galen's work also deserves a place in history as the longest unchallenged scientific work. The physiology described in this section was taught in medical schools throughout the world, and scientifically mostly unchallenged, for around 1400 years.

There was also a darker and more controversial side to Galen. He is widely believed to have been conceited, dogmatic and abusive of those criticising him.[6] *On the usefulness of the parts of the body* contains several prolonged and personal refutations of the ideas of his predecessors, for example, accusing *'Asclepiades, wisest of men'* of making errors *'no child would fail to recognise, not to mention a man so full of his own importance'*.

AFTER GALEN

When Galen died, the study of physiology and anatomy effectively ceased. The Roman Empire was in decline, and in 389AD Christian fanatics burned down the library in Alexandria, which contained many writings by the Greek philosopher-physicians.

Preservation of knowledge now fell to scholars of the Byzantine and Arabic empires. The latter embraced Galen's ideas with enthusiasm and translated many Greek works into Arabic, almost certainly adding their own refinements as they did so. The greatest of these Arabic scholars was Avicenna (circa 980–1037) whose canon was an impressive document pulling together and classifying all the available medical knowledge of the time, creating what has been described as a popular medical encyclopaedia of the medieval period. Some years later, Ibn Al Nafis[13] (1210–1288), a prolific Arabic writer on many subjects, studied Avicenna's writings and wrote his own treatise *Sharh Tashirh Al-Qanun* (Commentary on the Anatomy of the Canon of Avicenna). In this he challenged Galen's scheme of pores in the inter-ventricular septum through which blood passed, and instead suggested that blood passed through the lung substance where it permeated with the air.[5,13] This was an early breakthrough in explaining the true nature of the pulmonary circulation, but Ibn Al Nafis' work did not become well known for many more centuries.

THE RENAISSANCE

In the 12th and 13th centuries, scholastic pursuits began again with the foundation of many European universities, firstly Oxford, Cambridge and Bologna closely followed by Paris, Naples and Padua. Soon, many of the ancient documents were translated from Greek or Arabic into Latin, and human dissection began to be performed after many centuries of interdiction by the Pope. Knowledge of anatomy again began to advance, though interest in the function of the body only began again with Leonardo da Vinci in the 15th century.

LEONARDO DA VINCI (1452–1519)[4]

Leonardo exemplified the Renaissance trend for combining art with science. His anatomical drawings are both extensive and ingenious, being mostly surrounded by extensive explanatory notes.[14,15] These notes are written in Latin and in mirror writing, possibly simply because Leonardo was left-handed and received no formal schooling to correct this, or possibly to make his notes harder to read by uneducated persons described by him as 'bad company'.[4]

Although Leonardo is known to have dissected over 30 human cadavers, most of his drawings of the respiratory system are based on dissections of animals, including Figure 13.2 showing in beautiful detail the structure of the pig lung. In the commentary on this drawing, Leonardo considers the use of the 'substance' of the lung and extends Galen's protective function of the lung parenchyma when he states that *'the substance is interposed between these ramifications* [of the trachea] *and the ribs of the chest to act as a soft covering'*. Structures entering the chest cavity are labelled a–e and their functions described:

a. trachea, whence the voice passes
b. oesophagus, whence the food passes
c. apoplectic [carotid] arteries, whence the vital spirit passes
d. dorsal spine, whence the ribs arise
e. spondyles [spinous processes of the vertebrae], whence the muscles arise which end in the nape of the neck and elevate the face towards the sky.

Leonardo adhered to other Galenic ideas such as the presence of air in the pleural space, but was unsure how the air entered or left this space, and in his later drawings he was clearly beginning to doubt that air was always present. Leonardo's adherence to Galen's ideas was in some areas unshakable, in particular his depiction of the inter-ventricular pores in several drawings of the cardiovascular system.

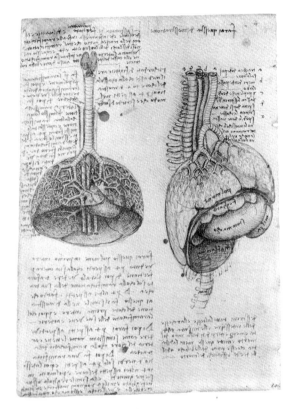

Fig. 13.2 Leonardo's drawing of the thoracic organs of a pig (c. 1508). The organs are labelled in mirror writing in Latin: *polmone*, lung; *feghato*, liver; *milza*, spleen; *stommacco*, stomach; *djaflamma*, diaphragm; *spina*, spine. See text for an explanation of labels a–e above the drawing on the right. (The Royal Collection © 2010, Her Majesty Queen Elizabeth II.)

He did however challenge some Galenic ideas by application of his engineering expertise. For example, he did not accept that the heart generated innate heat, instead writing that heat generation in the heart resulted from mechanical friction between the blood and the walls of the heart.[4] Similarly, his engineering knowledge made him intrigued by the actions of the chest wall and respiratory muscles, including the complexities of defining the different function of internal and external intercostal muscles. For the diaphragm, Leonardo described four functions – dilating the lung for inspiration; pressing the stomach to drive food into the intestine; contracting with the abdominal muscles to drive out abdominal superfluities; and to separate the spiritual (thoracic) organs from the natural (abdominal) ones. Finally, he considered in detail the movements of the trachea and bronchi on breathing, showing them to dilate and open wider at branches on inspiration as shown to the right of Figure 13.3.

Leonardo and the bronchial circulation. In Figure 13.3, Leonardo depicts in detail the relationship of the pulmonary circulation to a bronchus. Much of the commentary in the drawing is concerned with the superiority of drawings rather than words to describe such anatomical configurations. The figure clearly shows a dual blood supply to the lung, and suggests that the smaller of these two supplies is to '*nourish and vivify the trachea*'. From this drawing, many writers have credited Leonardo

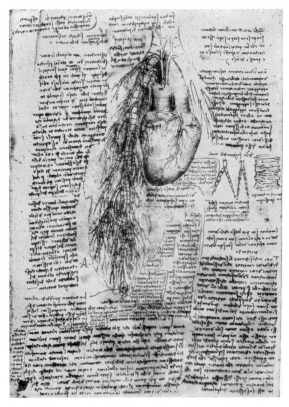

Fig. 13.3 Leonardo's drawing of the pulmonary circulation in relation to the bronchi (c. 1513). Pulmonary vessels arise from several parts of the heart, leading Leonardo to propose a dual blood supply to the lung. Coronary arteries and veins can be clearly seen on the heart. At the lower end of the main drawing, Leonardo has drawn a small circle containing the letter N. The notes describe the structure as having '*a crust, like a nutshell*' containing a '*dust and watery humour*' possibly representing his discovery of a lung cyst[16] or a tuberculous cavity.[14] (The Royal Collection © 2010, Her Majesty Queen Elizabeth II.)

with discovering the bronchial circulation, though this claim is disputed.[16,17] The drawing is believed to be based on an ox, a species recently shown to have distinct small pulmonary veins draining directly into the left atrium, which may be those found by Leonardo.

The possibility of artistic license in his drawings has caused disputes that will never be resolved, such as that of the bronchial circulation. For example, in Figure 13.2 the perfectly branching pattern of the bronchi on the lung surface is clearly not based on true observation of pig lungs. In Figure 13.3 of ox lungs, the right upper lobe bronchus that arises directly from the trachea in this species is absent. However, in spite of these misgivings regarding his drawings, Leonardo's genius in combining art, science and engineering in the study of physiology is undisputed.

ANATOMY IN THE RENAISSANCE

After Leonardo, the pursuit of medical knowledge in the universities continued, with anatomy in particular aided by the continuing resurgence of dissection and vivisection. Andreas Vesalius (1514–1564) is primarily remembered as the founder of modern anatomy, his dissections culminating in the publication in 1543 of *De Humanis Corporis Fabrica*, a book of seven volumes including over 250 anatomical illustrations (Figure 13.4).[18] His ideas met with resistance from his contemporaries whenever his views were at odds with those of Galen, and this eventually forced Vesalius to cease his study of anatomy and to return to work as a physician. Nevertheless, the *Fabrica* continued to gain acceptance and became the foundation for future anatomy texts. Vesalius was also a skilled physiologist. He was the first to describe an experiment reproduced much later, in which a section of the chest wall of an animal was carefully removed without breaching the pleura beneath, so enabling direct observation of lung movements through the transparent pleura.[6]

The pulmonary circulation.[19] Unaware of the earlier writings of Ibn Al Nafis, Servetus (1509–1553), in his religious treatise *Christianismi restitutio*,[20] again challenged the existence of Galen's interventricular pores. He wrote that rather than passing through the middle wall of the heart, '*blood is urged forward by a long course through the lung … and is poured from the pulmonary artery to the pulmonary vein*'.[21] He also commented that on passing through the lung the

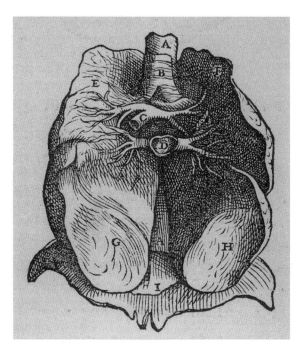

Fig. 13.4 Figure from Book VI of Vesalius's *Fabrica*,[18] showing an anterior view of the lungs after removal of the heart. A, oesophagus; B, trachea; C, pulmonary artery; D, pulmonary vein; I, diaphragm. E–H refer to the lobes of the lung – Vesalius's illustrations always showed each lung to have four lobes. (Reproduced by permission of the Special Collections, Leeds University Library.)

blood changed colour, becoming 'reddish-yellow', though an explanation for this observation was still two centuries away. Tragically, *Christianismi restitutio* was deemed to be heretical by the Christian church, and the book, along with its author, was burned at the stake in 1553. Only three copies of *Christianismi restitutio* are believed to exist today,[21] though more recent reprints are available.[22]

Just a few years later, Realdus Colombo (1516–1559) became the third physiologist to apparently independently describe the pulmonary circulation. Colombo, a pupil of Vesalius, posthumously published his account of anatomy, *De Re Anatomicae*, in which he clearly describes blood flowing through the lung whilst mixing with air.[23] There is a suspicion that Colombo had previously had access to Servetus's *Christianismi restitutio,* or that he knew of the writings of Ibn Al Nafis from 300 years earlier, causing confusion as to which of these eminent physiologists should be credited with the discovery of pulmonary blood flow.[5,19]

EXPERIMENTAL PHYSIOLOGY IN THE 17TH CENTURY

At the start of the 17th century the dominance of Italian universities with respect to medicine and anatomy subsided, and progress in the understanding of respiration moved to England, where a new approach of experimental philosophy was developing.[4]

DISCOVERIES TO ASSIST THE RESPIRATORY PHYSIOLOGISTS

Circulation. William Harvey (1578–1657) studied at Cambridge and Padua Universities, so was well placed to combine the Italian methods and knowledge of anatomy with the English approach of physiological experimentation engendered by Francis Bacon. The most notable of Harvey's teachers in Padua was Hieronymus Fabricius, who is credited with the discovery of the venous valves, including the simple demonstration in arm veins that valves prevent blood from flowing distally. In 1616 Harvey first presented his ideas of the blood circulating continuously in a lecture to the College of Physicians in London. After a further 12 years of experimentation, Harvey published *De Motu Cordis*, in which he describes the circular motion of the blood in both the lesser (pulmonary) and greater (systemic) circulation.[24,25] Harvey's comments on respiration in *De Motu Cordis* are sparse, and though he refers in several places to a future separate treatise on respiration, it seems this was never written.

Atmospheric pressure.[4] The Italian physicists Berti and Torricelli, both of whom were acquainted with Galileo, accidentally discovered air pressure in their search to create a vacuum. First Berti, with a water barometer built of lead pipe attached to his house in Rome, measured the height of the water column at 27 feet. Torricelli and a mathematician colleague Vivianni then made the first mercury barometer using mercury in a glass tube inverted over a bowl of mercury, and so allowed the height of the column to be visualised.

The microscope. Harvey and his numerous predecessors who described blood flowing through the lung tissue were not able to determine by what route this occurred or how the blood and air were mixed. Harvey thought it most likely that the blood and air came into contact through pores in the lung structures. Marcelus Malpighi (1628–1694) used a primitive microscope to observe lung tissue. His original communication in 1661, *De Pulmonibus*,[26,27] consisted of two letters to his friend Borrelli who was a professor of science in Pisa.[5] Malpighi used frogs for his studies, and describes in detail the lung preparations used, remarking that he had *'destroyed almost the whole race of frogs'* in the course of his work.[27] He described lung tissue to be *'an aggregate of very light and very thin membranes, which, tense and sinuous, form an almost infinite number of orbicular vesicles and cavities, such as we see in the honeycomb of bees'*. This first description of the alveoli was accompanied by a drawing of his preparation (Figure 13.5), and he went on to describe how the vesicles were all terminations of branches of the bronchi, and that under normal circumstances the blood and air were separated by them.

The mystery of the structure of lung tissue was now solved. Blood flowed from the right heart to the

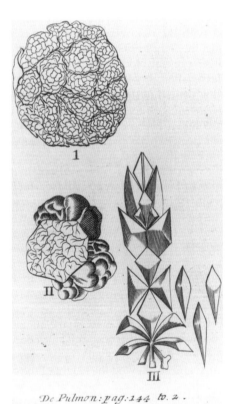

De Pulmon: pag: 144 to. 2.

Fig. 13.5 Drawing of Malpighi's preparation of frog lungs.[26] I, Seen from the surface of the lungs; II, showing the cut surface of the lung (including blood vessels on the surface of the vesicles [alveoli]); III, a schematic representation of the branching of the bronchi into vesicles. (Reproduced by permission of the Special Collections, Leeds University Library.)

lung, through Malpighi's 'smallest of vessels' past the air containing vesicles, and returned to the left heart. However, scientists were still no closer to discovering the purpose of this elaborate arrangement.

THE OXFORD PHYSIOLOGISTS AND THE 'USE OF BREATHING'[1,5,6]

In the mid-17th century a remarkable group of scientists happened upon each other in London, where the group held meetings to exchange ideas and discuss scientific topics, often holding the meetings in their lodgings. The group was initially referred to by its members in London as the 'Invisible College' but later, in Oxford, became the 'Experimental Philosophy Club'. After around 15 years in existence the club was granted a royal charter by the King and formed the Royal Society of London. Of the numerous notable club members, four are worthy of particular note here in view of their contribution to knowledge of respiration.

Robert Boyle (1627–1691).[28] Assisted by Hooke, Boyle constructed a 'new pneumatical engine' that was capable of pumping air out of closed containers to produce a vacuum. He soon demonstrated that flames were extinguished and animals died in the vacuum, and so began to believe there was some vital component present in air that was necessary for both combustion and animal life. Other experiments led Boyle away from the truth about the purpose of respiration. Enclosing a candle and a chick together, he observed that the chick survived much longer than the flame, indicating that combustion and respiration were different. Similarly, using a mercury gauge, observations that the pressure within closed vessels did not change when animals expired led Boyle to believe that the vital component was present in only tiny amounts. For a scientist so dedicated to experimentation, Boyle was often considered to be poor at interpreting their results,[4] often leaving this important task to his close friend Robert Hooke.

Robert Hooke (1635–1702).[29] A crucial partnership between Hooke and Boyle brought about the studies described in the previous paragraph. However, Hooke is best known in the area of respiration for a dramatic demonstration to the Royal Society in 1667.[30] Keeping animals alive by artificial ventilation with bellows had been demonstrated many times before by both Leonardo da Vinci and Vesalius. However in Hooke's demonstration, he used two pairs of bellows to provide a constant stream of air and ventilated a dog with part of the chest wall removed, and with '*numerous small holes pricked in the outer coat of the lungs*' (pleura). With this experiment he achieved successful apnoeic ventilation for well over an hour, and so conclusively demonstrated that '*bare motion of the lungs without fresh air contributes nothing to the life of the animal*'.

Richard Lower (1631–1691). Lower performed many animal experiments to investigate the known colour change of blood on exposure to air. Firstly he proved that the colour change occurred within the lungs, rather than in the heart, demonstrating the colour difference between blood from the pulmonary artery and vein. He then proceeded to show that the colour change occurred only when air was present within the lung, by, for example, ceasing artificial respiration of an animal and observing that blood in the pulmonary vein quickly turned blue.

John Mayow (1641–1679).[4] Mayow was the youngest of the Oxford physiologists, having studied with Lower and worked as Boyle's laboratory assistant. His major work on respiration, *Tractatus Quinque Medico-Physici*,[31] was published in 1674, a few years after Boyle, Lower and Hooke had moved on from their studies of respiration. *Tractatus Quinque* was an impressive treatise, bringing together in a single book the ideas of Mayow's eminent colleagues, supplemented with his own experimental work and ideas on chemistry and the physiology of respiration. His many experiments were illustrated with a single page drawing containing six figures (Figure 13.6). Mayow again showed that animal respiration and combustion had similar effects on the volume of air within the enclosed glasses. By good fortune, Mayow found a much greater change in volume than Boyles pressure changes. Mayow's use of water, and observations over a longer time period, allowed the carbon dioxide to be absorbed into the water and the temperature within the vessel to return to ambient. This led him to extend Boyle's ideas that air contained a vital component, which he named nitro-aerial spirit. When breathed in by animals nitro-aerial spirit combined with salino-sulphureous particles in the blood to produce a 'fermentation', which ultimately gave rise to muscular contraction. This last observation occurred from Mayow's appreciation of increased breathing during exercise.

Tractatus Quinque also contains excellent sections on respiratory mechanics. Mayow clearly understood that lung movement was brought about only by expansion and contraction of the chest wall. He demonstrated this by placing a bladder within a

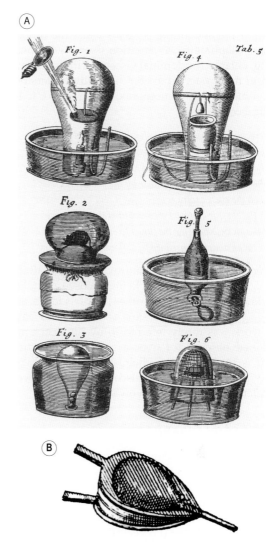

Fig. 13.6 Illustration of Mayow's experiments on respiration.[31] A, Combustible materials, ignited by a magnifying glass and the sun's heat (Fig. 1) or animal respiration (Fig. 6) cause the water to rise within the enclosed glass, or a moistened bladder to be drawn into the glass (Fig. 2). Chemical reactions were instituted within the closed glasses by for example adding iron to spirit of nitre (Fig. 4) directly or leaving globules of iron in the base of a glass in contact with diluted spirit of nitre. Fig. 5 shows Mayow's system for transferring air from one glass to another. B, drawing of the bladder in the bellows to demonstrate the passive expansion and contraction of the lungs by the chest wall.

pair of bellows fitted with a glass window to allow observation of the bladder inflating and deflating as the bellows were worked (Figure 13.6B). Mayow then applied his knowledge of physiology to pathology, by explaining that difficulty in breathing occurs if the abdominal contents resist the descent of the diaphragm, a situation seen with over-eating, enlarged abdominal viscera, orthopnoea and even in the 'hysteric passion'. He fully understood the problems of pneumothorax, giving advice to his surgical colleagues:

> Here, by the way, surgeons should be warned not to close the wound if the chest has been perforated except when the thorax is contracted to the utmost; for, otherwise, if the opening made by the wound is closed when the chest cavity is expanded it will be impossible for the chest to contract on account of the resistance of the air inside, or for the lungs to expand, except partially, and, in consequence, suffocation will occur.

Tractatus Quinque was controversial soon after it was written, with Mayow being accused of failing to acknowledge his use of other people's ideas, and *'clogging the work with absurd additions of his own'*. The work was rarely referred to by his peers, and remained obscure for over a century. In particular, it is likely that the chemists of the following century (see below) who discovered oxygen were completely unaware of Mayow's work.

PHYSIOLOGY HIBERNATES

After the death of Mayow, the study of respiratory physiology again halted, this time for about 100 years. The other Oxford scientists had already moved on to different pursuits such as physical chemistry (Boyle), architecture (Hooke) and lucrative private medicine (Lower). The other great centres of learning in Europe did not take up the mantle of respiratory research. The cause of this stagnancy is uncertain:[4] this was another politically turbulent period of history in Europe, and conditions may not have been conducive to academic study. There may even have been a sense that respiration was now effectively explained, considering that knowledge of other closely related scientific disciplines, particularly chemistry, was still at a very primitive stage.

CHEMISTRY AND RESPIRATION

DIFFERENT TYPES OF AIR

Phlogiston.[6] George Ernst Stahl (1660–1734) had begun to investigate the chemistry of combustion in the early 18th century and provided the scientific

community with a completely erroneous explanation, which was nevertheless widely accepted. Stahl proposed that all combustible substances were made up of two components: calx, combined with a fiery principle named phlogiston. On burning, the phlogiston was driven off from the substance leaving just the calx, or ash. Substances such as charcoal, which left very little ash, must have contained a greater proportion of phlogiston. Combustion in an enclosed space was extinguished when the air contained within became saturated with phlogiston. Calcination of metals (intense heating in air until oxidation occurs) was explained as driving off the phlogiston contained in the metal, whilst conversion of the metal oxide back to metal by heating with charcoal was achieved by the charcoal donating its phlogiston to recreate the metal. A powerful piece of evidence contradicted the phlogiston theory for metal calcination. Boyle, Mayow and others had all demonstrated that when metals were calcined, they gained weight, so could not have lost phlogiston. Stahl provided a very dubious explanation of this by explaining that on calcination the metal also lost some of its 'negative weight'.

Although the phlogiston theory was a complete inversion of what we now know to be true, it fitted with almost all known observations of combustion in the 18th century, with only the single exception already described. Stahl's views therefore became very enduring, and are believed to have impeded progress in understanding the chemistry of gases for many decades.

Fixed air and vitiated air. Joseph Black (1728–1799) was a Scottish chemist whose work focussed on the chemistry of alkalis, a group of substances widely used at the time for the treatment of kidney complaints. He demonstrated that heating chalk ($CaCO_3$) caused a gas to be liberated, and a reduction in weight to occur. To explain the large observed weight loss, Black believed the liberated gas to be air rather than phlogiston. After further experiments Black found that the same gas was produced by fermentation, by burning charcoal, and was present in expired air. From these observations he named it 'fixed air', believing that the gas made up all the non-respirable portion of air. Only a few years later in 1772, the discovery of 'vitiated air' (nitrogen) demonstrated that fixed air was present in only small quantities in air. Black's explanation of the chemical reactions of carbon dioxide did not involve phlogiston at all, which must have been surprising considering the fundamental place phlogiston held in the chemistry of the time, but the phlogiston theory continued unchallenged.

Dephlogisticated air. Two chemists independently demonstrated the concept of oxygen and respiration. Joseph Priestley[32] (1733–1804) in England carried out a range of experiments with respiratory gases. His work was published in *Experiments and observations on different kinds of air*,[33] which included an illustration of the equipment used (Figure 13.7). Initially described by Priestley as 'pure air', the gas produced by heating mercuric oxide was found to cause a candle to burn with *'a remarkably vigorous flame'* and allow a mouse to survive much longer than in 'common air'. Priestley tried breathing the pure air himself with no apparent ill effects. His experiments on plants led to the major discovery that vegetation, in particular fast growing species such as spinach, reversed the gaseous changes caused by respiration, burning candles or putrefaction within his closed vessels. He fully appreciated the import of this discovery on a global scale by commenting that air in the common atmosphere that has been reduced to a noxious state by respiration or combustion *'has never failed to be perfectly restored by vegetation, so that the growing vegetables with which the surface of the Earth is overspread, may be a cause of the purification of the atmosphere'*. An

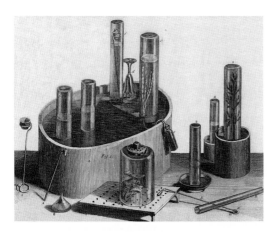

Fig. 13.7 Frontispiece from Priestley's *'Experiments and observations on different kinds of air'*,[33] showing the variety of apparatus used in his experiments. Mice can be seen contained within a beer glass (d) which allowed them to breathe for 20–30 minutes in 'common air', whilst others are held in receivers open at the top and bottom for use in later experiments (at the front of the illustration). Plants can be seen growing in the jar on the far right. (Reproduced by permission of the Special Collections, Leeds University Library.)

advocate of phlogiston, Priestley soon renamed his 'pure air' as 'dephlogisticated air'. He believed his experiments confirmed the phlogiston theory, i.e. the mercuric oxide removed phlogiston from the air so allowing candles to burn longer, or animals to respire longer, before the air became saturated with phlogiston.

Fire air. Carl Scheele[32] (1742–1786) studied chemistry and pharmacy in Sweden. Unaware of Priestley's work Scheele, using a variety of methods, also produced oxygen, which he named 'fire air'. He too demonstrated its effect on burning candles and animal respiration, but he also failed to use his results to challenge the phlogiston theory.

OXYGEN

Antoine-Laurent Lavoisier[35] (1743–1794) was born in Paris and graduated in science before the age of 20, specialising in chemistry soon after. In a very productive few years commencing around 1772 Lavoisier studied combustion and respiration, during which time he was visited by Priestley who discussed his own experiments with 'pure air'. Lavoisier approached chemistry differently, in effect introducing quantitative studies to the qualitative ones of his predecessors.[6] He showed that when metals were calcined in a closed jar the combined weight of apparatus, air and jar remained unchanged, so proving that it was air combining with the metal that increased their weight. In experiments with animals breathing nearly pure oxygen, he observed that the animals expired before all the oxygen was used up, and this led him to investigate the harmful effects of carbon dioxide in the atmosphere.

Respiratory experiments over acidified water allowed the CO_2 produced by respiration to be absorbed, and allowed quantification of oxygen consumption, which in a resting subject was measured by Lavoisier as 1200 cubic inches per hour ($\approx 330\,ml.min^{-1}$), a result very close to the modern value (page 203). However, it is Lavoisier's discovery that 'eminently respirable air' was a chemical element, and his naming of the element as oxygen, for which he is most remembered. Once again, the contribution made by the scientists of the time to this seminal discovery is controversial, for example Priestley was later irritated at Lavoisier's use of the ideas they discussed in 1774, and Mayow's work is never referred to in Lavoisier's writings in spite of him being aware of it at the time.[4] Lavoisier's interests were wider than his study of science, and he was closely involved in a French financial institution responsible for generating tax revenues, the Ferme Generale. Income from this clearly provided the resources for Lavoisier's extensive experiments, but also resulted in accusations of financial impropriety which led to his untimely death at the guillotine in 1794.[6] After Lavoisier's death, his friend Lagrange commented that *'It took but a second to cut off his head; a hundred years will not suffice to produce one like it'.*[34]

EARLY DEVELOPMENT OF CURRENT IDEAS OF RESPIRATORY PHYSIOLOGY

TISSUE RESPIRATION

Ancient ideas of some type of combustion in the heart to generate heat gave way in the 16th century to the suggestion that heat was generated by friction within the ever-moving blood. As chemistry developed, the similarities between combustion and respiration became progressively more compelling, but where this oxidation reaction took place eluded even Lavoisier who believed it occurred in the bronchi. The impetus to look beyond the lungs and heart to find the site of combustion in the body came from the discovery of calorimetry by Adair Crawford (1748–1795).[35] Measurements made by Crawford and Lavoisier of the heat generated by the body made it clear to Lavoisier's mathematician friend Lagrange, and his colleague Hassenfratz, that if all the heat were produced in the lungs their temperature *'would necessarily be raised so much that one would have reason to fear they would be destroyed'*[36]

In Italy, further experiments into where in the body combustion took place were performed by Lazzaro Spallanzani (1729–1799), though his work was only published posthumously in 1803.[37] He studied respiration in a huge variety of creatures including insects, reptiles, amphibians and mammals, and described how those creatures without lungs exchanged oxygen and carbon dioxide via their integument. That respiration still occurred in the absence of lungs led Spallanzani to his most important respiratory discovery when he showed that a variety of tissues from recently deceased creatures (including humans) continued to respire for some time, so showing that the tissues were the site of oxygen consumption.

In the 19th century, advances in science led to improved techniques for gas and temperature measurement. Heat production was measured in animals and humans and found to correlate with the specific heat capacity of the oxygen consumed and carbon dioxide produced. The respiratory quotient was measured at between 0.6 and 1.0, and found to depend on diet. Finally, with the birth of organic chemistry, and the foundation of the laws of conservation of energy, the modern account of energy metabolism was elucidated.[6]

BLOOD GASES

Once it was clear that oxygen metabolism occurred in the tissues, the search was on to find how the blood carried oxygen to, and returned carbon dioxide from, the tissues in sufficient quantities. However, other fundamental discoveries were needed before this question could be addressed in detail.

Partial pressure. John Dalton (1766–1844), whose law on partial pressures (page 516) is widely used today, first developed the concept that mixtures of gases could exist together irrespective of the pressure and temperature of the mixture. His description stated that the particles of each component gas had no interaction with those of the other gases and so *'arranged themselves just the same as in a void space'* whilst paradoxically occupying the whole space allotted to the mixture of gases. He illustrated this as shown in Figure 13.8.[38]

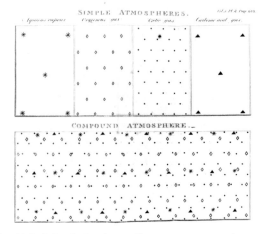

Fig. 13.8 Dalton's drawing to illustrate a compound atmosphere, made up of a mixture of simple atmospheres.[38] Two centuries after it was drawn, this diagram would be helpful to today's physiology students when first learning of Dalton's law of partial pressures. Aqueous vapour, water vapour; oxygenous gas, oxygen; azotic gas, nitrogen; carbonic acid gas, carbon dioxide. (Reproduced by permission of the Wellcome Library of the History of Medicine.)

Paul Bert (1833–1886), most famous for his studies of altitude physiology and medicine, also made a significant contribution to fundamental respiratory physiology by discovering that it was the partial pressure, rather than concentration, of respiratory gases that affected biological systems.[39,40] In an elegant series of experiments, he exposed animals to a variety of atmospheric pressures whilst maintaining the partial pressure of oxygen constant, with no ill effect on the animals. Whenever inspired Po_2 was reduced below that of air at atmospheric pressure, irrespective of the total pressure, the animal suffered the consequences of hypoxia. He repeated the experiments on humans in a large specially constructed chamber (Figure 13.9) and showed that by breathing supplementary oxygen, the harmful effects of low ambient pressure could be entirely alleviated.

Bert applied his knowledge to the recently discovered pastime of ballooning, and assisted his friend Gaston Tissandier to use oxygen to ascend to record new heights in his balloon. However, in his enthusiasm for altitude, M. Tissandier and two friends undertook a balloon flight with the specific aim of reaching 8000 m (26 200 feet) altitude, but in their enthusiasm they did not have time to consult Bert on the likely oxygen requirement. An unusually rapid ascent (Figure 13.10) resulted in confusion in all three balloonists, who were unable to breathe the oxygen and lost consciousness (page 280). Only Tissandier recovered sufficiently to record their altitude as 8600 m (28 200 feet), before battling with hypoxia to intermittently breathe oxygen and facilitate a controlled descent, during which the full tragedy of the flight unfolded, and he discovered that his two friends had died some time earlier in the flight.

Haemoglobin and its dissociation curve. Boyle and Mayow had both used a vacuum to extract gases from blood and surmised that this may have been air or nitro-aerial spirit (oxygen). In the 19th century the excellence of German chemists led them to dominate this field of research. Gustav Magnus (1802–1870) extracted oxygen and carbon dioxide from blood, showing that the former was more abundant in arterial blood and vice versa.[41] Lothar Meyer did similar experiments in 1857, but showed that the liberation of oxygen as pressure was reduced was not linear, so demonstrating that the oxygen was not simply dissolved in the blood.[42] Meanwhile, the red compound in blood was identified and soon

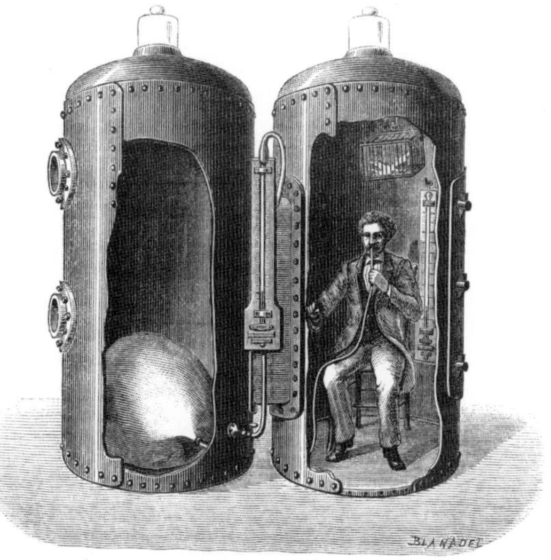

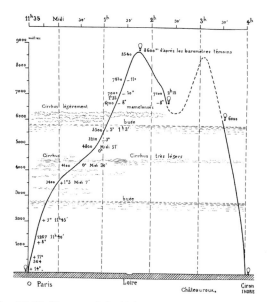

Fig. 13.9 Figure from *La pression barométrique*[39] showing Paul Bert breathing oxygen whilst sitting in the chamber at progressively sub-atmospheric pressure. Note the sparrow in the cage above the subject – the bird falls in its cage when the pressure reaches 450 mmHg, but Bert persists with the experiment down to 410 mmHg, maintained conscious by intermittently breathing oxygen. (Reproduced by permission of the Wellcome Library of the History of Medicine.)

Fig. 13.10 Diagram of the high altitude ascent of the balloon *Zenith* on April 15th 1875.[39] The dashed line indicates estimated altitude, as the only survivor of the flight Gaston Tissandier, was too hypoxic to make recordings of the altitude. (Reproduced by permission of the Wellcome Library of the History of Medicine.)

chemically found to be a combination of globulin proteins and an iron containing haematin. The affinity of this new 'haemoglobin' for oxygen was soon understood, and Hüfner quantified this binding by showing that 1.34 ml of oxygen combined with 1 g of crystallised haemoglobin, a remarkably accurate measurement (page 189).[43] By 1888, Hüfner had used haemoglobin solutions to record the relationship between the partial pressure of oxygen and haemoglobin saturation, and obtained a rectangular hyperbola.[5] Finally in 1904, Christian Bohr and colleagues showed that when fresh whole blood was used to measure the haemoglobin dissociation an S-shaped curve was found, and that the curve altered with varying partial pressures of carbon dioxide (Figure 13.11).[44]

The oxygen secretion controversy.[1,45] Measurement of the partial pressure of oxygen in arterial blood in the 19th century provoked a huge scientific controversy. In 1870, Bohr and colleagues developed a primitive aerotonometer and found arterial Po_2 to be around 80 mmHg (10.7 kPa), though in some measurements the arterial Po_2 was found to be slightly higher than the alveolar Po_2. At around this time, physiologists studying other body systems were discovering numerous active membrane transport systems in such places as the kidney and bowel. This led Bohr to suggest that active transport of oxygen may occur in the lung and he soon

had the support for this hypothesis from the eminent respiratory physiologist John Scott Haldane. In his laboratories in Oxford, Haldane devised a new technique for measuring arterial Po_2. His technique involved the subject breathing small concentrations of carbon monoxide, and then using direct colour matching of the subject's blood with standard samples to ascertain the carboxy-haemoglobin concentration from which the Po_2 could be calculated.[46] To standardise the light used for comparing colours, experiments had to be done during daylight, and by today's standards several aspects of the technique seem remarkably subjective, but nevertheless Haldane was an excellent scientist who applied rigorous methodology. Using his technique Haldane found the average arterial Po_2 to be 200 mmHg (26.7 kPa) so claiming to have proved that oxygen secretion was occurring in the lung.

A Danish husband and wife team, August and Marie Krogh,[47] became Haldane's adversaries over oxygen secretion. August Krogh, a former pupil of Bohr, continued to refine the technique of aerotonometry, using analysis of smaller volumes of gas from continuously flowing blood samples. His results always showed arterial Po_2 to be slightly less than alveolar Po_2 even when tested across a variety of inspired oxygen concentrations. Meanwhile his wife performed extensive investigations of the diffusing capacity of the lung for carbon monoxide to show that, in theory, the lung was easily able to passively absorb sufficient oxygen without the need for active secretion.

Following a bitter exchange of contradictory scientific papers over a period of 20 years, the Kroghs did begin to win the argument. By 1911, Haldane and his team seemed to accept that oxygen secretion may only be occurring when inspired oxygen levels were low. They demonstrated this, using their usual methodology, in an adventurous study of Po_2 measurements on the summit of Pikes Peak at an altitude of 4300 m (14 100 feet) where they again found arterial Po_2 to be higher than alveolar Po_2.[48]

Haldane never abandoned his faith in oxygen secretion, in spite of subsequent investigations in his lifetime by Barcroft who also found the phenomenon did not exist. Why a physiologist as brilliant as Haldane had such an unshakeable believe in an erroneous hypothesis remains unexplained, and for this reason the controversy continues. When a review of these events was published in the *Lancet* in 1987[45] the dispute over Haldane's contribution was reignited.[49,50]

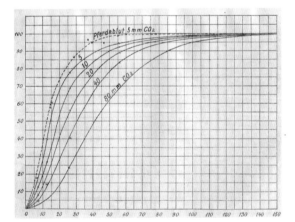

Fig. 13.11 The first publication (from 1904) showing the shape of the oxy-haemoglobin dissociation curve.[44] Note the effect of blood Pco_2 on the position and shape of the curve (page 192). Pferdeblut, horse blood. (Reproduced by permission of the Special Collections, Leeds University Library.)

LUNG MECHANICS[51]

Galen knew that inflation of the lungs was a passive phenomenon and occurred as a result of chest movement brought about by the respiratory muscles. However, the way in which this occurred was not understood for many centuries until the discovery of air pressure and therefore the existence of a vacuum, when it soon became clear that chest expansion would draw air into the lungs. Even then there were those who would not accept the scientific explanation; Rene Descartes proposed in 1662 that when the chest expanded, the air outside was pushed away from the chest, compressing adjacent air until the air near the mouth was forced into the lungs.[6] Mayow's elegant demonstration with the bladder within the bellows, described above, provided clear confirmation of the scientific theory.

Around 1500 years after Galen, Vesalius' experiments demonstrated that on puncturing the pleura, the lung retracted into the chest cavity. Many of his successors repeated this observation, Mayow commenting that *'the lungs, as if shrinking from observation, cease their movement and collapse at once on the first entrance of light and self-revelation'.*[31] It was another 160 years before further investigation of lung elasticity occurred. In 1820 Carson measured the pressure in the trachea (with a closed airway) when the chest was opened, and so made the first measurement of lung recoil pressure.[52] A short time later, Ludwig recorded a sub-atmospheric pressure in the pleura, leading to the proposal by Donders in 1849 that in the intact subject the recoil outwards by the chest wall is equal to the lung recoil inwards[4] (Chapter 3). Finally, John Hutchinson, whose work on lung volumes is described below, produced the first lung compliance curves in humans, obtained shortly after the subject's death.

Elasticity and surfactant. For some time lung recoil seems to have been adequately explained as simply resulting from the inherent elasticity of lung tissue. At the start of the 20th century the geometry and size of the alveoli was well known, and around 100 years had elapsed since Laplace had described the relationship between pressure, surface tension and the radii of curved surfaces (page 28). Yet the inherent instability of lung tissue based on these laws was not recognised until 1929, when Kurt von Neergard first questioned whether tissue elasticity alone was sufficient explanation for the properties of lung tissue.[53] von Neergard's experiments demonstrated that surface tension in alveoli was indeed

lower than expected by Laplace's law, and just a few years later Richard Pattle demonstrated that lung tissue contained an insoluble protein layer that reduced the surface tension of alveoli to almost zero,[54] and surfactant (page 29) was discovered.

Lung volumes. The first measurements of the volume of air contained in the lung were made in the 17th century by Borelli, who also raised the concept of a residual volume.[6] Following this, numerous scientists measured a confusing variety of lung volumes by various methods, such as estimating total lung capacity from plaster casts made in the chest cavity of cadavers. Measurement of lung volumes similar to those in modern use was first made by John Hutchinson in 1846, alongside his description of the first pulmonary spirometer.[55] Hutchinson's spirometer (Figure 13.12) differs little from the water spirometers used until very recently, with a volume measuring chamber over water counterbalanced with weights to offer minimal resistance to

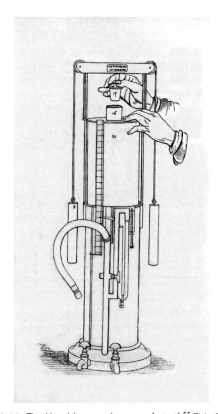

Fig. 13.12 The Hutchinson spirometer (1846).[55] This figure shows the operator removing the bung to reset the level of the spirometer before making another measurement. (Reproduced by permission of the Special Collections, Leeds University Library.)

the subject's breathing. Hutchinson described the following divisions of the air in the chest, with the modern equivalents (page 36) in parentheses:

Residual air – the quantity of air that remains in the lungs after the most violent muscular effort, and over which we have no control (residual volume)

Reserve air – the air in the lungs after a gentle respiratory movement, which may be thrown out if required (expiratory reserve volume)

Breathing air – the portion required to perform ordinary gentle inspiration and expiration (tidal volume)

Complemental air – the volume that can at will be drawn into the lungs by a violent exertion (inspiratory reserve volume)

Vital capacity – the last three divisions combined.

In the same paper,[55] Hutchinson reported his measurements of vital capacity in 1970 healthy subjects to establish normal values. He showed with great accuracy that vital capacity was directly related to subject height and age, and obtained measurements comparable with today, e.g. 188 in^3 at 60°F for a 55-year-old male subject 5 feet 4 inches tall (188 in^3 equals 3.31 L BTPS, compared with a modern predicted normal value of 3.64 L). He then measured vital capacity in 60 patients with phthisis (cough) from a variety of causes, and compared the results obtained with predicted normal values based on height and weight etc. and was able to use his results to demonstrate declining lung volumes as their respiratory disease progressed.

CONTROL OF VENTILATION

Galen's observations of gladiator injuries had shown that the brain was responsible for respiratory activity, and that the phrenic nerves were involved in bringing about this action.

More specific localisation of the respiratory centre did not begin until the 18th century, when the French physiologist Antoine Lorry (1725–1783) showed that in animals all parts of the brain above the brainstem could be removed before respiration ceased.[4] In 1812, the French physiologist Antoine Legallois published reports of similar, but more precise, experiments showing that rhythmic inspiratory movements ceased only when the medulla was removed.[56] During the next 150 years a long series of distinguished investigators carried out more detailed localisation of the neurones concerned in the control of respiration and studied their interaction.[4] These experiments resulted in

the description of anatomical regions which, when isolated in animals, caused a specific respiratory pattern, for example the apneustic and pneumotaxic centres. The complexity of respiratory control in the intact animal is such that this crude anatomical approach to unravelling the various interactions was limited, and human studies of function were mostly impossible until recent imaging techniques were developed (page 61).

The origin of rhythmicity in the respiratory centre received much attention from 19th century physiologists.[57] The role of afferent neural inputs into the respiratory centre, particularly those from the vagus nerve, were clearly demonstrated. In particular, Hering and Breuer described how lung inflation led to inhibition of inspiratory activity, and a 'deflation' reflex was also described (page 67). These observations gave rise to the basis of the *Selbsteuerung* (self-steering) hypothesis where rhythm generation was simply two alternating inhibitory reflexes.

Chemical control of breathing.[58] Rapid breathing followed by gasping and death had been observed by the Oxford physiologists in the 17th century in their experiments on animals in closed atmospheres. As the analysis of gases in blood improved, so the chemical control of breathing could be elucidated. In 1868, Pflüger performed a comprehensive study in dogs showing that both oxygen lack and carbon dioxide excess stimulated respiration, and that the former was the stronger stimulant.[59] Soon after, a fellow German physiologist Miescher-Rusch investigated the carbon dioxide response in humans to show that the respiratory system exerted very tight control over carbon dioxide concentrations and concluded that this, rather than oxygen, was the predominant chemical stimulus to breathing.[60] Leon Fredericq demonstrated in a series of very elegant experiments that the chemical control of breathing predominated over the vagal reflex control described in the previous paragraph.[61] He managed to cross connect the blood supply to and from the heads of two animals and, for example, produce apnoea in one dog by hyperventilating the other, the apnoea occurring even though the dog's lungs were not inflated to induce the Hering–Breuer reflex. Finally, at the start of the 20th century, further improvements in analytical chemistry led to the work of Haldane and Priestley, published in 1905, which involved meticulous quantitative analysis of the chemical control of breathing and the interactions between oxygen, carbon dioxide and exercise.[62]

References

*1. West JB. *Respiratory physiology: People and ideas*. Oxford: American Physiology Society & Oxford University Press; 1996.

2. West JB. A century of pulmonary gas exchange. *Am J Respir Crit Care Med*. 2004;169:897–902.

3. Macklem PT. A century of the mechanics of breathing. *Am J Respir Crit Care Med*. 2004;170:10–15.

4. Proctor DF. *A history of breathing physiology*. New York: Marcel Dekker; 1995.

5. Gottlieb LS. *A history of respiration*. Springfield, Illinois: Charles C Thomas; 1964.

6. Perkins JF. Historical development of respiratory physiology. In: Fenn WO, Rahn H, eds. *Handbook of Physiology. Section 3: Respiration*. Washington: American Physiological Society; 1964.

*7. Nunn JF. *Ancient Egyptian Medicine*. London: British Museum Press; 1996.

8. Bryan CP. *Ancient Egyptian medicine: the papyrus Ebers*. Chicago: Ares; 1974.

9. Ghalioungui P. *The Ebers papyrus. A new English translation, commentaries and glossaries*. Cairo: Academy of Scientific Research and Technology; 1987.

*10. May MT. *Galen – On the usefulness of the parts of the body*. New York: Cornell University Press; 1968.

11. Furley DJ, Wilkie JS. *Galen on respiration and the arteries*. Princeton NJ: Princeton University Press; 1984.

12. Singer C. *A short history of anatomy & physiology from the Greeks to Harvey*. New York: Dover Publications; 1957.

*13. West JB. Ibn al-Nafis, the pulmonary circulation, and the Islamic Golden Age. *J Appl Physiol*. 2008;105:1877–1880.

14. Leonardo da Vinci. *Anatomical drawings from the Royal Collection*. London: Royal Academy of Arts; 1977.

15. Clark K. *The drawings of Leonardo da Vinci in the collection of Her Majesty the Queen at Windsor Castle (Volume 3)*. London: Phaidon Press; 1969.

16. Mitzner W, Wagner E. On the purported discovery of the bronchial circulation by Leonardo da Vinci. *J Appl Physiol*. 1992;73:1196–1201.

17. Charan NB, Carvalho P. On the purported discovery of the bronchial circulation by Leonardo da Vinci: A rebuttal. *J Appl Physiol*. 1994;76:1836–1838.

18. Vesalius A. *De Humani Corporis Fabrica Libri Septem*. Venice: Basel; 1543.

19. Coppola ED. The discovery of the pulmonary circulation: A new approach. *Bull Hist Med*. 1957;31:44–77.

20. Servetus M. *Christianismi restitutio*. 1553

21. O'Malley CD. *Michael Servetus: A translation of his geographical, medical and astrological writings with introductions and notes*. Philadelphia: American Philosophical Society; 1953.

22. Servetus M. *Christianismi Restitutio*. Frankfurt: Minerva; 1966.

23. Colombo R. *De Re Anatomica libri XV*. Paris: Andreum Wechelum; 1572.

24. Harvey W. *De Motu Cordis*. Frankfurt: Wm Fitzeri; 1628.

25. Harvey W. *Movement of the heart and blood in animals*. Oxford: Blackwell Science; 1957.

26. Malpighi M. *De Pulmonibus*. Bologna, 1661.

27. Young J. Malpighi's 'De Pulmonibus'. *Proc R Soc Med Lond*. 1929;23:1–11.

28. West JB. Robert Boyle's landmark book of 1660 with the first experiments on rarified air. *J Appl Physiol*. 2005;98:31–39.

29. Harsch V. Robert Hooke, inventor of the vacuum pump and the first altitude chamber (1671). *Aviat Space Environ Med*. 2006;77:867–869.

30. Hooke R. An account of an experiment made by Mr Hook of preserving animals alive by blowing through their lungs with bellows. *Phil Trans R Soc Lond*. 1667;2(28):539–540.

31. Mayow J. *Medico-Physical works: Being a translation of Tractatus Quinque Medici-Physici*. Edinburgh: The Alembic Club; 1907.

*32. Severinghaus JW. Priestley, the furious free thinker of the enlightenment, and Scheele, the taciturn apothecary of Uppsala. *Acta Anesthesiol Scand*. 2002;46:2–9.

33. Priestley J. *Experiments and observations on different kinds of air*. London: J.Johnson; 1775.

34. Lusk G. Nutrition. Clio Medica: A series of primers on the history of medicin, Volume 10. New York: Hoeber Inc.; 1933.

35. Crawford A. *Experiments and observations on animal heat, and the inflammation of combustible bodies: being an attempt to resolve these phenomena into a general law of nature*. London: J. Johnson; 1788.

36. Hassenfratz JH. Mémoire sur la combinaison de l'oxygèn dans le sang et sur la manière dont la calorique se degage. *Ann Chim Paris*. 1791;9:261–274.

37. Spallanzani L. *Mémoire sur la respiration*. Geneva: Paschoud; 1803.

38. Dalton J. Experimental essays on the constitution of mixed gases; on the force of steam or vapour from water and other liquids in different temperatures, both

in a Torricellean vacuum and in air; on evaporation; and on the expansion of gases by heat. *Mem Lit Phil Soc, Manchester*. 1802;5:535–602.

39. Bert P. *La pression barométrique*. Paris: Masson; 1878.

40. Hitchcock MA, Hitchcock FA. *Paul Bert. Barometric Pressure. Researches in experimental physiology*. Columbus Ohio: College Book Company; 1943.

41. Magnus H. Ueber die im blute enthalten gase, sauerstoff stickstoff und kohlensäure. *Ann Phys Chem*. 1837;40:583–606.

42. Meyer L. Die gase des blutes. *Z Rat Med*. 1857;8:256.

43. Hüfner G. Ueber die quantität sauerstoff, welche 1 gramm hämoglobin zu binden vermag. *Z Phys Chem*. 1877;1(5):317–329.

44. Bohr C, Hasselbalch K, Krogh A. Ueber einen in biologischer beziehung wichtigen einfluss, den die kohlensäurespannung des blutes auf dessen sauerstoffbindung übt. *Skand Arch Physiol*. 1904;16:402–412.

*45. Milledge JS. The great oxygen secretion controversy. *Lancet*. 1985;2:1408–1411.

46. Haldane JS, Lorrain Smith J. The oxygen tension of arterial blood. *J Physiol*. 1891;20:497–520.

47. Schmidt-Nielsen B. August and Marie Krogh and respiratory physiology. *J Appl Physiol*. 1984;57:293–303.

48. Douglas CG, Haldane JS, Henderson Y, Schneider EC. Physiological observations made on Pike's Peak, Colorado, with special reference to adaptation to low barometric pressures. *Phil Trans R Soc Lond*. 1913;203:185–318.

49. Passmore R. Haldane and Barcroft. *Lancet*. 1986;1:443.

50. Cunningham DJC. The oxygen secretion controversy. *Lancet*. 1986;1:683.

51. Otis AB. History of respiratory mechanics. In: Fishman AP, Macklem PT, Mead JT, Geiger SR, eds. *Handbook of Physiology. Section 3: The respiratory system*. Bethesda: American Physiological Society; 1986.

52. Carson J. On the elasticity of the lungs. *Phil Trans R Soc Lond*. 1820;110:29–44.

53. von Neergard K. Neue auffassungen über einen grundbegriff der atemmechanik. Die retraktionkraft der lunge, abhängig von der oberflächenspannung in den alveolen. *Z Ges Exp Med*. 1929;66:1–22.

54. Pattle RE. Properties, function and origin of the alveolar lining layer. *Nature*. 1955;175:1125–1126.

55. Hutchinson J. On the capacity of the lungs, and on the respiratory functions, with a view of establishing a precise and easy method of detecting disease by the spirometer. *Med Chir Trans (Series 2)*. 1846;29:137–252.

56. Legallois C. *Experiences sur le principe de la vie*. Paris: d'Hautel; 1812.

57. Widdicombe J. Reflexes from the lungs and airways: historical perspective. *J Appl Physiol*. 2006;101:628–634.

58. Remmers JE. A century of control of breathing. *Am J Respir Crit Care Med*. 2005;172:6–11.

59. Pflüger E. Ueber die ursache der athembewegungen, sowie der dyspnoë und apnoë. *Arch Ges Physiol*. 1868;1:61–106.

60. Miescher-Rüsch F. Bemerkungen zur lehre von den atembewegungen. *Arch Anat u Physiol Leipzig*. 1885;6:355–380.

61. Fredericq L. Sur la cause de l'apnée. *Archiv Biol Liége*. 1900;17:561–576.

62. Haldane JS, Priestley JG. The regulation of lung ventilation. *J Physiol*. 1905;32:225–266.

PART 2

Applied physiology

Chapter 14

Pregnancy, neonates and children

KEY POINTS

- Hormonal changes of pregnancy stimulate breathing, causing an increase in tidal volume and hypocapnia.
- In late pregnancy the enlarged uterus reduces lung volume, particularly in the supine position.
- Human lung development is incomplete at birth with new alveoli continuing to form until around 3 years of age.
- Compared with adults, the respiratory system of a neonate has a very low compliance and a high resistance.
- In children, most measures of lung function are the same as adults provided the values are related to lung volume or height.

RESPIRATORY FUNCTION IN PREGNANCY[1]

Several physiological changes occur during pregnancy that affect respiratory function. Fluid retention resulting from increasing oestrogen levels causes oedema throughout the airway mucosa, and increases blood volume, substantially increasing oxygen delivery. Progesterone levels rise six-fold through pregnancy and have significant effects on the control of respiration and therefore arterial blood gases. Finally, in the last trimester of pregnancy, the enlarging uterus has a direct impact on respiratory mechanics. A summary of the changes for common respiratory measurements is shown in Table 14.1.

Table 14.1 Respiratory function throughout pregnancy				
VARIABLE	NON-PREGNANT	PREGNANT		
		1ST TRIMESTER	2ND TRIMESTER	3RD TRIMESTER
Tidal volume (l)	0.52	0.60	0.65	0.72
Respiratory rate (breaths per min)	18	18	18	18
Minute volume ($l.min^{-1}$)	9.3	11.0	11.8	13.1
Residual volume (l)	1.37	1.27	1.26	1.01
Functional residual capacity (l)	2.69	2.52	2.48	1.95
Vital capacity (l)	3.50	3.45	3.58	3.0
Oxygen consumption ($ml.min^{-1}$)	194	211	242	258
Arterial P_{O_2} (kPa)	12.6	14.2	13.7	13.6
(mmHg)	95	106	103	102
Arterial P_{CO_2} (kPa)	4.70	3.92	3.93	4.05
(mmHg)	35	29	29	31
CO_2 response slope ($l.min^{-1}.kPa^{-1}$)	11.6	15.0	17.3	19.8
Oxygen saturation response slope ($l.min^{-1}.\%^{-1}$)	0.64	1.04	1.13	1.33

Non-pregnant figures refer to normal subjects with an average body weight of 60 kg; pregnant figures refer to the end of each trimester of pregnancy. Derived from references 2 and 3.

DOI: 10.1016/B978-0-7020-2996-7.00014-3

Lung volumes. During the last third of pregnancy the diaphragm becomes displaced cephalad by the expansion of the uterus into the abdomen. This reduces both the residual volume (by about 20%) and expiratory reserve volume, such that functional residual capacity is greatly reduced (Table 14.1). This is particularly true in the supine position, and effectively removes one of the largest stores of oxygen available to the body, making pregnant women very susceptible to hypoxia during anaesthesia or with respiratory disease.

Vital capacity, forced expiratory volume in one second and maximal breathing capacity are normally unchanged during pregnancy.

Oxygen consumption. Oxygen consumption increases throughout pregnancy peaking at between 15% and 30% above normal at full term.[2,4] The increase is mainly attributable to the demands of the fetus, uterus and placenta, such that when oxygen consumption is expressed per kg of body weight there is little change.

Ventilation. Respiratory rate remains unchanged whilst tidal volume, and therefore minute volume of ventilation, increase by up to 40% above normal at full term. The increase in ventilation is beyond the requirements of the enhanced oxygen uptake or carbon dioxide production so alveolar and arterial $P\text{CO}_2$ are reduced to about 4 kPa (30 mmHg).[3] This must facilitate clearance of carbon dioxide by the fetus. There is also an increase in alveolar and arterial $P\text{O}_2$ of about 1 kPa (7.5 mmHg).

The hyperventilation is attributable to progesterone, and the mechanism is assumed to be a sensitisation of the central chemoreceptors. Pregnancy gives rise to a three-fold increase in the slope of a $P\text{CO}_2$/ventilation response curve.[2] The hypoxic ventilatory response is increased two-fold, most of the change occurring before the mid-point of gestation, at which time oxygen consumption has hardly begun to increase.[5]

Dyspnoea occurs in more than half of pregnant women, often beginning early in pregnancy, before the mass effect of the uterus becomes apparent. Dyspnoeic pregnant women, compared with non-dyspnoeic controls, show a greater degree of hyperventilation in spite of having similar plasma progesterone levels.[2] Dyspnoea early in pregnancy therefore seems to arise from a greater sensitivity of the chemoreceptors to the increase in progesterone levels. In the third trimester, when dyspnoea on mild exercise is almost universal, the extra effort required by the respiratory muscles to increase tidal volume is believed to be responsible for breathlessness rather than an altered perception of respiratory discomfort.[6]

THE LUNGS BEFORE BIRTH

EMBRYOLOGY

The lungs develop in four stages, under the control of a host of transcriptional factors:[7–11]

1. Pseudoglandular stage (5–17 weeks of gestation). A ventral outgrowth from the foregut first appears about 24 days after fertilisation, and around week 5 of gestation this begins to form the basic airway and vascular architecture, including the branching patterns of the adult lung. Dividing epithelial cells lengthen the airways, and their ability to do this is influenced by physical factors relating to the lung liquid and fetal breathing described below.

2. Canalicular stage (16–26 weeks gestation). The primitive pulmonary capillaries now become more closely associated with the airway epithelium and the connective tissue architecture of the lung is formed. Fibroblasts and other cells involved in morphogenesis of the lung undergo apoptosis, so reducing the wall thickness of the embryonic lung structures.

3. Saccular stage (24 weeks gestation to term). Distal airways now develop primitive alveoli in their walls to become respiratory bronchi (see Figure 2.5). Saccules form at the termination of airways, these being primitive pulmonary acini.

4. Alveolar stage. Saccules on embryonic bronchioles now expand, and septation occurs to form the groups of alveoli seen in adult pulmonary acini. This phase of development begins at 36 weeks gestation and in humans continues until around 3 years of age. In humans at full term all major elements of the lungs are therefore fully formed, but the number of alveoli present is only about 15% of the adult lung. This postnatal maturation of lung structure is only seen in altricial mammals (humans, mouse, rabbit) who have the luxury of being able to remain 'helpless' following birth. Precocial species such as range animals are born with a structurally mature lung, ready for immediate activity.[12]

The lungs begin to contain surfactant and are first capable of function by approximately 24–26 weeks, this being a major factor in the viability of premature infants.

LUNG LIQUID

Fetal lungs contain 'lung liquid' (LL) which is secreted by the pulmonary epithelial cells and flows out through the developing airway into the amniotic fluid or gastrointestinal tract, flushing debris from the airways as it does so. A more important function of LL seems to be to prevent the developing lung tissues from collapsing. It is thought that LL maintains the lung at a slight positive pressure relative to the amniotic fluid, and that this expansion is responsible for stimulating cell division and lung growth, particularly with respect to airway branching.[10] The respiratory tract in late pregnancy contains some 40 ml of LL, but its turnover is rapid, believed to be of the order of 500 ml per day. Its volume corresponds approximately with the functional residual capacity (FRC) after breathing is established.[9]

Fetal breathing movements also contribute to lung development. In humans they begin in the middle trimester of pregnancy, and are present for over 20 minutes per hour in the last trimester,[13] normally during periods of general fetal activity. During episodes of breathing, the frequency is about 45 breaths per minute and the diaphragm seems to be the main muscle concerned, producing an estimated fluid shift of about 2 ml at each 'breath'.

Maintenance of a positive pressure in the developing lung requires the upper airway to offer some resistance to the outflow of LL.[9] During apnoea, elastic recoil of the lung tissue and continuous production of LL are both opposed by intrinsic laryngeal resistance and a collapsed pharynx. Fetal inspiratory activity, as in the adult, includes dilation of the upper airway. With quiet breathing this would allow increased efflux of LL from the airway, but simultaneous diaphragmatic contraction opposes this. During vigorous breathing movements with the mouth open, pharyngeal fluid may be 'sucked' into the airway thus contributing to the expansion of the lungs. Thus fetal breathing movements are believed to contribute to maintaining lung expansion, and their abolition is known to impair lung development.[9]

LUNG DEVELOPMENT AND LUNG FUNCTION LATER IN LIFE

Complications of pregnancy such as maternal hypertension, pre-eclampsia or the use of antibiotics have all been shown to increase the incidence of wheezing in childhood.[14] Small abnormalities of lung development in utero or in the early post-natal phase can adversely affect lung function beyond childhood and into adult life.[10,15] For example, in genetically susceptible individuals maternal smoking causes irreversible abnormalities of airway calibre. Abnormalities of amniotic fluid turnover may impair normal lung development in utero, and premature birth alters the normal process of alveolar formation with long term impairment in lung function (see below).

THE FETAL CIRCULATION

The fetal circulation differs radically from the postnatal circulation (Figure 14.1). Blood from the right heart is deflected away from the lungs, partly through the foramen ovale and partly through the ductus arteriosus. Less than 10% of the output of the right ventricle reaches the lungs, the remainder passing to the systemic circulation and the placenta. Right atrial pressure exceeds left atrial pressure and this maintains the patency of the foramen ovale. Furthermore, because the vascular resistance of the pulmonary circulation exceeds that of the systemic circulation before birth, pressure in the right ventricle exceeds that in the left ventricle and these factors control the direction of flow through the ductus arteriosus.

The umbilical veins drain via the ductus venosus into the inferior vena cava, which therefore contains better oxygenated blood than the superior vena cava. The anatomy of the atria and the foramen ovale is such that the better oxygenated blood from the inferior vena cava passes preferentially into the left atrium and thence to the left ventricle and so to the brain. (This is not shown in Figure 14.1). Overall gas tensions in the fetus are of the order of 6.4 kPa (48 mmHg) for P_{CO_2} and 4 kPa (30 mmHg) for P_{O_2}. The fact that the fetus remains apnoeic for much of the time in utero with these blood-gas levels is probably in part attributable to central hypoxic ventilatory depression (page 74).

EVENTS AT BIRTH

Oxygen stores in the fetus are small and it is therefore essential that air breathing and oxygen uptake be established within a few minutes of birth. This requires radical changes in the function of both lungs and circulation.

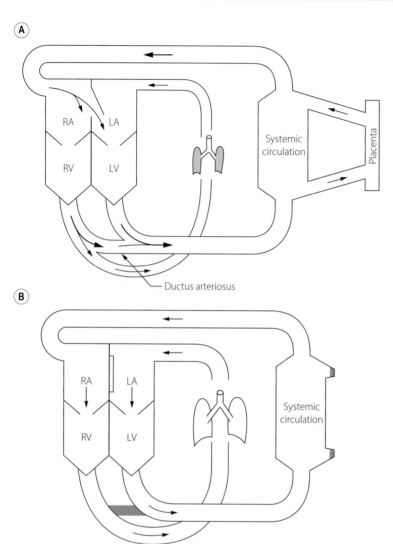

Fig. 14.1 Fetal circulation (A) compared with adult circulation (B). The foramen ovale is between right atrium (RA) and left atrium (LA). RV and LV, right and left ventricles.

FACTORS IN THE INITIATION OF BREATHING

Most infants take their first breath within 20 s of delivery, and rhythmic respiration is usually established within 90 s. Thoracic compression during vaginal delivery followed by recoil of the rib cage causes air to be drawn passively into the lungs. However, the major stimuli to breathing are probably the cooling of the skin and mechanical stimulation, both acting via the respiratory centre. Without this, babies born via Caesarean section would suffer greatly from immediate respiratory difficulties, which is not the case in practice. Hypoxaemia, resulting from apnoea or clamping of the cord, is unlikely to be a reliable respiratory stimulus at this time because of central hypoxic ventilatory depression (see above).

Fate of the fetal lung liquid. The volume of LL decreases just before and during labour. Some of the residual fluid may be expressed during a vaginal delivery but this is not thought to be a major factor. During in-utero life, the pulmonary epithelium actively secretes lung liquid but at birth this process reverses and the epithelial cells switch to absorption of fluid from the airway.[16] Absorption of fluid from airways and alveoli is an active process facilitated by a sodium channel (page 421). The sodium channels are primed during the third trimester by thyroid and steroid hormones, and at birth, fetal adrenaline and oxygen trigger the channels to become active. Aquaporin, a trans-membrane protein that facilitates water transport across membranes, is present in lungs at birth but its role remains uncertain.[16,17]

CHANGES IN THE CIRCULATION

The geometry of the circulation changes radically and quickly at birth. The establishment of spontaneous breathing causes a massive decrease in the vascular resistance of the pulmonary circulation, due partly to mechanical factors and partly to changes in blood gases. Simultaneously there is an increase in the resistance of the systemic circulation, due partly to vasoconstriction and partly to cessation of the placental circulation. As a result, the right atrial pressure falls below the left atrial pressure, to give the relationship that is then maintained throughout life. This normally results in closure of the foramen ovale (Figure 14.1), which is followed by closure of the ductus arteriosus as a result of active vasoconstriction of its smooth muscle layer in response to increased Po_2. The circulation is thus converted from the fetal mode, in which the lungs and the systemic circulation are essentially in parallel, to the adult mode in which they are in series.

Mechanism of reduced pulmonary vascular resistance at birth. Pulmonary vascular resistance declines due to a combination of ventilation of the lung and changes in blood gases, particularly increasing Po_2. Clearly this is a difficult area to study in humans, and most work has been performed in other mammals,[9] but there is no reason to expect humans to differ significantly. Removal of LL from the lung establishes an air–liquid interface that is responsible for a rapid increase in lung recoil pressure, which, possibly along with changes in chest wall compliance, results in a negative intrapleural pressure as in adult lungs. This creates the transmural pressure gradient between the alveoli and pleura, which physically dilates the pulmonary capillaries (page 104). These mechanical forces leading to a reduction in pulmonary vascular resistance are believed to account for over half of the observed changes at birth.

Further reductions in pulmonary vascular resistance as a result of increased Po_2 and decreased Pco_2 are believed to be endothelium dependent.[18] Though many mediators may be involved, prostaglandins, endothelin and nitric oxide are the most

widely studied. The first two groups have conflicting effects on the neonatal pulmonary circulation, with in vitro studies showing both vasodilating and vasoconstricting effects of different individual mediators. Prostacyclin seems to be involved in the in vivo vasodilation of pulmonary blood vessels at birth, but the effect is minor. In animals, inhibition of nitric oxide synthase prior to birth attenuates the reduction in pulmonary vascular resistance on delivery.

Persistent pulmonary hypertension of the newborn (PPHN)[19] occurs in about 1 in 1000 births. Pulmonary vascular resistance remains elevated, so right heart pressures remain high and a significant right-to-left shunt continues with resulting hypoxaemia. Although PPHN may occur with other parenchymal lung problems such as meconium aspiration or respiratory distress syndrome, it also occurs in isolation. Mechanical changes at birth leading to pulmonary vasodilation, as described above, still occur and are probably responsible for bringing about sufficient pulmonary blood flow for immediate survival. However, structural abnormalities of pulmonary vessels are common in PPHN, and may limit the vasodilation obtained by mechanical factors. There is undoubtedly an element of abnormal pulmonary vasoconstriction, or at least a failure of oxygen-stimulated vasodilation, in babies with PPHN and abnormalities of both endothelin and nitric oxide activity are implicated.

THE APGAR SCORE

The scoring system devised many years ago by Virginia Apgar is still widely accepted as an assessment of the overall condition of the neonate. This is based on scoring of a scale of 0–2 for five attributes, two of which are related to respiration (Table 14.2).[20] The total score is the sum of each of the five constituent scores and is best undertaken 1 and 5 minutes after delivery. Scores of 8–10 are regarded as normal.

NEONATAL LUNG FUNCTION

Mechanics of breathing. Functional residual capacity is about $30\,ml.kg^{-1}$ and total respiratory compliance $50\,ml.kPa^{-1}$ ($5\,ml.cmH_2O^{-1}$). Most of the impedance to expansion is due to the lung and depends primarily on the presence of surfactant in the alveoli. The chest wall of the neonate is highly compliant. This

Table 14.2 The Apgar scoring system

SCORE	0	1	2
Heart rate	Absent	Less than 100 per min	More than 100 per min
Respiratory effort	Absent	Slow, irregular	Good, crying
Colour	Blue, pale	Body pink, extremities blue	Completely pink
Reflex irritability	Absent	Grimace	Cough, sneeze
Muscle tone	Limp	Some flexion of extremities	Active motion

Add together scores for each section (maximum possible 10). Score at 1 and 5 minutes after delivery. After reference 20.

contrasts with the adult, in whom compliance of lung and chest wall are approximately equal. Total respiratory resistance is of the order of $7\,kPa.l^{-1}.s$ $(70\,cmH_2O.l^{-1}.s)$, most of which is in the bronchial tree. Compliance is about one-twentieth that of an adult and resistance about 15 times greater. At the first breath the infant is capable of generating a sub-atmospheric intra-thoracic pressure of the order of $7\,kPa$ $(70\,cmH_2O)$.

Ventilation and gas exchange. For a 3 kg neonate, the minute volume is about $0.6\,l.min^{-1}$, with a high respiratory frequency of 25–40 breaths per minute. Dead space is close to a half of tidal volume, giving a mean alveolar ventilation of about $0.3\,l.min^{-1}$ for a neonate of average size. There is a shunt of about 10% immediately after birth. However, distribution of gas is better than in the adult and there is, of course, a negligible hydrostatic pressure gradient in the vertical axis of the tiny lungs of an infant.

Oxygen consumption is of the order of 20–30 ml. min^{-1}, depending on weight in the range 2–4 kg. Arterial Pco_2 is close to $4.5\,kPa$ $(34\,mmHg)$ and Po_2 $9\,kPa$ $(68\,mmHg)$. Because of the shunt of 10%, there is an alveolar/arterial Po_2 gradient of about $3.3\,kPa$ $(25\,mmHg)$ compared with less than half of this in a young adult. Arterial pH is within the normal adult range.

Control of breathing. Animal studies have shown that, in the fetus, carotid chemoreceptors are active but at a much lower Po_2 than in adults; the ventilatory response curve is displaced far to the left compared with adults. Prolonged periods of apnoea seen in utero in spite of this carotid sinus activity occur because of brain stem inhibition of the respiratory centre. In contrast to this, cardiovascular responses to hypoxia are well developed in the fetus, bradycardia and vasoconstriction being well recognised responses to hypoxia in neonates as shown by the Apgar score. After birth, there is a very rapid transition towards the adult pattern of respiratory control. Brainstem hypoxic ventilatory depression ceases, and the carotid chemoreceptors 'reset' to adult values within a few weeks.[21] Ventilatory response to carbon dioxide appears to be similar to that in the adult if allowance is made for body size, although the response is depressed in REM sleep[22] and the apnoeic threshold (page 70) may be closer to the normal Pco_2 in neonates resulting in a susceptibility to apnoea.[23]

At birth, changes in respiratory pattern must, by necessity, be substantial as the long periods of apnoea seen in utero are incompatible with life in the outside world. Although most changes occur shortly after birth, complete transition to 'adult' respiration may take some weeks to complete, particularly in premature and small babies, and those with other respiratory problems that cause repeated periods of hypoxia.[24] In the meantime, newborn infants have a variety of breathing patterns. For example, 'periodic breathing' consists of slowly oscillating changes in respiratory rate and tidal volume size; 'periodic apnoea' consists of a series of respiratory pauses of over four seconds' duration with a few normal breaths in between. In normal babies aged under two months of age, there may be in excess of 200 apnoeic episodes and 50 minutes of periodic breathing per day,[25] and these may be associated with short lived reductions in saturation.[26] The proportion of time spent with regular breathing increases with age, such that, beyond three months old, periodic breathing and apnoeas are significantly less.[25] Moderate reductions in inspired oxygen (15%), similar to that seen during flying or at altitude (Chapter 17), cause a dramatic increase in the amount of time 3-month-old infants spend with periodic apnoea, indicating that adult hypoxic ventilatory responses are not fully developed.[27]

Haemoglobin. Children are normally born polycythaemic with a mean haemoglobin of about

$18 \, g.dl^{-1}$ and a haematocrit (packed cell volume) of 53%. Some 70% of the haemoglobin is HbF and the resultant P_{50} is well below the normal adult value (see Figure 11.9). Arterial oxygen content is close to the normal adult value in spite of the low arterial Po_2. The haemoglobin concentration decreases rapidly to become less than the normal adult value by 3 weeks of life. HbF gradually disappears from the circulation to reach negligible values by 6 months, by which time the P_{50} has already attained the normal adult value.

PREMATURE BIRTH AND THE LUNGS

RESPIRATORY DISTRESS SYNDROME (RDS)[28]

The syndrome comprises respiratory distress within a few hours of birth and occurs in 2% of all live births, but with a greatly increased incidence in premature infants. The essential lesion is a deficiency of surfactant, which is first detectable in the fetal lung at 20–24 weeks of gestation, but the concentration increases rapidly after the 30th week. Therefore, prematurity is a major factor in the aetiology of RDS, though male babies, Caesarean delivery, perinatal stress or birth asphyxia, and maternal diabetes are all additional risk factors for its development. There is believed to be a genetic susceptibility to developing RDS, possibly resulting from inherited variations in surfactant proteins A and B (page 29).

The disease presents with difficulty in inspiration against the decreased compliance due to the high surface tension of the surfactant-deficient alveolar lining fluid. This progresses to ventilatory failure, alveolar collapse, hyaline membrane deposit, pulmonary oedema leading to denaturing of surfactant, and ultimately interference with gas exchange, resulting in severe hypoxaemia. Increased pulmonary vascular resistance may raise right atrial pressure and reopen the foramen ovale, so increasing the shunt.

Principles of therapy. The physiological basis of therapy is to supplement surfactant activity and employ artificial ventilation as a temporary expedient to spare the infant the excessive work of breathing against stiff lungs.

Surfactant replacement therapy is difficult because endogenous surfactant is complex, consisting of phospholipids and protein components (page 29).[29,30] Exogenous surfactants may be either synthetic,

consisting mostly of phospholipids, or natural surfactant preparations, obtained from mammalian lungs, which contain both phospholipid and some of the surfactant proteins, though not necessarily of the same type and proportion as in humans. Surfactant proteins are important to facilitate spreading of the surfactant around the lung following administration by intra-tracheal instillation, and natural surfactants may therefore be more effective as therapeutic agents.[29] Surfactant replacement therapy has now been conclusively shown to improve survival and reduce complication rates in RDS, with greater efficacy when given earlier in the course of the disease.[31]

Artificial ventilation is considered in Chapter 32. A high respiratory frequency is required such that inspiratory and expiratory durations may be as little as 0.3 second, but inflation pressures are similar to those used in adults and do not usually exceed $3 \, kPa$ ($30 \, cmH_2O$). Both the compressible volume of the ventilator circuit and the apparatus dead space tend to be large in relation to the size of very small children so pressure generators are preferable to volume generators.

Extracorporeal membrane oxygenation (ECMO) is described in Chapter 32. In contrast to its use in adults, ECMO is of proven benefit in infants (page 487) reducing mortality and long term disability in severe neonatal respiratory failure from a variety of causes,[32] including RDS. Unfortunately, most cases of RDS cannot be treated with ECMO as a result of technical problems in babies of less than $2 \, kg$ weight or 35 weeks gestation.

Partial liquid ventilation with perflubron, a synthetic oxygen carrier (page 197), has been successfully used in neonates with severe RDS.[33] A volume of Perflubron approximately equal to the infant's FRC is instilled into the lungs, and positive pressure ventilation by conventional methods continued. The liquid improves lung function by replacing the alveolar air–liquid interface, by physically preventing alveolar collapse, and by increasing lung compliance allowing more effective ventilation. Chest radiographs show the extent to which partial liquid ventilation replaces normal gas-filled lung, and also shows that clearance of Perflubron by evaporation from the lung takes some time (Figure 14.2).

BRONCHOPULMONARY DYSPLASIA[30]

Bronchopulmonary dysplasia describes a condition in which a neonate requires oxygen therapy for more than 28 days because of poor lung function.

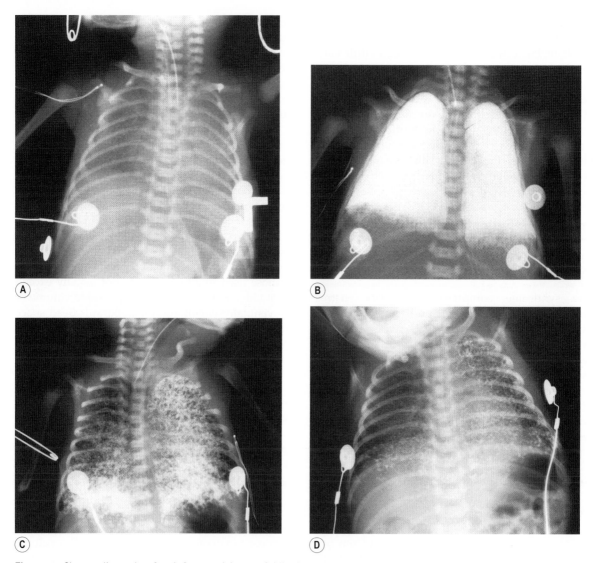

Fig. 14.2 Chest radiographs of an infant receiving partial liquid ventilation for severe respiratory distress syndrome. (A) Conventional ventilation for respiratory distress syndrome. (B) partial liquid ventilation with Perflubron. (C) 48 hours after termination of liquid ventilation, and (D) three weeks later. (After reference 33 with permission of the authors and the publishers of New England Journal of Medicine. Copyright © 1996 Massachusetts Medical Society. All rights reserved.)

It is a common complication of RDS, and may simply be a form of pulmonary barotrauma (page 482) in the ventilated neonate or may represent abnormal lung development as a result of prematurity. Airway damage, including smooth muscle hypertrophy, inflammation and fibrosis all occur, and the alveolar stage of lung development (page 250) may be abnormal. Long-term impairment of lung function results, at least into childhood and possibly throughout the patient's whole life.[30,34]

SUDDEN INFANT DEATH SYNDROME (SIDS)[35,36]

This is defined simply as the sudden death of an infant younger than 1 year of age that remains unexplained after review of the clinical history, examination of the circumstances of the death and a post-mortem examination. The peak incidence is at 2–3 months of age and there remains a multitude of theories regarding the aetiology, though the respiratory system is implicated in most. A triple risk hypothesis is proposed, which suggests that an infant must be vulnerable to SIDS, must be at a critical stage of development of homeostatic control and must receive a stressor such as an infection, parental smoking or sleeping in the prone position.[36]

Abnormal homeostatic control may include respiratory disturbances. The apnoea hypothesis remains popular, mainly because of the frequent periods of apnoea and desaturation observed in almost all babies under 3 months old (see above). The peak incidence of SIDS corresponds to the period of development when the fetal and adult systems for ventilatory control are swapping over, and it is believed that this may make the infant susceptible to respiratory disturbances. Normal patterns of arousal from sleep are altered in babies who subsequently become SIDS victims.[37] Post-mortem studies have found decreased binding of serotonin in several areas of the brain including an area which, in adults, is believed to be crucial in controlling arousal from sleep.[35] Despite the popularity of the apnoea hypothesis evidence that these episodes of periodic breathing or apnoeas contribute directly to SIDS is lacking.

Sleeping position. There is a substantial body of agreement that the prone sleeping position is commoner in infants dying of SIDS, though the mechanism remains uncertain. In the late 1980s and early 1990s many countries introduced national health educational policies to encourage the avoidance of the prone sleeping position, and the incidence of SIDS was reduced by 50–90%.

DEVELOPMENT OF LUNG FUNCTION DURING CHILDHOOD

The lungs continue to develop during childhood. Chest wall compliance, which is very high at birth, decreases rapidly for the first two years of life, when it becomes approximately equal to lung compliance as in the adult.[38] Below the age of 8 years, measurement of lung volumes is difficult, but beyond this age many studies of normal lung function are available. Because of large variations in the rate at which children grow, reference values are usually related to height rather than age or weight. Equations relating lung volumes to height are available,[39] and some are shown in graphical form in Figure 14.3.

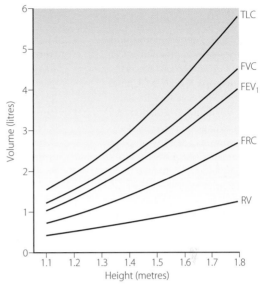

Fig. 14.3 Changes in lung volumes as a function of stature. When considering reference values for children, height in metres is used in preference to age to allow for large differences in growth rate. Each graph represents the mean for both boys and girls, though boys generally have greater values at equivalent heights.

Various indices of respiratory function are independent of age and body size so that adult values can be used. These include forced expiratory volume (1 second) as a fraction of vital capacity, functional residual capacity and peak expiratory flow rate as a fraction of total lung capacity, *specific* airway conductance and *specific* compliance (page 34) and probably dead space/tidal volume ratio.[39]

Blood gases and the control of breathing. Arterial Pco_2 and alveolar Po_2 do not change appreciably during childhood but arterial Po_2 increases from the neonatal value to reach a maximum of about 13 kPa (98 mmHg) at young adulthood. Much of this increase occurs during the first year of life. There are obvious difficulties in determining the normal arterial Po_2 in children. Ventilatory responses to both hypercapnia and hypoxia are at their highest in early childhood and decrease progressively into adulthood.[40] The changes are small for hypoxic responses, but quite marked for hypercapnia, and are believed to relate to the higher metabolic rate in children.

References

1. Elkus R, Popovich J. Respiratory physiology in pregnancy. *Clin Chest Med*. 1992;13:555–565.

2. Garcia-Rio F, Pino JM, Gomez L, Alvarez-Sala R, Villasnate C, Villamor J. Regulation of breathing and perception of dyspnoea in healthy pregnant women. *Chest*. 1996;110:446–453.

3. Templeton A, Kelman GR. Maternal blood-gases, ($P_{A_{O2}}$-Pa_{O2}), physiological shunt and V_D/V_T in normal pregnancy. *Br J Anaesth*. 1976;48:1001–1004.

4. Pernol ML, Metcalfe J, Schlenker TL, Welch JE, Matsumoto JA. Oxygen consumption at rest and during exercise in pregnancy. *Respir Physiol*. 1975; 25:285–292.

5. Moore LG, McCullough RE, Weil JV. Increased HVR in pregnancy: relationship to hormonal and metabolic changes. *J Appl Physiol*. 1987;62:158–163.

6. Jensen D, Webb KA, Davies GAL, O'Donnell DE. Mechanical ventilatory constraints during incremental cycle exercise in human pregnancy: implications for respiratory sensation. *J Physiol*. 2008;586:4735–4750.

7. Merkus PJFM, ten Have-Opbroek AAW, Quanjer PH. Human lung growth: A review. *Ped Pulmonol*. 1996;21:383–397.

*8. Jeffery PK. The development of large and small airways. *Am J Respir Crit Care Med*. 1998;157:S174–S180.

9. Harding R, Hooper SB. Regulation of lung expansion and lung growth before birth. *J Appl Physiol*. 1996;81:209–224.

*10. Shi W, Bellusci S, Warburton D. Lung development and adult lung diseases. *Chest*. 2007;132:651–656.

11. Maeda Y, Davé V, Whitsett JA. Transcriptional control of lung morphogenesis. *Physiol Rev*. 2007;87:219–244.

12. Massaro GD, Massaro D. Formation of pulmonary alveoli and gas-exchange surface area: Quantitation and regulation. *Annu Rev Physiol*. 1996;58:73–92.

13. Patrick J, Campbell K, Carmichael L, Natale R, Richardson B. Patterns of human fetal breathing during the last 10 weeks of pregnancy. *Obstet Gynecol*. 1980;56:24–30.

14. Rusconi F, Galassi C, Forastiere F, et al. Maternal complications and procedures in pregnancy and at birth and wheezing phenotypes in children. *Am J Respir Crit Care Med*. 2007;175:16–21.

15. Bush A, Annesi-Maesano I. Beam Me Up, Scotty!. *Am J Respir Crit Care Med*. 2007;175:1–2.

16. Barker PM, Olver RE. Clearance of lung liquid during the perinatal period. *J Appl Physiol*. 2002;93:1542–1548.

17. Verkman AS, Matthay MA, Song Y. Aquaporin water channels and lung physiology. *Am J Physiol Lung Cell Mol Physiol*. 2002;278:L867–L879.

18. Ziegler JW, Ivy DD, Kinsella JP, Abman SH. The role of nitric oxide, endothelin, and prostaglandins in the transition of the pulmonary circulation. *Clin Perinatol*. 1995;22:387–403.

19. Steinhorn RH, Millard SL, Morin FC. Persistent pulmonary hypertension of the newborn. *Clin Perinatol*. 1995;22:405–428.

20. McIntosh N. The newborn. In: Campbell AGM, McIntosh N, eds. *Forfar and Arneil's Textbook of Pediatrics*. Edinburgh: Churchill Livingstone; 1998.

21. Donnelly DF. Assisting Mother Nature in postnatal chemoreceptor maturation. *J Appl Physiol*. 2008;104:1260–1261.

22. Cohen G, Xu C, Henderson-Smart D. Ventilatory response of the sleeping newborn to CO_2 during normoxic rebreathing. *J Appl Physiol*. 1991;71:168–174.

23. Khan A, Qurashi M, Kwiatkowski K, Cates D, Rigatto H. Measurement of the CO_2 apneic threshold in newborn infants: possible relevance for periodic breathing and apnea. *J Appl Physiol*. 2005;98:1171–1176.

24. Greer J. Development of respiratory rhythm generation. *J Appl Physiol*. 2008;104:1211–1212.

25. Richards JM, Alexander JR, Shinebourne EA, de Swiet M, Wilson AJ, Southall DP. Sequential 22-hour profiles of breathing patterns and heart rate in 110 full-term infants during their first 6 months of life. *Pediatrics*. 1984;74:763–777.

26. Stebbens VA, Poets CF, Alexander JR, Arrowsmith WA, Southall DP. Oxygen saturation and breathing patterns in infancy. 1: Full term infants in the second month of life. *Arch Dis Child*. 1991;66:569–573.

27. Parkins KJ, Poets CF, O'Brien LM, Stebbens VA, Southall DP. Effect of exposure to 15% oxygen on breathing patterns and oxygen saturation in infants: interventional study. *BMJ*. 1998;316:887–894.

28. Copland IB, Post M. Understanding the mechanisms of infant respiratory distress and chronic lung disease. *Am J Respir Cell Mol Biol*. 2002;26:261–265.

29. Merrill JD, Ballard RA. Pulmonary surfactant for neonatal respiratory disorders. *Curr Opin Pediatrics*. 2003;15:149–154.

30. Baraldi E, Filippone M. Chronic lung disease after premature birth. *N Engl J Med*. 2007;357:1946–1955.

*31. Stevens TP, Sinkin RA. Surfactant replacement therapy. *Chest*. 2007;131:1577–1582.

32. UK Collaborative ECMO Trial Group. UK collaborative trial of neonatal extracorporeal membrane oxygenation. *Lancet*. 1996;348:75–82.

33. Leach CL, Greenspan JS, Rubenstein SD, et al. Partial liquid ventilation with perflubron in premature infants with severe respiratory distress syndrome. The LiquiVent study group. *N Engl J Med.* 1996;335:761–767.

34. Vrijlandt EJLE, Gerritsen J, Boezen HM, Grevink RG, Duiverman EJ. Lung function and exercise capacity in young adults born prematurely. *Am J Respir Crit Care Med.* 2006;173:890–896.

35. Hunt CE. Sudden infant death syndrome and other causes of infant mortality. Diagnosis, mechanisms, and risk for recurrence in siblings. *Am J Respir Crit Care Med.* 2001;164:346–357.

*36. Moon RY, Horne RSC, Hauck FR. Sudden infant death syndrome. *Lancet.* 2007;370:1578–1587.

37. Harper RM. Impaired arousals and sudden infant death syndrome. Pre-existing neuronal injury? *Am J Respir Crit Care Med.* 2003;168:1262–1263.

38. Papastamelos C, Panitch HB, England SE, Allen JL. Developmental changes in chest wall compliance in infancy and early childhood. *J Appl Physiol.* 1995;78:179–184.

39. Cotes JE, Chinn DJ, Miller MR. *Lung Function. Physiology, Measurement and Application in Medicine.* Oxford: Blackwell Publishing; 2006.

40. Marcus CL, Glomb WB, Basinski DJ, Davidson SL, Keens TG. Developmental pattern of hypercapnic and hypoxic ventilatory responses from childhood to adulthood. *J Appl Physiol.* 1994;76:314–320.

Chapter 15

Exercise

KEY POINTS

- Oxygen consumption increases linearly with the power expended during exercise.
- The extra tissue oxygen requirement is provided by increases in cardiac output and blood oxygen extraction.
- To accommodate these changes ventilation also increases linearly with exercise – this response occurs the moment exercise begins.
- As exercise intensity increases lactate is produced from anaerobic muscle metabolism and blood lactate levels increase, initially reaching a steady state, but continuing to rise with severe exercise.

The respiratory response to exercise depends on the level of exercise performed, which can be conveniently divided into three grades:

1. *Moderate exercise* is below the subject's anaerobic threshold (see below) and the arterial blood lactate is not raised. The subject is able to transport all the oxygen required and remain in a steady state.
2. *Heavy exercise* is above the anaerobic threshold. The arterial blood lactate is elevated but remains constant. This too may be regarded as a steady state.
3. *Severe exercise* is well above the anaerobic threshold and the arterial blood lactate continues to rise. This is an unsteady state and the level of work cannot long be sustained.

OXYGEN CONSUMPTION DURING EXERCISE

There is a close relationship between the external power that is produced and the oxygen consumption of the subject (Figure 15.1). The oxygen consumption at rest (the basal metabolic rate) is of the order of 200–250 ml.min^{-1}. As work is done, the oxygen consumption increases by approximately 12 ml.min^{-1} per watt. Exercise intensity is commonly described in terms of *metabolic equivalents* (METs), which refer to the number of multiples of the normal resting oxygen consumption. For example, walking briskly on the level requires an oxygen consumption of about 1 l.min^{-1} or 4 METs, whilst running at 12 km per hour (7.5 miles per hour) requires about 3 l.min^{-1} of oxygen and is rated as 12 METs of activity. Further examples are shown in Figure 15.1.

TIME COURSE OF THE INCREASE IN OXYGEN CONSUMPTION[1]

Oxygen consumption rises rapidly at the onset of a period of exercise, with an accompanying increase in carbon dioxide production and a small increase in blood lactate. With moderate exercise (Figure 15.2A) a plateau is quickly reached and the lactate level remains well below the normal maximum resting level (<3.5 mmol.l^{-1}). With heavy exercise $\dot{V}_{O_2}$, $\dot{V}_{CO_2}$ and lactate all increase more quickly, again

DOI: 10.1016/B978-0-7020-2996-7.00015-5

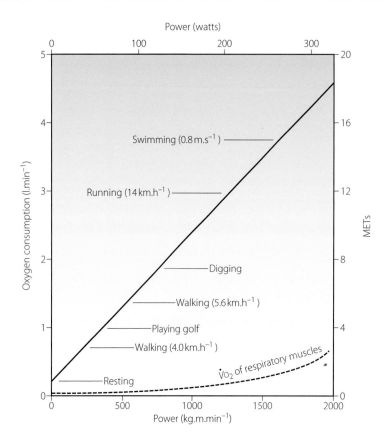

Fig. 15.1 Steady state oxygen consumption with varying degrees of exercise. The continuous straight line denotes whole body oxygen consumption as a function of the level of power developed. The broken curve is an estimate of the oxygen cost of breathing for the increasing hyperventilation of exercise.[1] MET, metabolic equivalent, which is the number of multiples of basal oxygen consumption required for different activities.

reaching constant levels within a few minutes, the magnitude of which relates to the power generated and the fitness of the subject (Figure 15.2B). If the level of exercise exceeds approximately 60% of the subject's maximal exercise ability (see below), there is usually a secondary 'slow component' to the increase in oxygen consumption, associated with a continuing increase in blood lactate level, which ultimately prevents the exercise from continuing (Figure 15.2C). There have been many explanations proposed for this slow component of $\dot{V}_{O_2}$, including increased temperature, the oxygen cost of breathing, lactic acidosis[1] and changes in muscle metabolism secondary to the use of differing fibre types with prolonged exercise.[2] The physiological mechanism underlying the linkage between oxygen requirement and its delivery during exercise, and the time course of this response, remain incompletely explained.[3]

MAXIMAL OXYGEN UPTAKE

Maximal oxygen uptake ($\dot{V}_{O_{2max}}$) refers to the oxygen consumption of a subject when exercising

as hard as possible for that subject. A fit and healthy young adult of 70 kg should be able to maintain a $\dot{V}_{O_{2max}}$ of about 3l.min^{-1}, but this decreases with age to about 2l.min^{-1} at the age of 70. A sedentary existence without exercise can reduce $\dot{V}_{O_{2max}}$ to 50% of the expected value. Conversely, $\dot{V}_{O_{2max}}$ can be increased by regular exercise, and athletes commonly achieve values of 5l.min^{-1}. The highest levels (over 6l.min^{-1}) are attained in rowers, who utilise a greater muscle mass than other athletes. For example elite oarsmen may attain, for a brief period, a mean oxygen consumption of 6.6l.min^{-1} on the treadmill.[4] This requires a minute volume of 200l.min^{-1} (tidal volume 3.29 litres at a frequency of 62 breaths per minute).

$\dot{V}_{O_{2max}}$ is commonly used in exercise physiology as a measure of cardiorespiratory fitness. Subjects undertake a period of graduated exercise while $\dot{V}_{O_2}$ is measured continuously by a spirometric method (page 211). In all but severe exercise, within a few minutes $\dot{V}_{O_2}$ reaches a plateau (Figure 15.2), which is the subject's $\dot{V}_{O_{2max}}$. At higher levels of exercise, as seen in athletes, defining when maximal oxygen uptake is reached may be difficult because of the slow component of oxygen consumption. Many varying definitions of $\dot{V}O_{2max}$ have therefore been used over the years,[5] none of which are universally accepted. Elite athletes rarely reach a satisfactory plateau in $\dot{V}O_2$, and secondary criteria such as high plasma lactate levels or a raised respiratory exchange ratio need to be used to define $\dot{V}O_{2max}$.[5]

At $\dot{V}O_{2max}$ in trained athletes, approximately 80% of the oxygen consumed is used by locomotor muscles. With the high minute volumes seen during exercise, the oxygen consumption of respiratory muscles also becomes significant, being around 5% of total $\dot{V}O_2$ with moderate exercise and 10% at $\dot{V}O_{2max}$ (Figure 15.1).[6,7]

RESPONSE OF THE OXYGEN DELIVERY SYSTEM

A 10- or 20-fold increase in oxygen consumption requires a complex adaptation of both circulatory and respiratory systems.

Oxygen delivery. This is the product of cardiac output and arterial oxygen content (page 202). The latter cannot be significantly increased, so an increase in cardiac output is essential. However, the cardiac output does not, and indeed could not, increase in proportion to the oxygen consumption. For example, an oxygen consumption of $4\,l.min^{-1}$ is a 16-fold increase compared with the resting state. A typical cardiac output at this level of exercise would be only $25\,l.min^{-1}$ (Figure 15.3), which is only five times the resting value. Therefore, there must also be increased extraction of oxygen from the blood. Figure 15.3 shows that the largest relative increase in cardiac output occurs at mild levels of exercise. At an oxygen consumption of $1\,l.min^{-1}$ cardiac output is already close to 50% of its maximal value.

Oxygen extraction. In the resting state, blood returns to the right heart with haemoglobin 70% saturated. This provides a substantial reserve of available oxygen and the arterial/mixed venous oxygen content difference increases progressively as oxygen consumption is increased, particularly in heavy exercise when the mixed venous saturation may be as low as 20% (Figure 15.3). This decrease in mixed venous saturation covers the steep part of the oxygen dissociation curve (Figure 11.9) and therefore the decrease in Po_2 is relatively less (5 to $2\,kPa$, or 37.5 to $15\,mmHg$). High levels of blood lactate seen during heavy exercise may

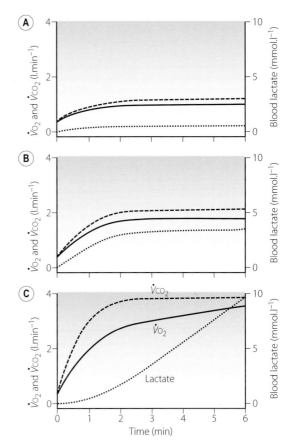

Fig. 15.2 Changes in oxygen consumption ($\dot{V}O_2$, solid line), CO_2 production ($\dot{V}CO_2$, dashed line) and blood lactate (dotted line) with the onset of varying levels of exercise. (A) Light to moderate exercise with little or no increase in lactate; (B) heavy exercise with an increase in lactate to an increased, but steady, level; (C) severe exercise, above the anaerobic threshold when levels continue to rise as exercise proceeds. Note that with severe exercise (C), the increase in oxygen consumption is biphasic with a second 'slow' component.

contribute to the increase in oxygen extraction by shifting the dissociation curve to the right at a capillary level.[1]

The additionally desaturated blood returning to the lungs and the greater volume of blood require that the respiratory system transport a larger quantity of oxygen to the alveoli. If there were no increased oxygen transport to the alveoli, the reserve oxygen in the mixed venous blood would be exhausted in one or two circulation times. Fortunately the respiratory system normally responds rapidly to this requirement.

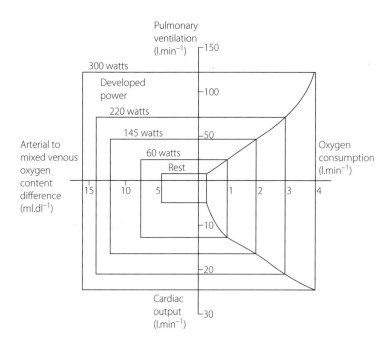

Fig. 15.3 Changes in ventilation, oxygen consumption, cardiac output and oxygen extraction at different levels of power developed.

ANAEROBIC METABOLISM

During heavy exercise, the total work exceeds the capacity for aerobic work, which is limited by oxygen transport (see below). The difference is made up by anaerobic metabolism, of which the principal product is lactic acid (see Figure 11.13), which is almost entirely ionised to lactate and hydrogen ions. The anaerobic threshold may be defined as the highest intensity of exercise at which measured oxygen uptake can account for the entire energy requirement.[8] Exercise intensity at the anaerobic threshold depends not only on the power produced but also on many other factors including environmental temperature, the degree of training undertaken by the subject and altitude. An additional factor is the muscle groups that are used to accomplish the work, as different skeletal muscle fibres, and therefore muscle groups, have different metabolic products.[1]

During severe exercise the lactate level continues to rise (Figure 15.2C) and begins to cause distress at levels above about $11\,mmol.l^{-1}$, 10 times the normal resting level. Lactate accumulation seems to be the limiting factor for sustained heavy work, and the progressive increase in blood lactate results in the level of work being inversely related to the time for which it can be maintained. Thus there is a reciprocal relationship between the record time for various distances and the speed at which they are run.

OXYGEN DEBT

The difference between the total work and the aerobic work is achieved by anaerobic metabolism of carbohydrates to lactate, which is ultimately converted to citrate, enters the citric acid cycle and is then fully oxidised (page 199). Like glucose, lactate has a respiratory quotient of 1.0. Although this process continues during heavy exercise, lactate accumulates and the excess is oxidised in the early stages of recovery. Oxygen consumption remains above the resting level during recovery for this purpose. This constitutes the 'repayment of the oxygen debt' and is related to the lactate level attained by the end of exercise.

Repayment of the oxygen debt is especially well developed in the diving mammals such as seals and whales. During a dive, their circulation is largely diverted to heart and brain, and the metabolism of the skeletal muscles is almost entirely anaerobic (page 298). On regaining the surface, very large quantities of lactate are suddenly released into the circulation and are rapidly metabolised while the animal is on the surface between dives.

Excess post-exercise oxygen consumption. Sustained heavy exercise results in an increased $\dot{V}O_2$ even when the subject's blood lactate remains only mildly elevated. Excess oxygen consumption may occur for several hours, and is related to both the intensity and duration of exercise undertaken.

Previous hypotheses put forward to explain the excess $\dot{V}_{O_2}$ included an increase in body temperature and increased fat metabolism, though proof of these is lacking. Exercise at around 75% of $\dot{V}_{O_2max}$ raises levels of catabolic hormones such as cortisol and catecholamines, which may explain the excess $\dot{V}_{O_2}$.[9]

THE VENTILATORY RESPONSE TO EXERCISE

Time course.[10] In the previous section it was seen that exercise without a rapid ventilatory response would be dangerous if not fatal. In fact, the respiratory system does respond with great rapidity (Figure 15.4). There is an instant increase in ventilation at, if not slightly before, the start of exercise (phase I). During moderate exercise, there is then a further increase (phase II) to reach an equilibrium level of ventilation (phase III) within about 3 minutes. With heavy exercise there is a secondary increase in ventilation that may reach a plateau, but ventilation continues to rise in severe work. At the end of exercise, the minute volume falls to resting levels within a few minutes. After heavy and severe exercise, return to the resting level of ventilation takes longer, as the oxygen debt is repaid and lactate levels return to normal.

The ventilation equivalent for oxygen. The respiratory minute volume is normally very well matched to the increased oxygen consumption, and the relationship between minute volume and oxygen consumption is approximately linear up to an oxygen consumption of about $2\,l.min^{-1}$ in the untrained subject and more following training (Figure 15.5). The slope of the linear part is the ventilation equivalent for oxygen and is within the range 20–$30\,l.min^{-1}$ ventilation per $l.min^{-1}$ of oxygen consumption. The slope does not appear to change with training.

In heavy exercise, above a critical level of oxygen consumption (Owles point), the ventilation increases above the level predicted by an extrapolation of the linear part of the ventilation/oxygen consumption relationship (Figure 15.5). This is surplus to the requirement for gas exchange and is accompanied by hypocapnia with arterial P_{CO_2} decreasing by levels of the order of $1\,kPa$ ($7.5\,mmHg$). The excess ventilation is probably driven by lactic acidosis, though other possible explanations exist such as a humoral agent from muscle metabolism affecting

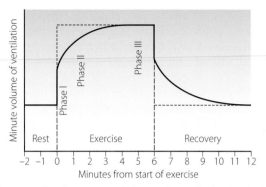

Fig. 15.4 The time course of changes in ventilation in relation to a short period of moderate exercise. Note the instant increase in ventilation at the start of exercise before the metabolic consequences of exercise have had time to develop.

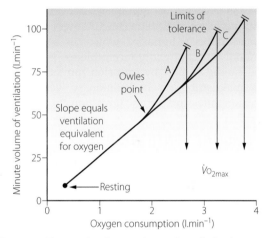

Fig. 15.5 Changes in minute volume of ventilation in response to the increased oxygen consumption of exercise. The break from linearity (Owles point) occurs at higher levels of oxygen consumption in trained athletes, who can also tolerate higher minute volumes. A to C shows progressive levels of training. Both mechanisms combine to enable the trained athlete to increase his maximum oxygen consumption.

the carotid body, possibly potassium.[11] In the trained athlete, the break from linearity occurs at higher levels of oxygen consumption. This together with improved tolerance of high minute volumes allows the trained athlete to increase his $\dot{V}_{O_2max}$ as shown in Figure 15.5.

Minute volume and dyspnoea. It is generally believed that the ventilatory system does not limit exercise in normal subjects, although the evidence for this view is elusive.[12] One study[13] found that 50–60% of maximal breathing capacity (MBC) was required for work at 80% of aerobic capacity. However, the breaking point of exercise is usually determined by breathlessness, which occurs when the exercise ventilation utilises a high proportion of the MBC. There is a close correlation between MBC and $\dot{V}O_{2max}$.

Minute volumes as great as 200 l.min^{-1} have been recorded during exercise although the normal subject cannot maintain a minute volume approaching MBC for more than a very short period. Tidal volume during maximal exercise is about half vital capacity, and 70–80% of MBC can normally be maintained, with difficulty, for 15 minutes by fit young subjects.[13] Ventilation approximates to 60% of MBC at maximal oxygen consumption. The usable fraction of the MBC can, however, be increased by training.

Diffusing capacity. Diffusion across the alveolar/capillary membrane does not normally limit the increased oxygen consumption at sea level but this is a limiting factor at altitude (see Chapters 9 and 17). Exercise-induced hypoxia, which is seen fairly commonly in elite endurance athletes, is believed to be caused in part by diffusion limitation along with maldistribution of pulmonary ventilation/perfusion ratios and airflow limitation.[14]

CONTROL OF VENTILATION

Elucidation of the mechanisms that underlie the remarkably efficient adaptation of ventilation to the demands of exercise has remained a challenge to generations of physiologists, and a complete explanation remains elusive.[10,15]

Neural factors. It has long been evident that neural factors play an important role, particularly as ventilation normally increases at or even before the start of exercise (phase I), when no other physiological variable has changed except cardiac output (Figure 15.4). There is evidence in humans that the phase I ventilatory response may be in part a 'learned' response to the onset of exercise.[16] Simply imagining exercising in an otherwise relaxed subject causes an increase in ventilation. Under these conditions, positron emission tomography shows activation of several areas of the cerebral cortex, again indicating that the early increase in ventilation with exercise is a behavioural response.[15]

Arterial blood gas tensions and the chemoreceptors. There is a large body of evidence that, during exercise at sea level with oxygen consumption up to about 3 l.min^{-1}, there is no significant change in either P_{CO_2} or P_{O_2} of arterial blood. In one study, even at the point of exhaustion (oxygen consumption 3.5 l.min^{-1}), the arterial P_{O_2} was the same as the resting value and P_{CO_2} was reduced. In healthy subjects, blood gas tensions do not therefore seem at first sight to be the main factor governing the increased minute volume. There is a caveat to this conclusion.

The P_{O_2}/ventilation response curve is known to be steeper during exercise (see Figure 5.7), so ventilation will respond to small fluctuations in normal arterial P_{O_2} under these circumstances. Carotid body resection[17] or administration of dopamine to inhibit carotid body activity[18] reduces the ventilatory response to exercise, particularly phase II (Figure 15.4). Thus it seems likely that the peripheral chemoreceptors are responsible for developing exercise-induced hyperpnoea, particularly during the non-steady state.[10,19] This response may not result from changes in P_{O_2}, but from oscillations in arterial P_{CO_2}.[20] Unlike in the resting state when gas flow within the alveolus is by diffusion (page 19) during the deep breathing that accompanies exercise, air flow into the alveoli becomes more tidal in nature, and the arterial P_{CO_2} rises and falls with each breath. The magnitude of these oscillations is believed to affect respiratory drive via the carotid bodies irrespective of the mean P_{CO_2} (to which the central chemoreceptors respond), an effect which is exaggerated under hypoxic conditions.

Humoral mechanisms. Humoral factors play a comparatively minor role in moderate exercise but are more important in heavy and severe exercise when metabolic acidosis is an important factor. Lactic acidosis contributes to excess ventilation during heavy and severe exercise (Figure 15.5), causing a slight reduction in arterial P_{CO_2}. Slight additional respiratory drive may result from hyperthermia.

FITNESS AND TRAINING

The definitions of moderate, heavy and severe exercise at the beginning of this chapter are not transferable between individuals. A given amount of energy expenditure that constitutes severe exercise to a sedentary unfit subject is likely to represent less than moderate exercise to a trained athlete. The linear relationship between power generated and $\dot{V}O_2$ (Figure 15.1) is remarkably consistent irrespective of fitness and training, but the distance a subject may progress along this line, that is their $\dot{V}O_{2max}$, is extremely variable.

In healthy untrained subjects, rapidly increasing lactate levels normally limit exercise tolerance.

Intracellular lactic acidosis in muscles gives rise to weakness and cramp, the respiratory stimulation rapidly takes the subject towards an intolerable minute ventilation, and exhaustion occurs. Training changes many aspects of exercise physiology. For example, improved cardiovascular fitness results in improved oxygen delivery, such that the $\dot{V}_{O_2}$ at which lactate rises is greatly increased. Muscle in trained athletes releases less lactate than in untrained subjects (see below), and animal studies indicate that training may improve the ability of the liver to remove circulating lactate.[1] Finally, trained athletes can tolerate much higher blood lactate levels, up to $20\,mmol.l^{-1}$, or twice that of untrained subjects. There are two respiratory aspects of training that merit further consideration.

Minute volume of ventilation. Maximal expiratory flow rate is limited by flow-dependent airway closure (page 49), and is relatively unaffected by training.[13] However, within the limits of MBC, it is possible to increase the strength and endurance of the respiratory muscles. It is therefore possible to improve the *fraction* of the MBC that can be sustained during exercise. Highly trained athletes may be able to maintain ventilations as much as 90% of their MBC.

Ventilation equivalent for oxygen. There is no evidence that training can alter the slope of the plot of ventilation against oxygen consumption (Figure 15.5). However, the upward inflection of the curve (Owles point) is further to the right in the trained subject. This permits the attainment of a higher oxygen consumption for the same minute volume. Prolongation of the straight part of the curve is achieved by improving metabolic processes in skeletal muscle to minimise the stimulant effect of lactic acid. There is ample evidence that training can improve the aerobic performance of muscles by many adaptations, including, for example, the increased density of the capillary network in the muscles. The consequent reduction in lactic acidosis and therefore the excess ventilation, together with

an increase in the tolerable minute volume, combine to increase the $\dot{V}_{O_{2max}}$ as shown in Figure 15.5. It would seem that the major factor in increasing the $\dot{V}_{O_{2max}}$ is improved performance of skeletal muscle and the cardiovascular system, rather than any specific change in respiratory function.

CARDIORESPIRATORY DISEASE[1,2,21]

Patients with cardiovascular or respiratory disease have poor exercise tolerance for three main reasons. First, the ventilatory response to exercise is more rapid so a greater minute volume is required to achieve a given $\dot{V}_{O_2}$. Secondly, the proportion of MBC that a patient can tolerate is reduced, and when combined with the previous observation this results in an extreme limitation of exercise tolerance before shortness of breath intervenes. Hypoxia or hypercapnia occur more commonly during exercise in patients with respiratory disease. Thirdly, a limited increase in cardiac output in response to exercise means that mixed venous oxygen levels will fall to low levels more quickly, and also causes inadequate muscle blood flow, impairing the function of respiratory and other muscles. Anaerobic metabolism therefore occurs much more quickly, leading to extra ventilatory requirements and exhaustion.

Cardiopulmonary exercise (CPX) testing. The limited respiratory response to exercise seen in patients with cardiorespiratory disease has led to the use of exercise testing as a means of quantifying the extent of their disease. During a progressively increasing workload a variety of measures may be made, including peak $\dot{V}_{O_2}$, anaerobic threshold ($\dot{V}_{O_2}$ at Owles point), and ventilation equivalent for oxygen ($\dot{V}/\dot{V}_{O_2}$) and carbon dioxide ($\dot{V}/\dot{V}_{CO_2}$). These measures are invariably reduced in patients with cardiac and/or respiratory disease, and have been shown to be predictive of poor outcomes in patients with heart failure[22] or those having major, high-risk surgery.[23]

References

1. Wasserman K. Coupling of external to cellular respiration during exercise: the wisdom of the body revisited. *Am J Physiol.* 1994;266:E519–E539.
2. Poole DC, Barstow TJ, Gaesser GA, Willis WT, Whipp BJ. $\dot{V}_{O_2}$ slow

component: physiological and functional significance. *Med Sci Sports Exer.* 1994;26:1354–1358.
3. Burnley M. Found in translation: the dependence of oxygen uptake kinetics on O_2 delivery

and O_2 utilization. *J Appl Physiol.* 2008;105:1387–1388.
4. Clark JM, Hagerman FC, Gelfand R. Breathing patterns during submaximal and maximal exercise in elite oarsmen. *J Appl Physiol.* 1983;55:440–446.

5. Howley ET, Bassett DR, Welch HG. Criteria for maximal oxygen uptake: review and commentary. *Med Sci Sports Exerc.* 1995;27:1292–1301.

6. Aaron EA, Seow KC, Johnson BD, Dempsey JA. Oxygen cost of exercise hyperpnea: implications for performance. *J Appl Physiol.* 1992;72:1818–1825.

7. Dempsey JA, Harms CA, Ainsworth DM. Respiratory muscle perfusion and energetics during exercise. *Med Sci Sports Exerc.* 1996;28:1123–1129.

8. Svedahl K, MacIntosh BR. Anaerobic threshold: The concepts and methods of measurement. *Can J Appl Physiol.* 2003;28:299–323.

9. Quinn TJ, Vroman NB, Kertzer R. Postexercise oxygen consumption in trained females: effect of exercise duration. *Med Sci Sports Exerc.* 1994;26:908–913.

10. Whipp BJ. Peripheral chemoreceptor control of exercise hyperpnea in humans. *Med Sci Sports Exerc.* 1994;26:337–347.

11. Cotes JE, Chinn DJ, Miller MR. *Lung Function. Physiology, Measurement and Application in Medicine.* Oxford: Blackwell Publishing; 2006.

12. Bye PTP, Farkas GA, Roussos C. Respiratory factors limiting exercise. *Annu Rev Physiol.* 1983;45:439–451.

13. Shephard RJ. The maximum sustained voluntary ventilation in exercise. *Clin Sci.* 1967;32:167–176.

14. Dempsey JA. Is the healthy respiratory system (always) built for exercise? *J Physiol.* 2006;576:339–340.

15. Thornton JM, Guz A, Murphy K, et al. Identification of higher brain centres that may encode the cardiorespiratory response to exercise in humans. *J Physiol.* 2001;533:823–836.

*16. Helbling D, Boutellier U, Spengler CM. Modulation of the ventilatory increase at the onset of exercise in humans. *Respir Physiol.* 1997;109:219–229.

17. Wasserman K, Whipp BJ, Koyal SN, Cleary MG. Effect of carotid body resection on ventilatory and acid-base control during exercise. *J Appl Physiol.* 1975;39:354–358.

18. Boetger CL, Ward DS. Effect of dopamine on transient ventilatory response to exercise. *J Appl Physiol.* 1986;61:2102–2107.

19. Forster HV, Pan LG. The role of carotid chemoreceptors in the control of breathing during exercise. *Med Sci Sports Exerc.* 1994;26:328–336.

*20. Collier DJ, Nickol AH, Milledge JS, et al. Alveolar P_{CO_2} oscillations and ventilation at sea level and at high altitude. *J Appl Physiol.* 2008;104:404–415.

*21. Epstein FH. Exercise limitation in health and disease. *N Engl J Med.* 2000;343:633–641.

22. Gitt AK, Wasserman K, Kilkowski C, et al. Exercise anaerobic threshold and ventilatory efficiency identify heart failure patients for high risk of early death. *Circulation.* 2002;106:3079–3084.

23. Carlisle J, Swart M. Mid-term survival after abdominal aortic aneurysm surgery predicted by cardiopulmonary exercise testing. *Br J Surg.* 2007;94:966–969.

Chapter 16

Sleep

KEY POINTS

- During normal sleep tidal volume is reduced, with maximal reduction in ventilation occurring during rapid eye movement sleep when breathing also becomes irregular.
- Reduction in the speed and strength of pharyngeal muscle reflexes causes increased airways resistance, leading to snoring in many normal individuals.
- Sleep-disordered breathing describes a continuum of abnormalities ranging from occasional snoring to frequent periods of airway obstruction and hypoxia during sleep.

NORMAL SLEEP

Sleep is classified on the basis of the electroencephalogram (EEG) and electro-oculogram (EOG) into rapid eye movement (REM) and non-REM (stages 1–4) sleep.

Stage 1 is dozing from which arousal easily takes place. The EEG is low voltage and the frequency is mixed but predominantly fast. This progresses to stage 2 in which the background EEG is similar to stage 1 but with episodic sleep spindles (frequency 12–14 Hz) and K complexes (large biphasic waves of characteristic appearance). Slow, large amplitude (delta) waves start to appear in stage 2 but become more dominant in stage 3 in which spindles are less conspicuous and K complexes become difficult to distinguish. In stage 4, which is often referred to as deep sleep, the EEG is mainly high voltage (more than 75 μV) and more than 50% slow (delta) frequency.

REM sleep has quite different characteristics. The EEG pattern is the same as in stage 1 but the EOG shows frequent rapid eye movements that are easily distinguished from the rolling eye movements of non-REM sleep. Dreaming occurs during REM sleep.

The stage of sleep changes frequently during the night, and the pattern varies between different individuals and on different nights for the same individual (Figure 16.1). Sleep is entered in stage 1 and usually progresses through 2 to 3 and sometimes into 4. Episodes of REM sleep alternate with non-REM sleep throughout the night. On average there are four or five episodes of REM sleep per night, with a tendency for the duration of the episodes to increase towards morning. Conversely, stages 3 and 4 predominate in the early part of the night.

RESPIRATORY CHANGES

Ventilation.[1] Tidal volume decreases with deepening levels of non-REM sleep and is minimal in REM sleep, when it is about 25% less than in the awake state. Respiratory frequency is generally unchanged, though breathing is normally irregular during REM sleep. Minute volume is progressively reduced in parallel with the tidal volume. These changes in ventilation are brought about by the same neurochemical changes that cause sleep. Increased activity of GABA secreting neurones during sleep has a direct depressant effect on the respiratory centre (see Figure 5.4) and activation of cholinergic neurones is thought to be responsible for the respiratory patterns seen during non-REM sleep.[1]

Arterial P_{CO_2} is usually slightly elevated by about 0.4 kPa (3 mmHg). In the young healthy adult,

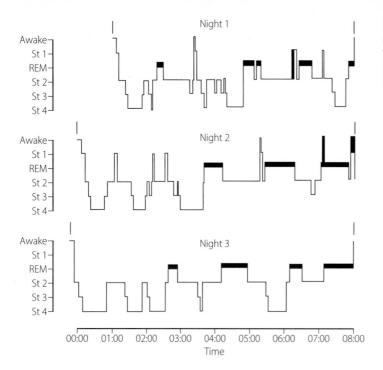

Fig. 16.1 Patterns of sleep on three consecutive nights in a young fit man aged 20. The thick horizontal bars indicate rapid eye movement (REM) sleep. (Record kindly supplied by Dr C Thornton)

arterial P_{O_2} decreases by about the same amount as the P_{CO_2} is increased, and therefore the oxygen saturation remains reasonably normal. Mean value for ribcage contribution to breathing (page 87) was found to be 54% in stage 1–2, decreasing slightly in stages 3–4.[2] However, in REM sleep, the value was reduced to 29%, which is close to the normal awake value in the supine position.

Chemosensitivity. In humans, the slope of the hypercapnic and hypoxic ventilatory responses are markedly reduced during sleep.[3,4] In both cases, the slope is reduced by approximately one-third during non-REM sleep, and even further reduced during REM sleep, but fortunately the responses are never abolished completely.

Effect of age. Compared with young subjects, the elderly have more variable ventilatory patterns when awake, which seems to result in more episodes of periodic breathing (page 76) and apnoea when asleep. Elderly subjects also have significant oscillations in upper airway resistance during sleep (see below),[5] which may contribute to the observed variations in ventilation. Thus as age advances, episodes of transient hypoxaemia occur in subjects who are otherwise healthy, with saturations commonly falling as low as 75% during sleep. Such

changes must be regarded as a normal part of the ageing process.

Pharyngeal airway resistance. Air flow through the sharp bends of the upper airway is normally laminar, but is believed to be very close to becoming turbulent even in normal subjects.[6] Pharyngeal muscles may play a crucial role in maintaining the optimum shape of the airway to maintain laminar flow, and the speed at which these control mechanisms can respond to changes in pharyngeal pressure (page 83) may be more critical than previously thought.[7] Any condition that attenuates or delays these reflexes even slightly, such as sleep or alcohol ingestion, will then have a major effect on airflow in the pharynx causing breakdown of the normally laminar flow.

The nasal airway is normally used during sleep, and upper airway resistance is consistently increased, especially during inspiration and in REM sleep. The main sites of increase are across the soft palate and in the hypopharynx.[8] Changes in pharyngeal muscle activity with sleep are complex. Muscles with predominantly tonic activity, such as tensor palati, show a progressive decrease in activity with deepening non-REM sleep,[9] reaching only 20–30% of awake activity in stage 4 sleep. This loss of tonic activity correlates very well with increased upper airway resistance.[9] Unlike in the awake state, tensor palati also fails to respond to an inspiratory resistive load. The activity of muscles with predominantly phasic inspiratory activity (e.g. geniohyoid and genioglossus) are influenced little by non-REM sleep. In spite of maintained phasic activity during non-REM sleep, tonic activity of geniohyoid is reduced whilst that of genioglossus is well preserved, and responds appropriately to resistive loading.[10] During REM sleep genioglossus activity is reduced.[11] It thus appears that the major effect is upon the tonic activity of nasopharyngeal muscles and the increase in hypopharyngeal resistance seems to be due to secondary downstream collapse.

The ventilatory response to increased airway resistance is important in normal sleep because of the increased pharyngeal resistance, and is generally well preserved. There are substantial and rapid increases in both diaphragmatic and genioglossal inspiratory activity following nasal occlusion in normal sleeping adults.[12]

SNORING

Snoring may occur at any age, but the incidence is bimodal, peaking in the first and the fifth to sixth decades of life. It is commoner in males than females, and linked to obesity. It may occur in any stage of sleep, becoming more pronounced as non-REM sleep deepens, though usually attenuated in REM sleep. As may be expected, snoring is less severe when sleeping in the lateral rather than supine position.[13] About one-quarter of the population are habitual snorers, but these vary from the occasional snorer (e.g. after alcohol or with an upper respiratory tract infection) to the habitual persistent and heavy snorer.

Snoring originates in the oropharynx and in its mildest form is due to vibration of the soft palate and posterior pillars of the fauces. However, in its more severe forms, during inspiration the walls of the oropharynx collapse and the tongue is drawn back as a result of the subatmospheric pressure generated during inspiration against more upstream airway obstruction. This may be at the level of the palate as described above or may be the result of nasal polyps, nasal infection or enlarged adenoids, which are the commonest cause of snoring in children.[14] As obstruction develops, the inspiratory muscles greatly augment their action and intrathoracic pressure may fall as low as $-7\,kPa$ ($-70\,cmH_2O$).

'Normal' snoring is not associated with either frequent arousal from sleep or apnoea, but is believed to precede the development of more serious sleep-related breathing disorders, with both increasing age and obesity making this progression more likely.[15]

SLEEP-DISORDERED BREATHING[16]

This term is used to describe a continuum of respiratory abnormalities seen during sleep, which affect around 20% of the population[16] and range from simple snoring to life-threatening obstructive sleep apnoea.[17,18,19] All are characterised by periods of apnoea, with or without episodes of airway narrowing or obstruction, that lead to repeated episodes of arterial hypoxia and arousal from sleep. Repeated arousals throughout the night give rise to excessive daytime sleepiness. Four syndromes are described, but there is considerable overlap between them:

Upper airway resistance syndrome[14] in which tidal volume and arterial oxygen saturation (Sa_{O_2}) remain normal, but at the expense of extensive respiratory effort, which causes over 15 arousals per hour.

Obstructive sleep hypopnoea involves frequent (>15 per hour) episodes of airway obstruction of sufficient severity to reduce tidal volume to less than 50% of normal for over 10 seconds. There may be small decreases in Sa_{O_2}.

Obstructive sleep apnoea is characterised by more than 5 episodes per hour of obstructive apnoeas lasting over 10 seconds and associated with severe decreases in Sa_{O_2}. In fact, durations of apnoea may be as long as 90 seconds and the frequency of the episodes as high as 160/hour. In severe cases, 50% of sleep time may be spent without tidal exchange.

The last two syndromes are commonly grouped together as sleep apnoea/hypopnoea syndrome (SAHS). Severity is quantified by recording the apnoea/hypopnoea index (AHI), which is simply the number of occurrences per hour of apnoeas or hypopnoeas lasting longer than 10 seconds. Milder forms of sleep-disordered breathing tend to progress to more severe forms as patients grow older and fatter. The prevalence of SAHS, defined as an AHI of over 5, is between 3.5% and 24% in men and between 1.5% and 9% in women depending on the population studied.[16,20,21]

Apnoea or hypopnoea may be central or obstructive. Differentiation between central and obstructive apnoea is conveniently made by recording rib cage and abdominal movements continuously during sleep (Figure 16.2). If, as a result of upper airway

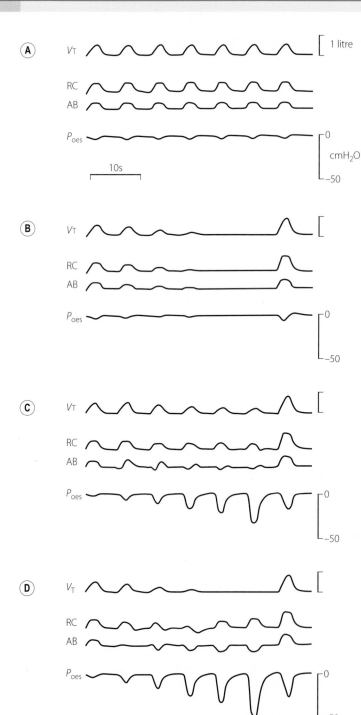

Fig. 16.2 Continuous records of breathing during differing types of apnoea and hypopnoea showing tidal volume (V_T), ribcage (RC) and abdominal (AB) contributions to breathing, and oesophageal pressure (P_{oes}). (A) normal; (B) central apnoea; (C) obstructive hypopnoea; (D) obstructive apnoea.

obstruction, abdominal and ribcage movements become uncoordinated (Figure 16.2C), hypopnoea results. When these movements are equal but opposite in phase, there is obstructive apnoea (Figure 16.2D). Obstructive apnoea may occur in REM or non-REM sleep but the longest periods of apnoea tend to occur in REM sleep. As for snoring, airway obstruction is less frequent when sleeping in the lateral, rather than supine, position.[13,22] Central apnoeas are more common in elderly patients.

Obesity hypoventilation syndrome (Pickwickian Syndrome) describes a combination of obesity, chronic hypercapnia (both nocturnal and daytime) and sleep-disordered breathing, usually severe OSA.[23,24] With increasing levels of obesity in the developing world this syndrome is likely to become more common. The syndrome has a poor prognosis without treatment, which usually involves non-invasive ventilation.

THE MECHANISM OF AIRWAY OBSTRUCTION[17,25,26]

Anatomical factors. There is now widespread agreement that, on average, patients with SAHS have anatomically narrower airways than controls, and that the airway shape differs. Anatomical airway narrowing is believed to relate to two main factors.

First, obesity influences pharyngeal airway size. A central pattern of obesity, commonly seen in males, includes extensive fat deposition in the neck tissues. This accounts for the association between SAHS and neck circumference.[24] Adipose tissue is best visualised using magnetic resonance imaging (MRI), and in patients with SAHS collections of fat are invariably seen lateral to the pharynx, between the pterygoid muscles and the carotid artery (Figure 16.3). Pharyngeal fat is increased above normal levels even in non-obese patients with SAHS (Figure 16.3C).[27] In addition, the quantity of adipose tissue seen correlates with the AHI, and weight loss predictably reduces both.

Secondly, facial structure may be different in some patients with SAHS, including micrognathia (small mandible) or retrognathia (posterior positioned mandible), both of which will tend to displace the tongue backwards, requiring extra genioglossus activity to maintain a normal-sized airway. This hypothesis raises the interesting possibility that SAHS may begin in early childhood, when enlarged adenoids and tonsils can influence facial bone development, and may also go some way to explaining familial 'aggregations' of SAHS and snoring.[14]

Pharyngeal dilator muscles are more active in awake subjects with SAHS when compared with controls, presumably as a physiological response to the anatomically abnormal airway. The activity is believed to originate from the usual reflex, stimulated by a negative pharyngeal pressure (page 83), which may be present to a greater extent in SAHS subjects even when awake. This requirement for increased pharyngeal muscle activity to maintain airway size may become impossible to maintain during sleep. Coupled with the normal loss of tonic activity of pharyngeal muscles (see above), sleep quickly results in airway obstruction.

Airway collapse occurs only in obstructive sleep apnoea, and normally results from increased upstream resistance behind the soft palate leading to secondary downstream collapse. The ease with which this collapse occurs is a function of the compliance (collapsibility) of the hypopharyngeal walls, opposed by the action of the pharyngeal dilator muscles. Collapse is more likely to occur when pharyngeal compliance is high and particularly when there is increased sub-mucosal fat in the pharynx, a situation that seems to occur more commonly in men than women.[28] Severe collapse of the hypopharynx occurs with the combination of enhanced diaphragmatic contraction, depressed pharyngeal dilator muscle activity and upstream obstruction.

RESPIRATORY CONTROL AND AROUSAL IN SAHS[29]

Instability of respiratory control systems also contributes to the pattern of respiration seen with OSA.[17,30] Multiple feedback loops are involved in controlling breathing (Chapter 5) such as the responses to P_{CO_2}, P_{O_2} and mechanical pharyngeal reflexes. A small alteration in the rate at which a feedback loop detects a physiological change, or responds to that change, will lead to instability of the overall system. Sleep is believed to cause sufficient disturbance of the feedback loops to cause this type of instability, and repetitive respiratory cycles are established, the simplest example being the normal periodic breathing (page 76) seen in old age, a more dramatic example being severe SAHS with long periods of apnoea, hypoxia and hypercarbia.

Apnoea or hypopnoea are terminated when the patient is aroused from sleep, though this arousal is normally subcortical; that is, the patient does not return to full consciousness. Arousal is followed by clearance of the pharyngeal airway, and this is crucially important for survival. In spite of the depressed ventilatory response curves, hypoxia and hypercapnia do contribute to arousal, probably alongside afferent input from pressure-sensitive pharyngeal receptors. Current opinion supports the view that a combination of all these factors results in increased respiratory drive, which brings about arousal.[31] Whatever the mechanism, arousal is often accompanied by significant sympathetic discharge.

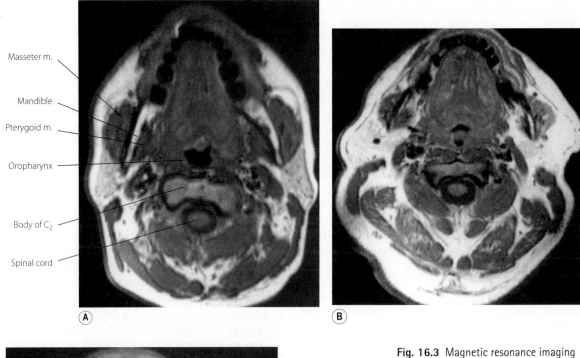

Masseter m.

Mandible

Pterygoid m.

Oropharynx

Body of C₂

Spinal cord

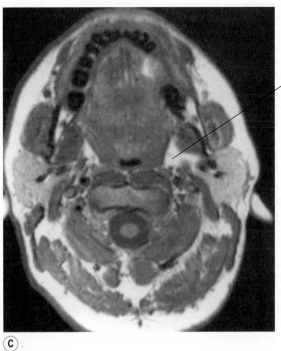

Parapharyngeal fat

Fig. 16.3 Magnetic resonance imaging scan of the neck at the level of the oropharynx. In this type of scan fat tissue appears white. (A) Normal, non-obese, subject. (B) Obese patient with obstructive sleep apnoea, showing deposits of adipose tissue throughout the neck (the uvula is seen in the pharynx). (C) Non-obese patient with sleep apnoea, showing fat deposits lateral to the pharynx with normal amounts of adipose tissue elsewhere. (I am indebted to Dr I Mortimore for providing the scans. Parts (A) and (C) reproduced from reference 27 by permission of the publishers of American Journal of Respiratory and Critical Care Medicine.)

MEDICAL EFFECTS OF SAHS[32]

The effects of the SAHS are not trivial and, over a period of years, morbidity and mortality in patients with SAHS is considerably higher than controls. There has been difficulty proving that this observation relates to the SAHS itself rather than the associated smoking, obesity and alcohol consumption, though the link with cardiovascular disease is now believed to be independent of these confounding variables, particularly with more severe forms of sleep disordered breathing.[32,33,34] There are two main causes of increased mortality:

Sleep deprivation. A night's sleep that is disturbed hundreds of times, even subconsciously, leaves the individual with severe daytime somnolence, with decrement of performance in many fields. The ability to drive is impaired, such that patients with SAHS have a much greater incidence of accidents than control subjects, with some studies finding a direct association between the AHI and likelihood of an accident.[35] Treatment with nasal continuous positive airways pressure (nCPAP, see below) reverses this observation.[36]

Cardiovascular effects. Each arousal is associated with significant secretion of catecholamines, and often an episode of hypoxia. These events, occurring many times each night, cause multiple adverse effects on the cardiovascular system acting via excessive production of reactive oxygen species (Chapter 26) and by amplification of inflammatory processes.[37] It is therefore unsurprising that SAHS is strongly implicated in the development of hypertension,[34] and also believed to contribute to the development of heart failure, ischaemic strokes, diabetes mellitus and hypercholesterolaemia.[33,38,39]

PRINCIPLES OF THERAPY[40]

Conservative treatment. Avoidance of alcohol, sedative drugs and the supine position during sleep will all improve the AHI. Weight loss is effective at reducing the AHI in obese patients with SAHS, and is believed to act by reducing peri-pharyngeal fat, so increasing airway diameter and reducing the tendency of the airway to collapse. There is some evidence that small amounts of weight loss are associated with large reductions in AHI. Many drug therapies for SAHS have been tried, including using respiratory stimulants, or drugs to reduce REM sleep or sympathetic tone, but none are currently recommended for routine use.[40]

Nasal continuous positive airway pressure (nCPAP)[41] aims to avoid the development of a sub-atmospheric pharyngeal pressure sufficient to cause downstream pharyngeal collapse. It requires a well-fitting nasal mask or soft plastic tubes that fit inside the external nares. Compressed air must then be provided at the requisite gas flow, preferably with humidification. nCPAP serves no useful purpose during expiration and systems have been developed to return airway pressure to atmospheric during expiration. In effect this provides a low level of intermittent positive pressure ventilation. Compliance with nCPAP is the only major limitation to its use, and the technique is now widely accepted as the most effective treatment for SAHS, including for the reduction of the daytime somnolence that has such a detrimental effect on the patient's life.

Oral appliances are available that can be maintained in the mouth at night to move either the tongue or the mandible forward so increasing the size of the airway. They are a non-invasive form of SAHS treatment that is less intrusive than nCPAP, but are also a less effective treatment, so are used mostly for patients who cannot use nCPAP.[42]

Surgical relief of obstruction. For snoring alone, the first approach is the removal of any pathological obstruction such as nasal polyps that cause downstream collapse, though this may not improve patients with SAHS. A variety of more radical operations are available, including uvulo-palatopharyngoplasty, which reduces the size of the soft palate and so dampens palatal oscillations and reduces pharyngeal collapse at this level. Non-obese patients with SAHS who have facial bone abnormalities may benefit from maxillofacial corrective surgery, usually involving advancement of the anterior mandible and/or maxilla. Tracheotomy (opened only at night) has been used in some cases as a last resort. The benefits of surgical treatment of SAHS remain uncertain and are now usually reserved for patients who have a specific anatomical abnormality of their airway as part of their SAHS.[40]

References

*1. Joseph V, Pequignot JM, Van Reeth O. Neurochemical perspectives on the control of breathing during sleep. *Respir Physiol Neurobiol*. 2002;130:253–263.

2. Millman RP, Knight H, Kline LR, Shore ET, Chung DC, Pack AI. Changes in compartmental ventilation in association with eye movements during REM sleep. *J Appl Physiol*. 1988;65:1196–1202.

3. Douglas NJ, White DP, Weil JV, Pickett CK, Zwillich CW. Hypercapnic ventilatory response in sleeping adults. *Am Rev Respir Dis*. 1982;126: 758–762.

4. Douglas NJ, White DP, Weil JV, et al. Hypoxic ventilatory response decreases during sleep in normal men. *Am Rev Respir Dis.* 1982;125:286–289.

5. Hudgel DW, Devadatta P, Hamilton H. Pattern of breathing and upper airway mechanics during wakefulness and sleep in healthy elderly humans. *J Appl Physiol.* 1993;74:2198–2204.

6. Shome B, Wang L-P, Prasad AK, Santere MH, Szeri AZ, Roberts D. Modeling of airflow in the nasopharynx with applications to sleep apnea. *J Biomech Eng.* 1998;120:416–422.

7. Roberts D. Invited editorial on 'Neuromechanical interaction in human snoring and upper airway obstruction'. *J Appl Physiol.* 1999;86:1757–1758.

8. Hudgel DW, Hendricks C. Palate and hypopharynx – sites of inspiratory narrowing of the upper airway during sleep. *Am Rev Respir Dis.* 1988;138:1542–1547.

9. Tangel DJ, Mezzanotte WS, White DP. Influence of sleep on tensor palatini EMG and upper airway resistance in normal men. *J Appl Physiol.* 1991;70:2574–2581.

10. Henke KG. Upper airway muscle activity and upper airway resistance in young adults during sleep. *J Appl Physiol.* 1998;84:486–491.

11. Eckert DJ, Malhotra A, Lo YL, White DP, Jordan AS. The influence of obstructive sleep apnea and gender on genioglossus activity during rapid eye movement sleep. *Chest.* 2009;135:957–964.

12. Kuna ST, Smickley J. Response of genioglossus muscle activity to nasal airway occlusion in normal sleeping adults. *J Appl Physiol.* 1988;64:347–353.

13. Nakano H, Ikeda T, Hayashi M, Ohshima E, Onizuka A. Effects of body position on snoring in apneic and nonapneic snorers. *Sleep.* 2003;2:169–172.

14. Rappai M, Colop N, Kemp S, deShazo R. The nose and sleep-disordered breathing. What we know and what we do not know. *Chest.* 2003;124:2309–2323.

15. Berger G, Berger R, Oksenberg A. Progression of snoring and obstructive sleep apnoea: the role of increasing weight and time. *Eur Respir J.* 2009;33:338–345.

16. Jennum P, Riha RL. Epidemiology of sleep apnoea/hypopnoea syndrome and sleep-disordered breathing. *Eur Respir J.* 2009;33:907–914.

*17. Patil SP, Schneider H, Schwartz AR, Smith PL. Adult obstructive sleep apnea: pathophysiology and diagnosis. *Chest.* 2007;132:325–337.

18. Bradley TD. Respiratory sleep medicine. A coming of age. *Am J Respir Crit Care Med.* 2008;177:363–364.

19. Stradling JR, Davies RJO. Obstructive sleep apnoea/hypopnoea syndrome: definitions, epidemiology, and natural history. *Thorax.* 2004;59:73–78.

20. Strohl KP, Redline S. Recognition of obstructive sleep apnea. *Am J Respir Crit Care Med.* 1996;154:279–289.

21. Ohayon MM, Guilleminault C, Priest RG, Caulet M. Snoring and breathing pauses during sleep: telephone interview survey of United Kingdom population sample. *BMJ.* 1997;314:860–863.

22. Akita Y, Kawakatsu K, Hattori C, Hattori H, Suzuki K, Nishimura T. Posture of patients with sleep apnea during sleep. *Acta Otolaryngol Supp.* 2003;550:41–45.

23. Mokhlesi B, Tulaimat A. Recent advances in obesity hypoventilation syndrome. *Chest.* 2007;132:1322–1336.

*24. Crummy F, Piper AJ, Naughton MT. Obesity and the lung: 2. Obesity and sleep disordered breathing. *Thorax.* 2008;63:738–746.

25. Ryan CM, Bradley TD. Pathogenesis of obstructive sleep apnea. *J Appl Physiol.* 2005;99:2440–2450.

26. Sanders MH. The upper airway and sleep-disordered breathing. Getting the big picture. *Am J Respir Crit Care Med.* 2003;168:509–515.

27. Mortimore IL, Marshall I, Wraith PK, Sellar RJ, Douglas NJ. Neck and total body fat deposition in nonobese and obese patients with sleep apnea compared with that in control subjects. *Am J Respir Crit Care Med.* 1998;157:280–283.

28. O'Donnell CP, Schwartz AR, Smith PL. Upper airway collapsibility. The importance of gender and adiposity. *Am J Respir Crit Care Med.* 2000;162:1606–1607.

29. Younes M. Role of respiratory control mechanisms in the pathogenesis of obstructive sleep disorders. *J Appl Physiol.* 2008;105:1389–1405.

30. White DP. Pathogenesis of obstructive and central sleep apnea. *Am J Respir Crit Care Med.* 2005;172:1363–1370.

31. Cherniack NS. If I die before I wake: not a worry for sleep apnea patients. *J Appl Physiol.* 2007;103:1919–1920.

32. McNicholas WT, Bonsignore MR and the Management Committee of EU COST ACTION B26. Sleep apnoea as an independent risk factor for cardiovascular disease: current evidence, basic mechanisms and research priorities. *Eur Respir J.* 2007;29:156–178.

33. Bradley TD, Floras JS. Obstructive sleep apnoea and its cardiovascular consequences. *Lancet.* 2009;373:82–93.

34. Logan A. Sleep-disordered breathing and hypertension. *Am J Respir Crit Care Med.* 2009;179:1082–1083.

35. Stradling J. Driving and obstructive sleep apnoea. *Thorax.* 2008;63:481–483.

36. Mazza S, Pépin J-L, Naëgelé B, et al. Driving ability in sleep apnoea patients before and after CPAP treatment: evaluation on a road safety platform. *Eur Respir J.* 2006;28:1020–1028.

37. Gozal D, Kheirandish-Gozal L. Cardiovascular morbidity in obstructive sleep apnea: oxidative stress, inflammation, and much more. *Am J Respir Crit Care Med*. 2008;177:369–375.

38. Murray BJ. Brain death by a thousand hypoxic cuts in sleep. *Am J Respir Crit Care Med*. 2007;175:528–529.

39. Lorenzi-Filho G, Drager LF. Obstructive sleep apnea and atherosclerosis: A new paradigm. *Am J Respir Crit Care Med*. 2007;175:1219–1221.

*40. Ryan CF. Sleep 9: An approach to treatment of obstructive sleep apnoea/hypopnoea syndrome including upper airway surgery. *Thorax*. 2005;60:595–604.

41. Gordon P, Sanders MH. Sleep 7: Positive airway pressure therapy for obstructive sleep apnoea/hypopnoea syndrome. *Thorax*. 2005;60:68–75.

42. Chan ASL, Lee RWW, Cistulli PA. Dental appliance treatment for obstructive sleep apnea. *Chest*. 2007;132:693–699.

Chapter 17

High altitude and flying

KEY POINTS

- The low inspired oxygen partial pressure at altitude causes immediate hyperventilation, which increases further with acclimatisation to produce hypocapnia and improve oxygen levels.
- The rate of ascent and altitude achieved are determinants of altitude-related illnesses, which vary from mild acute mountain sickness to potentially lethal high altitude pulmonary oedema.
- High altitude populations have adaptations to their environment such as lesser degrees of hyperventilation compensated for by a greater lung surface area for gas exchange.
- Commercial aircraft cabins are pressurised to an equivalent altitude of below 2400 m (8000 ft) and so represent a level of hypoxia similar to breathing 15% oxygen at sea level.

With increasing altitude, the barometric pressure falls, but the fractional concentration of oxygen in the air (0.21) and the saturated vapour pressure of water at body temperature (6.3 kPa or 47 mmHg) remain constant. The P_{O_2} of the inspired air is related to the barometric pressure as follows:

$$\text{Inspired gas } P_{O_2} = 0.21 \times (\text{Barometric pressure} - 6.3) \text{ kPa}$$

or

$$\text{Inspired gas } P_{O_2} = 0.21 \times (\text{Barometric pressure} - 47) \text{ mmHg}$$

The influence of the saturated vapour pressure of water becomes relatively more important until, at

an altitude of approximately 19 000 m or 63 000 feet, the barometric pressure equals the water vapour pressure, and alveolar P_{O_2} and P_{CO_2} become zero.

Table 17.1 is based on the standard table relating altitude and barometric pressure. However, there are important deviations from the predicted barometric pressure under certain circumstances, particularly at low latitudes.[1] At the summit of Everest, the actual barometric pressure was found to be 2.4 kPa (18 mmHg) greater than predicted, and this was crucial to reaching the summit without oxygen. The uppermost curve in Figure 17.1 shows the expected P_{O_2} of air as a function of altitude, while the crosses indicate observed values in the Himalayas that have been consistently higher than expected.

EQUIVALENT OXYGEN CONCENTRATION

The acute effect of altitude on inspired P_{O_2} may be simulated by reduction of the oxygen concentration of gas inspired at sea level (Table 17.1). This technique is extensively used for studies of hypoxia and for clinical assessment of patients before flying (see below), but there are theoretical reasons why the same inspired P_{O_2} at normal and low barometric pressure may have different physiological effects. These include the density of the gas being breathed and different P_{N_2} values in the tissues.[4]

Up to 10 000 m (33 000 ft), it is possible to restore the inspired P_{O_2} to the sea level value by an appropriate increase in the oxygen concentration of the inspired gas (also shown in Table 17.1). Lower inspired P_{O_2} values may be obtained between 10 000 and 19 000 m, above which body fluids boil.

DOI: 10.1016/B978-0-7020-2996-7.00017-9

Table 17.1 Barometric pressure relative to altitude

ALTITUDE		BAROMETRIC PRESSURE		INSPIRED GAS P_{O_2}		EQUIVALENT OXYGEN % AT SEA LEVEL	PERCENTAGE OXYGEN REQUIRED TO GIVE SEA LEVEL VALUE OF INSPIRED GAS P_{O_2}
feet	metres	kPa	mmHg	kPa	mmHg		
0	0	101	760	19.9	149	20.9	20.9
2000	610	94.3	707	18.4	138	19.4	22.6
4000	1220	87.8	659	16.9	127	17.8	24.5
6000	1830	81.2	609	15.7	118	16.6	26.5
8000	2440	75.2	564	14.4	108	15.1	28.8
10000	3050	69.7	523	13.3	100	14.0	31.3
12000	3660	64.4	483	12.1	91	12.8	34.2
14000	4270	59.5	446	11.1	83	11.6	37.3
16000	4880	54.9	412	10.1	76	10.7	40.8
18000	5490	50.5	379	9.2	69	9.7	44.8
20000	6100	46.5	349	8.4	63	8.8	49.3
22000	6710	42.8	321	7.6	57	8.0	54.3
24000	7320	39.2	294	6.9	52	7.3	60.3
26000	7930	36.0	270	6.3	47	6.6	66.8
28000	8540	32.9	247	5.6	42	5.9	74.5
30000	9150	30.1	226	4.9	37	5.2	83.2
35000	10700	23.7	178	3.7	27	3.8	–
40000	12200	18.8	141	2.7	20	2.8	–
45000	13700	14.8	111	1.8	13	1.9	–
50000	15300	11.6	87	1.1	8	1.1	–
63000	19200	6.3	47	0	0	0	–

100% oxygen restores sea level inspired P_{O_2} at 10000 m (33000 ft)

RESPIRATORY SYSTEM RESPONSES TO ALTITUDE[1]

Ascent to altitude presents three main challenges to the respiratory system, resulting from progressively reduced inspired P_{O_2}, low relative humidity, and, in outdoor environments, extreme cold. Hypoxia is by far the most important of these, and requires significant physiological changes to allow continuation of normal activities at altitude. The efficiency of these changes depends on many factors such as the normal altitude at which the subject lives, the rate of ascent, the altitude attained and the health of the subject.

ACUTE EXPOSURE TO ALTITUDE

Transport technology now permits altitude to be attained quickly and without the exertion of climbing. Within a few hours, rail, air, cable car or motor transport may take a passenger from near sea level to as high as 4000 m (13100 ft).

Ventilatory changes. At high altitude the decrease in inspired gas P_{O_2} reduces alveolar and therefore arterial P_{O_2}. The actual decrease in alveolar P_{O_2} is mitigated by hyperventilation caused by the hypoxic drive to ventilation. However, on acute exposure to altitude, the ventilatory response to hypoxia is very short lived due to a combination of the resultant hypocapnia and hypoxic ventilatory decline (page 73 and Figure 5.6). During the first few days at altitude, this disadvantageous negative feedback is reversed by acclimatisation (see below).

Signs and symptoms. Impairment of night vision is the earliest sign of hypoxia, and may be detected as low as 1200 m (4000 ft). However, the most serious aspect of acute exposure to altitude is impairment of mental performance, culminating in loss of consciousness, which usually occurs on acute exposure to altitudes in excess of 6000 m (about 20000 ft). The time to loss of consciousness varies with altitude and is of great practical importance to pilots in the event of loss of pressurisation (Figure 17.2).

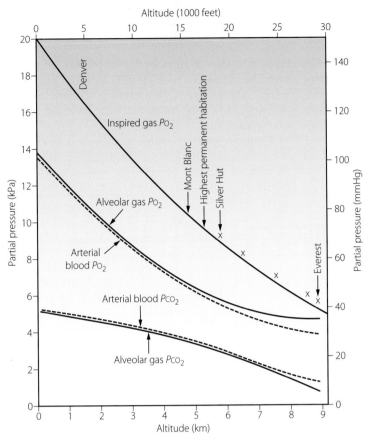

Fig. 17.1 Inspired, alveolar and arterial gas partial pressures at rest, as a function of altitude. The curve for inspired P_{O_2} is taken from standard data in Table 17.1, but the crosses show actual measurements in the Himalayas. The alveolar gas data are from reference 2, and agree remarkably well with the arterial blood data from the simulated ascent of Everest.[3]

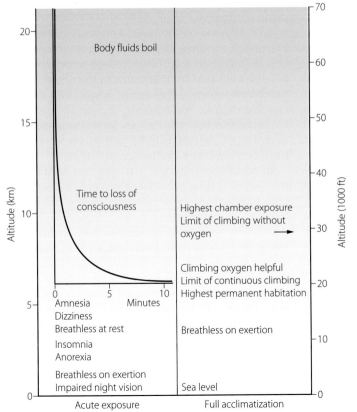

Fig. 17.2 Symptoms of acute and chronic exposure to altitude.

The shortest possible time to loss of consciousness (about 15 seconds) applies above about 16000 m (52000 ft) and is governed by lung-to-brain circulation time and the capacity of high energy phosphate stores in the brain (page 363). Impaired mental function as a result of hypoxia is due to both a direct effect of hypoxia on brain tissue and from cerebral vasoconstriction from the resulting hypocapnia.[5]

ACCLIMATISATION TO ALTITUDE

Acclimatisation refers to the processes by which tolerance and performance are improved over a period of hours to weeks after an individual who normally lives at relatively low altitude ascends to a much higher area. Everest has been climbed without oxygen by well-acclimatised lowlanders, although the barometric pressure on the summit would cause rapid loss of consciousness without acclimatisation (Figure 17.2). Adaptation to altitude (described below) refers to physiological differences in permanent residents at high altitude and is quite different from acclimatisation.

Earlier studies of acclimatisation took place in the attractive, though somewhat hostile, environment of high altitude expeditions in many mountain ranges. Technical limitations in these conditions led to two experiments, named Operation Everest II and III, in which volunteers lived in a decompression chamber in which an ascent to the summit of Everest was simulated.[6,7] These conditions permitted extensive physiological research to be undertaken at rest and during exercise.

Ventilatory control. Prolonged hypoxia results in several complex changes in ventilation and arterial blood gases, which are shown in Figure 17.3.[8] The initial hypoxic drive to ventilation on acute exposure is short lived, and after about 30 minutes ventilation returns to only slightly above normoxic levels with P_{CO_2} just below control levels (Figure 17.3). This poor ventilatory response causes significant arterial hypoxaemia and results in many of the symptoms seen during the first few hours and days at altitude. Over the next few days, ventilation slowly increases with an accompanying reduction of P_{CO_2} and increase in arterial P_{O_2}. This increase in P_{O_2} is of relatively small magnitude and can never correct P_{O_2} to normal (sea level) values, but it does seem to be enough to ameliorate most of the symptoms of exposure to acute altitude.

There are significant differences between species in the rate at which acclimatisation takes place, being just a few hours in most animals, and several days or weeks in humans.[4] Both the rate of ascent and the altitude attained influence the speed at which ventilatory acclimatisation occurs, but in humans, most subjects are fully acclimatised within one week.

There are many possible mechanisms to explain the ventilatory changes seen with acclimatisation.[8,9] In spite of the low blood P_{CO_2}, stimulation of the central chemoreceptors almost certainly plays a part in the hyperventilation that occurs with acclimatisation. It was first suggested, in 1963, that the restoration of cerebrospinal fluid (CSF) pH, by means of bicarbonate transport, might explain this acclimatisation of ventilation to altitude.[10] Shortly afterwards Severinghaus and his colleagues measured their own CSF pH during acclimatisation to altitude and showed that it did indeed tend to return towards its initial value of 7.2.[10] Subsequent work showed that the time course of changes in CSF pH did not match changes in ventilation,[8] with most studies finding a persistent increase in CSF pH during continued exposure to hypoxia.[9] Changes in CSF pH therefore seem unlikely to represent an important mechanism of acclimatisation. Other studies, mainly in animals, indicate that acclimatisation represents an increase in the responsiveness of the respiratory centre to hypoxia from both direct effects of prolonged hypoxia on the central nervous system and prolonged maximal afferent input from the peripheral chemoreceptors. This increased responsiveness may be mediated by alterations in the sensitivity to neurotransmitters involved in respiratory control (see Figure 5.4). For example, increased sensitivity to glutamate will directly increase ventilation, or decreasing GABA sensitivity will effectively reduce hypoxic ventilatory decline (page 73).[9]

In addition to changes affecting the central chemoreceptors, there is evidence that peripheral chemoreceptor sensitivity is increased during prolonged hypoxia, so contributing to the progressive hyperventilation seen with acclimatisation. In humans, the acute hypoxic ventilatory response is increased during the first few days at altitude and for several days after return to sea level. The mechanism of this increased sensitivity to hypoxia is not known, but is independent of changes in P_{CO_2},[11] and may reside either with increased sensitivity of the carotid bodies themselves or with the increased responsiveness of the respiratory centre described in the previous paragraph.[8,9]

Respiratory alkalosis at altitude is counteracted, over the course of a few days, by renal excretion of

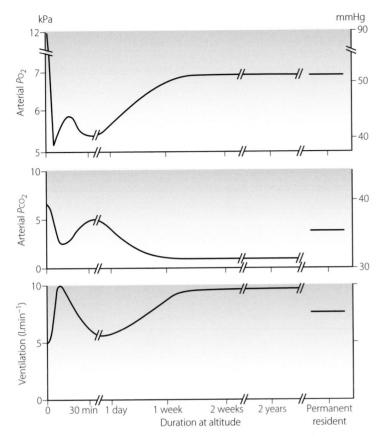

Fig. 17.3 Effects of prolonged hypoxia (equivalent to 4300 m, 14 100 ft) on ventilation and blood gases. The first section of the graph shows the acute hypoxic response and hypoxic ventilatory decline described in Chapter 5. Acclimatisation then takes place, partially restoring Po_2 by means of long-term hyperventilation and hypocapnia, a situation that is maintained indefinitely while remaining at altitude. Individuals who reside throughout life at this altitude maintain similar Po_2 values with lesser degrees of hyperventilation, but still have a minute ventilation greater than sea level normal. (After reference 8.)

bicarbonate, resulting in a degree of metabolic acidosis that will tend to increase respiratory drive (see Figure 5.5). This was formerly thought to be the main factor in the ventilatory adaptation to altitude but it now appears to be of minor importance compared to the changes in the central and peripheral chemoreceptors.

Blood gas tensions. Figure 17.3 shows the time course of blood gas changes during acclimatisation and Figure 17.1 shows changes in alveolar gas tensions with altitude in fully acclimatised mountaineers. Alveolar Po_2 was found to be unexpectedly well preserved at extreme altitude, and above 8000 m (26 000 ft) tended to remain close to 4.8 kPa (36 mmHg).[2] Operations Everest II and III found arterial Po_2 values of 3.62 and 4.08 kPa (27 and 31 mmHg) at a pressure equivalent to the summit of Everest (Table 17.2), with an alveolar/arterial Po_2 difference of less than 0.3 kPa (2 mmHg) at rest.[12] The recent Caudwell Extreme Everest expedition obtained arterial blood samples at 8400 m (27 559 ft) with an average Po_2 of 3.28 kPa (24.6 mmHg). There was also a significant alveolar to arterial Po_2

difference of 0.72 kPa (5.4 mmHg) which the authors suggested may have resulted from a diffusion barrier to oxygen at such low levels, possibly as a result of sub-clinical pulmonary oedema.[13]

Haemoglobin concentration and oxygen affinity. An increase in haemoglobin concentration was the earliest adaptation to altitude to be demonstrated. The recent data from subjects at 8400 m (27 559 ft) reported an increase from 14.8 to 19.3 g.dl^{-1} which, at the resting value of 54% saturation, maintained an arterial oxygen content of almost 15 ml.dl^{-1}.[13] Plasma erythropoietin levels begin to increase within a few hours at altitude, reaching a maximum at 24–48 hours and then declining.[16]

The haemoglobin dissociation curve at altitude is affected by changes in both pH and 2,3-diphosphoglycerate (DPG) concentration (page 193). 2,3-DPG concentrations increased from 1.7 to 3.8 mmol.l^{-1} on Operation Everest II.[3] It has been estimated that the resultant effect is a leftward shift at extreme altitude, where oxygen loading in the lung takes priority over maintaining Po_2 at the point of release.[1]

Table 17.2 Cardiorespiratory data obtained at rest and during exercise at extreme reduction of ambient pressure during the simulated ascent of Everest in a low pressure chamber

	SEA LEVEL EQUIVALENT		EXTREME ALTITUDE EQUIVALENT	
Ambient pressure (kPa)	101		33.7	
(mmHg)	760		253	
Haemoglobin concentration (g.dl^{-1})	13.5		17.0	
$\dot{V}_{O_2max}$ (ml.min^{-1}, STPD)	3980		1170	

STATE	REST	EXERCISE	REST	EXERCISE
Exercise intensity (watts)	0	281	0	90
Ventilation (l.min^{-1}, BTPS)	11	107	42.3	157.5
$\dot{V}_{O_2}$ (ml.min^{-1}, STPD)	350	3380	386	1002
Ventilation equivalent	31	32	110	157
Arterial P_{O_2} (kPa)	13.2	12.0	4.0	3.7
(mmHg)	99.3	90.0	30.3	27.7
Arterial P_{CO_2} (kPa)	4.5	4.7	1.5	1.3
(mmHg)	33.9	35.0	11.2	10.1
Arterial/venous O_2 content difference (ml.dl^{-1})	5.7	15.0	4.6	6.7
Mixed venous P_{O_2} (kPa)	4.7	2.6	2.9	1.9
(mmHg)	35.1	19.7	22.1	14.3
Cardiac output (l.min^{-1})	6.7	27.2	8.4	15.7
Pulmonary arterial pressure (mean, mmHg)	15	33	33	48

Notes
1. Actual ambient pressure at simulated high altitude was 32 kPa (240 mmHg) but leakage of oxygen from masks worn by investigators had caused the oxygen concentration in the chamber to rise to 22%, the equivalent of 33.7 kPa at 21%, which is equivalent to the summit of Everest.
2. Study 14 reported cardiovascular data for a mean exercise intensity of 90 watts at the highest altitude. Data from other studies have been interpolated to give values corresponding to the same exercise intensity in order to achieve compatibility.
(Data from references 3, 14 and 15.)

ADAPTATION TO ALTITUDE[1,17]

Adaptation refers to physiological and genetic changes that occur over a period of years to generations by those who have taken up permanent residence at high altitude. There are qualitative as well as quantitative differences between acclimatisation and adaptation but each is remarkably effective. High altitude residents have a remarkable ability to exercise under grossly hypoxic conditions, but their adaptations show many striking differences from those in acclimatised lowlanders. Residents in different high altitude areas of the world have differing adaptations.[18]

Long-term residence at altitude leads to a reduced ventilatory response to hypoxia, the magnitude of which relates to the product of altitude level and years of residence there.[8] This results in a reduction of ventilation compared with an acclimatised lowlander, and a rise in P_{CO_2}, though neither of these returns to sea level values (Figure 17.3). High altitude residents maintain similar arterial P_{O_2} values as

acclimatised lowlanders in spite of the reduced ventilation and therefore lower alveolar P_{O_2}. Pulmonary diffusing capacity must therefore be increased, and depends on anatomical pulmonary adaptations increasing the area available for diffusion by the generation of greater numbers of alveoli and associated capillaries. This adaptation seems not to be inherited, but occurs in children and infants who spend their formative years at altitude. In humans, the development of alveoli by septation of saccules formed in utero occurs mostly after birth (page 250), and it is this process that must be stimulated by hypoxia, though the mechanism of this stimulation remains unknown.[19] An adult moving permanently to high altitude will therefore never achieve the same degree of adaptation as a native of the area, so explaining the ability of high altitude residents to exercise to a much greater degree than their non-resident visitors.

Research has found that residents of high altitude areas of the Andes hyperventilate less than residents at equivalent altitude in Tibet.[18] This higher ventilation in Tibetans may explain their reduced susceptibility, in comparison with populations in the Andes, to chronic mountain sickness (see below) and some complications of pregnancy that are normally associated with high altitude life.[20] Human occupation of Tibet is believed to have begun earlier than other high-altitude areas of the world, and these differences in Tibetan physiology could represent a more advanced genetic adaptation to the physiologically hostile environment.

Polycythaemia is normal and influenced by altitude, population and sex,[21] for example male subjects of the Chinese Han population residing at 5200 m (17 060 ft) on the Tibetan plateau have an average haemoglobin concentration of 19.6 g.dl^{-1}. Another major adaptation to altitude by long-term residents appears to be increased vascularity of heart and striated muscles, a change that is also important for the trained athlete. For the high altitude resident, increased perfusion appears to compensate very effectively for the reduced oxygen content of the arterial blood.

Recent data regarding the mortality of climbers attempting to reach the summit of Mount Everest illustrates how effective adaptations to altitude are compared with acclimatised lowlanders. Sherpa residents had a mortality of only 0.4%, compared with 2.7% amongst climbers.[22]

Chronic mountain sickness (Monge's disease).[1] A small minority of those who dwell permanently at very high altitude develop this dangerous illness. It is characterised by an exceptionally poor ventilatory response to hypoxia resulting in low arterial P_{O_2} and high P_{CO_2}. There is cyanosis, high haematocrit, finger clubbing, pulmonary hypertension, right heart failure, dyspnoea and lethargy.

EXERCISE AT HIGH ALTITUDE[23,24]

The summit of Everest was attained without the use of oxygen in 1978 by Messner and Habeler, and by many other climbers since that date. Studies of exercise have been made at various altitudes up to and including the summit, and on the simulated ascents in Operations Everest II and III. Of necessity, these observations are largely confined to very fit subjects.

Capacity for work performed. There is a progressive decline in the external work that can be performed as altitude increases. On Operation Everest II, 300–360 watts was attained at sea level, 240–270 watts at 440 mmHg pressure (equivalent to 4300 m, 14 000 ft) and 120 watts at 280 mmHg (Everest summit), very

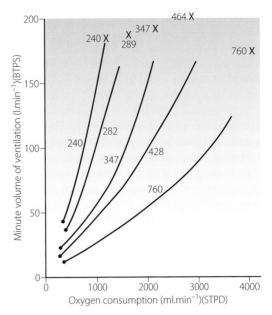

Fig. 17.4 The relationship between minute volume of ventilation and oxygen consumption at rest and during exercise at altitude. The relationship is radically changed at altitude primarily because ventilation is reported at body temperature and pressure (saturated), whereas oxygen consumption is reported at standard temperature and pressure (dry). Numbers in the figure indicate barometric pressure. •, resting points; ×, values at $\dot{V}_{O_{2}max}$ from reference 15. (Data from reference 3.)

close to the results obtained on Everest.[25] $\dot{V}_{O_{2}max}$ declined in accord with altitude to 1177 ml.min^{-1} at 240 mmHg pressure.[15] Resting cardiac output is unchanged at moderate altitude and only slightly increased at extreme altitude. During exercise, for a given power expenditure, the increase in cardiac output at altitude is the same as at sea level.[3]

Ventilation equivalent of oxygen consumption. Figure 15.5 shows that ventilation as a function of $\dot{V}_{O_2}$ is comparatively constant. The length of the line increases with training but the slope of the linear portion remains the same. With increasing altitude, the slope and intercept are both dramatically increased up to four times the sea level value[3,15] with maximal ventilation approaching 200 l.min^{-1} (Figure 17.4). This is because ventilation is reported at body temperature and pressure saturated (BTPS) and oxygen consumption at standard temperature and pressure dry (STPD) – see Appendix C.

Fortunately, the density of air is reduced in proportion to the barometric pressure at altitude.

Resistance to turbulent flow is decreased and therefore the work of breathing at a particular minute volume of respiration is less. Even with this mitigation, the extra ventilation needed to deliver the oxygen requirement at altitude means that the energy expenditure upon breathing for a given intensity of exercise is considerably higher than at sea level.

Pco_2 and Po_2. During exercise at altitude, alveolar Pco_2 falls and alveolar Po_2 rises.[3,26] Arterial Pco_2 falls with alveolar Pco_2 but the alveolar/arterial Po_2 difference increases more than the alveolar Po_2 rises[26] and there is a consistent decrease in arterial Po_2 during exercise at altitude, leading to very low values for Po_2. The lower alveolar to pulmonary capillary Po_2 gradient, along with a faster pulmonary capillary transit time during exercise, causes diffusion-limitation of oxygen uptake. There is also some evidence that ventilation perfusion inequality occurs during exercise at altitude, and adversely affects oxygenation.[23]

ALTITUDE ILLNESS[27,28,29]

ACUTE MOUNTAIN SICKNESS

Acute mountain sickness (AMS) is characterised by headache, nausea, fatigue, anorexia, dyspnoea, difficulty in sleeping (see below) and impaired climbing performance (Figure 17.2). Symptoms normally begin to occur at above 2000 m (6600 ft), with an abrupt increase in the incidence above 4500 m (14 760 ft), affecting about half of trekkers at this altitude.[30] The unacclimatised subject has extreme dyspnoea on exertion at this level and has dyspnoea at rest. Severity varies greatly from a mild inconvenient headache to a severe life threatening illness involving cerebral and pulmonary oedema.

The likelihood of developing AMS relates to altitude (particularly sleeping altitude), the rate of ascent and the degree of exertion. The mountaineer is therefore affected by altitude in a manner that differs from that of the aviator because his physical exertion is much greater and the time course of exposure is different. Rate of ascent seldom exceeds 2000 m (6500 ft) per day from sea level, decreasing to only 300 m (1000 ft) per day at very high altitude.

HIGH ALTITUDE PULMONARY OEDEMA (HAPE)[1,31]

A small amount of sub-clinical pulmonary oedema probably occurs in all subjects at high altitude, but in a few percent the oedema becomes progressive

and life-threatening.[1] As for AMS, the proportion of subjects who develop HAPE depends on the altitude, the speed of ascent, the amount of strenuous exercise performed, and an individual susceptibility to the condition.[28,31] It is most commonly seen in the unacclimatised and overambitious climber. Clinical features include cough, dyspnoea and hypoxia with clinical and radiological signs of pulmonary oedema. Untreated, HAPE has a mortality rate of almost 50%, but with appropriate treatment this is normally less than 3%.

The pathophysiology of HAPE is complex.[27,31,32] Subjects with HAPE have significant pulmonary hypertension secondary to hypoxia, and low pulmonary capillary wedge pressures indicating normal left ventricular function. Subjects who are susceptible to HAPE seem to have an excessive hypoxic pulmonary vasoconstriction response to hypoxia, and this may in part be due to impaired release of endothelial relaxing factors such as nitric oxide (page 107). Compared with subjects who are not susceptible to HAPE, susceptible subjects exhaled lower concentrations of nitric oxide during a high-altitude trip.[33] Pulmonary vasoconstrictors such as endothelin-1 are found in higher concentrations in HAPE susceptible subjects, who also have greater sympathetic responses to hypoxia. Pulmonary shadows on chest X-rays with HAPE are typically patchy, indicating that pulmonary vasoconstriction is non-uniform, such that some areas of lung have little blood flow whilst others have greatly increased blood flow. High capillary flow in some areas is postulated to lead to 'stress failure' of capillaries. This mechanism would explain the association between exercise and HAPE, with increased cardiac output causing huge blood flows through less vasoconstricted regions of lung. Magnetic resonance imaging of the lung during hypoxia has shown that hypoxic pulmonary vasoconstriction is patchy in all subjects, but the uneven vasoconstriction is more pronounced in HAPE-susceptible subjects.[34] Although inflammation is not believed to be a primary event in the pathogenesis of HAPE, it does occur in severe cases and explains why coincidental lung inflammation from, for example, lower respiratory tract infections, may exacerbate or even cause HAPE.

OTHER RESPIRATORY PROBLEMS AT ALTITUDE

Cerebral oedema is also potentially lethal and is manifest in the early stages by ataxia, irritability and irrational behaviour and may progress to hallucinations, drowsiness and coma. Pulmonary and cerebral forms of severe acute mountain sickness may both be present in the same patient, but a common aetiology has not been found. Mild, or localised, brain swelling is thought to occur in all people ascending to high altitudes, but it is unclear whether this always represents cerebral oedema.[27]

Following return to low altitude, cerebral disturbance may persist. Investigations up to 30 days after expeditions to very high altitudes have shown a variety of impairments, including visual long-term memory.[35]

Cough.[36] Almost half of trekkers in Nepal complain of a cough, which may be severe. Coughing normally develops after a few days at altitude and airway sensitivity to irritants is increased as a result of hyperventilation of low humidity cold air. Development of a cough may however be the first manifestation of impending HAPE.

Sleep disturbance.[1] Periodic breathing (page 76) occurs in most individuals during the first few nights above about 4000 m (13 000 ft). There are cyclical changes in tidal volume, often associated with central (rather than obstructive) apnoeas, with or without arousal from sleep (see Figure 16.2). Apnoeas may result in considerable additional hypoxaemia at high altitude. A study at 4500 m (15 000 ft) found nocturnal reductions in saturation of 8% which reduced median nocturnal saturation to just 50%.[37] The primary problem is an abnormality of respiratory control, with arousal occurring at the end of a period of apnoea, presumably secondary to hypoxia. The severity of periodic breathing is related to the strength of the subject's hypoxic ventilatory drive, and it is seldom seen in high altitude residents, who have a much attenuated hypoxic drive. The onset of sleep disturbance and severe nocturnal hypoxia may also contribute to the symptoms of AMS, and subjects developing HAPE have lower oxygen saturations during sleep.[37]

THERAPY FOR ALTITUDE–INDUCED ILLNESS[28,38]

For any severe form of AMS, administration of oxygen and descent to a lower altitude are the first essentials. Without these simple interventions, patients with cerebral oedema or HAPE will have a high mortality. Nifedipine is now an established treatment for HAPE, and when used prophylactically prevents HAPE developing in susceptible individuals.[27,28] It is an effective drug for treating pulmonary hypertension, and the convenience of administration by oral or sublingual route makes it a popular choice for mountaineers.

People with milder degrees of AMS do not need to be removed from high altitude. With acclimatisation, most symptoms of AMS will resolve but, if time is limited or symptoms interfere with planned activities, acetazolamide may be useful.[39] This carbonic anhydrase inhibitor (page 161) interferes with the transport of carbon dioxide out of cells, causing an intracellular acidosis that includes the cells of the medullary chemoreceptors and so drives respiration, in effect accelerating acclimatisation. Acetazolamide also improves sleep-induced periodic breathing, possibly by an effect on the carotid body responses to hypoxia, and via its renal effects also induces a metabolic acidosis that may further drive respiration via the central chemoreceptors.[39]

Sildenafil is a pulmonary vasodilator that acts via inhibition of phosphodiesterase (page 112) and may be taken orally. Sildenafil has been shown to be effective at reducing the hypoxia induced rise in pulmonary arterial pressure at altitude, and therefore has potential as a useful treatment for HAPE.[40]

FLYING

Only a very small number of people will ever visit places of high enough altitude to induce any of the respiratory changes described in this chapter so far. However, worldwide, almost 2 billion people per year fly in commercial aircraft, so it is useful to consider the respiratory effects of aviation.[41]

ALTITUDE EXPOSURE[42]

For reasons of fuel economy and avoidance of weather systems, commercial aircraft operate at between 9000–12 000 m (30–40 000 ft). The passenger cabin must therefore be pressurised, and a typical design aims for a cabin pressure equivalent to less than 2400 m (8000 ft), often referred to as the 'cabin altitude'.[43] Cabin pressure is maintained by indrawing and compression of external air whilst limiting cabin air outflow to maintain the desired pressure. In practice, a differential pressure is established, which represents the absolute pressure difference between the outside and inside of the aircraft. Differential pressure is increased as the aircraft climbs, and vice versa. Thus cabin pressure changes in parallel with altitude, but to a much lesser degree than the external pressure.

Supersonic flight requires much higher operating altitude to reduce air resistance, for example Concorde's cruise altitude was 18300 m (60000 ft). The differential pressure must therefore be greater to sustain a normal cabin environment at this altitude, which was facilitated in Concorde by the significantly more powerful engines from which compressed air was drawn. Military aircraft fly prolonged reconnaissance missions at an altitude of 22400 m (73500 ft), with the cockpit pressurised to an equivalent altitude of 9000 m (30000 ft). Pilots must therefore breathe 100% oxygen by mask to maintain an inspired P_{O_2} close to sea level to facilitate the required mental performance. At this altitude, military pilots are also at risk of altitude decompression sickness, which is discussed on page 300.

In theory, cabin altitudes of below 2400 m (8000 ft) should represent a minimal physiological challenge to healthy individuals resulting in a drop of only a few per cent in oxygen saturation. In practice, a study of healthy cabin crew during normal flight patterns showed that over half had saturation drops to less than 90%.[43] The effects of this degree of hypoxia on performance are controversial, though impaired night vision or colour recognition may occur at this altitude (page 280).[37] For passengers, average oxygen saturation during a flight is approximately 92%, though this may be worse during exercise and sleep (Figure 17.5).[44,45]

Depressurisation. Loss of cabin pressure at altitude either through equipment failure or accident is extremely rare. In the case of slow loss of cabin pressure, oxygen is provided for passengers as an interim measure until the aircraft can descend: 100% oxygen provides adequate protection from loss of consciousness up to an altitude of about 12000 m (40000 ft), where the atmospheric pressure is roughly equal to the sea level atmospheric P_{O_2}.

There are sporadic reports of stowaway passengers undertaking long haul flights in the wheel well of modern aircraft.[46] This environment affords little protection against the cold and severe hypoxia of altitude levels well above that of Everest. That half of these stowaways die is not surprising, but it is remarkable that half of them survive. Severe hypothermia is believed to protect them against the effects of hypoxia.

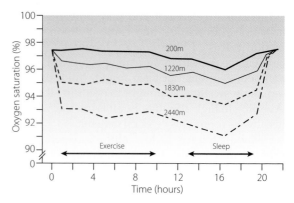

Fig. 17.5 Oxygen saturation in healthy subjects breathing air in a hypobaric chamber simulating four different altitudes: 200 m (650 ft), 1220 m (4000 ft), 1830 m (6000 ft) and 2440 m (8000 ft), the last of which is the highest 'cabin altitude' used in commercial flying. During the exercise period subjects walked on a treadmill for 10 minutes in each hour; during the sleep period subjects slept in coach class aircraft seats. (After reference 45 with permission. Copyright © 2007 Massachusetts Medical Society. All rights reserved.)

AIR TRAVEL IN PATIENTS WITH RESPIRATORY DISEASE[47,48]

To patients with respiratory disease flying may present a significant problem, particularly if arterial hypoxaemia already exists at sea level, and careful preflight assessment is required. A variety of preflight clinical evaluations and investigations have been recommended to determine whether an individual patient would require supplemental oxygen during flight. British Thoracic Society guidelines[47] have provided recommendations for assessing patients with respiratory disease, a summary of which is shown in Table 17.3. For patients with an oxygen saturation whilst breathing air of less than 92%, or in those with Sa_{O_2} of 92–95% with other risk factors (Table 17.3), then a hypoxic challenge test is recommended. This test involves measurement of arterial P_{O_2} whilst simulating flying conditions by using a hypoxic gas mixture, usually 15% oxygen. This inspired P_{O_2} equates to a cabin altitude of 2400 m (8000 ft) and represents the lowest oxygen tension that should be experienced during a commercial flight (Table 17.1).

CABIN AIR QUALITY[42,49]

Aircraft ventilation systems deliver 4–8 l.sec^{-1} of air per passenger during flight. However, compression and temperature regulation of fresh air from outside

Table 17.3 British Thoracic Society recommendations on assessing the need for in-flight supplemental oxygen in patients with respiratory disease[47]

ASSESSMENT RESULT	ACTION
Screening:	
$Sao_2 > 95\%$	Oxygen not required
Sao_2 92–95% and no risk factor[†]	Oxygen not required
Sao_2 92–95% and additional risk factor[†]	Hypoxic challenge test
$Sao_2 < 92\%$	In-flight oxygen
Hypoxic challenge test:	
$Pao_2 > 7.4$ kPa (>55 mmHg)	Oxygen not required
Pao_2 6.6–7.4 kPa (50–55 mmHg)	Borderline – walk test may be helpful
$Pao_2 < 6.6$ kPa (<50 mmHg)	In-flight oxygen

Screening test is oxygen saturation whilst breathing air at sea level. Hypoxic challenge test is arterial oxygen tension after breathing 15% oxygen for 20 minutes.
[†], Additional risk factors include hypercapnia; FEV_1 <50% of predicted; lung cancer; restrictive lung disease involving the parenchyma, chest wall (kyphoscoliosis) or respiratory muscles; ventilator support, cerebrovascular or cardiac disease; within 6 weeks of discharge for an exacerbation of chronic lung or cardiac disease.

is expensive in energy terms, and more recent designs of aircraft incorporate cabin air recirculation systems.[50] Total air delivered remains the same, but up to 50% may be recirculated rather than fresh. This recirculation of cabin air has caused concerns about the potential transmission of airborne pathogens between passengers. These fears seem to be unfounded: recirculated air passes through a high efficiency particulate air filter before re-entering the cabin,[49] and studies comparing passengers travelling on aircraft with recirculated compared with 100% fresh air ventilation systems found no difference in the likelihood of developing a common cold after the flight.[50]

Carbon dioxide concentration in aircraft often exceeds the generally accepted 'comfort' level of 1000 ppm, and would be expected to be higher in aircraft with greater amounts of recirculation air-conditioning. Concentrations observed in aircraft vary between around 700 and 1700 ppm,[51] and are highest when the aircraft is occupied, but on the ground, and lowest whilst flying at cruise altitude. Carbon dioxide itself does not cause respiratory problems at these levels, but is used more as a marker of the adequacy of ventilation.

Humidity is invariably low in aircraft, with most studies finding relative humidity to average 14–19% during flight compared with in excess of 50% in most sea level environments.[52] Like carbon dioxide, cabin humidity is maximal when on the ground and minimal at cruise altitude.[51] The low humidity occurring in aircraft is responsible for many minor symptoms such as irritation of the eyes and upper airway, though these symptoms are unusual with less than 3–4 hours of exposure.[52]

With the exception of low humidity, there is therefore little evidence that the cabin air of aircraft poses any threat to healthy passengers. The numerous symptoms reported following air travel almost certainly have their origins in other activities associated with air travel, in particular the consumption of alcohol and differing time zones.

THE RESPIRATORY SYSTEM OF BIRDS[53–55]

Many species of birds fly at high altitude, including bar-headed geese that fly over the Himalayas twice each year on their migration, though the highest recorded bird is a Rüppell's griffon vulture that unfortunately collided with a commercial airliner at 11 285 m (37 900 ft). Compared with mammals, birds have a higher body temperature (40°C) and are generally more active, and so expend more energy per unit body mass. The activity of flying is strenuous, with oxygen consumption in a flying bird reaching 13–30 times resting values depending on conditions. To supply this high oxygen consumption whilst at altitude requires the architecture of the avian respiratory system to be fundamentally different to that of mammals, and evolution of birds led to the development of a lung-air-sac system.

Much of a bird's body volume consists of air sacs, which can be inflated or deflated by the muscles of the body cavities. The air sacs are fundamental to a bird's breathing, but also have numerous other functions such as reducing body weight and voice production by the passage of air through the syrinx. Avian lungs make up a much smaller proportion of a bird's body than in mammals, and are almost rigid, being firmly fixed to the ribs. Rather than the tidal breathing used by mammals, in birds the various air sacs are used to pass gas through the lungs, in the same direction, during both inspiration and expiration so the lungs are, in effect, simply acting as a passive gas exchanger. This is achieved with two main groups of air sacs, which vary widely between bird species, but may be approximately divided into caudal and cephalad

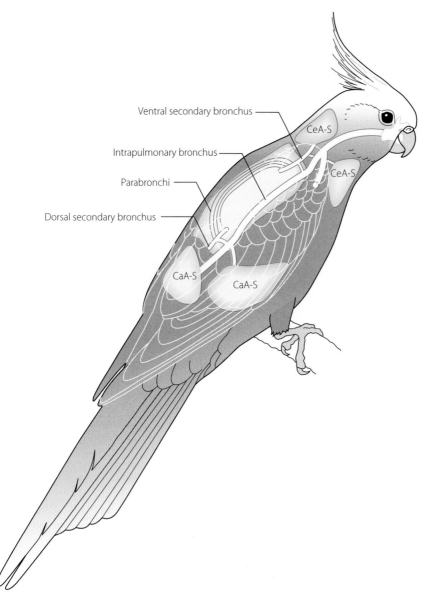

Fig. 17.6 Schematic diagram of the respiratory system of a bird. See text for details. CeA-S, cephalad air sacs; CaA-S, caudal air sacs.

Ventral secondary bronchus

Intrapulmonary bronchus

Parabronchi

Dorsal secondary bronchus

CeA-S

CeA-S

CaA-S

CaA-S

groups (Figure 17.6). During inspiration, inspired air passes through the larynx and syrinx into each primary intrapulmonary bronchus, from which some air enters the dorsal secondary bronchus and the remainder inflates the caudal air sacs. From the secondary bronchus air passes through the numerous parabronchi, where gas exchange occurs, and on through the ventral secondary bronchus into the cephalad air sacs. On expiration, the caudal air sacs empty into the dorsal secondary bronchus, the air passing through the lung and being expired through the primary bronchus whilst at the same

time the cephalad air sacs empty, the gas also being expired. As a result of this pattern of breathing there is an almost continuous flow of inspired air through the lung in a caudad to cephalad direction, whilst pulmonary blood flow is in a cephalad to caudad direction, providing an efficient counter-current gas exchange system.

Other features of the avian respiratory system further increase its gas exchange efficiency. At a microscopic level within the avian lung, the blind ending air capillaries (equivalent to a mammalian alveolus, but more tubular in shape) that arise from the parabronchi are structurally arranged with the blood capillaries to provide a further counter current system. Finally, the blood–gas barrier in avian lungs is much thinner than in mammals because the lack of repetitive movement required by tidal breathing requires less structural strength.[55] Two separate counter-current gas exchange systems and the reduced blood–gas barrier mean that in birds the P_{O_2} of inspired gas and pulmonary venous blood are almost equal.

References

*1. West JB, Schoene RB, Milledge JS. *High Altitude Medicine and Physiology*. London: Hodder Arnold; 2007.

2. West JB, Hackett PH, Maret KH, et al. Pulmonary gas exchange on the summit of Mount Everest. *J Appl Physiol*. 1983;55:678–687.

3. Sutton JT, Reeves JT, Wagner PD, et al. Operation Everest II: oxygen transport during exercise at extreme simulated altitude. *J Appl Physiol*. 1988;64:1309–1321.

4. Conkin J, Wessell JH. Critique of the equivalent air altitude model. *Aviat Space Environ Med*. 2008;79:975–982.

5. van Dorpe E, Los M, Dirven P, et al. Inspired carbon dioxide during hypoxia: effects on task performance and cerebral oxygen saturation. *Aviat Space Environ Med*. 2007;78:666–672.

6. Houston CS, Sutton JR, Cymerman A, Reeves JT. Operation Everest II: man at extreme altitude. *J Appl Physiol*. 1987;63:877–882.

7. Richalet JP, Robach P, Jarrot S, et al. Operation Everest III (COMEX '97): effects of prolonged and progressive hypoxia on humans during a simulated ascent to 8848 m in a hypobaric chamber. *Adv Exp Med Biol*. 1999;474:297–317.

8. Bisgard GE, Forster HV. Ventilatory responses to acute and chronic hypoxia. In: Fregly MJ, Blatteis CM, eds. *Handbook of Physiology, Section 4: Environmental Physiology*. New York & Oxford: Oxford University Press; 1996:1207–1239.

*9. Powell FL, Huey KA, Dwinell MR. Central nervous system mechanisms of ventilatory acclimatisation to hypoxia. *Respir Physiol*. 2000;121:223–236.

10. Severinghaus JW, Mitchell RA, Richardson BW, Singer MM. Respiratory control at high altitude suggesting active transport regulation of CSF pH. *J Appl Physiol*. 1963;18:1155–1166.

11. Tansley JG, Fatemian M, Howard LSGE, Poulin MJ, Robbins PA. Changes in respiratory control during and after 48 h of isocapnic and poikilocapnic hypoxia in humans. *J Appl Physiol*. 1998;85:2125–2134.

12. Wagner PD, Sutton JT, Reeves JT, Cymerman A, Groves BM, Malconian MK. Operation Everest II: pulmonary gas exchange during a simulated ascent of Mt. Everest. *J Appl Physiol*. 1987;63:2348–2359.

13. Grocott MPW, Martin DS, Levett DZH, et al. Arterial blood gases and oxygen content in climbers on mount Everest. *N Engl J Med*. 2009;360:140–149.

14. Groves BM, Reeves JT, Sutton JT, et al. Operation Everest II: elevated high-altitude pulmonary resistance unresponsive to oxygen. *J Appl Physiol*. 1987;63:521–530.

15. Cymerman A, Reeves JT, Sutton JT, et al. Operation Everest II: maximal oxygen uptake at extreme altitude. *J Appl Physiol*. 1989;66:2446–2453.

16. Ward MP, Milledge JS, West JB. *High Altitude Medicine and Physiology*. London: Chapman and Hall; 1995.

17. Ramirez G, Bittle PA, Rosen R, Rabb H, Pineda D. High altitude living: genetic and environmental adaptation. *Aviat Space Environ Med*. 1999;70:73–81.

18. Moore LG. Comparative human ventilatory adaptation to high altitude. *Respir Physiol*. 2000;121:257–276.

19. Massaro D, Massaro GD. Pulmonary alveoli: formation, the 'call for oxygen', and other regulators. *Am J Physiol Lung Cell Mol Physiol*. 2002;282: L345–L348.

*20. Moore LG, Armaza F, Villena M, Vargas E. Comparative aspects of high-altitude adaptation in human populations. *Adv Exp Med Biol*. 2000;475:45–62.

21. Wu T, Wang X, Wei C, et al. Hemoglobin levels in Qinghai-Tibet: different effects of gender for Tibetans vs. Han. *J Appl Physiol*. 2005;98:598–604.

22. Firth PG, Zheng H, Windsor JS, et al. Mortality on Mount Everest, 1921–2006: descriptive study. *BMJ*. 2008;337:a2654.

23. Schoene RB. Limits of human lung function at high altitude. *J Exp Biol*. 2001;204:3121–3127.

24. Schoene RB. Limits of respiration at high altitude. *Clin Chest Med*. 2005;26:405–414.

25. West JB, Boyer SJ, Graber DJ, et al. Maximal exercise at extreme altitudes on Mount Everest. *J Appl Physiol*. 1983;55:688–698.

26. Pugh LGCE, Gill MB, Lahiri S, Milledge JS, Ward MP, West JB. Muscular exercise at great altitudes. *J Appl Physiol*. 1964;19:431–440.

27. Basnyat B, Murdoch DR. High-altitude illness. *Lancet*. 2003;361:1967–1974.

28. Schoene RB. Illnesses at high altitude. *Chest*. 2008;134:402–416.

29. Maloney JP, Broeckel U. Epidemiology, risk factors, and genetics of high-altitude-related pulmonary disease. *Clin Chest Med*. 2005;26:395–404.

30. Vardy J, Vardy J, Judge K. Acute mountain sickness and ascent rates in trekkers above 2500 m in the Nepali Himalaya. *Aviat Space Environ Med*. 2006;77:742–744.

31. Bärtsch P, Mairbäurl H, Maggiorini M, Swenson ER. Physiological aspects of high-altitude pulmonary edema. *J Appl Physiol*. 2005;98:1101–1110.

32. Jerome EH, Severinghaus JW. High-altitude pulmonary edema. *N Engl J Med*. 1996;334:662–663.

33. Duplain H, Sartori C, Lepori M, et al. Exhaled nitric oxide in high-altitude pulmonary edema. Role in the regulation of pulmonary vascular tone and evidence for a role against inflammation. *Am J Respir Crit Care Med*. 2000;162:221–224.

34. Dehnert C, Risse F, Ley S, et al. Magnetic resonance imaging of uneven pulmonary perfusion in hypoxia in humans. *Am J Respir Crit Care Med*. 2006;174:1132–1138.

35. Hornbein TH, Townes BD, Schoene RB, Sutton JR, Houston CS. The cost to the central nervous system of climbing to extremely high altitude. *N Engl J Med*. 1989;321:1714–1719.

36. Barry PW, Mason NP, Riordan M, O'Callaghan C. Cough frequency and cough-receptor sensitivity are increased in man at altitude. *Clin Sci*. 1997;93:181–186.

37. Eichenberger U, Weiss E, Riemann D, Oelz O, Bärtsch P. Nocturnal periodic breathing and the development of acute high altitude illness. *Am J Respir Crit Care Med*. 1996;154:1748–1754.

38. Luks AM, Swenson ER. Medication and dosage considerations in the prophylaxis and treatment of high-altitude illness. *Chest*. 2008;133:744–755.

39. Leaf DE, Goldfarb DS. Mechanisms of action of acetazolamide in the prophylaxis and treatment of acute mountain sickness. *J Appl Physiol*. 2007;102:1313–1322.

40. Richalet J-P, Gratadour P, Robach P, et al. Sildenafil inhibits altitude-induced hypoxemia and pulmonary hypertension. *Am J Respir Crit Care Med*. 2005;171:275–281.

41. Silverman D, Gendreau M. Medical issues associated with commercial flights. *Lancet*. 2008;373:2067–2077.

42. Harding RM, Mills FJ. *Aviation Medicine*. London: BMJ Publishing Group; 1993.

43. Cottrell JJ, Lebovitz BL, Fennell RG, Kohn GM. Inflight arterial saturation: continuous monitoring by pulse oximetry. *Aviat Space Environ Med*. 1995;66:126–130.

44. Kelly PT, Swanney MP, Frampton C, Seccombe LM, Peters MJ, Beckert LE. Normobaric hypoxia inhalation test vs. response to airline flight in healthy passengers. *Aviat Space Environ Med*. 2006;77:1143–1147.

45. Muhm JM, Rock PB, McMullin DL, et al. Effect of aircraft-cabin altitude on passenger discomfort. *N Engl J Med*. 2007;357:18–27.

46. Veronneau SJH, Mohler SR, Pennybaker AL, Wilcox BC, Sahiar F. Survival at high altitudes: Wheel-well passengers. *Aviat Space Environ Med*. 1996;67:784–786.

47. British Thoracic Society Standards of Care Committee. Managing passengers with respiratory disease planning air travel: British Thoracic Society recommendations. *Thorax*. 2002;57:289–304.

48. Dine CJ, Kreider ME. Hypoxia altitude simulation test. *Chest*. 2008;133:1002–1005.

*49. Rayman RB. Cabin air quality: an overview. *Aviat Space Environ Med*. 2002;73:211–215.

50. Zitter JN, Mazonson PD, Miller DP, Hulley SB, Balmes JR. Aircraft cabin air recirculation and symptoms of the common cold. *JAMA*. 2002;288:483–486.

51. Lindgren T, Norbäck D. Cabin air quality: indoor pollutants and climate during intercontinental flights with and without tobacco smoking. *Indoor Air*. 2002;12:263–272.

52. Nagda NL, Hodgson M. Low relative humidity and aircraft cabin air quality. *Indoor Air*. 2001;11:200–214.

53. Maina JN. Development, structure, and function of a novel respiratory organ, the lung-air sac system of birds: to go where no other vertebrate has gone. *Biol Rev*. 2006;81:545–579.

54. Brown RE, Brain JD, Wang N. The avian respiratory system: a unique model for studies of respiratory toxicosis and for monitoring air quality. *Environ Health Perspect*. 1997;105:188–200.

55. West JB, Watson RR, Fu Z. The human lung: did evolution get it wrong? *Eur Respir J*. 2007;29:11–17.

Chapter 18

High pressure and diving

KEY POINTS

- When diving in water the increased density of inhaled gases and immersion in water cause an increase in the work of breathing, which can impair gas exchange during exercise.
- Above about 4 atmospheres absolute pressure nitrogen has anaesthetic effects and divers must breathe helium, which also overcomes the problem of increased gas density.
- On ascent from a dive expansion of gases in closed body spaces and bubble formation in the tissues and blood can cause pulmonary barotrauma and decompression sickness.

Humans have sojourned temporarily in high-pressure environments since the introduction of the diving bell. The origin of this development is lost in antiquity but Alexander the Great was said to have been lowered to the seabed in a diving bell.

The environment of the diver is often, but not invariably, aqueous. Saturation divers spend most of their time in a gaseous environment in chambers that are held at a pressure close to that of the depth of water at which they will be working. Tunnel and caisson workers may also be at high pressure in a gaseous environment. Those in an aqueous environment also have the additional effect of different gravitational forces applied to their trunks, which influence the mechanics of breathing and other systems of the body. Workers in both environments share the physiological problems associated with increased ambient pressures and partial pressures of respired gases.

In this field, as in others, we cannot escape from the multiplicity of units, and some of these are set out in Table 18.1. Note particularly that 'atmosphere gauge' is relative to ambient pressure. Thus 2 atmospheres absolute (ATA) equals 1 atmosphere gauge relative to sea level. Throughout this chapter atmospheres of pressure refer to absolute and not gauge.

EXCHANGE OF OXYGEN AND CARBON DIOXIDE[1]

EFFECT OF PRESSURE ON ALVEOLAR P_{CO_2} AND P_{O_2}

Pressure has complicated and very important effects on P_{CO_2} and P_{O_2}. The alveolar concentration of CO_2 equals its rate of production divided by the alveolar ventilation (page 167). However, both gas volumes must be measured under the same conditions of temperature and pressure. Alveolar CO_2 concentration at 10 ATA will be about one tenth of sea level values, i.e. 0.56% compared with 5.3% at sea level. When these concentrations are multiplied by pressure to give P_{CO_2}, values are similar at sea level and 10 atmospheres. Thus, as a rough approximation, alveolar CO_2 concentration decreases inversely to the environmental pressure, but the P_{CO_2} remains near its sea level value.

Effects on the P_{O_2} are slightly more complicated but no less important. The difference between the inspired and alveolar oxygen *concentrations* equals the ratio of oxygen uptake to inspired alveolar ventilation. This fraction, like the alveolar CO_2 concentration, decreases inversely with the increased

Table 18.1 Pressures and Po_2 values at various depths of sea water

| DEPTH OF SEA WATER | | PRESSURE (ABSOLUTE) | | Po_2 BREATHING AIR | | | | PERCENTAGE OXYGEN TO GIVE SEA LEVEL INSPIRED Po_2 |
| | | | | INSPIRED | | ALVEOLAR | | |
metres	feet	atm.	kPa	kPa	mmHg	kPa	mmHg	
0	0	1	101	19.9	149	13.9	104	20.9
10	32.8	2	203	41.2	309	35.2	264	10.1
20	65.6	3	304	62.3	467	56.3	422	6.69
50	164	6	608	126	945	120	900	3.31
Usual limit for breathing air								
100	328	11	1 110					1.80
200	656	21	2 130					0.94
Usual limit for saturation dives								
Threshold for high pressure nervous syndrome								
500	1640	51	5 170					0.39
1000	3280	101	10 200					0.20
Depth reached by sperm whale								
2000	6560	201	20 400					0.098
2500	8200	251	25 400					0.078
Pressure reached by non-aquatic mammals with pharmacological amelioration of high pressure nervous syndrome								

Notes: 10 metres sea water = 1 atmosphere (gauge). Alveolar Po_2 is assumed to be 6 kPa (45 mmHg) less than inspired Po_2.

pressure. However, the corresponding *partial pressure* will remain close to the sea level value, as does the alveolar Pco_2. Therefore the difference between the inspired and alveolar Po_2 will remain roughly constant, and the alveolar Po_2, to a first approximation, increases by the same amount as the inspired Po_2 (Figure 18.1). However, these considerations only take into account the direct effect of pressure on gas partial pressures. There are other, more subtle, effects on respiratory mechanics and gas exchange which must now be considered.

EFFECT ON MECHANICS OF BREATHING[2,3,4]

Two main factors must be considered. First, there is the increased density of gases at pressure, although this can be reduced by changing the composition of the inspired gas. The second factor is the pressure of water on the body, which alters the gravitational effects to which the respiratory system is normally exposed.

Gas density is increased in direct proportion to pressure. Thus air at 10 atmospheres has 10 times the density of air at sea level, which increases the resistance to turbulent gas flow (page 45) and limits

the maximal breathing capacity (MBC) that can be achieved. In fact, it is usual to breathe a helium/oxygen mixture at pressures in excess of about 6 atmospheres because of nitrogen narcosis (see below). Helium has only one-seventh the density of air and so is easier to breathe. Furthermore, lower inspired oxygen concentrations are both permissible and indeed desirable as the pressure increases (Table 18.1). Therefore, at 15 atmospheres it would be reasonable to breathe a mixture of 98% helium and 2% oxygen. This would more than double the MBC that the diver could attain while breathing air at that pressure. Hydrogen has even lower density than helium, and has been used in gas mixtures for dives to more than 500 metres deep.[5]

The effect of immersion is additional to any change in the density of the respired gases. In open-tube snorkel breathing, the alveolar gas is close to normal atmospheric pressure but the trunk is exposed to a pressure depending on the depth of the subject, which is limited by the length of the snorkel tube. This is equivalent to a standing subatmospheric pressure applied to the mouth and it is difficult to inhale against a 'negative' pressure loading of more than about 5 kPa (50 cmH$_2$O). This corresponds to

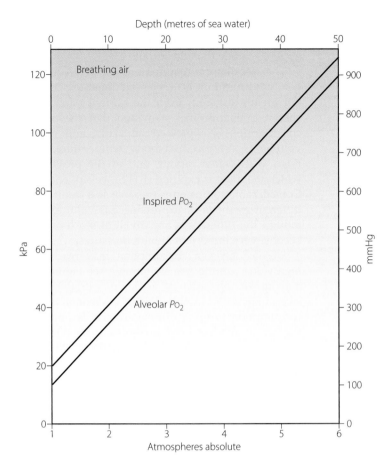

a mean depth of immersion of only 50 cm, and it is therefore virtually impossible to use a snorkel tube at a depth of 1 metre. However, the normal length of a snorkel tube assures that the swimmer is barely more than awash, and so these problems should not arise.

'Negative' pressure loading is prevented by supplying gas to the diver's airway at a pressure that is close to the hydrostatic pressure surrounding the diver. This may be achieved by providing an excess flow of gas with a pressure-relief valve controlled by the surrounding water pressure. Such an arrangement was used for the traditional helmeted diver supplied by an air pump on the surface. Free-swimming divers carrying their own compressed gas supply rely on inspiratory demand valves, which are also balanced by the surrounding water pressure.

These arrangements supply gas that is close to the hydrostatic pressure surrounding the trunk. However, the precise 'static lung loading' depends on the location of the pressure-controlling device in relation to the geometry of the chest. Minor differences result from the various postures that the diver may assume. Thus, if he is 'head-up' when using a valve at mouthpiece level, the pressure surrounding the trunk is higher than the airway pressure by a mean value of about 3 kPa (30 cmH₂O). If he is 'head-down', airway pressure is greater than the pressure to which the trunk is exposed. The head-down position thus corresponds to positive pressure breathing and the head-up position to negative pressure breathing. The latter causes a reduction of functional residual capacity (FRC) of about 20–30% but breathing is considered to be easier head-up than head-down.[1]

Apart from these considerations, immersion has relatively little effect on respiratory function, and the additional respiratory work of moving extracorporeal water does not seem to add appreciably to the work of breathing.

EFFECT ON EFFICIENCY OF GAS EXCHANGE[4]

Dead space/tidal volume ratio in divers increases with greater depth.[2,6] Changes are seen at relatively low pressures, for example, in one study dead space/tidal volume ratio increased from 37% at sea level to 42% at 2.8 ATA.[2] During exercise at this pressure, values decreased to around 20%.

The best measure of the efficiency of oxygenation of the arterial blood is the alveolar/arterial Po_2 gradient. Measurement of arterial blood gas tensions presents formidable technical difficulties at high pressures. However, studies at 2.8, 47 and 66 ATA have reported only small increases in alveolar/arterial Po_2 gradient.[2,6] Since it is customary to supply deep divers with an inspired oxygen tension of at least 0.5 ATA, arterial hypoxaemia is unlikely to occur either from hypoventilation or from maldistribution of pulmonary ventilation and perfusion in healthy subjects.[6]

The position as regards arterial Pco_2 is less clear. Hypercapnia is a well-recognised complication of diving, and divers are known to have a blunted Pco_2/ventilation response, though the cause of this is unknown.[1] Hypercapnia in divers at rest is uncommon, but during exercise elevated end-tidal and arterial Pco_2 levels are described. Arterial Pco_2 during exercise at 2.8 ATA were around 5 kPa (37 mmHg),[2] but at pressures of 47 and 66 ATA were in the range 6.2–8.3 kPa (47–62 mmHg).[6] This is potentially hazardous because 9 kPa is approaching the level at which there may be some clouding of consciousness, and that is potentially dangerous at depth. High gas density at depth causing increased work of breathing is believed to be responsible for the inadequate ventilation during exercise.

OXYGEN CONSUMPTION

The relationship between power output and oxygen consumption at pressures up to 66 ATA, whether under water or dry, is not significantly different from the relationship at normal pressure[6] shown in Figure 15.1. Oxygen consumption is expressed under standard conditions of temperature and pressure, dry (STPD, see Appendix C) and therefore represents an absolute quantity of oxygen. However, this volume, when expressed at the diver's environmental pressure, is inversely related to the pressure. Thus, an oxygen consumption of 1 l.min^{-1} (STPD) at a pressure of 10 atmospheres would be only 100 ml.min^{-1} when expressed at the pressure to which the diver is exposed. Similar considerations apply to carbon dioxide output.

The ventilatory requirement for a given oxygen consumption at increased pressure is also not greatly different from the normal relationship shown in Figure 15.5, provided that the oxygen consumption is expressed at STPD, and minute volume is expressed at body temperature, saturated with water vapour, and at the pressure to which the diver is exposed (BTPS, see Appendix C). Considerable confusion is possible as a result of the different methods of expressing gas volumes, and though the differences are trivial at sea level they become very important at high pressures.

Exercise.[5] Oxygen consumption may reach very high values during free swimming (see Figure 15.1) and are of the order of 2–3 l.min^{-1} (STPD) for a swimming speed of only 2 km h^{-1}. Maximal oxygen consumption (Vo_{2max}) during exercise is improved slightly at modest high pressures (<20 ATA), an observation that results from hyperoxia (0.3 ATA oxygen) normally used at this depth. With deeper dives, there is a progressive reduction in exercise capacity, irrespective of the oxygen pressure, as a result of respiratory limitation secondary to higher gas density.

EFFECTS ATTRIBUTABLE TO THE COMPOSITION OF THE INSPIRED GAS

AIR

Oxygen. When breathing air at a pressure of 6 ATA, the inspired Po_2 will be about 126 kPa (945 mmHg) and the alveolar Po_2 about 120 kPa (900 mmHg). This is below the threshold for oxygen convulsions of about 2 ATA, but above the threshold for pulmonary oxygen toxicity if exposure is continued for more than a few hours (see Chapter 26).[1,3]

Nitrogen. It is actually nitrogen that limits the depth to which air may be breathed. It has three separate undesirable effects.

First, nitrogen is an anaesthetic and, in accord with its lipid solubility, can cause full surgical anaesthesia at a partial pressure of about 30 ATA. The narcotic effect of nitrogen is first detectable when breathing air at about 4 ATA and there is usually serious impairment of performance at 10 atmospheres. This effect is known as nitrogen narcosis or 'the rapture of the deep'. It is a general rule that nitrogen narcosis precludes the use of air at depths greater than 100 metres of sea water (11 ATA pressure) and, in fact, air is not used today at pressures greater than 6 ATA. Helium is the preferred substitute at higher pressures and has no detectable narcotic properties up to at least 100 ATA.

The second problem attributable to nitrogen at high pressures is its density, which causes greatly increased hindrance to breathing at high pressure (see above). Helium has only one-seventh of the density of nitrogen and this is the second reason for its choice.

The third problem with nitrogen is its solubility in body tissues, with the resultant formation of bubbles on decompression. This is discussed in more detail below. Other inert gases, particularly helium, are less soluble in body tissues and this is the third reason for the use of helium at high pressures.

HELIUM/OXYGEN MIXTURES (HELIOX)

For the three reasons outlined in the previous section, helium is the preferred diluent inert gas at pressures above 6 ATA. The concentration of oxygen required to give the same inspired gas Po_2 as at sea level is shown in Table 18.1. In fact, it is usual practice to provide an inspired Po_2 of about 0.5 ATA (50 kPa or 375 mmHg) to give a safety margin in the event of error in gas mixing and to provide protection against hypoventilation or defective gas exchange. This level of Po_2 appears to be below the threshold for pulmonary oxygen toxicity, even during prolonged saturation dives.

A special problem of helium is its very high thermal conductivity, which tends to cause hypothermia unless the diver's environment is heated. Heat loss from radiation and evaporation remain generally unchanged, but convective heat loss from the respiratory tract and skin is greatly increased.[5] It is usual for chambers to be maintained at temperatures as high as 30–32°C during saturation dives on helium/oxygen mixtures.

HELIUM/OXYGEN/NITROGEN MIXTURES (TRIMIX)

The pressure that can be attained while breathing helium/oxygen mixtures is currently limited by the high pressure nervous syndrome (HPNS).[5,7] This is a hyperexcitable state of the central nervous system which appears to be due to hydrostatic pressure per se and not to any changes in gas tensions. It becomes a serious problem for divers at pressures in excess of about 50 ATA, but is first apparent at about 20 ATA.

Various treatments can mitigate this effect and so increase the depth at which a diver can operate safely. The most practicable is the addition of 5–10% percent nitrogen to the helium oxygen mixture. This in effect reverses HPNS with partial nitrogen narcosis, whilst the HPNS reverses the narcosis that would be caused by the nitrogen. Trimix containing 5% nitrogen allows divers to function normally at depths of over 600 metres.[5]

TYPES OF DIVING ACTIVITY AND THEIR RESPIRATORY EFFECTS

Snorkelling is the simplest form of human diving but, as described above, respiratory effects limit the diver to the top 50 cm of water. Many other forms of diving have therefore evolved.

BREATH–HOLD DIVING[8,9,10]

The simplest method of diving is by breath holding, and this is still used for collecting pearls, sponges and food from the sea bed. After breathing air, breath holding time is normally limited to 60–75 seconds, and the changes in alveolar gas tensions are shown in Figure 5.9. Astonishingly, the depth record is currently 214 metres.[11] Many remarkable mechanisms interact to make this possible.

Lung volume. As pressure increases lung volume decreases by Boyle's law (page 515). Thus at 10 ATA, an initial lung volume of 6 litres would be reduced to about 600 ml, well below residual volume (RV), and with the loss of 5.4 kg of buoyancy. During descent a point is reached when the body attains neutral buoyancy and the body will sink below that depth. To increase lung volume before diving, breath-hold divers have developed a technique called glossopharyngeal insufflation, in which air is taken into the oropharynx and compressed before being forced into the already fully inflated lung.[12] Pulmonary pressure is increased above atmospheric and lung volumes increased above normal total lung capacity by 2 litres or more. A similar procedure, glossopharyngeal exsufflation, allows the divers to practice reducing their lung volumes below residual volume. For dives to 200 m depth the lungs must be almost totally collapsed, and must be reinflated on the return ascent, and the ability of a human to perform this manoeuvre contradicts much of what we currently understand about lung mechanics.[11]

Alveolar Po_2. increases with greater depth as the alveolar gas is compressed, providing a doubling of Po_2 at about 8 metres deep. More of the alveolar oxygen is therefore available at depth. Conversely, during ascent, alveolar Po_2 decreases due partly to oxygen consumption, but mainly to decreasing pressure. There is thus danger of hypoxia just before reaching the surface. However, when the alveolar Po_2 falls below the mixed venous Po_2, there is a paradoxical transfer of oxygen from mixed venous blood to alveolar gas, and the arterial Po_2 is maintained above the very low partial pressure that would otherwise occur in the alveoli. This may be an important factor in preventing loss of consciousness in the final stages of ascent.

Alveolar Pco_2. By a similar mechanism, alveolar Pco_2 is greater during a breath-hold dive than during a simple breath hold at sea level. At an environmental pressure of only 12 kPa (90 mmHg) gauge, the alveolar Pco_2 will be increased above the mixed venous Pco_2, and there will be a paradoxical transfer of carbon dioxide from alveolus to arterial blood. Fortunately there is a limited quantity of carbon dioxide in the alveolar gas, and the process is reversed during late descent and ascent.

Adaptations in the diving mammals.[13] Diving mammals rely on breath holding for dives and have adaptations that permit remarkably long times under water and the attainment of great depths. For example, Sperm whales can attain depths of 1000 metres and Weddell seals can reach 500 metres and remain submerged for 70 minutes. Such feats depend on a variety of biochemical, cardiovascular and respiratory adaptations. It seems likely that the lungs of the Weddell seal collapse completely at depths between 25 and 50 metres, thus preventing the partial pressure of nitrogen increasing above the level of 320 kPa (2400 mmHg) which has been recorded at depths between 40 and 80 metres.

Many diving mammals use the spleen as a reservoir for oxygenated blood during dives. In some diving species, the spleen represents over 10% of body mass, and contains a much more muscular capsule than terrestrial animals. Splenic contraction is the probable cause of an increase of haemoglobin concentration from 15 to 25 g.dl^{-1} during long dives.[14] Furthermore, these animals have twice the blood volume per kilogram body weight relative to humans, so oxygen stored in blood for a dive is proportionately about three times that of humans.

LIMITED DURATION DIVES

Most dives are of relatively brief duration and involve a rapid descent to operating depth, a period spent at depth, followed by an ascent, the rate of which is governed by the requirement to avoid release of inert gas dissolved in the tissues. The profile and the duration of the ascent are governed by the depth attained, the time spent at depth and the nature of the diluent inert gas.

The diving bell. The simplest and oldest technique was the diving bell. Air was trapped on the surface but the internal water level rose as the air was compressed at depth. Useful time at depth was generally no more than 20–30 minutes. More recently, additional air was introduced into the bell under pressure from the surface.

The helmeted diver. From about 1820 until recent times, the standard method of diving down to 100 metres has been by a helmeted diver supplied with air pumped from the surface into the helmet and escaping from a relief valve controlled by the water pressure. This gave much greater mobility than the old diving bell and permitted the execution of complex tasks.

SCUBA diving.[15] There was for some years a desire to move towards free-swimming divers carrying their own gas supply (SCUBA – self-contained underwater breathing apparatus), first achieved in 1943. The system is based on a demand valve that is controlled by both the ambient pressure and the inspiration of the diver. Air-breathing SCUBA dives are usually restricted to depths of 30 metres. Greater depths are possible but special precautions must then be taken to avoid decompression sickness. SCUBA divers are far more mobile than helmeted divers and can work in almost any body position.

Caisson and tunnel working. Since 1839, tunnel and bridge foundations have been constructed by pressurising the work environment to exclude water. The work environment is maintained at pressure, normally of less than 4 ATA, with staff entering and leaving by air locks. Entry is rapid but exit requires adherence to the appropriate decompression schedule if the working pressure is in excess of 2 ATA.

Free submarine escape. It is possible to escape from a submarine by free ascent from depths down to about 100 metres. The submariner first enters an escape chamber which is then pressurised to equal the external water pressure. He then opens a hatch communicating with the exterior and leaves the chamber. During the ascent, the gas in his lungs expands according to Boyle's law. It is therefore imperative that he keeps his glottis and mouth open, allowing gas to escape in a continuous stream. If gas is not allowed to escape, barotrauma is almost certain to occur (see below). In an uneventful escape, the time spent at pressure is too short for there to be any danger of decompression sickness. Thorough training is necessary and all submariners are trained in a vertical tank of 100 feet depth.

SATURATION DIVES

When prolonged and repeated work is required at great depths, it is more convenient to hold the divers in a dry chamber, kept on board a ship or oil rig, and held at a pressure close to the pressure of their intended working depth. Divers transfer to a smaller chamber at the same pressure, which is lowered to depth as and when required. The divers then leave the chamber for work, without any major change in pressure, but remaining linked to the chamber by an umbilical. On return to the chamber, they can be raised to the surface where they wait, still at pressure, until they are next required. A normal tour of duty is about 3 weeks, the whole of which is spent at operating pressure, currently up to about 20 atmospheres breathing helium/oxygen mixtures. During the long period at pressure, tissues are fully saturated with inert gas at the chamber pressure and prolonged decompression is then required which may last for several days.

RESPIRATORY ASPECTS OF DECOMPRESSION ILLNESS[3]

Returning to the surface following a dive is a hazardous procedure, and can give rise to a variety of complications variously known as 'bends', 'chokes' or caisson disease. In its mildest form, subjects have short-lived joint pain, but more serious presentations include pulmonary barotrauma or neurological deficit that can result in permanent disability. In the late 19th century, before decompression illness was understood, the effects on caisson workers were severe. For example, of the 600 men involved in building the underwater foundations of the St Louis Bridge in the USA, 119 of them had serious decompression illness and 14 died.[16] Nowadays some form of decompression illness is thought to affect 1 in 3500–10 000 recreational dives,[17] and one in 500–1000 commercial dives.[16] Nomenclature of

the many syndromes associated with decompression is confusing, but there are two main ways in which illness arises.

BAROTRAUMA

Barotrauma as a result of change in pressure will affect any closed body space containing gas, and tends to occur during ascent when the gas expands. The ears, sinuses and teeth are the most commonly affected areas, but pulmonary barotrauma, although rare, is much more dangerous. Pulmonary barotrauma may occur during rapid ascent in untrained subjects, for example during submarine escape training (see above) when the subject forgets to exhale during ascent.[18] Barotrauma results in disruption of the airway or alveolar wall, and air may enter either the pulmonary vessels or interstitial tissue, from where it spreads to the pleura, mediastinum or subcutaneous tissues. Mediastinal or pleural air pockets continue to expand during ascent, until chest pain or breathing difficulties occur within a few minutes of surfacing.

Some divers develop barotrauma during relatively shallow dives, and efforts have been made to identify which divers are at risk.[19] In this case, barotrauma is believed to result from expansion of air trapped in the periphery of the lung by small airway closure. Subjects with reduced expiratory flow rates at low lung volume, including some asthmatics, are therefore at a theoretically greater risk.[19] There is currently only weak evidence that this is a practical problem in asthmatic patients taking part in recreational diving.[20]

DECOMPRESSION SICKNESS

Tissue bubble formation[1,16,21] occurs when tissues become 'supersaturated' with an inert gas, usually nitrogen. As decompression occurs, tissue P_{N_2} becomes greater than the ambient pressure, and bubbles form, exactly as occurs when opening a carbonated drink. The increase in tissue P_{N_2} during descent and the decrease in P_{N_2} on ascent are both exponential curves. Tissues poorly perfused with blood have the slowest half-time for both uptake and elimination, hence on decompression tissue P_{N_2} decreases most slowly in poorly perfused tissues such as cartilage, giving rise to the 'bends'.

Arterial gas embolism. Venous bubbles occur commonly during decompression, and the filtration provided by the lung is extremely effective. Overload of the filtration system may result in arterial gas embolism, but this is only believed to be the case in severe decompression sickness. There is an increasing body of evidence that arterial gas embolism follows shunting of blood containing air bubbles from the right to left sides of the heart through an otherwise asymptomatic atrial septal defect (page 217).[17] Whatever the origins, arterial gas embolism is believed to be the major factor causing the neurological deficits of decompression sickness, and may be contributing to long-term neurological damage in professional divers.[22]

Treatment of decompression sickness is best achieved by avoidance. Detailed and elaborate tables have been prepared to indicate the safe rate of decompression depending on the pressure and time of exposure. Administration of oxygen will reduce the blood P_{N_2} and so accelerate the resorption of bubbles in both blood and tissue. In severe cases, including all divers with neurological deficits, urgent recompression in a chamber is required, followed by slow decompression with oxygen and other therapeutic interventions.[23]

ALTITUDE DECOMPRESSION SICKNESS[24,25]

Flying at high altitude by military aircraft exposes the pilots to significant degrees of decompression, a cabin altitude of 9000 m (30 000 ft) being equivalent to approximately 0.3 ATA (see Chapter 16). During actual flights, symptoms of decompression sickness tend to be under-reported because these elite pilots may fear restrictions on their flying activities. However, during their careers, three-quarters of pilots experience problems, and almost 40% of trainee pilots develop symptoms during hypobaric chamber testing to normal cabin altitudes.[25] Joint pain is predictably the most common symptom, whilst the 'chokes' (sub-sternal pain, cough and dyspnoea) occurs in 1–3% of cases. Breathing oxygen prior to altitude exposure is likely to significantly ameliorate the symptoms seen, and is required by the US Air Force prior to altitude exposure.

Flying in the partially pressurised cabin (page 287) of commercial aircraft shortly after underwater diving increases the risk of decompression sickness. The likelihood of developing symptoms is increased by both greater depth of the last dive and shorter duration of time between the dive and flying. Dives to less than 18.5 m deep, and leaving over 24 hours between diving and flying, are generally accepted as resulting in a minimal, but not zero, risk of decompression sickness.[26]

References

1. Lundgren CEG, Harabin A, Bennett PB, Van Liew HD, Thalmann ED. Gas physiology in diving. In: Fregly MJ, Blatteis CM, eds. *Handbook of Physiology, Section 4: Environmental physiology*. New York & Oxford: Oxford University Press; 1996:999–1019.

2. Mummery HJ, Stolp BW, Dear GdeL, et al. Effects of age and exercise on physiological dead space during simulated dives at 2.8 ATA. *J Appl Physiol*. 2003;94:507–517.

3. Tetzlaff K, Thorsen E. Breathing at depth: physiologic and clinical aspects of diving while breathing compressed gas. *Clin Chest Med*. 2005;26:355–380.

4. Moon RE, Cherry AD, Stolp BW, Camporesi EM. Pulmonary gas exchange in diving. *J Appl Physiol*. 2009;106:668–677.

5. Hong SK, Bennett PB, Shiraki K, Lin Y-C, Claybaugh JR. Mixed gas saturation diving. In: Fregly MJ, Blatteis CM, eds. *Handbook of Physiology, Section 4: Environmental Physiology*. New York & Oxford: Oxford University Press; 1996:1023–1045.

6. Salzano JV, Camporesi EM, Stolp BW, Moon RE. Physiological responses to exercise at 47 and 66 ATA. *J Appl Physiol*. 1984;57:1055–1068.

7. Halsey MJ. The effects of high pressure on the central nervous system. *Physiol Rev*. 1982;62:1341–1377.

8. Ferretti G. Extreme human breath-hold diving. *Eur J Appl Physiol*. 2001;84:254–271.

9. Muth C-M, Ehrmann U, Radermacher P. Physiological and clinical aspects of apnea diving. *Clin Chest Med*. 2005;26:381–394.

*10. Lindholm P, Lundgren CE. The physiology and pathophysiology of human breath-hold diving. *J Appl Physiol*. 2009;106:284–292.

11. Fahlman A. The pressure to understand the mechanism of lung compression and its effect on lung function. *J Appl Physiol*. 2008;104:907–908.

12. Whittaker LA, Irvin CG. Going to extremes of lung volume. *J Appl Physiol*. 2007;102:831–833.

*13. Butler PJ, Jones DR. Physiology of diving of birds and mammals. *Physiol Rev*. 1997;77:837–895.

14. Qvist J, Hill RD, Schneider RC, et al. Hemoglobin concentrations and blood gas tensions of free-diving Weddell seals. *J Appl Physiol*. 1986;61:1560–1569.

15. Lynch PR. Historical and basic perspectives of SCUBA diving. *Med Sci Sports Exerc.* 1996;28:570–572.

16. Moon RE, Vann RD, Bennett PB. The physiology of decompression illness. *Sci Am Aug.* 1995;273:54–61.

*17. Foster PD, Boriek AM, Butler BD, Gernhardt ML, Bove AA. Patent foramen ovale and para-doxical systemic embolism: a bibliographic review. *Aviat Space Environ Med.* 2003;74: B1–B40.

18. Broome CR, Jarvis LJ, Clark RJ. Pulmonary barotrauma in submarine escape training. *Thorax.* 1994;49:186–187.

19. Bove AA. Pulmonary barotrauma in divers: can prospective pulmonary function testing identify those at risk? *Chest.* 1997;112:576–578.

20. Koehle M, Lloyd-Smith R, McKenzie D, Taunton J. Asthma and recreational SCUBA diving. *Sports Med.* 2003;33:109–116.

21. Barak M, Katz Y. Microbubbles: pathophysiology and clinical implications. *Chest.* 2005;128:2918–2932.

22. Wilmshurst P. Brain damage in divers. *BMJ.* 1997;314:689–690.

23. Moon RE, Sheffield PJ. Guidelines for treatment of decompression illness. *Aviat Space Environ Med.* 1997;68:234–243.

24. Bendrick GA, Ainscough MJ, Pilmanis AA, Bisson RU. Prevalence of decompression sickness among U-2 pilots. *Aviat Space Environ Med.* 1996;67:199–206.

25. Balldin UI, Pilmanis AA, Webb JT. Pulmonary decompression sickness at altitude: early symptoms and circulating gas emboli. *Aviat Space Environ Med.* 2002;73:996–999.

26. Freiberger JJ, Denoble PJ, Pieper CF, Uguccioni DM, Pollock NW, Vann RD. The relative risk of decompression sickness during and after air travel following diving. *Aviat Space Environ Med.* 2002;73:980–984.

Chapter 19

Respiration in closed environments and space

KEY POINTS

- Environments in which a closed atmosphere suitable for breathing is maintained include closed-circuit anaesthesia, submarines and space vehicles.
- Problems of maintaining acceptably low carbon dioxide concentrations and low levels of inhaled contaminants are common to all these environments.
- In the microgravity of space static lung volumes are reduced, ventilation and perfusion are better matched, and airway obstruction during sleep is uncommon.
- For atmospheric regeneration in long-term space missions of the future, a combination of physicochemical and biological systems is likely to be needed.

The fascination of the human race with exploration has taken humans well beyond the high altitude and underwater environments described in Chapters 17 and 18. Our ability to maintain life in space, the most hostile of environments yet explored, was developed as a result of techniques used to sustain breathing in other seemingly unrelated environments on Earth. All these environments share the problems common to maintaining respiration while separated from the Earth's atmosphere.

CLOSED-SYSTEM ANAESTHESIA

This may not represent the most dramatic example of closed-environment breathing but it is by far the most common. Careful control of the composition of respired gas is the hallmark of inhalational anaesthesia. The anaesthetist must maintain safe concentrations of oxygen and carbon dioxide in the patient's lungs, while controlling with great precision the dose of inhaled anaesthetic. It was recognised over 100 years ago that anaesthesia could be prolonged by allowing the patient to rebreathe some of their expired gas, including the anaesthetic vapour.[1] Provided oxygen is added and carbon dioxide removed, other gases can be circulated round a breathing system many times, providing beneficial effects such as warm and humid inspired gas. More recently, rebreathing systems have become popular as a method of reducing both the amount of anaesthetic used and pollution of the operating theatre environment.

A totally closed system during anaesthesia means that all expired gases are recirculated to the patient, with oxygen added only to replace that consumed and anaesthetic agent added to replace that absorbed by the patient. In practice, low-flow anaesthesia, in which over half of the patient's expired gases are recirculated, is much more commonly used.[1] In each case, carbon dioxide is absorbed by chemical reaction with combinations of calcium, sodium, potassium or barium hydroxides, resulting in the formation of the respective carbonate and water. The reaction cannot be reversed, and the absorbent must be discarded after use.

Widespread use of closed-circuit anaesthesia is limited by perceived difficulties with maintaining adequate circuit concentrations of gases that the patient is consuming, such as oxygen and anaesthetic agent. However, gas-monitoring systems are now almost universally used with low-flow and closed circuit anaesthesia, allowing accurate control of circuit gas composition.

DOI: 10.1016/B978-0-7020-2996-7.00019-2

ACCUMULATION OF OTHER GASES IN CLOSED CIRCUITS

Closed-circuit systems with a constant inflow and consumption of oxygen will allow retention of other gases entering the circuit either with the fresh gas or from the patient. This affects the patient in two quite distinct ways. First, essentially inert gases such as nitrogen and argon may accumulate to such an extent that they dilute the oxygen in the system. Secondly, small concentrations of more toxic gases may arise within the breathing system.

Nitrogen enters the circuit from the patient at the start of anaesthesia. Body stores of dissolved nitrogen are small, but air present in the lungs may contain 2–3 litres of nitrogen, which will be transferred to the circuit in the first few minutes. If nitrogen is not intended to be part of the closed-circuit gas mixture, the patient must 'denitrogenate' by breathing high concentrations of oxygen before being anaesthetised, or higher fresh gas flow rates must be used initially to flush the nitrogen from the closed circuit.

Argon is normally present in air at a concentration of 0.93%. Oxygen concentrators effectively remove nitrogen from air, and so concentrate argon in similar proportions to oxygen, resulting in argon concentrations of around 5%. In a study of closed-circuit breathing in volunteers using oxygen from an oxygen concentrator, argon levels in the circuit reached 40% after only 80 minutes.[2] Cylinders of medical grade oxygen and hospital supplies from liquid oxygen evaporators contain negligible argon, so the risk of significant accumulation is low.

Methane is produced in the distal colon by anaerobic bacterial fermentation and is mostly excreted directly from the alimentary tract. Some methane is, however, absorbed into the blood, where it has low solubility so is rapidly excreted by the lung, following which it will accumulate in the closed circuit. There is a large variation between subjects in methane production and, therefore, the concentrations seen during closed-circuit anaesthesia. Mean levels in the circle system in healthy patients reached over 900 ppm, well below levels regarded as unacceptable in other closed environments, but sufficient to cause interference with some anaesthetic gas analysers.[3]

Acetone, ethanol and carbon monoxide all have high blood solubility, so concentrations in the closed circuit remain low, but rebreathing causes accumulation in the blood. Levels achieved are generally low,[3] but acetone accumulation may be associated with postoperative nausea.[4] Closed-circuit anaesthesia is not recommended in patients with increased excretion of acetone or alcohol, such as uncontrolled diabetes mellitus, recent alcohol ingestion or during prolonged starvation.[1]

SUBMARINES

Submersible ships have been used for almost 100 years, almost exclusively for military purposes until the last few decades when they have become more widespread for undersea exploration and industrial use. Atmospheric pressure in the submarine remains approximately the same as at surface level during a dive, the duration of which is limited by the maintenance of adequate oxygen and carbon dioxide levels for the crew in the ship.

Diesel powered. Submarines were used extensively during both world wars, and were powered by diesel engines like surface-based warships. Clearly, the oxygen requirement of the engines precluded them from use during dives and battery-powered engines were used, thus limiting the duration of dives to just a few hours. A more significant limitation to dive duration was atmospheric regulation. No attempt was made to control the internal atmosphere, and, after ventilation at the surface, the submarine dived with only the air contained within. After approximately 12 hours the atmosphere contained 15% oxygen, 5% carbon dioxide and a multitude of odours and contaminants. The need to return to the surface was apparent when the submariners became short of breath and were unable to light their cigarettes due to low levels of oxygen.[5]

Nuclear powered. Short dive duration severely limited the use of diesel-powered submarines. The development of nuclear power allowed submarines to generate an ample supply of heat and electricity completely independent of oxygen supply, and so allowed prolonged activity underwater. Atmospheric regeneration was therefore needed. Current nuclear-powered submarines have a crew of up to 180, and routinely remain submerged for weeks.

Atmosphere regeneration.[5,6] The plentiful supply of sea water and electricity make hydrolysis of water the obvious method for oxygen generation. Sea water must first have all electrolytes removed by a combination of evaporation and de-ionisation. Theoretically, one litre of water can yield 620 litres of oxygen, so, even with less than 100% efficient electrolysis, large volumes of oxygen are easily produced. Submarine atmosphere oxygen concentration is maintained at $21 \pm 2\%$.

Atmospheric CO_2 in submarines is absorbed by passage through monoethanolamine, which chemically combines with CO_2 to produce carbonates. When fully saturated, the absorber can either be replaced or be regenerated by heating with steam, when the CO_2 is released and can be vented into the sea. This method maintains the CO_2 concentration in submarines at 0.5–1.5%, and though further reduction is possible, the energy cost of doing so is prohibitive.

Atmospheric contamination during prolonged submarine patrols is well recognised, many hundreds of substances entering the atmosphere, originating from both machinery and crew. These substances include volatile hydrocarbons such as benzene, oil droplets, carbon monoxide, cadmium, and microbial organisms, with varying concentrations in different parts of the submarine. Continuous monitoring of many compounds is now routine, and maximum allowable levels during prolonged patrols are defined.[7] Submarine air-conditioning units include catalytic burners that oxidise carbon monoxide, hydrogen and other hydrocarbons to CO_2 and water, and charcoal absorbers to absorb any remaining contaminants. The health risks from submarine occupation are therefore believed to be extremely small.[5,7,8]

PHYSIOLOGICAL EFFECTS OF PROLONGED HYPERCAPNIA

Definition of a 'safe' level of atmospheric CO_2 over long periods has concerned submarine designers for some years. The respiratory response to inhalation of low concentrations of CO_2 ($< 3\%$) is similar to that at higher levels (page 69), but compensatory acid–base changes seem to be quite different.

Respiratory changes.[9,10] Atmospheric CO_2 levels of 1% cause an elevation of inspired P_{CO_2} of 1 kPa (7.5 mmHg), which results in an average increase in minute ventilation of 2–3 l.min^{-1}. However, the degree of hyperventilation is highly variable between subjects, and presumably relates to their central chemoreceptor sensitivity to CO_2 (page 69). Measurements of arterial blood gases in submariners show that the elevated minute volume limits the increase in arterial P_{CO_2} to an average of only 0.14 kPa (1 mmHg). After a few days, the increase in ventilation declines, and minute volume returns towards normal, allowing arterial

P_{CO_2} to increase further to reflect the inspired P_{CO_2}. The time course of the decline in ventilation is too short to result from blood acid–base compensation (see below), and is believed to reflect a small attenuation of the central chemoreceptor response. On return to the surface, ventilation may be temporarily reduced following withdrawal of the CO_2 stimulus.

Calcium metabolism.[9,11] Elevation of arterial P_{CO_2} causes a respiratory acidosis, which is normally, over the course of one or two days, compensated for by the retention of bicarbonate by the kidney (page 359). The changes in pH seen when breathing less than 3% CO_2 appear to be too small to stimulate measurable renal compensation, and pH remains slightly lowered for some time. During this period, CO_2 is deposited in bone as calcium carbonate, and urinary and faecal calcium excretion is drastically reduced to facilitate this. Serum calcium levels also decrease, suggesting a shift of extracellular calcium to the intracellular space.[11] After about three weeks, when bone stores of CO_2 are saturated, renal excretion of calcium and hydrogen ions begins to increase and pH tends to return to normal. Abnormalities of calcium metabolism have been demonstrated with inspired CO_2 concentrations as low as 0.5%.

Some other effects of low levels of atmospheric CO_2 during space travel are described below (page 307).

SPACE[6,12–14]

Space represents the most hostile environment into which humans have sojourned. At 80 km (50 miles) above Earth there is insufficient air to allow aerodynamic control of a vehicle, and at 200 km (125 miles) there is an almost total vacuum. True space begins above 700 km (435 miles), where particles become so scarce that the likelihood of a collision between two atoms becomes negligible. Even under these conditions, there are estimated to be 10^8 particles (mainly hydrogen) per cubic metre compared with 10^{25} on the Earth's surface. Maintenance of a respirable atmosphere in these circumstances is challenging, and both American and Soviet space pioneers lost their lives during the development of suitable technology. Current experience is based on expeditions in close proximity to Earth, involving Earth orbit or travel to the moon. This means that the raw materials for atmosphere regeneration can be repeatedly supplied from Earth.

ATMOSPHERE COMPOSITION

A summary of manned space missions and the atmospheres used is shown in Table 19.1. Spacecraft have an almost totally sealed, closed-circuit system of atmospheric control, and early Soviet space vehicles aimed to be completely sealed environments. Their designers had such confidence in the structure that emergency stores of oxygen were considered unnecessary until Soyuz 11 depressurised on re-entry in 1971, tragically killing all three cosmonauts. American Apollo missions leaked approximately 1 kg of gas per day in space, even with a lower atmospheric pressure (Table 19.1).

The use of a total pressure of 34.5 kPa (259 mmHg) in early US space vehicles required a high atmospheric oxygen concentration to provide an adequate inspired Po_2 (Table 19.1). Because of the fatal fire on the launch pad in 1967, the composition of the atmosphere during launch was changed from 100% oxygen to 64% oxygen in 36% nitrogen at the same pressure, which still gave an inspired Po_2 in excess of the normal sea level value. Previous Soviet designs were all based on maintaining normal atmospheric pressure, and space vehicles in current use continue to do so with inspired oxygen concentrations of near 21%. Extravehicular activity in space presents a particular problem. In order to maintain a functionally acceptable flexibility of the space suit in the vacuum of space, the internal pressure is only 28 kPa (212 mmHg). This entails the use of 100% oxygen after careful decompression and denitrogenation of the astronaut.

OXYGEN SUPPLY

Storage of oxygen and other gases in space presents significant problems. The weight of the containers used is critical during launch, and storage of significant quantities of oxygen requires high pressures and therefore strong, heavy tanks. Liquid oxygen presents a greatly improved storage density, but the behaviour of stored liquids in weightless conditions is complex.

Chemical generation of oxygen has been used mainly by Soviet space missions. Potassium superoxide releases oxygen on exposure to moisture, a reaction that generates potassium hydroxide as an intermediate and so also absorbs carbon dioxide:

$$4KO_2 + 3H_2O + 2CO_2 \rightarrow 2K_2CO_3 + 3H_2O + 3O_2$$

One kilogram of KO_2 can release over 200 litres of oxygen, but the reaction is irreversible and the used canisters must be discarded. Sodium chlorate candles release oxygen when simply ignited, and were used for emergency oxygen generation in Soviet space missions and are still used for atmospheric regeneration in disabled submarines.[15]

Electrolysis of water is an efficient way to produce oxygen in space where solar panels provide the electricity supply. In contrast to submarines, water

Table 19.1 Summary of manned space missions and their respiratory environments

MISSIONS	PERIOD OF USE	NUMBER OF CREW	HABITABLE VOLUME (m³)	CABIN PRESSURE		OXYGEN CONC. (%)	ATMOSPHERE REGENERATION METHODS	
				kPa	mmHg		O₂ SUPPLY	CO₂ REMOVAL
Vostok	1961–65	1	2.5	100	760	100	KO_2	KO_2
Mercury	1961–63	1	1.6	34	258	100	Pressurised O_2	LiOH
Gemini	1965–66	2	2.3	34	258	100	Liquid O_2	LiOH
Soyuz	1967–	2/3	–	100	760	22	KO_2	KO_2/LiOH
Apollo	1968–72	3	5.9	34	258	100*	Liquid O_2	LiOH
Salyut	1971–86	5	100	100	760	21	KO_2	KO_2/LiOH
Skylab	1973–74	3	361	34	258	72	Liquid O_2	Molecular sieve
Shuttle	1981–	7	74	100	760	21	Liquid O_2	LiOH
Mir	1986–01	6	150	100	760	23	Electrolysis/Chemical	Molecular sieve
ISS	2001–	Variable	401/1217†	100	760	21	Electrolysis/Chemical	Molecular sieve

*Oxygen concentration reduced to 60% during launch to reduce fire risk.
†Current/projected habitable volumes. All missions, except early Soyuz launches, carry emergency oxygen supplies as pressurised or liquid oxygen. (Data from references 6, 12 and 13.)

is scarce in space vehicles, again because of weight considerations at launch. In the International Space Station oxygen is generated by electrolysis using waste water from the occupants, though this alone does not produce sufficient oxygen for a reasonably active astronaut.

CARBON DIOXIDE REMOVAL

Chemical absorption by lithium hydroxide has been the mainstay of the US space program, whilst the Soviet program used KO_2 as described above. Reversible chemical reactions such as those used in submarines have been adapted for space use, and can be regenerated by exposure to the vacuum of space.

Molecular sieves allow CO_2 to be adsorbed into a chemical matrix without undergoing any chemical reaction. When saturated with CO_2, exposure to the space vacuum causes release of the adsorbed gas. Use of two- or four-bed molecular sieves allows continuous CO_2 removal by half the processors whilst the others are regenerated.

Maintenance of low levels of CO_2 on prolonged future space missions is likely to have unacceptable costs in terms of energy and consumables.[16] This fact led to three space agencies worldwide undertaking a joint research programme to study the effects of 1.2% and 0.7% atmospheric CO_2 on a wide range of physiological systems. The study involved normal volunteers spending 22 days in a closed mock 'space station' on the ground.[16] Some of the results have already been described above (page 305).[10,11] Effects at 0.7% atmospheric CO_2 were generally concluded to be minimal.[17] At 1.2% however, changes in respiration and calcium metabolism were significant and, more important, mental performance was impaired with a loss of alertness and visuomotor performance.[18]

ATMOSPHERIC CONTAMINATION

Chemical contamination within space vehicles is mainly from within the habitable area of the vehicle, with external contamination from propellants etc. being very rare.[12] The greatest contribution to atmospheric contamination is the astronauts themselves, but the compounds released such as carbon monoxide, ammonia, methane and indole are easily dealt with by standard methods. More complex chemicals may be released into the atmosphere by a process called off-gassing. Almost any non-metallic substance, but particularly plastics, release small quantities of volatile chemicals for many months and years after manufacture. This is more likely to occur at low atmospheric pressure as on the earlier space missions. Within a closed environment, these chemicals may accumulate to toxic levels and air-conditioning units similar to those described for submarines (page 305) are required.

LONG-TERM SPACE TRAVEL

Manned space travel to planets more distant than the moon requires expeditions of years' duration with no access to supplies from Earth. For example, the journey time to Mars is around 6 months, so the minimum realistic mission duration would be 2 years. The estimated mass of provisions required to sustain 6 crew members for this duration would be over 45 tons, which far exceeds the capacity of current space vehicles.[19] Regenerative life support systems have, therefore, been studied extensively in recent years and aim to reverse the effects of animal metabolism on a closed atmosphere. Biological solutions are believed by many to be the only feasible option, and biospheres are discussed below. Physico-chemical methods are, however, now realistic options, and are likely to act as valuable backup systems.

CO_2 reduction reactions convert carbon dioxide back into oxygen, and two main methods are described.[20] The Sabatier reaction requires hydrogen to produce methane and water:

$$CO_2 + 4H_2 \rightarrow CH_4 + 2H_2O$$

Methane can then be converted to solid carbon and hydrogen gas, which re-enters the Sabatier reactor. The Bosch reaction produces solid carbon in one stage:

$$CO_2 + 2H_2 \rightarrow 2H_2O + \text{solid C}$$

Electrolysis of water generates oxygen and hydrogen gas, and the latter enters the Bosch or Sabatier reactions and the water produced is recycled. Both reactions ultimately generate solid carbon, which must be removed from the reactors periodically: current hardware can convert CO_2 into oxygen for 60 person-days before the carbon deposits must be emptied.[20]

In-situ resource utilisation on Mars.[21] The atmosphere of Mars is composed of 95.3% CO_2, 2.7% N_2, 1.6%

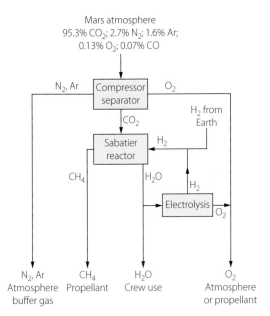

Mars atmosphere
95.3% CO_2; 2.7% N_2; 1.6% Ar;
0.13% O_2; 0.07% CO

Fig. 19.1 In-situ resource utilisation on Mars. Using a series of simple physicochemical processes, the atmosphere of Mars, supplemented by hydrogen transported from Earth, may be used to provide buffer gas and oxygen for the space vehicle atmosphere, methane as propellant for the vehicle and water for use by the crew or for generation of oxygen. (After reference 21.)

Ar, 0.13% O_2 and 0.07% CO. For any mission to Mars, these gases could be used for atmospheric regeneration as shown in Figure 19.1. Separation of the gases in the atmosphere will produce a small amount of oxygen, and larger volumes of nitrogen and argon, which may be used as buffer gas in the atmosphere. On prolonged missions, loss of buffer gas from the vehicle by leakage and from activation of airlocks is a substantial problem. The abundant CO_2 on Mars can enter a Sabatier reactor and the methane produced may then be used as a propellant for the mission, the water used either by the crew or to provide oxygen for the life support systems and the hydrogen can re-enter the Sabatier reactor.

MICROGRAVITY[22,23]

All bodies with mass exert gravitational forces on each other, so *zero* gravity is theoretically impossible. Once in space, away from the large mass of Earth or other planets, gravitational forces become negligible and are referred to as microgravity. Space vehicles in orbit around Earth are still subject to its considerable gravitational forces, but

these are matched almost exactly by the centrifugal force from the high tangential velocity of the space vehicle.[13] Occupants of orbiting space vehicles are normally subject to a gravitational force of approximately 10^{-6} times that on Earth's surface.

Chapter 8 contains numerous references to the effect of gravity on the topography of the lung and the distribution of perfusion and ventilation. Microgravity may therefore be predicted to have significant effects on respiratory function.

The first studies of short-term microgravity used a Lear jet flying in a series of Keplerian arcs, which gave 20–25 seconds of weightlessness. Unfortunately, between each period of microgravity the subject is exposed to a similar duration of increased gravitational forces (2G) as the jet pulls out of the free-fall portion of the flight,[24] and this may influence the results of physiological studies. Sustained microgravity has been studied in space. In 1991 an extended series of investigations on seven subjects was undertaken in Spacelab SLS-1, which was carried into orbit by the space shuttle for a nine day mission, and studies of prolonged microgravity on the International Space Station are now being published.[25]

Lung volumes. Chest radiography in the sitting position during short-term microgravity showed no striking changes other than a tendency for the diaphragm to be slightly higher in some of the subjects at functional residual capacity (FRC).[26] This accords with a 413 ml reduction in FRC also measured in Keplerian arc studies on seated subjects.[24] Abdominal contribution to tidal excursion was increased at microgravity in the seated position, probably because of loss of postural tone in the abdominal muscles,[24] an observation now confirmed in space studies.[27]

During sustained microgravity subdivisions of lung volume were again found to be intermediate between the sitting and supine volumes at 1G, except for residual volume which was reduced below that seen in any position at 1G (Figure 19.2).[28] The FRC was reduced by 750 ml compared with preflight standing values. These changes in lung volume are ascribed to altered respiratory mechanics and increased thoracic blood volume.

Topographical inequality of ventilation and perfusion.[22] Early results in the Lear jet, using single-breath nitrogen washout (page 123), indicated a substantial reduction in topographical inequality of ventilation and perfusion during weightlessness, as expected.[29] However, the more detailed studies

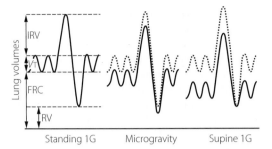

Fig. 19.2 Static lung volumes during sustained microgravity after nine days in Earth orbit. Dotted line shows the normal standing values on Earth for comparison. Volumes at microgravity are generally intermediate between standing and supine values at 1G, except residual volume, which is further reduced. FRC, functional residual capacity; IRV, inspiratory reserve volume; RV, residual volume; V_T, tidal volume.

in Spacelab showed that a surprising degree of residual inequality of blood flow[30] and ventilation[31] persisted despite the major improvement at zero gravity. Ventilatory inequality with microgravity is believed to result from continued airway closure at low lung volume,[31] airway closure possibly occurring in a patchy fashion.[32] The most likely explanation for the continued perfusion inequality is the central to peripheral 'radial' gradient within each horizontal slice of lung (page 124), which is mostly overshadowed at 1G by the large vertical perfusion gradient.

Breathing during sleep in space.[33] Snoring and airway obstruction during sleep are common, and many factors are involved in their initiation (page 271). Reduced activity of pharyngeal dilator muscles and increased compliance of pharyngeal structures both encourage the normal gravitational force on Earth to initiate obstruction. This important contribution of gravity to sleep-disordered breathing has been confirmed by studies of astronauts sleeping in the orbiting space shuttle.[34] Compared with sleeping at 1G before the mission, in microgravity there were dramatic reductions in their apnoea-hypopnoea index (page 271) and snoring was virtually eliminated.

BIOSPHERES[13]

A biosphere is defined as 'a closed space of two or more connected ecosystems in equilibrium with their environment'.[35] Only energy enters and leaves a biosphere. Earth is the largest and most successful known

biosphere, though the equilibrium between its ecosystems is almost certainly changing (Chapter 1). Attempts to create smaller biospheres have mostly been driven by the prospect of long-term space travel.[36] Physico-chemical methods of sustaining life, as described above, have many limitations whereas a biological system has numerous advantages. Plants perform the complex CO_2-reduction chemistry using chlorophyll, and at the same time, rather than generating carbon, they produce varying amounts of food.[37] Plants also act as efficient water-purification systems via transpiration.

SMALL SCALE BIOLOGICAL ATMOSPHERIC REGENERATION

The first report of prolonged biological atmosphere regeneration was described in 1961 when a single mouse was maintained in a closed chamber for 66 days.[38] Air from the chamber was circulated through a second chamber containing four litres of *Chlorella* alga solution illuminated with artificial light. Over the course of the experiment, oxygen concentration in the chamber increased from 21% to 53%, and carbon dioxide concentrations remained below 0.2%. Subsequent experiments by both American and Soviet researchers demonstrated the feasibility of human life support by *Chlorella*, culminating in a 30-day closure of a single researcher in a 4.5 m³ room, maintained by just 30 litres of alga solution. Algae alone are unsuitable for long-term life support.[13] Their excellent atmospheric regeneration properties result from a very fast rate of growth but *Chlorella* is generally regarded as inedible, and so presents a significant disposal problem in a totally closed system. In addition, if the algal solution becomes acidic for any reason, such as bacterial contamination, algae produce carbon monoxide in unacceptable quantities.

Unknown to the scientific community at large, from 1963 the Soviet Union ran a 'Bios' research centre at the Institute of Biophysics in Krasnoyarsk, Siberia.[13,39] A whole series of progressively more complex biospheres were constructed. In 1983, two researchers successfully spent five months in a biosphere (Bios 3), which provided all their atmospheric regeneration needs and over three-quarters of their food.[39] In these studies, plants were grown hydroponically – that is, without soil with their roots bathed in carefully controlled nutrient solution. Light was provided with continuous xenon lighting to maximise growth, to such an extent that, under these conditions, wheat can be harvested six times per year. An estimated $13\,m^2$ of planted area will then produce enough oxygen for one human, though over $30\,m^2$ is probably required to produce almost enough food as well. Beds of *Chlorella* algae were also used to maximise oxygen production and, along with larger planted areas, resulted in excess oxygen. This was reduced by incineration of the non-edible portion of the plants, and so enabled the researchers to exercise some control over the balance between oxygen and carbon dioxide concentration within the biosphere.

American research of controlled ecological life support systems (CELSS) began in 1977 and has focused on basic plant physiology.[13] Plant species, light, humidity, nutrients and atmospheric gas concentrations all have profound effects on the design of a CELSS. Atmospheric regeneration is usually the easiest problem to overcome, whilst the plant species used has important implications for the dietary intake and psychological well-being of the CELSS inhabitants.[37,39] In contrast to this American project, the European Space Agency is developing a life-support system for long-term space travel centred around micro-organisms, which are more versatile biochemically.[40] For example, bacteria may be used to compost crew waste and inedible plant components into nitrogenous compounds to enhance the plant growth.

atmospheric air is pumped through the soil where bacterial action provides an adaptable and efficient purification system.[13] A CO_2 'scrubber' system was included in biosphere 2 to control atmospheric CO_2 levels, particularly during winter when shorter days reduce photosynthetic activity. Also, the amount of O_2-consuming biomass relative to atmosphere volume was known to be high, and therefore small increases in CO_2 levels were anticipated.

Biosphere 2 aimed, wherever possible, to use ecological engineering. By the inclusion of large numbers of species (3800 in total), it was hoped that there would be sufficient flexibility between systems to respond to changes in the environment. In particular, microbial diversity is believed to be extremely important in maintaining biosphere 1 (Earth), and multiple habitats were established to facilitate this type of diversity in biosphere 2.

Outcome from the two-year closure. Concentrations of oxygen and carbon dioxide in biosphere 2 were very unstable (Figure 19.3), and after 16 months, oxygen concentration had fallen to only 14%. Extensive symptoms were reported by the human inhabitants, including significantly reduced work capacity, and external oxygen had to be added to the atmosphere. Carbon dioxide levels did increase slightly during winter months (Figure 19.3) when the CO_2 was removed by the scrubber system.

BIOSPHERE 2[13]

Small-scale biosphere experiments never attained a totally closed system, particularly with respect to food supplies and waste disposal, and always struggled with the accumulation of toxic atmospheric compounds. With these problems in mind, an ambitious series of biosphere experiments were established in Arizona, USA, culminating in the biosphere 2 project in 1991.

A totally sealed complex, covering 3.15 acres (1.3 hectares) was purpose built with a stainless steel underground lining and principally glass cover. Two flexible walls, or 'lungs', were included to minimise pressure changes within the complex with expansion and contraction of the atmosphere. A two-year closure was planned, with the complex containing a wide range of flora and fauna, including eight humans. Soil was chosen as the growing medium for all plants in preference to hydroponic techniques used previously. This was to facilitate air purification by soil bed reactors, in which

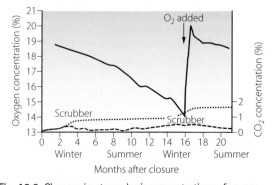

Fig. 19.3 Changes in atmospheric concentrations of oxygen (solid line) and carbon dioxide (dashed line) during the two-year closure of biosphere 2. Less daylight during winter months reduces photosynthesis causing increased levels of CO_2. Carbon dioxide was therefore removed using a CO_2 'scrubber' system, during the periods shown. Even when CO_2 absorption by the scrubbers is taken into account (dotted line), it can clearly be seen that the reduction in O_2 concentration exceeds the increase in CO_2 concentration; after 16 months, O_2 had to be added to the biosphere. See text for details. (Data from references 13 and 38.)

It was never expected that all species introduced into biosphere 2 would survive, and extinction of some species was seen as a natural response to stabilisation of the ecosystem. However, after 21 months, extinct species were numerous, including 19 of 25 vertebrates and most insects, including all pollinators.[41] In contrast, ants and cockroaches thrived.

The success of biosphere 2 as a closed ecosystem was therefore limited, and, in contrast to the smaller biospheres previously used, basic atmospheric regeneration was a significant problem. Any increase in CO_2 concentration should be matched by an equivalent decrease in O_2 concentration, as biological reactions between CO_2 and O_2 are generally equimolar. Even when the CO_2 removed by the recycling system is taken into account, it can clearly be seen from Figure 19.3 that oxygen losses were much greater. The explanation for this is believed to be two-fold.[42] First, oxygen depletion occurred due to respiration in the biosphere proceeding faster than photosynthesis, most likely as a result of excessive microbial activity in the soil. Secondly, much of the CO_2 produced by this respiration was lost from the atmosphere by chemical reaction with the concrete from which the biosphere complex was built.

We remain some way away from being able to establish a long-term habitable atmosphere away from Earth.

References

1. Baum JA, Aitkenhead AR. Low-flow anaesthesia. *Anaesthesia*. 1995;50(supp):37–44.

2. Parker CJR, Snowdon SL. Predicted and measured oxygen concentrations in the circle system using low fresh gas flows with oxygen supplied by an oxygen concentrator. *Br J Anaesth*. 1988;61:397–402.

3. Versichelen L, Rolly G, Vermeulen H. Accumulation of foreign gases during closed-system anaesthesia. *Br J Anaesth*. 1996;76:668–672.

4. Strauß JM, Hausdörfer J. Accumulation of acetone in blood during long-term anaesthesia with closed systems. *Br J Anaesth*. 1993;70:363–364.

5. Knight DR, Tappan DV, Bowman JS, O'Neill HJ, Gordon SM. Submarine atmospheres. *Toxicol Lett*. 1989;49:243–251.

6. Wieland PO. *Designing for human presence in space: an introduction to environmental control and life support systems*. NASA Reference Publication 1324. National Aeronautics and Space Administration 1994.

7. Dean MR. Benzene exposure in Royal Naval submarines. *J R Soc Med*. 1996;89:286P–288P.

8. Lambert RJW. Environmental problems in nuclear submarines. *Proc R Soc Med*. 1972;65:795–796.

9. Pingree BJW. Acid-base and respiratory changes after prolonged exposure to 1% carbon dioxide. *Clin Sci Mol Med*. 1977;52:67–74.

10. Elliott AR, Prisk GK, Schöllmann C, Hoffmann U. Hypercapnic ventilatory response in humans before, during, and after 23 days of low level CO_2 exposure. *Aviat Space Environ Med*. 1998;69:391–396.

11. Drummer C, Friedel V, Börger A, et al. Effects of elevated carbon dioxide environment on calcium metabolism in humans. *Aviat Space Environ Med*. 1998;69:291–298.

12. Nicogossian AE, Huntoon CL, Pool SL. *Space physiology and medicine*, 3rd ed Philadelphia: Lea & Febiger; 1994.

13. Churchill SE. *Fundamentals of space life sciences*. Malabar, Florida: Krieger Publishing; 1997.

14. West JB. Historical aspects of the early Soviet/Russian manned space program. *J Appl Physiol*. 2001;91:1501–1511.

15. Risberg J, Österberg C, Svensson T, et al. Atmospheric changes and physiological responses during a 6-day "disabled submarine" exercise. *Aviat Space Environ Med*. 2004;75:138–149.

16. Wenzel J, Luks N, Plath G, Wilke D, Gerzer R. The influence of CO_2 in a space-like environment: study design. *Aviat Space Environ Med*. 1998;69:285–290.

17. Frey MAB, Sulzman FM, Oser H, Ruyters G. The effects of moderately elevated ambient carbon dioxide levels on human physiology and performance: A joint NASA-ESA-DARA study – overview. *Aviat Space Environ Med*. 1998;69:282–284.

18. Manzey D, Lorenz B. Effects of chronically elevated CO_2 on mental performance during 26 days of confinement. *Aviat Space Environ Med*. 1998;69:506–514.

19. Grigoriev AI, Kozlovskaya IB, Potapov AN. Goals of biomedical support of a mission to Mars and possible approaches to achieving them. *Aviat Space Environ Med*. 2002;73:379–384.

20. Noyes GP. Carbon dioxide reduction processes for spacecraft ECLSS: A comprehensive review. *Proceedings of the 18th intersociety conference on environmental systems*, paper 881042. San Francisco: July 1988.

21. Sridhar KR, Finn JE, Kliss MH. In-situ resource utilisation technologies for Mars life support systems. *Adv Space Res*. 2000;25:249–255.

*22. Prisk GK. Microgravity and the lung. *J Appl Physiol*. 2000;89:385–396.

*23. Prisk GK. The lung in space. *Clin Chest Med*. 2005;26:415–438.

24. Paiva M, Estenne M, Engel LA. Lung volumes, chest wall configuration, and pattern of breathing in microgravity. *J Appl Physiol*. 1989;67:1542–1550.

25. Prisk GK, Fine JM, Cooper TK, West JB. Vital capacity, respiratory muscle strength, and pulmonary gas exchange during long-duration exposure to microgravity. *J Appl Physiol*. 2006;101:439–447.

26. Michels DB, Friedman PJ, West JB. Radiographic comparison of human lung shape during normal gravity and weightlessness. *J Appl Physiol*. 1979;47:851–857.

27. Wantier M, Estenne M, Verbanck S, Prisk GK, Paiva M. Chest wall mechanics in sustained microgravity. *J Appl Physiol*. 1998;84:2060–2065.

28. Elliott AR, Prisk GK, Guy HJB, West JB. Lung volumes during sustained microgravity on Spacelab SLS-1. *J Appl Physiol*. 1994;77:2005–2014.

29. Michels DB, West JB. Distribution of pulmonary ventilation and perfusion during short periods of weightlessness. *J Appl Physiol*. 1978;45:987–998.

30. Prisk GK, Guy HJB, Elliott AR, West JB. Inhomogeneity of pulmonary perfusion during sustained microgravity on SLS-1. *J Appl Physiol*. 1994;76:1730–1738.

31. Guy HJB, Prisk GK, Elliott AR, Deutschman RA, West JB. Inhomogeneity of pulmonary ventilation during sustained microgravity as determined by single breath washouts. *J Appl Physiol*. 1994;76:1719–1729.

32. Dutrieue B, Verbanck S, Darquenne C, Prisk GK. Airway closure in microgravity. *Respir Physiol Neurobiol*. 2005;148:97–111.

33. Dinges DF. Sleep in space flight. Breath easy – sleep less. *Am J Respir Crit Care Med*. 2001;164:337–340.

34. Elliott AR, Shea SA, Dijk D-J, et al. Microgravity reduces sleep-disordered breathing in humans. *Am J Respir Crit Care Med*. 2001;164:478–485.

35. Walford RL, Bechtel R, MacCallum T, Paglia DE, Weber LJ. 'Biospheric medicine' as viewed from the two-year first closure of biosphere 2. *Aviat Space Environ Med*. 1996;67:609–617.

36. Schwartzkopf SH. Human life support for advanced space exploration. *Adv Space Biol Med*. 1997;6:231–253.

37. Mitchell CA. Bioregenerative life-support systems. *Am J Clin Nutr*. 1994;60:820S–824S.

38. Bowman RO, Thomae FW. Long-term nontoxic support of animal life with algae. *Science*. 1961;134:55–56.

39. Ivanov B, Zubareva O. To mars and back again on board Bios. *Soviet Life*. April 1985:22–25.

40. Hendrickx L, De Wever H, Hermans V, et al. Microbial ecology of the closed artificial ecosystem MELiSSA (Micro-Ecological Life Support System Alternative): Reinventing and compartmentalising the Earth's food and oxygen regeneration system for long-haul space exploration missions. *Res Microbiol*. 2006;157:77–86.

41. Cohen JE, Tilman D. Biosphere 2 and biodiversity: the lessons so far. *Science*. 1996;274:1150–1151.

42. Severinghaus JP, Broecker WS, Dempster WF, MacCallum T, Wahlen M. Oxygen loss in biosphere 2. *EOS*. 1994;75:33–40.

Chapter 20

Drowning

KEY POINTS

■ Immersion in thermoneutral water activates protective airway reflexes and aspiration does not occur until lung oxygen stores have been used up and hypoxia causes the airway to open.

■ In cold water, the cold shock reflex causes gasping and hyperventilation under water, with inhalation of large quantities of water and rapid, severe hypoxia.

It is estimated that there were more than 400 000 victims of drowning worldwide in the year 2000.[1] In several countries drowning is a major cause of accidental death, particularly amongst children. Drowning is more common in low- or middle-income countries than high-income countries,[1] and is around three times more common in men than women. Alcohol is a major aetiological factor.[2] For each victim of death by drowning, there are estimated to be between several cases of 'near-drowning' that are severe enough to require hospital admission, and probably hundreds of other less severe incidents.[2] Death from pulmonary complications ('secondary drowning') may occur a considerable time after the accident, in patients who were initially normal.

The essential feature of drowning is asphyxia, but many of the physiological responses depend on whether aspiration of water occurs and upon the substances that are dissolved or suspended in the water. The temperature of the water is crucially important, and hypothermia following drowning in very cold water is a major factor influencing survival, though the mechanism underlying this observation remains controversial.

PHYSIOLOGY OF IMMERSION[2,3]

The hydrostatic pressure exerted on the body during immersion can be substantial. As a result there is a huge increase in venous return, causing increased pulmonary blood volume, cardiac output and, soon afterwards, a significant diuresis. Cephalad displacement of the diaphragm from raised abdominal pressure coupled with direct chest compression increases the work of breathing by about 65%. Three reflexes affect the respiratory system and come into play in drowning:

Airway irritant reflexes play a major part in drowning. Aspiration of water into the mouth initially stimulates swallowing followed by coughing, glottic closure and laryngospasm. If water penetrates deeper into the respiratory tract, below the vocal folds, bronchospasm results.

Cold shock describes a combination of several cardiovascular and respiratory reflexes that occur in response to sudden total-body immersion in cold water.[4] Sudden immersion in water below 25°C is a potent stimulant to respiration and causes an initial large gasp followed by substantial hyperventilation. The stimulus is increased with colder temperatures, reaching a maximum at 10°C.[2] Functional residual capacity is acutely increased, and individuals may find themselves breathing almost at total lung capacity, giving a sensation of dyspnoea. Breath-hold time is severely reduced, often to less than 10 seconds, which impairs the ability of victims to escape from a confined space underwater or to orientate themselves before seeking safety.

Diving reflex. In response to cold water stimulation of the face and eyes, the diving reflex produces bradycardia, peripheral vasoconstriction and apnoea in most mammals. It is particularly well developed in diving mammals, to reduce oxygen consumption and facilitate long duration dives. The reflex is present in humans,[5] though of small magnitude compared with other species, and is believed to be more significant in infants than adults.[2]

PHYSIOLOGICAL MECHANISMS OF DROWNING

Glottic closure from inhaled water, pulmonary aspiration, cold shock and the diving response all influence the course of events following submersion in water; the relative importance of each depends, amongst many other factors, on the age of the victim and the temperature of the water. Conflicting influences on the heart from activation of both the parasympathetic (diving reflex) and sympathetic (cold shock) systems are believed to contribute to death from cardiac dysrhythmia in some victims.[2,4]

DROWNING WITHOUT ASPIRATION OF WATER

This occurs in less than 10% of drowning victims.[6] In thermoneutral water, when cold-stimulated reflexes will be minimal, the larynx is firmly closed during submersion and some victims will lose consciousness before water is aspirated. The rate of decrease of alveolar, and therefore arterial, Po_2 depends on the lung volume and the oxygen consumption. Oxygen stored in the alveolar gas after a maximal inspiration is unlikely to exceed 1 litre, and an oxygen consumption of $3 l.min^{-1}$ would not be unusual in a subject either swimming or struggling. Loss of consciousness from decreased alveolar Po_2 usually occurs very suddenly and without warning.

In cold water, hypoxia secondary to glottic closure may still occur. In addition, the cold shock and diving reflexes both leave the victim vulnerable to cardiovascular complications such as arrhythmias and sudden circulatory failure leading to death before aspiration can occur. This is likely to be more common in elderly individuals.

DROWNING WITH ASPIRATION OF WATER

Almost 90% of drowning victims have aspirated significant volumes of water. Following sudden immersion in cold water the cold shock response is believed to be more common than the diving reflex, and hyperventilation rapidly leads to aspiration. In thermoneutral water, glottic closure may either be overcome by the conscious victim or will eventually subside due to hypoxia, and in both circumstances aspiration is likely to continue. Once aspiration occurs, reflex bronchospasm quickly follows, further worsening respiratory function.

Fresh water. Aspiration of fresh water further down the bronchial tree causes rapid and profound changes to the alveolar surfactant, leading to loss of the normal elastic properties of the alveoli and a disturbed ventilation/perfusion ratio. In fresh water drowning, alveolar water is quickly absorbed, resulting in alveolar collapse and a pulmonary shunt, this being in addition to the changes resulting from dilution of surfactant. A significant shunt is therefore quickly established, with resulting hypoxia. Some studies indicate that neurogenic pulmonary oedema due to cerebral hypoxia might coexist with alveolar flooding from aspirated water.[7] The pulmonary changes caused by immersion appear to be quickly reversible,[7] with good prospects of return to normal pulmonary function in those who survive near-drowning.

A substantial volume of water may be absorbed from the lungs, and profound hyponatraemia, leading to fits, has been described in infants drowned in fresh water.[8] However, most human victims absorb only small quantities of water and redistribution rapidly corrects the blood volume. Hypovolaemia is the more common problem following near-drowning.[8]

Sea water. Sea water is hypertonic, having more than three times the osmolarity of blood. Consequently, sea water in the lungs is not initially absorbed and, on the contrary, draws fluid from the circulation into the alveoli. Thus, in laboratory animals that have aspirated sea water, it is possible to recover from the lungs 50% more than the original volume that was inhaled.[9] This clearly maintains the proportion of flooded alveoli and results in a persistent shunt with reduction in arterial PO_2.

POST-MORTEM TESTS OF DROWNING

There appears to be no conclusive test for aspiration of either fresh or sea water. Tests based on differences in specific gravity and chloride content of plasma from the right and left chambers of the heart are unreliable. The demonstration of diatoms in bone marrow tissue is also controversial. For example, to improve the accuracy of the diatom test the species, morphology and number of diatoms found at post-mortem need to be compared with those in a sample of the water in which the victim allegedly drowned.[10]

THE ROLE OF HYPOTHERMIA[2,3]

Some degree of hypothermia is usual in near-drowned victims and body temperature is usually in the range 33–36°C. Hypothermia induced reduction in cerebral metabolism is protective during hypoxia and is believed to contribute to the numerous reports of survival after prolonged immersion in cold water, particularly in children. There have been reports of survival of near-drowned children and adults trapped for periods as long as 80 minutes beneath ice.[8] However, for the reasons outlined above, arterial hypoxia is believed to develop very quickly, and there is controversy surrounding how body temperature can decrease quickly enough to provide any degree of cerebral protection. Surface cooling is not believed to allow a rapid enough fall in temperature as normal physiological responses to cold such as peripheral vasoconstriction and shivering limit the decline in temperature. Even so, the greater body surface area of children relative to their body size will theoretically result in more rapid cooling by heat conduction from the body surface.[3]

Absorption of cold water either from the lungs or stomach will contribute to hypothermia during prolonged immersion, but quantitatively the volumes required are unlikely to be absorbed, particularly in sea water. Heat loss from the flushing of cold water in and out of the respiratory tract, without absorption occurring, is another possible explanation. Animal studies have shown that airway flushing with cold water reduces carotid artery blood temperature by several degrees within a few minutes,[11] which is sufficient to produce a useful reduction in cerebral oxygen requirement. Finally, repeated aspiration of cold water may directly cool deep areas of the brain through conductive heat loss to the nasopharynx.[3]

In spite of these potential benefits, hypothermia in most drowning victims probably does more harm than good. Consciousness is lost at around 32°C, making further aspiration almost inevitable, and ventricular fibrillation or asystole commonly occur at temperatures below 28°C. Once rescued, near-drowned patients often cool further before arrival at hospital.

PRINCIPLES OF THERAPY FOR NEAR-DROWNING

There is a high measure of agreement on general principles of treatment.[2,6,8]

IMMEDIATE TREATMENT

Circulatory failure and loss of consciousness may occur when a patient is lifted from the water in a vertical position, as for example by a helicopter winch. This is probably due to the loss of water pressure resulting in relative redistribution of blood volume into the legs. It is now recommended that victims are removed from the water in the prone position wherever possible.

At the scene of the drowning, it can be very difficult to determine whether there has been cardiac or even respiratory arrest. However, there are many records of apparently dead victims who have recovered without evidence of brain damage after long periods of total immersion. It is therefore essential that cardiopulmonary resuscitation be undertaken in all victims until fully assessed in hospital, no matter how hopeless the outlook may appear at the scene.

Early treatment of near-drowning is crucial and this requires efficient instruction in resuscitation for those who may be available in locations where drowning is likely to occur. The normal priorities of airway clearance, artificial ventilation and cardiac massage should be observed. Out of hospital, mouth-to-mouth ventilation is the method of choice, but high inflation pressures are usually required when there has been flooding of the lungs. Attempts to drain water from the lungs by postural drainage or an abdominal thrust (the Heimlich manoeuvre) are generally unsuccessful. These manoeuvres are likely to cause regurgitation of stomach contents with possible aspiration, and will delay the institution of artificial ventilation. Tracheal intubation should be performed as soon as possible to protect the airway from aspiration. Most survivors will breathe spontaneously within 1–5 minutes after removal from the water. The decision to discontinue resuscitation should not be taken until assessment in hospital, particularly if the state of consciousness is confused by hypothermia.

HOSPITAL TREATMENT

On arrival at hospital, patients should be triaged into the following categories:

1. Awake.
2. Impaired consciousness (but responsive).
3. Comatose.

There should be better than 90% survival in the first two categories, but patients should still be admitted for observation and followed up after discharge. Late deterioration of pulmonary function may occur and is known as 'secondary drowning', which is a form of acute lung injury (see Chapter 31). This can develop in any patient who has aspirated water, and the onset is usually within 4 hours of the aspiration.[3] Patients who are comatose or hypoxic will require admission to a critical care unit. Treatment follows the general principles for hypoxic cerebral damage and aspiration lung injury. If spontaneous breathing does not result in satisfactory levels of arterial Po_2 and Pco_2, continuous positive airway pressure (CPAP) may be tried and is frequently useful. If this is unsuccessful, or in a patient with neurological impairment, artificial ventilation is required (Chapter 32).

References

1. Hyder AA, Borse NN, Blum L, Khan R, El Arifeen S, Baqui AH. Childhood drowning in low- and middle-income countries: urgent need for intervention trials. *J Paediatr Child H*. 2008;44:221–227.
2. Golden FStC, Tipton MJ, Scott RC. Immersion, near-drowning and drowning. *Br J Anaesth*. 1997;79:214–225.
3. Giesbrecht GG. Cold stress, near drowning and accidental hypothermia: a review. *Aviat Space Environ Med*. 2000;71:733–752.
*4. Datta A, Tipton M. Respiratory responses to cold water immersion: neural pathways, interactions, and clinical consequences awake and asleep. *J Appl Physiol*. 2006;100:2057–2064.
5. Schagatay E, Holm B. Effects of water and ambient air temperatures on human diving bradycardia. *Eur J Appl Physiol*. 1996;73:1–6.
6. Modell JH. Drowning. *N Engl J Med*. 1993;328:253–256.
7. Rumbak MJ. The etiology of pulmonary edema in fresh water near drowning. *Am J Emerg Med*. 1996;14:176–179.
*8. Harries M. Near drowning. *BMJ*. 2003;327:1336–1338.
9. Modell JH, Calderwood HW, Ruiz BC, Downs JB, Chapman R. Effects of ventilatory patterns on arterial oxygenation after near-drowning in sea water. *Anesthesiology*. 1974;40:376–384.
10. Hurlimann J, Feer P, Elber F, Niederberger K, Dirnhofer R, Wyler D. Diatom detection in the diagnosis of death by drowning. *Int J Legal Med*. 2000;114:6–14.
11. Conn AW, Miyassaka K, Katayama M, et al. A canine study of cold water drowning in fresh versus salt water. *Crit Care Med*. 1995;23:2029–2036.

Chapter 21

Smoking and air pollution

KEY POINTS

- A quarter of the UK population smoke tobacco, most taking up the habit in their teenage years.
- Smoking involves the regular inhalation of a variety of toxic compounds that stimulate airway irritant receptors and activate inflammatory pathways in the lung.
- The effects of passive smoking begin in utero when lung development is impaired leaving the infant susceptible to lower airway illness for the first few years of life.
- Air pollution with carbon monoxide, ozone, nitrogen dioxide, and particulate matter can occur either indoors or outside, and is associated with a variety of respiratory diseases and symptoms.

The air we breathe is rarely a simple mixture of oxygen, nitrogen and water vapour. For much of the world's population air also contains a variety of other, more noxious, gases and particles. In addition, a substantial proportion of people choose to further contaminate the air that they, and others, breathe with tobacco smoke.

TOBACCO SMOKE

In the Americas tobacco was used for medicinal purposes for many centuries before being introduced from the New World into Europe in the 16th century. Through his acquaintance with Queen Elizabeth I, Sir Walter Raleigh made smoking tobacco an essential fashionable activity of every gentleman. Thereafter the practice steadily increased in popularity until the explosive growth of the habit following the First World War (1914–1918).

There have always been those opposed to smoking and King James I (1603–1625) described it as 'a custom loathsome to the eye, hateful to the nose, harmful to the brain and dangerous to the lungs'. However, firm evidence to support his last conclusion was delayed by some 350 years. Only relatively recently did it become clear that smokers had a higher mortality and that the causes of the excess mortality included many respiratory diseases.[1,2] The proportion of the population who smoke has generally declined since evidence of serious health consequences emerged, though in the UK the proportion of the adult population who smoke is falling only slowly, reaching 24% in 2005. The global health costs of tobacco smoking are enormous: a third of people who smoke will die as a result of their habit, and it is estimated that smoking will cause 1000 million premature deaths worldwide in this century.[3]

CONSTITUENTS OF TOBACCO SMOKE

More than 2000 potentially noxious constituents have been identified in tobacco smoke, some in the gaseous phase and others in the particulate or tar phase. The particulate phase is defined as the fraction eliminated by passing smoke through a filter of pore size $0.1\,\mu m$. This is not to be confused with the 'filter tip', which allows passage of considerable quantities of particulate matter.

There is great variation in the yields of the different constituents between different brands and different types of cigarettes. This is achieved by using leaves of different species of plants, by varying the conditions of curing and cultivation, and by using filter tips. Ventilated filters have a ring of small holes in the paper between the filter tip and

DOI: 10.1016/B978-0-7020-2996-7.00021-0

the tobacco. These holes admit air during a puff and dilute all constituents of the smoke. By these means, it is possible to have wide variations in the different constituents of smoke, which do not bear a fixed relationship to one another.

The gaseous phase. Carbon monoxide is present in cigarette smoke at a concentration issuing from the butt of the cigarette during a puff of around 1–5%, which is far into the toxic range. A better indication of the extent of carbon monoxide exposure is the percentage of carboxyhaemoglobin in blood. For nonsmokers, the value is normally less than 1.5% but is influenced by exposure to air pollution and other people's cigarette smoke (see below). Typical values for smokers range from 2% to 12%. The value is influenced by the number of cigarettes smoked, the type of cigarette and the pattern of inhalation of smoke.

Tobacco smoke also contains very high concentrations (about 400 parts per million) of nitric oxide (page 382) and trace concentrations of nitrogen dioxide, the former being slowly oxidised to the latter in the presence of oxygen. The toxicity of these compounds is well known. Nitrogen dioxide hydrates in alveolar lining fluid to form a mixture of nitrous and nitric acids. In addition, the nitrite ion converts haemoglobin to methaemoglobin.

Other constituents of the gaseous phase include hydrocyanic acid, cyanogen, aldehydes, ketones, nitrosamines and volatile polynuclear aromatic hydrocarbons.

The particulate phase. The material removed by a Cambridge filter is known as the 'total particulate matter', with aerosol particle size in the range 0.2–1 μm. The particulate phase comprises water, nicotine and 'tar'. Nicotine ranges from 0.05 to 2.5 mg per cigarette and 'tar' from 0.5 to 35 mg per cigarette.

INDIVIDUAL SMOKE EXPOSURE

Individual smoke exposure is a complex function of the quantity of cigarettes that are smoked and the pattern of inhalation.

The quantity of cigarettes smoked. Exposure is usually quantified in 'pack years'. This equals the product of the number of packs (20 cigarettes) smoked per day, multiplied by the number of years that that pattern was maintained. The totals for each period are then summated for the lifetime of the subject.

The pattern of inhalation. There are very wide variations in patterns of smoking. Air is normally drawn through the cigarette in a series of 'puffs' with a volume of about 25–50 ml per puff. The puff

may be simply drawn into the mouth and rapidly expelled without appreciable inhalation. However, the habituated smoker will either inhale the puff directly into the lungs or, more commonly, pass the puff from the mouth to the lungs by inhaling air either through the mouth or else through the nose while passing the smoke from the mouth into the pharynx by apposing the tongue against the palate and so obliterating the gas space in the mouth. The inspiration is often especially deep, to flush into the lung any smoke remaining in the dead space.

It will be clear that the quantity of nicotine, tar and carbon monoxide obtainable from a single cigarette is highly variable, and the number and type of cigarettes smoked are not the sole determinants of effective exposure. There is good evidence that the habituated smoker adjusts his smoking pattern to maintain a particular blood level of nicotine.[4] For example, after changing to a brand with a lower nicotine yield, it is common practice to modify the pattern of inhalation to maximise nicotine absorption.

RESPIRATORY EFFECTS OF SMOKING

Cigarette smoking has extensive effects on respiratory function and is clearly implicated in the aetiology of a number of respiratory diseases, particularly chronic obstructive pulmonary disease (COPD) and bronchial carcinoma, which are discussed in Chapters 28 and 30 respectively. Why only around one-fifth of smokers go on to develop COPD remains uncertain, but possibly relates to a genetic susceptibility to the effects of tobacco smoke.[5] For example smokers who have developed COPD have different patterns of expression of oxidant/antioxidant pathway genes compared with smokers who have not developed COPD.[6]

Airway mucosa.[7] There are conflicting reports regarding the sensitivity of airway reflexes in smokers, with increased sensitivity demonstrated in response to inhalation of small concentrations of ammonia vapour,[8] and decreased sensitivity in response to capsaicin.[9] The same workers also found different effects of smoking cessation on the cough reflex.[8,10] The reasons for these varied results are unclear, but there are multiple ways in which smoking could alter cough reflexes, for example by desensitisation of stimulant receptors or by covering of the receptors with the excessive mucus present in the airways of smokers.

Ciliary function is inhibited by both particulate and gas phase compounds in vitro, but in-vivo studies have shown contradictory results, with some studies showing increased ciliary activity in response to cigarette smoke.

There is agreement that mucous production is increased in long-term smokers, who have hyperplasia of submucosal glands and increased numbers of goblet cells even when asymptomatic. In spite of the inconsistent findings regarding ciliary activity, mucus clearance is universally found to be impaired in smokers, which, coupled with increased mucus production and airway sensitivity, gives rise to the normally productive smoker's cough. Three months after smoking cessation, many of these changes are reversed except in those patients who have developed airway damage from long-term airway inflammation.

Airway diameter. Airway diameter is reduced acutely with smoking as a result of reflex bronchoconstriction in response to inhaled particles and the increased mucus production already described. Airway narrowing is greatest in those subjects with known bronchial hypersensitivity such as asthmatics. Long-term small airway inflammation causes chronic airway narrowing that has a multitude of effects on lung function. Airway narrowing promotes premature airway closure during expiration, which results in an increase in closing volume and disturbed ventilation/perfusion relationships. Distribution of inspired gas as indicated by the single-breath nitrogen test (page 123) is therefore often abnormal in smokers. Small airway narrowing over many years gives rise to a progressive reduction in the forced expiratory volume in one second (FEV_1) described below. Many of these changes are at an advanced stage before smokers develop respiratory symptoms.

Ventilatory capacity.[11] FEV_1 normally reaches a peak in early adulthood, remains constant for some years, and then declines steadily as the subject grows older (Figure 21.1). Longitudinal studies of FEV_1 in smokers reveal a very different picture, illustrated in Figure 21.1. Most smokers begin smoking in early adulthood, and the rate of increase of FEV_1 immediately slows, resulting in a delayed and lower plateau. The plateau in FEV_1 is also shorter, before a more rapid decline begins. Smoking cessation is followed by a small improvement in FEV_1, followed by a return to the normal rate of decline, but rarely demonstrates a return to non-smoker values. Eventually, this decline in lung function results in lung pathology, with one in every five smokers developing COPD.

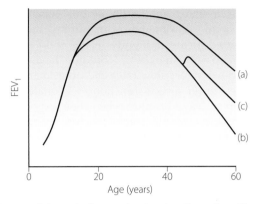

Fig. 21.1 Schematic diagram showing the effects of smoking on normal lifelong changes in the forced expiratory volume in one second (FEV_1). (a) Normal changes; (b) smoking begins at age 16 years; (c) smoking stopped at 45 years of age. See text for details.

PASSIVE SMOKING

A non-smoker is exposed to all the constituents of tobacco smoke whilst indoors in the presence of smokers. Exposure varies with many factors, including size and ventilation of the room, number of people smoking and absorption of smoke constituents on soft furnishings and clothing. Carbon monoxide concentrations of 20 ppm have been reported, which is above the recommended environmental concentration (see below). 'Side-stream' smoke from a smouldering cigarette stub produces greater quantities of potentially noxious substances than 'main-stream' smoke produced when a cigarette burns in a stream of air drawn through it during a puff. On average, 'side-stream' smoke is generated during 58 seconds in each minute of cigarette smoking and this is not included in the measured yield of a cigarette.

Evidence for adverse health effects of passive smoking is now convincing: passive smoking by adults has been linked to lung cancer, cardiovascular disease, asthma and COPD.[12]

Maternal smoking. Infants whose mothers smoke during pregnancy have low birthweight, are more likely to be born prematurely and are at greater risk of sudden infant death syndrome (page 256). Up to two years of age, infants with smoking parents are more prone to lower respiratory tract illnesses and episodes of wheezing, and when older they have reduced lung volumes, higher carboxyhaemoglobin levels and a greater likelihood of developing asthma.[11,13] It is uncertain whether this results from passive smoking in utero or from post-natal exposure to tobacco smoke in the home, but evidence for an in utero contribution is mounting, mediated by reduced innate immunity in the child born to a mother who smokes.[12,13] Studies have found reduced expiratory flow rates and other markers of impaired lower airway function in neonates even before they leave hospital when their exposure to atmospheric cigarette smoke begins.[14] The same finding in neonates born on average 7 weeks before their expected date[15] indicates that maternal smoking adversely affects lung development at a crucial stage when terminal airways and alveoli are being formed (page 250). The increased risk of lower respiratory tract illness in passive-smoking infants is believed to result from smaller airway calibre at birth causing a greater propensity to airway closure with the normal infective or allergic challenges of infancy.[14] After a few years of normal growth, airway size increases sufficiently to reduce symptoms, and the child 'grows out' of their susceptibility to respiratory illness, though their lung function remains worse than children who did not have lower airways disease in early life.[16]

SMOKING AND PERIOPERATIVE COMPLICATIONS[17,18,19]

The increased sensitivity of the airway to inhaled irritants seen in smokers causes a greater incidence of adverse events such as cough, breath hold or laryngospasm on induction of general anaesthesia, even in passive smokers.[20] These complications are not necessarily associated with decreases in oxygen saturation, though episodes of desaturation in the recovery period may be more common in smokers, or even in passively smoking children.[21] It is worth noting that commercially available pulse oximeters record carboxyhaemoglobin as if it were oxyhaemoglobin (page 210), and so will consistently overestimate oxygen saturation in recent smokers.

There is ample evidence that smokers have an increased incidence of postoperative pulmonary complications (PPCs), which in comparison to non-smokers are several times more common in smokers,[19,22] depending on the definitions used and type of surgery undertaken. This is attributable both to increased secretion and impaired clearance of mucus and to small airway narrowing. Almost all studies of the perioperative effects of smoking have been undertaken in patients having major surgery, usually coronary artery revascularisation or upper abdominal surgery. The high incidence

of respiratory complications in this group makes them an ideal study population, but there remains little information regarding the respiratory effects of perioperative smoking and more minor surgery.

Preoperative smoking cessation is vital. Nicotine, which is responsible for many untoward cardiovascular changes, has a half-life of only 30 minutes, whilst carboxyhaemoglobin has a half-life of 4 hours when breathing air. A smoking fast of just a few hours will therefore effectively remove the risks associated with carbon monoxide and nicotine. The duration of smoking abstinence required to reduce the high incidence of PPCs is controversial.[18,19] Some studies, mostly in patients having cardiac surgery, found a greater incidence of PPC in patients who stopped smoking for less than 8 weeks compared with those who continued smoking until the day before surgery. Other studies have failed to demonstrate this effect, and there are concerns that the original investigations had insufficient statistical power to conclusively prove a benefit to continuing to smoke before major surgery.[18] Current advice is therefore that smokers should always strive to stop smoking preoperatively, and that the longer the period of cessation the greater will be the benefit in terms of avoiding PPCs.

MECHANISMS OF SMOKING RELATED LUNG DAMAGE[23]

Many of the compounds present in cigarette smoke have direct irritant and toxic effects on the lungs. There are three other mechanisms by which lung damage occurs.

OXIDATIVE INJURY[24]

There is compelling evidence that oxidative injury, including peroxidation of membrane lipids, is an important component of the pulmonary damage caused by cigarette smoke.

Direct oxidative damage. The tar phase contains quinone, the semiquinone free radical and hydroquinone in a polymeric matrix, and the gas phase contains nitric oxide. These compounds can reduce oxygen in the body, to yield the superoxide free radical and thence the highly damaging hydroxyl free radical (Figure 26.3).

Cell-mediated oxidative damage. This results from smoking-induced activation of, or enhancement of, neutrophil and macrophage activity in the respiratory tract. Bronchoalveolar lavage in humans has shown that smokers have larger numbers of intra-alveolar macrophages and also significant numbers of neutrophils that are not normally present in non-smokers.[25] It is the particulate component of smoke that is responsible for the recruitment and activation of neutrophils in the alveoli. This suggests that the interaction of particulate matter and alveolar macrophages releases a neutrophil chemattractant and that neutrophils are subsequently activated to release either proteases or reactive oxygen species. This activation may be a direct response to cigarette smoke or may represent excessive reactive oxygen species production in response to minor infective challenge in smokers.

Evidence of in vivo oxidative stress in smokers is based mainly on measures of antioxidant activity in both the lungs and blood. Compared with non-smokers, human smokers have reduced levels of vitamin E in alveolar fluid, reduced plasma concentrations of vitamin C, and greatly increased superoxide dismutase and catalase activity in alveolar macrophages. These abnormalities of oxidant-antioxidant activity are being used to try and find therapeutic agents that may mitigate the damage done by smoking.[24]

CARCINOGENESIS

Smoking contributes to the development of cancer in many organs, but the respiratory tract clearly receives the greatest exposure to tobacco smoke carcinogens, and this topic is described in more detail on page 439. There are two groups of compounds with carcinogenic activity, found mostly in the tar of the particulate phase. Some hydrocarbons, in particular polynuclear aromatic hydrocarbons (PAH), are carcinogenic, whilst others such as aromatic phenols (phenol, indole and catechol) are cocarcinogens and tumour promoters, without which the carcinogenic compounds are relatively innocuous. Tobacco-related nitrosamines and nicotine derivatives are also carcinogenic and, because of their ease of absorption into the blood, are responsible for cancer formation not only in the respiratory tract and oesophagus but also in more distant organs such as the pancreas. Knowledge about these carcinogens has led to many attempts to reduce their concentration in smoke by modifying the cigarette, and tar levels in cigarettes have declined almost threefold since 1955. However, these changes have had little impact on the incidence of lung cancer (page 438) and smoking cessation remains the best way of avoiding all smoking-related cancers.

IMMUNOLOGICAL ACTIVATION[26]

Smokers have elevated serum IgE levels compared with non-smokers, the cause of which is uncertain but may be two-fold. Direct toxicity and oxidative cell damage result in greater airway mucosal cell permeability, allowing better access for allergens to underlying immunologically active cells. Smoking also increases the activity of some T-lymphocyte subsets that are responsible for producing interleukin-4, a cytokine well known for stimulating IgE production, and is known to produce a long term systemic inflammatory response.

AIR POLLUTION[27]

Detrimental effects of air pollution were first recognised in the 13th century, though it is only in the last 50 years that effective control of pollution has been achieved. In spite of these controls, increased overall energy requirements and the internal combustion engine have ensured that air pollution remains a current problem. At the same time as levels of pollutants have been reduced in many parts of the world evidence of their harmful effects on health has increased, and air pollution remains a global problem.[28] Many of the pollutants described below, like tobacco smoke, create oxidative stress systemically[29] and therefore have effects not only on the lungs but are also implicated in causing cardiovascular diseases.[30] Recent epidemiological research has found significant effects of air pollution on lung function in children, showing that the closer children live to busy roads the slower is the rate at which their forced expiratory volume in one second (FEV_1) increases as they grow,[31] and the more likely they are to develop respiratory disease, including asthma.[32,33,34] Similar observations have been made relating lung function in adults with proximity to road traffic.[35] Fine particulate matter (see below) seems to be the main pollutant responsible for the increased mortality,[36] and recent work has found that some individuals are genetically susceptible to these effects on long term health.[34,37] These recent developments have led to renewed calls to further reduce 'acceptable' levels of all air pollutants.[38]

SOURCES OF POLLUTANTS

Primary pollutants are substances that are released into the atmosphere directly from the polluting source, and are mostly derived from the combustion of fossil fuels. Petrol engines that ignite the fuel in an oxygen-restricted environment produce varying quantities of carbon monoxide, nitrogen oxides and hydrocarbons such as benzene and polycyclic aromatic compounds. All of these pollutants are reduced by the use of a catalytic converter. In contrast, diesel engines burn fuel with an excess of oxygen and so produce little carbon monoxide but more nitrogen oxides and particulate matter. Burning of coal and oil is now restricted almost entirely to power generation, and the pollutants produced depend on the type of fuel used and the amount of effort expended on 'cleaning' the emissions. However, particulates and nitrogen oxides are invariably produced, and this remains the major source of sulphur dioxide.

Secondary pollutants are formed in the atmosphere from chemical changes to primary pollutants. Nitric oxide produced from vehicle engines is quickly converted to nitrogen dioxide, and in doing so may react with ozone, reducing the atmospheric concentration of the latter. Alternatively, when exposed to sunlight in the lower atmosphere both NO and NO_2 react with oxygen to produce ozone (O_3).

Meteorological conditions influence air pollution. In conditions of strong wind, pollutants are quickly dispersed; in cloudy weather the development of secondary pollutants is unlikely. Ground level pollution in urban areas is exacerbated by clear, calm weather when 'temperature inversion' can occur. On a clear night, heat is lost from the ground to the atmosphere by radiation and the ground level air cools dramatically (Figure 21.2A). At dawn the ground is quickly heated by the sun's radiation and warms the air, which lifts a blanket of cool air to approximately 50–100 m high. Because in still conditions mixing of air masses is slow to occur, the relatively cold air sits on top of the warm air below. In the meantime, the morning rush hour produces large amounts of pollutants that are unable to disperse and become trapped near the ground (Figure 21.2B).

RESPIRATORY EFFECTS OF POLLUTANTS[27,39]

Recommended maximum levels of common pollutants are shown in Table 21.1. The extent to which these levels are achieved varies greatly between different countries and from year to year.

Carbon monoxide (CO) is found in the blood of patients, in trace concentrations, as a result of its production in the body, but mainly as a result of smoking and air pollution. The amount of carboxyhaemoglobin

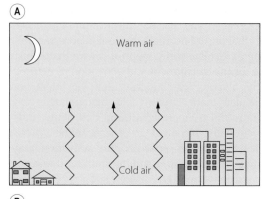

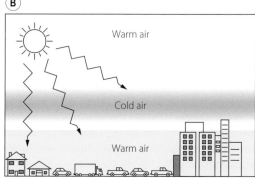

Fig. 21.2 Temperature inversion producing pollution in the morning rush hour. (A) At night, the ground loses heat to the atmosphere by radiation and ground level air cools. (B) In the morning, with strong sun and still conditions, the ground heats up quickly and displaces the blanket of cold air upwards, so preventing effective air mixing and trapping vehicular pollution at ground level.

formed when breathing air polluted with CO will depend on the subject's minute volume. One study reported carboxyhaemoglobin levels of 0.4–9.7% in London taxi drivers but the highest level in a non-smoking driver was 3%.[41] Recommended levels shown in Table 21.1 are calculated to result in a carboxyhaemoglobin concentration of less than 2.5% even during moderate exercise. Carbon monoxide levels similar to those seen in smokers are only likely to occur during severe outdoor pollution episodes, though indoor pollution with CO may be more common (see below).

Nitrogen dioxide is mainly a primary pollutant, but a small amount is produced from nitric oxide. In the UK, about half of atmospheric NO_2 is derived from vehicles. Indoor levels of NO_2 commonly exceed outdoor levels, and the respiratory effects of NO_2 are therefore described in the next section.

Table 21.1 World Health Organization air quality guidelines[40]

POLLUTANT	DURATION OF EXPOSURE		
	SHORT (≤ 1 HOUR)	MODERATE (8–24 HOURS)	ANNUAL
Ozone		$100 \mu g.m^{-3}$	
Particulate PM_{10}	$50 \mu g.m^{-3}$		$20 \mu g.m^{-3}$
Particulate $PM_{2.5}$	$25 \mu g.m^{-3}$		$10 \mu g.m^{-3}$
Sulphur dioxide	$500 \mu g.m^{-3}$	$20 \mu g.m^{-3}$	
Nitrogen dioxide	$200 \mu g.m^{-3}$		$40 \mu g.m^{-3}$
Carbon monoxide	25–87 ppm	10 ppm	

ppm, parts per million.

Ozone is a secondary pollutant formed by the action of sunlight on nitrogen oxides, and therefore highest levels tend to occur in rural areas downwind from cities and roads. In all areas, the dependence on sunlight means that ozone levels slowly increase throughout the day reaching peak levels shortly after the evening rush hour. Ozone is toxic to the respiratory tract, with effects being dependent on both concentration and duration of exposure. Exposure to concentrations of $200 \mu g.m^{-3}$ for just a few hours commonly causes throat irritation, chest discomfort and cough, resulting from both direct stimulation of irritant receptors in the airway and activation of inflammatory pathways. Bronchoconstriction may occur accompanied by a decrease in FEV_1, and exercise capacity is limited. There is a large variability between individuals in their spirometric response to ozone, with approximately 10% of subjects having a severe response. This variability in response is partly a result of differing genetic susceptibility.[27] It is interesting that laboratory studies have failed to demonstrate that asthmatic subjects are more susceptible to ozone-induced pulmonary symptoms. Even so, there is good evidence that high ozone concentrations are associated with increased hospital attendance, respiratory problems (particularly in children[42]) and with an increased risk of death from respiratory causes.[43]

Sulphur dioxide. Declining use of coal has substantially reduced the production of sulphur dioxide in recent years, and two-thirds of production in the UK now originates from oil-burning power stations. Normal atmospheric levels have no short-term effect on healthy subjects, but asthmatic patients may develop bronchoconstriction at between 100 and 250 ppb.

Particulate matter consists of a mixture of soot, liquid droplets, recondensed metallic vapours and organic debris. The disparate nature of particulate pollution reflects its very varied origins, but in the urban environment, diesel engines are a major source. Only particles of less than $10 \mu m$ diameter are considered to be 'inhalable' into the lung (page 220), so particulate pollution is measured as the concentration of particles less than this diameter, known as PM_{10}. Particulate matter is further subdivided into:

- Coarse particles, between $2.5–10 \mu m$ diameter, make up a smaller proportion of PM_{10} than the other particles and are less well studied, but are still believed to contribute significantly to the adverse health effects of particulate pollution.[44]
- Fine particles, or $PM_{2.5}$, are less than $2.5 \mu m$ in diameter, the most numerous particle present in air pollution, and responsible for most of the respiratory effects of particulate pollution.
- Ultrafine particles are carbon particles less than $0.1 \mu m$ in size.[45] Their small size means they should be breathed in and out without being trapped by the airway lining fluid (page 220). However, some particles are retained in the lung, where they remain in the long term, probably contained within macrophages, and without any evidence of systemic absorption. Their contribution to the health effects of particulate pollution is uncertain.

Acute effects of particles on lung function again include airway irritation and small reductions in lung volumes such as FEV_1 and FVC.[46] It is, however, associations between PM_{10} levels and overall mortality that have been the focus of much research. Even when smoking habits are taken into account, particulate pollution is associated with an increased risk of death from lung cancer or other cardiopulmonary diseases.[27] Particulate pollution has widespread pro-inflammatory effects on lung epithelial cells and alveolar macrophages, causing inflammatory responses both locally, in the lung, and in distant sites where activation of clotting pathways may explain PM_{10}-induced increases in death from cardiovascular disease.

INDOOR AIR POLLUTION[47]

Worldwide, the most common form of indoor air pollution is smoke produced by fires used for cooking. Burning biomass fuels produces large amounts of particulate matter, containing smaller particle sizes than diesel engines. As for the outdoor pollution described above these pollutants are associated with the development of COPD,[48] and also respiratory infections in children.[49]

In the developed world energy-efficient homes have become the norm in recent years, with effective heating systems and extensive insulation. This has led to dramatic changes in indoor air quality, including warmer temperatures, higher humidity levels and reduced ventilation. It is estimated that most people spend in excess of 80% of their time indoors, so indoor air pollution may have a considerable impact on public health. The respiratory effects of passive smoking are described above (page 319), and the impact of environmental radon exposure on lung cancer are discussed on page 439.

Indoor air quality generally reflects that of the outdoor air except that ozone levels are invariably low indoors due to the rapid reaction of ozone with the synthetic materials that make up much of the indoor environment. In addition to pollutants from outside, there are three specific indoor pollutants.

Allergens. Warm moist air, poor ventilation and extensive floor coverings provide ideal conditions for house dust mite infestation and the retention of numerous other allergens. This is believed to contribute to the recent upsurge in the prevalence of atopic diseases such as asthma, and is discussed in Chapter 28.

Carbon monoxide.[50] Malfunctions of heating equipment in the home may release CO into the indoor environment. Acute CO poisoning from this cause is common, but the occurrence of prolonged low-level exposure to indoor CO may be underestimated. Headache, malaise and flu-like symptoms are all features of long-term CO poisoning, though these symptoms are believed to be completely reversible once the exposure to CO is stopped. Smokers, who have permanently elevated carboxyhaemoglobin levels, appear to be resistant to these symptoms.

Nitrogen dioxide. Gas-fired cookers, stoves and boilers all produce NO_2, the amount being dependent on the arrangements for waste gas exclusion.[51] In this respect, gas cookers are the worst culprits as they are rarely associated with chimneys and flues, and normally discharge their waste gases directly into the kitchen atmosphere. During cooking, NO_2 levels may reach over $750\,\mu g.m^{-3}$, which is well in excess of outdoor pollution targets (Table 21.1). Mild airway irritant effects are seen at levels of around $550\,\mu g.m^{-3}$ in asthmatic subjects, or at $1800\,\mu g.m^{-3}$ in non-asthmatic subjects,[52] so acute effects are probably uncommon. However, long-term exposure does seem to be clinically significant by, for example, causing worsening of asthma symptoms in children.[53]

References

1. Doll R, Hill AB. Smoking and carcinoma of the lung. *BMJ.* 1950;2:739–748.
2. Anderson DO, Ferris BG. Role of tobacco smoking in the causation of chronic respiratory disease. *N Engl J Med.* 1962;267:787–794.
*3. Frieden TR, Bloomberg MR. How to prevent 100 million deaths from tobacco. *Lancet.* 2007;369:1758–1761.
4. Ashton H, Stepney R, Thompson PW. Self-titration by cigarette smokers. *BMJ.* 1979;2:357–360.
5. Anthonisen NR. "Susceptible" smokers? *Thorax.* 2006;61:924–925.
6. Pierrou S, Broberg P, O'Donnell RA, et al. Expression of genes involved in oxidative stress responses in airway epithelial cells of smokers with chronic obstructive pulmonary disease. *Am J Respir Crit Care Med.* 2007;175:577–586.
7. Wanner A, Salathe M, O'Riordan TG. Mucociliary clearance in the airways. *Am J Respir Crit Care Med.* 1996;154:1868–1902.
8. Erskine RJ, Murphy PJ, Langton JA. Sensitivity of upper airway reflexes in cigarette smokers: effect of abstinence. *Br J Anaesth.* 1994;73:298–302.
9. Dicpinigaitis PV. Cough reflex sensitivity in cigarette smokers. *Chest.* 2003;123:685–688.
10. Dicpinigaitis PV, Sitkauskiene B, Stravinskaite K, Appel DW, Negassa A, Sakalauskas R. Effect of smoking cessation on cough reflex sensitivity. *Eur Respir J.* 2006;28:786–790.
11. Samet JM, Lange P. Longitudinal studies of active and passive smoking. *Am J Respir Crit Care Med.* 1996;154:S257–S265.
12. Eisner MD, Forastiere F. Passive smoking, lung function, and public health. *Am J Respir Crit Care Med.* 2006;173:1184–1185.
13. Le Souëf PN. Adverse effects of maternal smoking during pregnancy on innate immunity in infants. *Eur Respir J.* 2006;28:675–677.
14. Morgan WJ, Martinez FD. Maternal smoking and infant lung function: Further evidence for an in utero effect. *Am J Respir Crit Care Med.* 1998;158:689–690.

15. Hoo AF, Henschen M, Dezateux C, Costeloe K, Stocks J. Respiratory function among preterm infants whose mothers smoked during pregnancy. *Am J Respir Crit Care Med*. 1998;158:700–705.

16. Martinez FD, Wright AL, Taussig LM, et al. Asthma and wheezing in the first six years of life. *N Engl J Med*. 1995;332:133–138.

17. Nel MR, Morgan M. Smoking and anaesthesia revisited. *Anaesthesia*. 1996;51:309–311.

*18. Warner DO. Perioperative abstinence from cigarettes. Physiologic and clinical consequences. *Anesthesiology*. 2006;104:356–367.

19. Tønnesen H, Nielsen PR, Lauritzen JB, Møller AM. Smoking and alcohol intervention before surgery: evidence for best practice. *Br J Anaesth*. 2009;102:297–306.

20. Schwilk B, Bothner U, Schraag S, Georgieff M. Perioperative respiratory events in smokers and nonsmokers undergoing general anaesthesia. *Acta Anaesthesiol Scand*. 1997;41:348–355.

21. Lyons B, Frizelle H, Kirby F, Casey W. The effect of passive smoking on the incidence of airway complications in children undergoing general anaesthesia. *Anaesthesia*. 1996;51:324–326.

22. Møller AM, Maaløe R, Pedersen T. Postoperative intensive care admittance: The role of tobacco smoking. *Acta Anaesthesiol Scand*. 2001;45:345–348.

23. Yanbaeva DG, Dentener MA, Creutzberg EC, Wesseling G, Wouters EFM. Systemic effects of smoking. *Chest*. 2007;131:1557–1566.

24. Kinnula VL. Focus on antioxidant enzymes and antioxidant strategies in smoking related airway diseases. *Thorax*. 2005;60:693–700.

25. Hunninghake GW, Crystal RG. Cigarette smoking and lung destruction. Accumulation of neutrophils in the lungs of cigarette smokers. *Am Rev Respir Dis*. 1983;128:833–838.

26. Villar MTA, Holgate ST. IgE, smoking and lung function. *Clin Exp Allergy*. 1995;25:206–209.

*27. Brunekreef B, Holgate ST. Air pollution and health. *Lancet*. 2002;360:1233–1242.

28. Thurston G. Air pollution, human health, climate change and you. *Thorax*. 2007;62:748–749.

29. Romieu I, Castro-Giner F, Kunzli N, Sunyer J. Air pollution, oxidative stress and dietary supplementation: a review. *Eur Respir J*. 2008;31:179–196.

30. Dockery DW, Stone PH. Cardiovascular risks from fine particulate air pollution. *N Engl J Med*. 2007;356:511–513.

31. Gauderman WJ, Vora H, McConnell R, et al. Effect of exposure to traffic on lung development from 10 to 18 years of age: a cohort study. *Lancet*. 2007;369:571–577.

32. Jerrett M. Does traffic-related air pollution contribute to respiratory disease formation in children? *Eur Respir J*. 2007;29:825–826.

33. Morgenstern V, Zutavern A, Cyrys J, et al. Atopic diseases, allergic sensitization, and exposure to traffic-related air pollution in children. *Am J Respir Crit Care Med*. 2008;177:1331–1337.

34. Sandström T, Kelly FJ. Traffic-related air pollution, genetics and asthma development in children. *Thorax*. 2009;64:98–99.

35. Holguin F. Traffic related exposures and lung function in adults. *Thorax*. 2007;62:837–838.

36. Pope CA, Ezzati M, Dockery DW. Fine-particulate air pollution and life expectancy in the United States. *N Engl J Med*. 2009;360:376–386.

37. Baccarelli A. Breathe deeply into your genes! Genetic variants and air pollution effects. *Am J Respir Crit Care Med*. 2009;179:431–432.

38. Gauderman WJ. Air pollution and children – an unhealthy mix. *N Engl J Med*. 2006;355:78–79.

39. Committee on the Medical Effects of Air Pollution. *The Quantification of the Effects of Air Pollution on Health in the United Kingdom*. London: The Stationery Office; 1998.

40. World Health Organization. *WHO Air Quality Guidelines for Particulate Matter, Ozone, Nitrogen Dioxide and Sulfur Dioxide*. Global update 2005. Summary of risk assessment. Geneva: WHO; 2006.

41. Jones RD, Commins BT, Cernik AA. Blood lead and carboxyhaemoglobin levels in London taxi drivers. *Lancet*. 1972;2:302–303.

42. Pinkerton KE, Balmes JR, Fanucchi MV, Rom WN. Ozone a malady for all. *Am J Respir Crit Care Med*. 2007;176:107–112.

43. Jerrett M, Burnett RT, Pope CA, et al. Long-term ozone exposure and mortality. *N Engl J Med*. 2009;360:1085–1095.

44. Brunekreef B, Forsberg B. Epidemiological evidence of effects of coarse airborne particles on health. *Eur Respir J*. 2005;26:309–318.

45. Möller W, Felten K, Sommerer K, et al. Deposition, retention, and translocation of ultrafine particles from the central airways and lung periphery. *Am J Respir Crit Care Med*. 2008;177:426–432.

46. Lippmann M. Health effects of airborne particulate matter. *N Engl J Med*. 2007;357:2395–2397.

*47. Samet JM, Spengler JD. Indoor environments and health: Moving into the 21st century. *Am J Public Health*. 2003;93:1489–1493.

48. Liu Y. Where there's smoke there's lung disease. *Thorax*. 2007;62:838–839.

49. Emmelin A, Wall S. Indoor air pollution. A poverty-related cause of mortality among the children of the world. *Chest*. 2007;132:1615–1623.

50. Townsend CL, Maynard RL. Effects on health of prolonged exposure to low concentrations of carbon monoxide. *Occup Environ Med*. 2002;59:708–711.

51. Fuhlbrigge A, Weiss S. Domestic gas appliances and lung disease. *Thorax*. 1997;52 (supp 3):S58–S62.

52. Committee on the Medical Effects of Air Pollutants. *Handbook on Air Pollution and Health*. London: The Stationery Office; 1997.

53. Belanger K, Gent JF, Triche EW, Bracken MB, Leaderer BP. Association of indoor nitrogen dioxide exposure with respiratory symptoms in children with asthma. *Am J Respir Crit Care Med*. 2006;173:297–303.

Chapter 22

Anaesthesia

KEY POINTS

- All anaesthetic drugs reduce ventilation and impair the ventilatory response to both hypercapnia and hypoxia.
- Upper airway muscle function is inhibited by anaesthesia leading to airway obstruction, usually at the level of the soft palate.
- Functional residual capacity is reduced within a few minutes of induction of anaesthesia as a result of altered respiratory muscle activity causing changes to the shape and volume of the thoracic cavity.
- Most patients develop small areas of atelectasis during anaesthesia, re-expansion of which requires high lung inflation pressures.
- Oxygenation is impaired by these changes, with wider scatter of ventilation/perfusion ratios along with increased alveolar dead space and pulmonary shunt.

Only 12 years after the first successful public demonstration of general anaesthesia in 1846, John Snow reported the pronounced changes that occur in respiration during the inhalation of chloroform.[1] Subsequent observations have confirmed that anaesthesia has profound effects on the respiratory system. However, these effects are diverse and highly specific, some aspects of respiratory function being profoundly modified while others are scarcely affected at all.

CONTROL OF BREATHING[2]

UNSTIMULATED VENTILATION

It is well known that anaesthesia diminishes pulmonary ventilation, and hypercapnia is commonplace if spontaneous breathing is preserved. Reduced minute volume is due partly to a reduction in metabolic demand but mainly to interference with the chemical control of breathing, in particular a reduced sensitivity to CO_2 as described below. In an uncomplicated anaesthetic there should not be sufficient resistance to breathing to affect the minute volume. However, the minute volume may be greatly decreased if there is respiratory obstruction.

At lower concentrations of inhaled anaesthetics, minute volume may remain unchanged, but smaller tidal volumes with higher respiratory frequency often occur resulting in reduced alveolar ventilation and an increase in $P\text{co}_2$. With higher concentrations of anaesthetic, breathing becomes slower and spontaneous minute volume may decrease to very low levels, particularly in the absence of surgical stimulation. This will inevitably result in hypercapnia, and end-expiratory $P\text{co}_2$ commonly rises to 10 kPa (75 mmHg). Clearly there is no limit to the rise that may occur if the anaesthetist is prepared to tolerate gross hypoventilation.

There are anaesthetists in many parts of the world who do not believe that temporary hypercapnia during anaesthesia is harmful to a healthy patient. Many hundreds of millions of patients must have been subjected to this transient physiological trespass since 1846 and there seems to be no convincing evidence of harm resulting from it – except perhaps increased surgical bleeding. In other parts of the world the departure from physiological normality is regarded with concern and it is usual either to assist spontaneous respiration by manual compression of the reservoir bag or, more commonly, to paralyse and ventilate artificially as a routine.

DOI: 10.1016/B978-0-7020-2996-7.00022-2

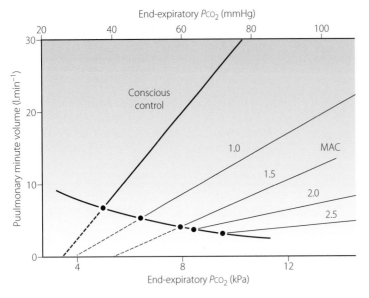

Fig. 22.1 Displacement of the $P\text{co}_2$/ventilation response curve with different end-expiratory concentrations of halothane. The curve sloping down to the right indicates the pathway of $P\text{co}_2$ and ventilation change resulting from depression without the challenge of exogenous carbon dioxide. The broken lines indicate extrapolation to apnoeic threshold $P\text{co}_2$. MAC; minimum alveolar concentration. The curves have been constructed from the data of reference 3.

Quite different conditions apply during anaesthesia with artificial ventilation. The minute volume can then be set at any level that seems appropriate to the anaesthetist, and in the past there was a tendency to hyperventilate patients, resulting in hypocapnia. Now that monitoring of end-expiratory $P\text{co}_2$ is routine artificial ventilation can be adjusted to maintain the target $P\text{co}_2$ selected by the anaesthetist.

EFFECT ON $P\text{co}_2$/VENTILATION RESPONSE CURVE

Progressive increases in the alveolar concentration of all inhalational anaesthetic agents decrease the slope of the $P\text{co}_2$/ventilation response curve and, at deep levels of anaesthesia, there may be no response at all to $P\text{co}_2$. Furthermore, the anaesthetised patient, as opposed to the awake subject, always becomes apnoeic if the $P\text{co}_2$ is reduced below this intercept, which is known as the apnoeic threshold $P\text{co}_2$ (page 70). In Figure 22.1, the flat curve rising to the left represents the starting points for various $P\text{co}_2$/ventilation response curves. Without added carbon dioxide in the inspired gas, deepening anaesthesia is associated with a decreasing ventilation and a rising $P\text{co}_2$, points moving progressively down and to the right. At intervals along this curve are shown $P\text{co}_2$/ventilation response curves resulting from adding carbon dioxide to the inspired gas.

At equivalent depth of anaesthesia, currently available inhaled anaesthetics depress the ventilatory

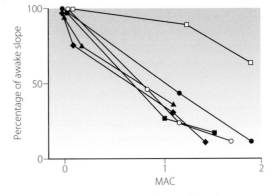

Fig. 22.2 Relative depression of the ventilatory response to CO_2 by different inhalational anaesthetics as a function of minimum alveolar concentration (MAC). ●, halothane; ▲, enflurane; ■, isoflurane; ◆, sevoflurane; ○, desflurane; □, diethylether. (Data from references 5, 6 and 7.)

response to $P\text{co}_2$ by a similar amount. This is conveniently shown by plotting the slope of the $P\text{co}_2$/ventilation response curve against equi-anaesthetic concentrations of different anaesthetics (Figure 22.2), shown as multiples of minimum alveolar concentration (MAC), although the validity of using MAC multiples in this way has been questioned. The currently used halogenated agents do not differ greatly from one another but diethyl ether is exceptional in having little effect up to 1 MAC. With low doses of inhaled anaesthetics (= 0.2 MAC) there is almost no depression of the hypercapnic ventilatory response,[4] in contrast to the response to hypoxia described below.

Surgical stimulation antagonises the effect of anaesthesia on the Pco_2/ventilation response curve (Figure 22.3). It may easily be observed that in a spontaneously breathing patient a surgical incision increases the ventilation whatever the depth of anaesthesia. During prolonged anaesthesia without surgical stimulation, there is no progressive change in the response curve up to 3 hours. With the exception of ketamine, intravenous anaesthetics have similar effects on ventilation to the inhalational anaesthetics.

EFFECT ON Po_2/VENTILATION RESPONSE CURVE[9,10]

The normal relationship between Po_2 and ventilation has been described on pages 71 et seq. It was long believed that this reflex was the ultima moriens and, unlike the Pco_2/ventilation response curve, unaffected by anaesthesia. This doctrine was a source of comfort to many generations of anaesthetists in the past. Little attention was given to the observation of Gordh in 1945 that ether anaesthesia nearly abolished the ventilatory response to hypoxaemia while the response to carbon dioxide was still present.[11]

Over 30 years later, halothane anaesthesia was shown to reduce the acute hypoxic ventilatory response (AHVR) in humans.[12] Shortly afterwards in 1978, Knill & Gelb[13] showed that not only was the hypoxic response affected by inhalational anaesthetics but it was also, in fact, exquisitely sensitive (Figure 22.4). Hypoxic drive was markedly attenuated at 0.1 MAC, a level of anaesthesia that would not be reached for a considerable time during recovery

from anaesthesia. Similar effects were found with all the currently used inhalational agents,[9] and with the intravenous anaesthetic propofol.[14]

These findings were widely accepted for some years, until a study by Temp et al[15] in 1992 showed that AHVR was only diminished in hypercapnic conditions. This study initiated a great deal of further research. A summary of the findings of these and many other studies are shown in Figure 22.5.

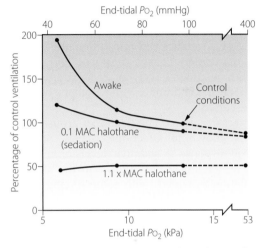

Fig. 22.4 Effect of halothane anaesthesia on the ventilatory response to hypoxia. The data shown in this figure have now been challenged; see text for details. (After reference 13.)

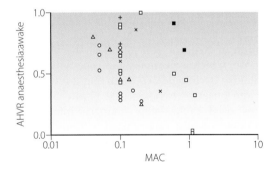

Fig. 22.5 Summary of studies of the acute hypoxic ventilatory response (AHVR) and inhalational anaesthesia or sedation. The ordinate is the ratio of the increase in minute volume with hypoxia during anaesthesia or sedation and the awake (control) response. Thus a ratio of unity represents no depression of the response and zero represents a completely abolished response. All studies were performed under isocapnic conditions except the two solid squares which used poikilocapnia with isoflurane. See text for details. ○, halothane; △, enflurane; □, isoflurane; ◇, sevoflurane; ×, nitrous oxide; +, desflurane.

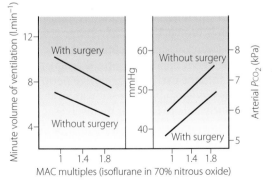

Fig. 22.3 Respiratory depression by isoflurane with and without surgery at different multiples of minimum alveolar concentration (MAC) required for anaesthesia. (Data from reference 8.)

The most notable feature of these results is their diversity, with, for example, different studies of similar concentrations of isoflurane, particularly at sedative levels, resulting in completely opposite results. However, for the other agents there does seem to be a generally dose-dependent depression of the hypoxic ventilatory response, though at 0.1 MAC considerable variation remains. There are many possible explanations for these results, mostly relating to methodological differences between studies:

Anaesthetic agent. Differences between anaesthetic agents in their effects on AHVR are not obvious from Figure 22.5. However, a recent quantitative review of 37 studies did find differences, with the least depression of the response by low-dose sevoflurane, progressively increasing depression by isoflurane and enflurane, with halothane having the greatest effect.[9]

Subject stimulation. The degree of arousal of subjects is known to affect the AHVR. Studies of hypoxic response at 'sedative' levels of anaesthesia (0.2 MAC or less) have differed in the amount of stimulation provided, with some forcing the subjects to remain awake[15] and others leaving subjects undisturbed. One study comparing awake and asleep subjects with 0.1 MAC isoflurane found no depression of the hypoxic response in the awake group.[16] However, the same review described in the previous paragraph did find subject stimulation to be a significant factor in determining the degree of depression of AHVR, and that this effect may be influenced by the specific anaesthetic agent used.[9]

Hypoxic challenge. The rate of onset, degree and duration of hypoxia will all affect the ventilatory response, which is normally biphasic with hypoxic ventilatory decline (HVD) occurring a few minutes after the onset of hypoxia (see Figure 5.6). Some studies used rapid 'step' changes into hypoxic conditions,[17] whilst others used a 'ramp' onset of hypoxia over 8–10 min.[18] In the latter situation, the response under study will be a combination of AHVR and HVD.[15] These differences do not seem to be of practical importance. One study addressing different patterns of hypoxic onset on AHVR found no difference between the two,[19] and a recent review did not find the hypoxic stimulus to be a major factor.[9] Hypoxic ventilatory decline seems to be uninfluenced by anaesthesia.[15,20]

Subject selection. The magnitude of the AHVR differs greatly between individuals (page 72). Some studies have been performed using only subjects found to have a 'brisk' ventilatory response to hypoxia,[17] and these results cannot therefore be extrapolated to a broader range of patients.

Carbon dioxide concentration may be maintained at normal, pre-hypoxic, levels (isocapnia) or allowed to find its own level (poikilocapnia). This has a large effect in the awake subject, with the hypoxic response being greatly attenuated during poikilocapnia (see Figure 5.6). During anaesthesia with up to 0.85 MAC isoflurane, the hypoxic ventilatory response during poikilocapnia is essentially maintained;[21] that is, the increase in ventilation with hypoxic challenge is the same when asleep as when awake. This has led to the suggestion that anaesthesia has less effect on the hypoxic ventilatory response itself, but may reduce the normally additive interaction between the ventilatory responses to hypoxia and hypercapnia (see Figure 5.7).[15,21]

It is generally agreed that the effect of anaesthetics on AHVR is on the peripheral chemoreceptors, possibly exclusively so at sedative levels.[22] Anaesthesia also impairs the ventilatory response to doxapram, which acts on the peripheral chemoreceptors (page 78).[13]

IMPLICATIONS OF THE DEPRESSION OF AHVR BY ANAESTHETIC AGENTS

There are four important practical implications of the attenuation of AHVR by anaesthesia:

1. Patients cannot act as their own hypoxia alarm by responding with hyperventilation.
2. Patients who have already lost their sensitivity to P_{CO_2} (e.g. some patients with chronic respiratory failure) may stop breathing after induction of anaesthesia has abolished their hypoxic drive.
3. Anaesthesia may be dangerous at very high altitude or in other situations where survival depends on hyperventilation in response to hypoxia (Chapter 17).
4. Because hypoxic drive is obtunded at subanaesthetic concentrations, this effect will persist into the early postoperative period after patients have regained consciousness and are apparently able to fend for themselves.

Recent uncertainty about the effect of subanaesthetic concentrations on AHVR has cast doubt on the validity of extrapolating the results of earlier studies to patients recovering from anaesthesia. The degree of stimulation of the patient is likely to affect their AHVR response, which will therefore be affected by many factors such as pain control and the amount of activity in their surroundings. A patient should behave like a poikilocapnic subject, and so depression of AHVR will be minimal.[9,21] Finally, patients recovering from an anaesthetic will frequently be hypercapnic secondary to opioid administration, sometimes compounded by airway obstruction. Under these circumstances the ventilatory response to the combination of hypoxia and hypercapnia is almost certainly reduced to less than that seen when awake.

There is little doubt that more research is needed to understand the complex effects of anaesthesia on ventilatory responses.[9,10,23] Though recent work may have cast some doubt on the earlier studies of Knill et al[13] (Figure 22.4), there remains plenty of evidence that a sleeping patient in the recovery room is at risk of failing to mount a suitable ventilatory response to hypoxia.

PATTERN OF CONTRACTION OF RESPIRATORY MUSCLES

One of the most remarkable examples of the specificity of anaesthetic actions is on the muscles associated with respiration. Many of these effects could hardly have been predicted but, nevertheless, have great clinical importance and underlie many of the secondary effects described later in this chapter.

THE PHARYNX

Anaesthesia usually causes obstruction of the pharyngeal airway unless measures are taken for its protection. Figure 22.6 shows changes in the sagittal geometry of the pharynx immediately after induction of anaesthesia with thiopentone in the supine position.[24] The soft palate falls against the posterior pharyngeal wall, occluding the nasopharynx in almost every patient, presumably due to interference with the action of some or all of tensor palati, palatoglossus or palatopharyngeus (page 83). Similar findings are also reported using magnetic resonance imaging, when the mean anteroposterior diameter of the pharynx at the level of the soft palate decreased from 6.6 mm when awake to 2.7 mm during propofol anaesthesia.[25] Radiographic studies have shown considerable posterior movement of tongue and epiglottis, but usually not sufficient to occlude the oral or hypopharyngeal airway (Figure 22.6). In animals, there is marked interference with genioglossus activity during anaesthesia,[26] and human observations

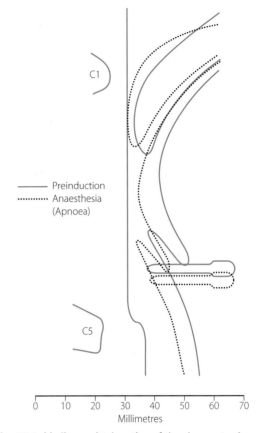

Fig. 22.6 Median sagittal section of the pharynx to show changes between the conscious state (continuous lines) and following induction of anaesthesia (broken lines). The most consistent change was occlusion of the nasopharynx. (Reproduced from reference 24 by permission of the Editor of the British Journal of Anaesthesia and Oxford University Press.)

have shown that thiopentone decreases the electromyographic (EMG) activity of genioglossus and the strap muscles.[27] Nevertheless, Nandi et al[24] showed that the posterior movement of the palate was not caused by pressure from the tongue.

Secondary changes occur when the patient attempts to breathe. Upstream obstruction then often causes major passive downstream collapse of the entire pharynx (Figure 22.7), a mechanism with features in common with the sleep apnoea hypopnoea syndrome (page 271). This secondary collapse of the pharynx is due to interference with the normal action of pharyngeal dilator muscles, particularly genioglossus. The epiglottis may be involved in hypopharyngeal obstruction during anaesthesia,[28]

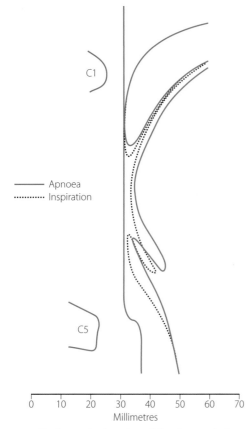

C1

——— Apnoea
·········· Inspiration

C5

0   10   20   30   40   50   60   70
Millimetres

Fig. 22.7 Median sagittal section of the pharynx during anaesthesia to show changes between the apnoeic state (continuous lines, corresponding to the broken lines in Figure 22.6) and following attempted inspiration (broken lines). Upstream obstruction in the nasopharynx results in downstream collapse of the oro- and hypopharynx. (Reproduced from reference 24 by permission of the Editor of the British Journal of Anaesthesia and Oxford University Press.)

and posterior movement is clearly seen in Figures 22.6 and 22.7.

Protection of the pharyngeal airway. Extension of the neck moves the origin of genioglossus anteriorly by 1–2 cm and usually clears the hypopharyngeal airway.[29] Protrusion of the mandible, originally proposed by Heiberg in 1874,[30] moves the origin of genioglossus still further forward. The use of a pharyngeal airway, such as that of Guedel, is frequently helpful, but the tip may become lodged in the valecula, or the tongue may be pushed downwards and backwards to obstruct the tip of the airway.[31] Developed by Brain in 1983,[32] the laryngeal mask airway provides an airtight seal around the laryngeal

perimeter allowing spontaneous ventilation. Use of a laryngeal mask does not prevent regurgitated gastric contents gaining access to the larynx, and with high airway pressures inspired gas may pass into the oesophagus or stomach during intermittent positive pressure ventilation (IPPV). For the most reliable maintenance of airway patency a tracheal tube is used, which requires the use of either 'deep' anaesthesia or muscle relaxants.

THE INSPIRATORY MUSCLES[2]

John Snow's early observations of respiration during anaesthesia describe that a decrease in thoracic respiratory excursion may be used as a sign of deepening anaesthesia. The effect was first quantified by Miller in 1925[33] and more precisely related to depth of anaesthesia with halothane in 1979.[34] Selective depression of some inspiratory ribcage muscles does occur. Electromyography of the parasternal intercostal muscles in humans shows their activity to be consistently abolished by 1 MAC of anaesthesia, and absent in some subjects at just 0.2 MAC.[35,36] Thiopentone decreases the EMG activity of sternothyroid, sternohyoid and the scalene muscles.[27] In contrast, diaphragmatic function seems to be well preserved during anaesthesia, particularly phasic EMG activity during inspiration. This combination of changes in muscle activity commonly gives rise to paradoxical inspiratory movements whereby diaphragmatic contraction causes expansion of the lower ribcage and abdomen whilst the upper ribcage is drawn in due to the negative intrathoracic pressure and a lack of support from upper ribcage respiratory muscles. This pattern of breathing is seen commonly in children, who have a more compliant chest wall than adults, and in adults when respiratory resistance is increased causing a greater fall in intrathoracic pressure. Some studies have, however, found no reduction in ribcage movement with, for example, isoflurane at 1 MAC[37] or ketamine.[38] It is possible that changes in spinal curvature during anaesthesia have caused earlier studies of ribcage movement to overestimate the changes.[35,39] Also, spontaneous ventilation via a tracheal tube is associated with greater airway resistance than other methods such as a laryngeal mask, which may contribute to less ribcage expansion during anaesthesia.[40] Thus earlier descriptions of selective depression of ribcage movement should not be regarded as an invariable feature of anaesthesia with spontaneous ventilation, particularly at the depth of anaesthesia used clinically and with a low-resistance, unobstructed airway.

The resting position and dimensions of the ribcage and diaphragm during anaesthesia are described below.

THE EXPIRATORY MUSCLES[41]

General anaesthesia causes expiratory phasic activity of the abdominal muscles, which are normally silent in the conscious supine subject. Anaesthetic agents, opioids and hypercapnia are all involved in stimulating the expiratory muscle activity. This activity begins in some subjects at only 0.2 MAC of halothane,[35] and is very difficult to abolish as long as spontaneous breathing continues.[42] Activation of expiratory muscles seems to serve no useful purpose and does not appear to have any significant effect on the change in functional residual capacity.[43]

Respiratory muscle co-ordination often becomes disturbed during anaesthesia with spontaneous ventilation.[37,40] Paradoxical movements between the upper and lower chest wall, and the chest and abdominal muscles, are accompanied by changes in respiratory timing between inspiratory and expiratory muscle groups. These are believed to originate in selective effects of anaesthesia on different respiratory neuronal groups in the central pattern generator,[36] and are more marked when airway resistance is higher.[40] The most usual pattern seen is a phase delay between abdominal and ribcage movement as illustrated in Figure 22.8.

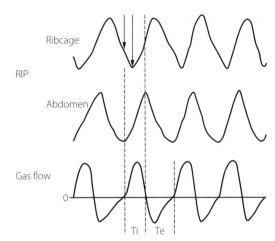

Fig. 22.8 Respiratory inductance plethysmography (RIP) tracings of ribcage and abdominal movements during 1.5 MAC halothane anaesthesia, and the accompanying respiratory gas flows. Note the phase delay between abdominal and ribcage movements, indicated by solid arrows, which in the example shown is approximately 30% of the inspiratory time. Ti, inspiratory time; Te, expiratory time. (After reference 44 with permission of the authors and the publishers of Anesthesiology.)

CHANGE IN FUNCTIONAL RESIDUAL CAPACITY

Bergman in 1963 was the first to report a decrease of functional residual capacity (FRC) during anaesthesia.[45] The reduction in FRC is now known to have the following characteristics:[43,46,47]

- FRC is reduced during anaesthesia with all anaesthetic drugs that have been investigated, by a mean value of about 16–20% of the awake FRC in the supine position. However, there is considerable individual variation and changes range from about +19% to −50%.
- FRC is reduced immediately on induction of anaesthesia, reaches its final value within the first few minutes, and does not seem to fall progressively throughout anaesthesia. It does not

return to normal until some hours after the end of anaesthesia.

- FRC is reduced to the same extent during anaesthesia whether the patient is paralysed or not.
- The reduction in FRC has a weak but significant correlation with the age of the patient.

THE CAUSE OF THE REDUCTION IN FRC[48]

There is general agreement that three factors may contribute to the reduced FRC, as follows.

Chest shape. Earlier studies that measured antero-posterior and lateral diameters, or the circumference, of the external chest wall gave conflicting results regarding changes in internal chest volume with anaesthesia. However, the introduction of fast computed tomography (CT) scanners led to the conclusion that there is a reduction in the cross-sectional area of the rib cage corresponding to a decrease in lung volume of about 200 ml.[49,50] A dynamic spatial reconstructor (DSR) technique allows scans of half the chest to be obtained in just 0.3 s, following which a three-dimensional picture of all chest structures can be generated and analysed.[35] This has confirmed that changes in chest wall shape account for a reduction in FRC of about 200 ml. There is less agreement about why the chest wall changes shape, possible explanations including the changes in respiratory muscle activity already described, diaphragmatic position and activity, or spinal curvature.

Diaphragm position. In the conscious subject in the supine position there is evidence of residual end-expiratory tone in the diaphragm,[51] which prevents the weight of the viscera pushing the diaphragm too far into the chest in the supine position. This diaphragmatic end-expiratory tone may be lost during anaesthesia. Such a change would result in the diaphragm moving cephalad during anaesthesia, which was reported in early studies.[50,52] However, other investigators found no consistent cephalad movement of the diaphragm during anaesthesia. Studies using DSR and fast computed tomography have provided good evidence that diaphragm *shape* alters during anaesthesia.[48,53] Although there is a large variation between subjects, these studies have consistently shown a cephalad movement of the dependent regions of the diaphragm, with little or no movement of the non-dependent regions.[35] One study found a significantly greater cephalad shift of the diaphragm in patients who were paralysed,[53] though this had not been observed in earlier studies. The change in FRC that can be ascribed to changes in diaphragm shape is on average less than 30 ml.[35] A summary of the changes in chest wall and diaphragm positions during anaesthesia is shown in Figure 22.9.

Thoracic blood volume. A shift of blood from the peripheral circulation into the chest during anaesthesia has been postulated as a cause of reduced FRC,[43] and one CT study seemed to demonstrate this.[54] However, this observation has not been confirmed,[35,50,55] and is currently regarded as an unlikely contributory factor to the reduced FRC.

ATELECTASIS DURING ANAESTHESIA[48]

'Miliary atelectasis' during anaesthesia was first proposed by Bendixen et al in 1963 as an explanation of the increased alveolar/arterial P_{O_2} difference during anaesthesia.[56] Conventional radiography, however, failed to show any appreciable areas of collapse, presumably due to most atelectasis being behind the diaphragm on anteroposterior radiographs (see below). Hedenstierna's group in Sweden were the first to demonstrate pulmonary opacities on CT scans of subjects during anaesthesia. These opacities usually occurred in the dependent areas of lung just above the

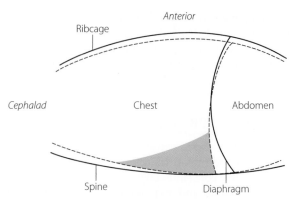

Fig. 22.9 Schematic diagram showing a mid-sagittal section of the chest wall and diaphragm awake (solid line) and during anaesthesia (dashed line). Note the reduction in rib cage volume, increased spinal curvature and change in diaphragmatic position. The shaded area shows where atelectasis usually occurs during anaesthesia.

diaphragm and were termed 'compression atelectasis' (Figure 22.10). Their extent correlated very strongly with the calculated intra-pulmonary shunt, and animal studies showed that the areas of opacity had a typical histological appearance of collapsed lung.[55]

Atelectasis occurs in between 75% and 90% of healthy individuals having general anaesthesia with muscle paralysis.[47,58] It occurs more commonly in children[59] because of their compliant chest wall, but is unrelated to age in adults. Atelectasis is most easily quantified from a single CT scan slice, taken immediately above the dome of the right diaphragm, and expressed as the percentage of the cross-sectional area containing atelectasis. The percentage of atelectasis during anaesthesia recorded in this way seems small, usually around 3%, but the atelectatic areas contain many more alveoli per unit volume than aerated lung, and this 3% of cross-sectional area equates to around 10% of lung tissue.[60]

CAUSES OF ATELECTASIS

There are three mechanisms involved, all closely interrelated, and it is likely that all three are involved in the formation of atelectasis in vivo.

Airway closure as a result of the reduced FRC may lead to atelectasis. In the supine position, the expiratory reserve volume has a mean value of approximately 1 litre in males and 600 ml in females. Therefore, the reduction in FRC following

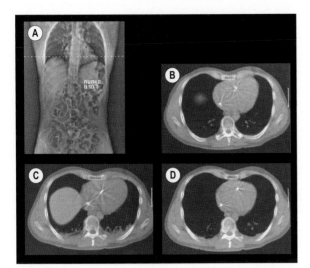

Fig. 22.10 Computed tomography of transverse sections of the thoracic cage (supine position) at the level shown in the scout view (A). (B) Control (awake) view. (C) Anaesthesia with zero end-expiratory pressure. Note the development of atelectasis in the dependent region of lung and some ascent of the right dome of the diaphragm. (D) The same patient with positive end-expiratory pressure, which reduces the amount of atelectasis. (Scans (A) and (B) are reproduced from reference 57 with the permission of the authors and the editors and publishers of Acta Anesthesiologica Scandinavica. I am indebted to the authors for supplying the other two scans.)

the induction of anaesthesia will bring the lung volume close to residual volume. This will tend to reduce the end-expiratory lung volume below the closing capacity (CC), particularly in older patients (see Figure 3.11), and so result in airway closure and collapse of lung. Pulmonary atelectasis can easily be demonstrated in conscious subjects who voluntarily breathe oxygen close to residual volume,[61] and Figure 22.11 shows the effect on arterial Po_2 of simulating the reduction in FRC that occurs during anaesthesia. Even if lung collapse does not occur, for example in younger patients, the airway narrowing caused by reduced lung volume creates areas with low ventilation/perfusion ($\dot{V}/\dot{Q}$) ratios that contribute to impaired gas exchange.[62]

An important aspect of this problem is whether CC remains constant during anaesthesia or whether it changes with FRC. Earlier studies by Hedenstierna and colleagues suggested that CC remained constant.[64] However, two other studies provided convincing evidence that FRC and CC are both reduced in parallel following the induction of anaesthesia.[65,66] It is possible that bronchodilatation caused by the anaesthetic counteracts the reduction in airway calibre that would be expected to result from the reduction in FRC (see below). The results of the last two studies suggest that there should be no increased tendency towards airway closure

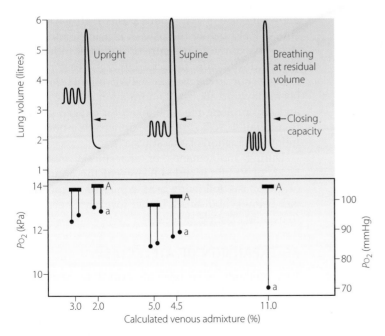

Fig. 22.11 Changes in tidal excursion relative to vital capacity in Dr Nunn when aged 45; arrows indicate the closing capacity. Ideal alveolar (A) Po_2 is shown by the horizontal bar and arterial (a) Po_2 by the black circles. Venous admixture was calculated on the assumption of an arterial/mixed venous oxygen content difference of 5 ml.dl^{-1}. (Reproduced from reference 63 by permission of the Editors of Acta Anaesthesiologica Scandinavica.)

during anaesthesia, but this is clearly at variance with Hedenstierna's work.[62]

Compression atelectasis may occur because of changes in chest wall and diaphragm position, which lead to the transmission of high intra-abdominal pressure to the chest and compression of areas of lung. As shown in Figure 22.9 the predominantly caudal distribution of atelectasis also points to a role for changes in the position of the dependent regions of the diaphragm.

Absorption atelectasis[67] develops when an airway becomes partially or totally closed and the gas contained within the pulmonary units distal to the airway is absorbed into the blood. Absorption of gas does not in itself cause atelectasis, but in effect accelerates collapse should airway closure occur from either of the preceding mechanisms. The rapid uptake of oxygen into the blood makes an important contribution to the development of absorption atelectasis (see below). The role of absorption in anaesthesia induced atelectasis is disputed.[67]

PREVENTION OF ATELECTASIS[68]

Recognition of atelectasis during anaesthesia has led to great interest in ways to prevent its occurrence. Several interesting findings have emerged.

Inspired oxygen concentration. Administration of high concentrations of oxygen during anaesthesia would be expected to promote atelectasis, and there is increasing evidence for this at a variety of stages during a general anaesthetic.

- Preoxygenation. An $F_{I_{O_2}}$ of 1.0 immediately prior to induction of anaesthesia leads to significantly more atelectasis than in patients with an $F_{I_{O_2}}$ of 0.3 or 0.21 during induction.[69,70] The crucial $F_{I_{O_2}}$ for worsening atelectasis seems to be above 0.6, as a study comparing an $F_{I_{O_2}}$ of 1.0, 0.8 or 0.6 found cross-sectional areas of atelectasis on CT scans following induction of 5.6%, 1.3% and 0.2% respectively.[71]
- Maintenance. Following re-expansion of atelectasis during anaesthesia (see below), a high inspired oxygen concentration causes a more rapid recurrence of atelectasis.[72,73] However, a study comparing an $F_{I_{O_2}}$ of 0.8 or 0.3 in nitrogen throughout anaesthesia and the early post-operative period did not find any differences in oxygenation post-operatively.[74]
- Before extubation. Use of a $F_{I_{O_2}}$ of 1.0 before removal of the tracheal tube at the completion of surgery is associated with more CT-

demonstrated atelectasis in the immediate post-operative period.[75]

Using 100% inspired oxygen before, during and at the conclusion of a general anaesthetic seems to be associated with greater severity of pulmonary atelectasis. These observations have led to the suggestion that it is time to challenge the routine use of 100% oxygen during anaesthesia.[76,77] Anaesthetists use 100% oxygen before induction and extubation to provide a longer time period before hypoxia occurs should there be difficulty in maintaining a patent airway. However, this safety period will be shortened only slightly by preoxygenating with an $F_{I_{O_2}}$ of 0.8, the use of which may significantly reduce the amount of atelectasis that occurs.[71]

Nitrous oxide. Mathematical modelling of the rate at which absorption atelectasis occurs suggests that using N_2O rather than N_2 with oxygen is unimportant.[78] Looking at diffusion of gases into and out of a closed lung unit, this model finds that the diffusion of N_2O into the lung unit from the mixed venous blood is faster than the diffusion of N_2 out of the lung unit, so its volume is maintained and collapse prevented. The in vivo situation is clearly more complex, and clinical studies of N_2O have given conflicting results.[79,80] Partial pressures of N_2O in lung units and blood are rarely in a steady state, and the time at which lung units become closed will vary, so causing unpredictable effects of N_2O on atelectasis (page 432).

Positive airway pressures. Application of a tight fitting face mask to the patient before induction allows the use of continuous positive airways pressure (CPAP) before the patient is asleep, and positive end expiratory pressure (PEEP) after induction. Using CPAP before induction may increase patient anxiety, but low levels of CPAP (6 cmH$_2$O) have been shown to abolish the formation of atelectasis[81] and also prolong the time taken for oxygen saturation to fall to 90% during the apnoea that normally follows induction of anaesthesia.[82]

During maintenance of anaesthesia moderate levels of PEEP (10 cmH$_2$O) prevent the occurrence of atelectasis following a re-expansion manoeuvre (see below),[83] but much higher levels are needed to re-expand existing atelectasis.

RE-EXPANSION OF ATELECTASIS

Two methods have been described to re-expand collapsed areas of lung, and these are shown in Figure 22.12.

Vital capacity manoeuvres. The first technique reported to re-expand atelectasis consisted of a series of hyperinflation manoeuvres using three breaths to an airway pressure of $30 \, cmH_2O$ followed by a final breath to $40 \, cmH_2O$, each sustained for 15 seconds (Figure 22.12A).[84] Between these large breaths normal IPPV is continued for 3–5 minutes. Computerised tomography assessment during this manoeuvre shows that the first hyperinflation of $30 \, cmH_2O$ reduces the area of atelectasis by half, and the subsequent inflations to $30 \, cmH_2O$ have little additional effect, but the final breath to $40 \, cmH_2O$ completely re-expands the atelectasis. Subsequent work by the same group showed that the inflation pressure of $40 \, cmH_2O$ did not need to be sustained for 15 seconds, with half of the atelectasis re-expanded after only 2 seconds, and all the atelectasis re-expanded after 7–8 seconds in three quarters of patients.[86]

PEEP. High levels of PEEP are required to re-expand atelectasis. Also, resolution of atelectasis is not complete and collapse recurs within minutes when PEEP is discontinued.[87] In addition, high levels of PEEP cause significant changes to $\dot{V}/\dot{Q}$ relationships within the lung and so may not improve oxygenation of the patient. Increasing levels of PEEP are more useful if used in conjunction with large

tidal volumes. One proposed technique involves increasing PEEP levels to $15 \, cmH_2O$, and then tidal volume is increased until peak airway pressures of $40 \, cmH_2O$ are achieved (Figure 22.12B).[85] This study did not use CT assessment but inferred re-expansion of atelectasis from improved arterial Po_2.

In both these techniques for re-expansion of atelectasis, airway pressures reach $40 \, cmH_2O$. An airway pressure this high is not without risk during anaesthesia, including the possibility of cardiovascular disturbances and pulmonary barotrauma (Chapter 32). In a similar fashion to PEEP, these recruitment manoeuvres reduce intrapulmonary shunt, but increase $\dot{V}/\dot{Q}$ mismatch such that there is often only a small improvement in oxygenation (see below).[84,85]

RESPIRATORY MECHANICS[88]

CALIBRE OF THE LOWER AIRWAYS[89]

Effect of reduced FRC. Figures 4.5 and 22.13 both show the hyperbolic relationship between lung volume and airway resistance. Figure 22.13 clearly shows that the curve is steep in the region of FRC

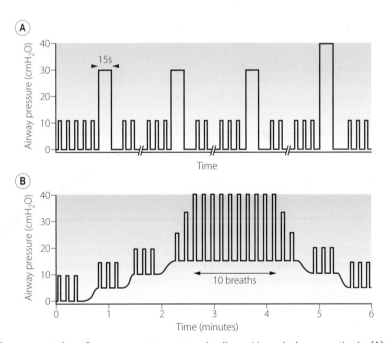

Fig. 22.12 Schematic representation of manoeuvres to re-expand collapsed lung during anaesthesia. (A) Vital capacity manoeuvre involving three large breaths sufficient to achieve airway pressures of $30 \, cmH_2O$ followed by a single breath to $40 \, cmH_2O$, each sustained for 15 seconds. The breaks on the abscissa represent 3–5 minutes of intermittent positive pressure ventilation with normal tidal volume. (B) Positive end-expiratory pressure (PEEP) and large tidal volumes showing progressive application of PEEP up to $15 \, cmH_2O$, followed by increased tidal volume until a peak airway pressure of $40 \, cmH_2O$ or tidal volume of $18 \, ml.kg^{-1}$ is achieved, which is then maintained for 10 breaths. (After references 84 and 85 by permission of the authors and Oxford University Press.)

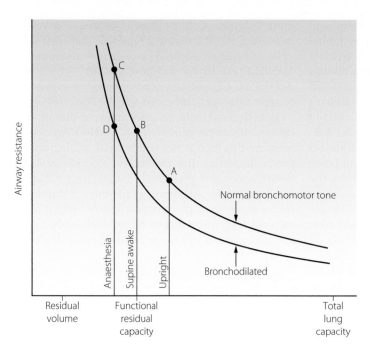

Fig. 22.13 Airway resistance as a function of lung volume with normal bronchomotor tone and when bronchodilated. A = upright and awake; B = supine and awake; C = supine and anaesthetised without bronchodilatation; D = supine, anaesthetised and with the degree of bronchodilatation that normally occurs during anaesthesia. Note that the airway resistance is similar at B and D, bronchodilatation approximately compensating for the decrease in FRC.

Table 22.1 Respiratory mechanics during anaesthesia

COMPLIANCE (STATIC)	ANAESTHETISED		AWAKE NORMAL RANGE	
	$l.kPa^{-1}$	$ml.cmH_2O^{-1}$	$l.kPa^{-1}$	$ml.cmH_2O^{-1}$
Respiratory system	0.81	81	0.5–1.9	47–190
Lungs	1.5	150	0.9–4.0	90–400
Chest wall	2.0	203	1.0–3.5	100–350
RESISTANCE	$kPa.l^{-1}.s$	$cmH_2O.l^{-1}.s$	$kPa.l^{-1}.s$	$cmH_2O.l^{-1}.s$
Respiratory system	0.48	4.8	0.12–0.44	1.2–4.4
Lung tissue/airway	0.35	3.5	0.07–0.24	0.7–2.4
Chest wall	0.13	1.3	0.05–0.20	0.5–2.0

Data during anaesthesia are in the supine position from reference 91.

in the supine position and therefore the reduction in FRC that occurs during anaesthesia might be expected to result in a marked increase in airway resistance. However, most anaesthetics are bronchodilators, as outlined in the following paragraphs, and, at least with halothane, this effect almost exactly offsets the effect of reduction in lung volume.[90] Thus total respiratory system resistance during anaesthesia is only slightly greater than in the awake supine subject, most of the change occurring in the lung/airway components rather than the chest wall (Table 22.1).[91] As would be expected, resistance increases

with increasing flow rate and decreases with increasing inflation volume during anaesthesia.[92]

Inhalational anaesthetics. All inhalational anaesthetics investigated have shown bronchodilator effects. Suppression of airway vagal reflexes, direct relaxation of airway smooth muscle[93] and inhibition of release of bronchoconstrictor mediators combine to cause an increase in airway conductance. In clinical concentrations, halothane reduces the amount of acetylcholine released from nerve terminals in response to nerve stimulation,[94] and suppresses the increase in both airway and tissue resistance following vagal

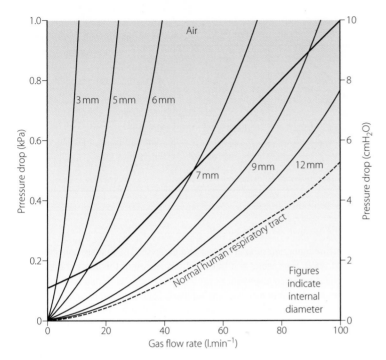

Fig. 22.14 Flow rate/pressure drop plots of a range of tracheal tubes, with their connectors and catheter mounts. The heavy line is the author's suggested upper limit of acceptable resistance for an adult. Pressure drop does not quite increase according to the fourth power of the radius because the catheter mount offered the same resistance throughout the range of tubes. With 70% N_2O/30% O_2, the pressure drop is about 40% greater for the same gas flow rate when flow is turbulent, but little different when the flow is chiefly laminar.

stimulation.[90] This appears to be more important than the direct effect of clinical concentrations of halothane on airway smooth muscle or histamine release from mast cells.[89]

Intravenous anaesthetics have similar effects to the inhalational anaesthetics. Their direct effects on smooth muscle are mostly weak in comparison with inhaled agents, and in clinical practice their ability to attenuate neural reflex bronchoconstriction predominates.

OTHER SITES OF INCREASED AIRWAY RESISTANCE

Breathing systems. Excessive resistance or obstruction may arise in apparatus such as breathing systems, valves, connectors and tracheal tubes. The tubes may be kinked, the lumen blocked or the cuff may herniate and obstruct the lower end, which may also abut against the carina or the side wall of the trachea. A reduction in diameter of a tracheal tube greatly increases its resistance, the pattern of flow being intermediate between laminar and turbulent for the conditions shown in Figure 22.14. Resistance imposed by a laryngeal mask airway is less than that of a corresponding size of tracheal tube.[95]

The pharynx and larynx. The pharynx is commonly obstructed during anaesthesia by the mechanisms described earlier in this chapter, unless active steps are taken to preserve patency. Reflex laryngospasm is still possible at depths of anaesthesia that suppress other airway protective reflexes. In most cases the spasm eventually resolves spontaneously, but it may be improved by application of CPAP or terminated by neuromuscular blockade.

COMPLIANCE

Total respiratory system compliance is reduced during anaesthesia to a figure approaching the lower end of the normal range (Table 22.1).[91] Both static and dynamic measurements (page 38) are reduced compared with the awake state.[92] Compliance seems to be reduced very early in anaesthesia and the change is not progressive.

Figure 22.15 summarises the effect of anaesthesia on the pressure/volume relationships of the lung and chest wall. The diagram shows the major differences between the conscious state and anaesthesia. There are only minor differences between anaesthesia with and without paralysis. The left-hand section shows the relationship for the whole respiratory system comprising lungs plus chest wall. The curves obtained during anaesthesia clearly show the reduction in FRC (lung volume with zero pressure gradient from alveoli to ambient).

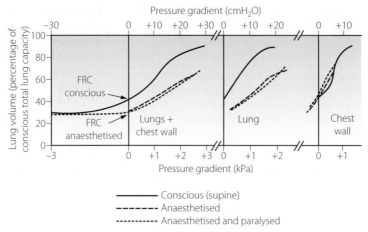

Fig. 22.15 Pressure/volume relationships before and after the induction of anaesthesia and paralysis. The first section shows the relationship for the respiratory system (lungs and chest wall). The second and third sections represent the lungs and the chest wall respectively. There are only insignificant differences between observations during anaesthesia with and without paralysis. There are, however, major differences in pressure volume relationships of the lung and total respiratory system following the induction of anaesthesia. Arrows indicate the FRC, which, during anaesthesia, is only slightly greater than the residual volume. (After reference 96.)

Application of a positive pressure as high as 30cmH$_2$O (3kPa) to the airways expands the lungs to barely 70% of the preoperative total lung capacity, which implies a reduced overall compliance. Table 22.1 and the two sections on the right of Figure 22.15 show that the major changes are in the lung rather than the chest wall.

The cause of this observed reduction in lung compliance has been difficult to explain. There is no convincing evidence that anaesthesia affects pulmonary surfactant in humans at clinically used concentrations. A more likely explanation is that the reduced lung compliance is simply the consequence of breathing at reduced lung volume. Strapping the chest of volunteers, thereby decreasing their lung volume, results in a decrease in pulmonary compliance that can be restored to normal by taking a maximal inspiration.[97] This suggests that pulmonary atelectasis is the explanation, and that ventilation with normal tidal volumes to a smaller lung volume will inevitably reduce the lung compliance.

GAS EXCHANGE

Every factor influencing gas exchange may be altered during anaesthesia, and many of the changes must be considered as normal features of the anaesthetised state. These 'normal' changes usually pose no threat to the patient, since their effects can easily be overcome by such simple means as increasing the concentration

of oxygen in the inspired gas and the minute volume. The 'normal' changes may be contrasted with a range of pathological alterations in gas exchange that may arise during anaesthesia from such circumstances as airway obstruction, apnoea, bronchospasm or pneumothorax. These may be life threatening and require urgent action for their correction.

The major changes that adversely affect gas exchange during anaesthesia are reduced minute volume of ventilation (described above), increased dead space and shunt (considered in terms of the three compartment model described on page 126 and in Figure 8.8) and altered distribution of ventilation and perfusion in relation to ventilation/perfusion ($\dot{V}/\dot{Q}$) ratios.

DEAD SPACE (see page 128)

The increase in physiological dead space during anaesthesia was first observed in 1958.[98] With allowance for the apparatus dead space of the tracheal tube and its connections, the dead space/tidal volume ratio *from carina downwards* averages 32% during anaesthesia with either spontaneous or artificial ventilation.[99] This is approximately equal to the ratio for the normal conscious subject *including trachea, pharynx and mouth* (approximately 70 ml). Physiological dead space equals the sum of its anatomical and alveolar components, and the sub-carinal anatomical dead space is not normally

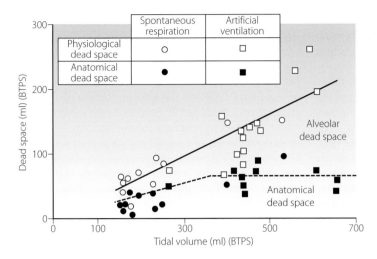

Fig. 22.16 Data and regression lines for physiological and anatomical dead space (the difference indicating alveolar dead space) as a function of tidal volume. There were no significant differences between anaesthesia with and without paralysis. Note the range over which physiological dead space appeared to be a constant fraction of tidal volume. Anatomical dead space was constant above a tidal volume of 350 ml, resulting in increased alveolar dead space. (After reference 99 by permission of the Editor and publishers of the Journal of Applied Physiology.)

increased. Therefore, the increase in sub-carinal physiological dead space during anaesthesia must be in the alveolar component.

Anatomical dead space. In the study of Nunn & Hill[99] (Figure 22.16), sub-carinal anatomical dead space was always significantly less than physiological, reaching a maximum of about 70 ml at tidal volumes above 350 ml. This roughly accords with the expected geometric dimensions of the lower respiratory tract. At smaller tidal volumes, the anatomical dead space was less than the expected geometric volume. Values of less than 30 ml were recorded in some patients with tidal volumes of less than 250 ml. This is attributed to axial streaming and the mixing effect of the heart beat, and is clearly an important and beneficial factor in patients with depressed breathing.

Alveolar dead space increases with tidal volume so that the sum of anatomical and alveolar (= physiological) dead space remains about 32% of tidal volume (Figure 22.16). The cause of the increase in alveolar dead space during uncomplicated general anaesthesia is not immediately obvious. There is no evidence that it is due to pulmonary hypotension causing development of a zone 1 (page 105) and the reduced vertical height of the lung in the supine position would mitigate against this. The alternative explanation is maldistribution with overventilation of *relatively* underperfused alveoli. Studies of ventilation/perfusion relationships outlined below give some support to this view, but such patterns of maldistribution have not invariably been observed during anaesthesia.

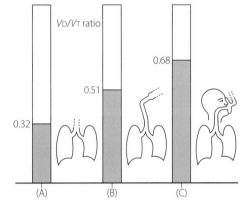

Fig. 22.17 Physiological plus apparatus dead space (where applicable) as a fraction of tidal volume in anaesthetised patients: (A) from carina downwards; (B) including tracheal tube or laryngeal mask airway and connector; and (C) including upper airway, facemask and connector.

Apparatus dead space. Use of a tracheal tube or laryngeal mask airway (LMA) will bypass much of the normal anatomical dead space arising in the mouth and pharynx. However, for practical purposes the apparatus dead space of the tracheal tube or LMA[100] and their connections must be included for the purpose of calculating alveolar ventilation during anaesthesia. The total dead space then increases to about 50% of tidal volume (Figure 22.17). When using a facemask, it is necessary to add the volume of the mask and its connections to the physiological dead space, which now also includes trachea, pharynx and mouth. The total dead space then amounts to about two-thirds of the tidal volume.[101] Thus, a seemingly adequate minute volume of 6l.min^{-1} may be expected to result in an alveolar ventilation of only 2l.min^{-1}, which would almost inevitably result in hypercapnia.

Compensation for increased dead space may be made by increasing the minute volume to maintain the alveolar ventilation. In artificially ventilated anaesthetised patients the problem hardly exists. The patient may have a large dead space, but the high minute volumes that are usually selected provide more than adequate compensation. Thus the alveolar ventilation is almost always greater than necessary for carbon dioxide homoeostasis. With monitoring of end-expiratory $P\text{CO}_2$, there is seldom any difficulty in maintaining a normal value. However, the existence of an alveolar dead space means that the arterial $P\text{CO}_2$ during anaesthesia is usually 0.5–1kPa (3.8–7.5mmHg) greater than the end-expiratory $P\text{CO}_2$.

In the case of the hypoventilating patient who is allowed to breathe spontaneously during anaesthesia, the reduction in dead space at smaller tidal volumes shown in Figure 22.16 prevents some of the alveolar hypoventilation that would be expected if the *volume* of the dead space remained constant. This, together with the reduced metabolic rate, results in the hypercapnia being much less than the values for minute volume sometimes observed during anaesthesia might lead one to expect. No doubt, over the years, many patients have owed their lives to these factors.

SHUNT

Magnitude of the change during anaesthesia. In the conscious healthy subject, the shunt or venous admixture amounts to only 1–2% of cardiac output (page 133). This results in an alveolar/arterial $P\text{O}_2$ gradient of less than 1kPa (7.5mmHg) in the young healthy subject breathing air, but the gradient increases with age and lung disease. During anaesthesia, the alveolar/arterial $P\text{O}_2$ difference is usually increased to a value that corresponds to an average shunt of about 10%. Formal measurements of pulmonary venous admixture, taking into account the mixed venous oxygen content, have also been made and these concur with shunts being of the order of 10%. This provides an acceptable basis for predicting arterial $P\text{O}_2$ during an uncomplicated anaesthetic and it also permits calculation of the concentration of oxygen in the inspired gas that will provide an acceptable arterial $P\text{O}_2$. Some 30–40% inspired oxygen is usually adequate in an uncomplicated anaesthetic.

The cause of the venous admixture during anaesthesia. About half of the observed venous admixture is true shunt through the areas of atelectasis described above. There is a very strong correlation between the shunt (measured as perfusion of alveoli with a $\dot{V}/\dot{Q}$ ratio of less than 0.005) and the area or volume of atelectasis seen on CT scans.[47,49] Studies using isotope techniques have demonstrated intrapulmonary shunting in the same areas of lung where atelectasis is seen on CT scans.[102] However, the venous admixture during anaesthesia also contains components due to dispersion of the $\dot{V}/\dot{Q}$ distribution, and to perfusion of alveoli with low $\dot{V}/\dot{Q}$ ratios (0.005–0.1).

VENTILATION/PERFUSION RELATIONSHIPS[103]

The three-compartment model of the lung (page 126) provides a definition of lung function in terms of dead space and shunt, parameters that are easily measured, reproducible and provide a basis for corrective therapy. Nevertheless, it does not pretend to provide a true picture of what is going on in the lung. A far more sophisticated approach is provided by the analysis of the distribution of pulmonary ventilation and perfusion in terms of $\dot{V}/\dot{Q}$ ratios by the multiple inert gas elimination technique (page 126), and studies during anaesthesia have been reported.[49,62,103]

During general anaesthesia and paralysis both ventilation and perfusion are found to be distributed to a wider range of $\dot{V}/\dot{Q}$ ratios than when awake (Figure 22.18).[69,104] Other studies have also found substantial $\dot{V}/\dot{Q}$ mismatch during anaesthesia and paralysis, with ventilation being preferentially distributed to ventral areas and vice versa for perfusion.[102] In the healthy young subject shown in Figure 22.18, the true intrapulmonary shunt had a mean value of less than 1% during anaesthesia, but the alveolar/arterial $P\text{O}_2$ gradient was slightly increased and this was attributed to the increased spread of the distribution of perfusion to areas of poorer ventilation (lower $\dot{V}/\dot{Q}$ ratio). Anatomical dead space was reduced, largely because of tracheal intubation, but alveolar dead space was increased, partly due to increased spread of distribution of ventilation to areas of poorer perfusion (higher $\dot{V}/\dot{Q}$ ratio).

Effect of age on $\dot{V}/\dot{Q}$ ratios during anaesthesia. In awake subjects, increasing age causes a widening of the distribution of $\dot{V}/\dot{Q}$ ratios, and the distribution widens still further with anaesthesia.[49] It would thus be expected that intrapulmonary shunt during anaesthesia would also increase with age, but studies

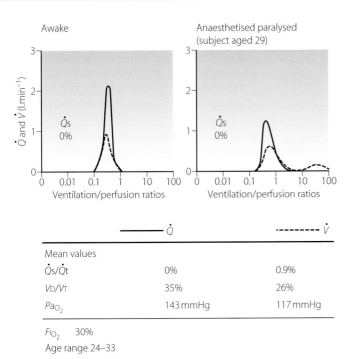

Fig. 22.18 Distribution of ventilation and perfusion as a function of ventilation/perfusion ratios in the awake and anaesthetised paralysed subject. (Adapted from reference 104 and reproduced from reference 105 by permission of the publishers.)

Mean values		
$\dot{Q}s/\dot{Q}t$	0%	0.9%
V_D/V_T	35%	26%
Pa_{O_2}	143 mmHg	117 mmHg

$F_{I_{O_2}}$ 30%

Age range 24–33

of this effect have produced conflicting results. One study involving typical surgical patients with ages ranging from 37 to 64 found that the true intrapulmonary shunt was increased during anaesthesia.[106] However, the shunt calculated from the alveolar/arterial P_{O_2} gradient according to the three-compartment lung model would be larger still, and the difference would be due to perfusion of areas of low $\dot{V}/\dot{Q}$ ratio. A second study of elderly patients (mean age 60) who all had some deterioration in pulmonary function showed wide variations in pulmonary shunt.[107] The results of this study can most easily be appreciated by considering the patients in three groups (Figure 22.19). In the first, there was only a small increase in the true shunt following the induction of anaesthesia but there appeared a 'shelf' of perfusion of regions with very low $\dot{V}/\dot{Q}$ ratios in the range 0.01–0.1. In the second group, this 'shelf' was less prominent but there was a substantial increase in true shunt. Finally, in the third group, there was both a 'shelf' and an increase in true shunt. All of these changes are compatible with a decrease in FRC below closing capacity.

Finally, a study by Gunnarsson et al[49] involved 45 patients of age range 23–69 years. They reached the surprising conclusion that atelectasis (as seen with CT) and true intrapulmonary shunt (determined by multiple inert gas elimination technique as alveoli with $\dot{V}/\dot{Q}$ ratio less than 0.005) did not relate to age.

However, both were substantially increased during anaesthesia and correlated with each other. It is difficult to reconcile the lack of correlation between age and shunt with the striking differences seen in previous studies. Nevertheless, this study confirmed the enhanced decline in arterial P_{O_2} with increasing age during anaesthesia, and venous admixture (calculated as for the three-compartment model) was increased significantly from a mean value of 5.5% of cardiac output before anaesthesia, to 9.2% during anaesthesia. Venous admixture increased steeply with age (0.17% per year), and this was attributed to an age-dependent increase in the spread of $\dot{V}/\dot{Q}$ ratios (Figure 22.20) and to greater perfusion of alveoli with low $\dot{V}/\dot{Q}$ ratios (0.005–0.1).

Effect of PEEP. It has long been known that, in contrast to the situation in intensive care, PEEP often does little to improve the arterial P_{O_2} during anaesthesia.[108] There are two reasons why PEEP is not associated with improved oxygenation. First, the decrease in cardiac output associated with PEEP reduces the saturation of the blood traversing the remaining shunt and so reduces arterial P_{O_2}.[106] Secondly, PEEP increases ventilation of alveoli with high $\dot{V}/\dot{Q}$ ratio, so further increasing overall $\dot{V}/\dot{Q}$ mismatch. The essential difference from the patient undergoing critical care is probably the lack of protection of intrathoracic blood vessels from raised

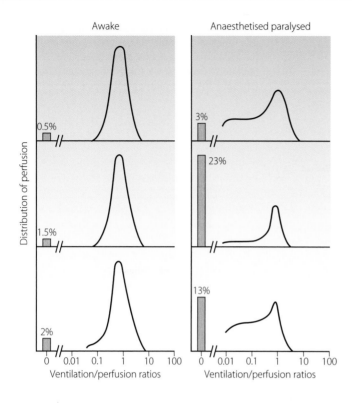

Awake   Anaesthetised paralysed

Fig. 22.19 Changes in pulmonary perfusion as a function of ventilation/perfusion ratios following induction of anaesthesia in elderly patients. Numbers to the left of each block indicate the shunt. (Adapted from reference 107 and reproduced from reference 105 by permission of the publishers.)

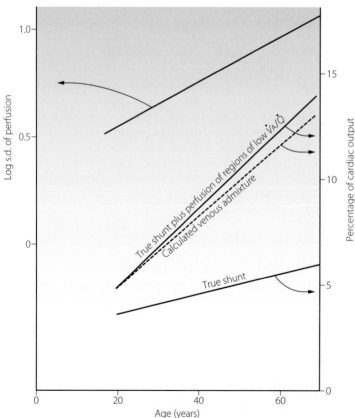

Fig. 22.20 Age-dependence of various factors influencing alveolar/arterial P_{O_2} difference during anaesthesia.[49] The logarithm of standard deviation of distribution of perfusion is significantly greater during anaesthesia (shown) than when awake (not shown) and has a significant regression against age under both circumstances. True shunt is significantly increased almost tenfold compared with before anaesthesia, but the correlation with age is not significant. Perfusion of areas of poorly ventilated regions ($0.005 < \dot{V}/\dot{Q} < 0.1$) was significantly increased compared with before anaesthesia and correlated with age in both circumstances. Venous admixture here refers to the value obtained from the shunt equation (page 132) and agrees well with the sum of shunt and perfusion of regions of low $\dot{V}/\dot{Q}$.

airway pressure that is afforded by stiff lungs in most patients requiring critical care.

Other factors affecting $\dot{V}/\dot{Q}$ ratio during anaesthesia. Hypoxic pulmonary vasoconstriction (HPV) contributes to maintaining a normal $\dot{V}/\dot{Q}$ ratio by reducing perfusion to underventilated alveoli (page 108). Inhalational anaesthetics inhibit HPV (page 346) and so in theory may worsen $\dot{V}/\dot{Q}$ mismatch during anaesthesia. There is some evidence from animal studies that this is the case,[103] and one human study of anaesthesia with intravenous barbiturates, which are believed to have less effect on HPV, demonstrated only a small amount of intrapulmonary shunting.[109] High concentrations of inspired oxygen will inhibit HPV by maintaining alveolar P_{O_2} at a high level even in poorly ventilated alveoli. Some work has shown that lower inspired oxygen concentrations during anaesthesia (30%) are associated with less $\dot{V}/\dot{Q}$ scatter than when breathing 100% oxygen.[69]

SUMMARY

These studies of $\dot{V}/\dot{Q}$ relationships during anaesthesia complement one another and give us greatly increased insight into the effect of anaesthesia on gas exchange. We are now in a position to summarise the effect of anaesthesia on gas exchange as follows:

- Uniformity of distribution of ventilation and perfusion is decreased by anaesthesia. The magnitude of the change is age-related and may be affected by the inspired oxygen concentration and anaesthetic agents used.
- The increase in alveolar dead space appears to be due to increased distribution of ventilation

to areas of high (but not usually infinite) $\dot{V}/\dot{Q}$ ratios.

- Venous admixture is increased in anaesthesia to a mean value of about 10%, but the change is markedly affected by age, being minimal in the young.
- The increased venous admixture during anaesthesia is due partly to an increase in true intrapulmonary shunt (due to atelectasis), and partly to increased distribution of perfusion to areas of low (but not zero) $\dot{V}/\dot{Q}$ ratios. The latter component increases with age.
- The major differences are between the awake and the anaesthetised states. Paralysis and artificial ventilation do not greatly alter the parameters of gas exchange in spite of the different spatial distribution of ventilation.
- Both PEEP and lung hyperinflation manoeuvres reduce the shunt, but the beneficial effect on arterial P_{O_2} is offset by greater $\dot{V}/\dot{Q}$ mismatch and a decrease in cardiac output which reduces the mixed venous oxygen content.

Typical values for the various factors discussed are shown in Table 22.2.

OTHER EFFECTS OF GENERAL ANAESTHESIA ON THE RESPIRATORY SYSTEM

RESPONSE TO ADDED RESISTANCE

The preceding sections would lead one to expect that anaesthesia would cause grave impairment of the

Table 22.2 Changes in factors influencing gas exchange after induction of anaesthesia				
	AWAKE	**ANAESTHETISED**		
		SPONTANEOUS VENTILATION	**IPPV**	**IPPV + PEEP**
$F_{I_{O_2}}$	0.21	0.4	0.4	0.4
$\dot{Q}s/\dot{Q}t$ (%)	1.6	6.2	8.6	4.1
V_D/V_T (%)	30	35	38	44
Cardiac output (l.min^{-1})	6.1	5.0	4.5	3.7
Pa_{O_2} (kPa)	10.5	17.6	18.8	20.5
Pa_{O_2} (mmHg)	79	132	141	153
$\dot{V}$ – mean $\dot{V}/\dot{Q}$	0.81	1.3	2.20	3.03
$\dot{Q}$ – mean $\dot{V}/\dot{Q}$	0.47	0.51	0.83	0.55
Adapted from reference 106 and reproduced from reference 105 by permission of the publishers.				

ability of a patient to increase their work of breathing in the face of added resistance. Surprisingly, this is not the case and anaesthetised patients preserve a remarkable ability to overcome added resistance.[110,111] The anaesthetised patient responds to inspiratory loading in two phases. First, there is an instant augmentation of the force of contraction of the inspiratory muscles, mainly the diaphragm, during the first loaded breath.[51] Detection of the inspiratory resistance may be mediated by either airway or lung receptors, and is only slightly inhibited by anaesthesia.[112] The second response is much slower and overshoots when the loading is removed, and the time course suggests that this is mediated by an increase in P_{CO_2}.[110] In combination, these two mechanisms enable the anaesthetised patient to achieve good compensation with inspiratory loading up to about 0.8 kPa (8 cmH$_2$O). Even more remarkable is the preservation of the elaborate response to expiratory resistance (see Figure 4.10), with a large *increase* in minute volume occurring with expiratory resistive loading during enflurane anaesthesia.[113]

HYPOXIC PULMONARY VASOCONSTRICTION[114,115]

The contribution to $\dot{V}/\dot{Q}$ mismatch of disturbed HPV during anaesthesia has already been described above, but the effects of anaesthesia on HPV merit further discussion. Early animal studies using isolated lungs found that several inhalational anaesthetics inhibit HPV, but no such effect was found with intravenous anaesthetics. Although in vitro studies gave clear evidence that inhalational anaesthetics depressed HPV, in vivo studies were inconsistent. One cause of this inconsistency was found to be the concomitant depression of cardiac output by inhalational anaesthetics.[114] In Chapter 7 it was explained how hypoxia influences pulmonary vascular resistance not only by the alveolar P_{O_2} but also, in part, by the mixed venous P_{O_2}. A reduction in cardiac output must decrease the mixed venous P_{O_2} if oxygen consumption remains unchanged, and this would intensify pulmonary vasoconstriction. Thus, on the one hand, an inhalational anaesthetic will inhibit HPV by direct action while, on the other hand, it may intensify HPV by reducing mixed venous P_{O_2} as a result of decreasing cardiac output. Thus most investigators' results are consistent with the view that inhalational anaesthetics depress HPV provided that allowance is made for the effect of concomitant changes of cardiac output.[114] An example of when HPV may be relevant in clinical anaesthesia is during one-lung ventilation which is described on page 498.

SPECIAL CONDITIONS ARISING DURING ANAESTHESIA

One-lung ventilation during anaesthesia is described on page 498.

OBESITY

Obese patients already have a small FRC when supine, and the further reduction with anaesthesia results in an exponential decrease in FRC during anaesthesia with increasing body mass index.[116] Similarly, with increasing obesity there is a greater fall in lung compliance and increase in lung resistance under anaesthesia.[116] Obese patients develop larger amounts of atelectasis during anaesthesia, and re-expansion manoeuvres as described above are particularly effective in these patients, often leading to a sustained improvement in oxygenation.[73,84] Although PEEP may not be particularly useful in preventing the respiratory changes with anaesthesia in non-obese subjects, in morbidly obese patients (BMI = 40 kg m^{-2}) modest levels of PEEP (10 cmH$_2$O) improve elastance and oxygenation.[117,118]

PATIENT POSITION

Lateral. In Chapter 8 it was explained that, in the lateral position, there is preferential distribution of inspired gas to the lower lung (see Table 8.1) and this accords approximately with the distribution of pulmonary blood flow. This favourable distribution of inspired gas is disturbed by anaesthesia whether respiration is spontaneous or artificial in the paralysed patient, with preferential ventilation of the non-dependent (upper) lung and continued preferential perfusion of the dependent lung. This predictably leads to a greater spread of $\dot{V}/\dot{Q}$ ratios and a further fall in P_{O_2} compared with the supine position.[119] Atelectasis seen on CT scanning forms only in the dependent lung, but the overall amount of atelectasis and the intrapulmonary shunt are similar to that seen when anaesthetised and paralysed when supine (see page 499 and Figure 33.3).[119]

Prone. A patient anaesthetised in the prone position should have the upper chest and pelvis supported, to allow free movement of the abdomen and lower chest. In subjects anaesthetised and paralysed in this position, respiratory mechanics are only minimally affected, and both FRC and arterial P_{O_2} are greater than when supine.[91] A study using the DSR showed that with anaesthesia in the prone position, motion of non-dependent areas of the diaphragm predominates, leading the authors to suggest a difference in the anatomical structure between dorsal and ventral areas of the diaphragm.[120] Other explanations for improved oxygenation when prone include more uniform lung perfusion and less ventilation of, or atelectasis formation in, dependent areas of lung that are reduced in volume by the presence of the mediastinum and heart.[91]

LAPAROSCOPIC SURGERY[121,122]

In comparison with open surgery, the benefits of many laparoscopic procedures are now well established and have led to an expansion in the number of surgical procedures carried out via laparoscopy. As confidence in, and understanding of, the technique improves, procedures become more complex, more prolonged, and are attempted in less fit patients.

Absorption of gas from the peritoneal cavity depends on the partial pressure of gas present and its solubility in peritoneal tissue. Gas mixtures are rarely used, so the partial pressure is normally equal to the insufflation pressure. Insoluble gases such as helium or nitrogen would be absorbed to a much smaller extent, but would also be more disastrous during the rare complication of gas embolus. Air, oxygen and nitrous oxide all support combustion so prevent the use of diathermy which is fundamental to laparoscopic surgery. Thus carbon dioxide remains the usual gas used for the erroneously named 'pneumoperitoneum'. Laparoscopic operations involve the insufflation of CO_2 into the peritoneum to a pressure of 10–15 mmHg, and normally also involve positioning the patient head-up (for upper abdominal surgery) or head-down (for lower abdominal and pelvic procedures). These procedures have two adverse effects on respiration.

Respiratory mechanics. In addition to the changes already described for general anaesthesia, the increased intra-abdominal pressure during laparoscopy causes further restriction of the diaphragm and lower chest wall. Respiratory system compliance is significantly reduced,[121] sometimes accompanied by increased airway resistance, particularly in obese patients.[123] An increase in airway pressures invariably occurs. The head-up position may alleviate some of these changes, but patients in the head-down position during laparoscopy have a further cause for substantially reduced compliance. In healthy patients, these significant changes in respiratory system mechanics have only a small effect on $\dot{V}/\dot{Q}$ distribution. A study of nine healthy patients using MIGET to characterise $\dot{V}/\dot{Q}$ ratios found only a transient reduction in pulmonary shunt and no significant changes in alveolar dead space or in areas of abnormally high or low $\dot{V}/\dot{Q}$ ratios.[124]

Carbon dioxide absorption.[125] Transperitoneal absorption of CO_2 into the blood begins within a few minutes of commencing a laparoscopic procedure, and is estimated to be 30–50 ml.min^{-1}. If ventilation remains unchanged, this will quickly increase arterial $P\text{CO}_2$, and CO_2 will begin diffusing into the medium and slow compartments of the body's huge CO_2 stores (see page 170 and Figure 10.10). After a prolonged procedure, with elevated Pa_{CO_2}, hypercapnia may be present for many hours post-operatively as the CO_2 stores empty.[121] Unfortunately, this is a period when the patient is no longer receiving artificial ventilation and is recovering from a general anaesthetic and so may struggle to meet the increased ventilatory requirement. Increasing the minute volume during surgery should allow the maintenance of a normal Pa_{CO_2} to prevent this scenario developing. In patients who are obese or have respiratory disease, the changes in compliance described previously will further impair the excretion of CO_2 and require an even larger minute volume. End-tidal CO_2 monitoring may be used to estimate the required ventilation, but in many patients $\dot{V}/\dot{Q}$ disturbances mean that there may be a large, and unpredictable, end-tidal to arterial $P\text{CO}_2$ gradient,[121] and measurement of Pa_{CO_2} may be required.

REGIONAL ANAESTHESIA

Epidural or spinal anaesthesia may be expected to influence the respiratory system, either by a central effect of drugs absorbed from the spinal canal or by affecting the pattern or strength of contraction of respiratory muscle groups.[126] These affects are generally small, but of great importance in view of the tendency to use regional anaesthetic techniques in patients with respiratory disease or in obstetric practice when respiratory function is already abnormal (Chapter 14).

CONTROL OF BREATHING

Thoracic epidural anaesthesia may cause a small reduction in resting tidal volume as a result of reduced rib cage movement.[127,128] Predictably this does not occur following lumbar epidural anaesthesia.[129] Studies of hypercapnic and hypoxic ventilatory responses during epidural anaesthesia have produced conflicting results. Thoracic anaesthesia may reduce the ventilatory response to hypercapnia by inhibition of intercostal muscle activity. Lumbar epidurals have been reported to *increased* the response to hypercapnia,[127,130] which is believed to be stimulated by anxiety (the study was performed immediately prior to surgery),[127] or because of a direct stimulant effect of lignocaine on the respiratory centre.[130] The acute hypoxic ventilatory response is unaffected by thoracic epidural anaesthesia, but lumbar epidurals may increase ventilation in response to hypoxia by a poorly understood mechanism.[127,128]

Respiratory muscle function has been extensively studied using EMGs and the DSR during high lumbar (block up to T1 dermatome) epidural anaesthesia,[131] and confirmed the reduced contribution of the rib cage to resting ventilation. Functional residual capacity was increased by 300 ml as a result of both caudad movement of the diaphragm and reduced thoracic blood volume. In spite of these changes, most respiratory function measurements remain essentially unchanged during epidural anaesthesia with only small changes in forced vital capacity and peak expiratory flow rate.[132] The situation is quite different in late pregnancy, when regional anaesthesia is commonly employed. Significant reductions in forced vital capacity and peak expiratory flow have been reported after spinal anaesthesia,[133] with lesser changes following epidural anaesthesia.[134] Peak expiratory pressure, a measure of abdominal muscle activity, was also decreased after lumbar epidural for Caesarean section, particularly when bupivacaine was used.[135]

Oxygenation during epidural anaesthesia is largely unaffected. In a study by Hedenstierna's group, lumbar epidural anaesthesia produced no changes in $\dot{V}/\dot{Q}$ relationships or pulmonary shunt, and no CT evidence of atelectasis except in one subject with a higher than normal body mass index in the lithotomy position.[136]

RESPIRATORY FUNCTION IN THE POSTOPERATIVE PERIOD[137]

EARLY POST-ANAESTHETIC RECOVERY

In the first few minutes of recovery, alveolar Po_2 may be reduced by elimination of nitrous oxide, which dilutes alveolar oxygen (diffusion hypoxia) and carbon dioxide, but this effect is usually transient. Hypoxia is very common during transfer to the recovery room when monitoring is often interrupted.[138] Airway obstruction, often associated with residual muscle paralysis, is a common potential cause of hypoxia shortly after anaesthesia. This may be compounded by the residual effects of anaesthetic agents on ventilatory control that have been described above. Both reduced FRC and the increased alveolar/arterial Po_2 gradient observed during anaesthesia usually return to normal during the first few hours after minor operations.

LATE POSTOPERATIVE RESPIRATORY CHANGES

Following major surgery, the restoration of a normal alveolar/arterial Po_2 gradient may take several days, and episodes of hypoxia are common. There are several contributory factors.

Lung volume and atelectasis. There is a continued reduction in FRC, usually reaching its lowest value 1–2 days postoperatively, before slowly returning to normal values within a week.[139] Reduction of the FRC is greatest in patients having surgery near the diaphragm, that is, upper abdominal or thoracic incisions,[140] but is less following laparoscopic surgery in the upper abdomen.[141] Atelectasis seen on CT scans during anaesthesia persists for at least 24 hours in patients having major surgery.[142] The effects of these changes on $\dot{V}/\dot{Q}$ relationships and oxygenation will be similar to those seen during anaesthesia, but the provision of adequate inspired oxygen concentration is now far less reliable.

Effort-dependent lung function tests such as forced vital capacity, forced expiratory volume in one second and peak expiratory flow rate are all reduced significantly following surgery, particularly if pain control is inadequate. Laparoscopic surgery is again associated with lesser, but still significant, reductions in lung function, and the degree of change is again related to the site of surgery.[139]

Respiratory muscles.[143] Diaphragmatic dysfunction is a term that has been used to describe changes in the pattern of contraction of respiratory muscles in patients following major surgery. Impairment of diaphragmatic contraction is believed to result from reflex inhibition of phrenic nerve output in response to surgical trauma. Changes are independent of the level of pain control, and are only improved by thoracic epidural which is believed to result in neural blockade of the inhibitory reflex.[139] The existence of diaphragmatic dysfunction has been challenged, mainly on the grounds that methods used to study diaphragm function are largely indirect, and greatly affected by changes in other respiratory muscle groups.[143] For example, there are well described increases in expiratory abdominal muscle activity following surgery[144] that may be interpreted as changes in diaphragm activity.

Sputum retention occurs in many patients following surgery. General anaesthesia, particularly with a tracheal tube, causes impairment of mucociliary transport in the airways,[145] an effect that may persist into the postoperative period. This, coupled with reduced FRC, residual atelectasis and an ineffective cough, is likely to contribute to the development of chest infections including pneumonia. Many of these factors are more pronounced in smokers, who are known to be more susceptible to chest complications following major surgery (page 320).

References

1. Snow J. *On Chloroform and Other Anaesthetics: Their Action and Administration*. London: Churchill; 1858.
2. Nunn JF. Effects of anaesthesia on respiration. *Br J Anaesth*. 1990;65:54–62.
3. Munson ES, Larson CP, Babad AA, Regan MJ, Buechel DR, Eger EI. The effects of halothane, fluroxene and cyclopropane on ventilation: a comparative study in man. *Anesthesiology*. 1966;27: 716–728.
4. Pandit JJ. Effect of low dose inhaled anaesthetic agents on the ventilatory response to carbon dioxide in humans: a quantitative review. *Anaesthesia*. 2005;60:461–469.
5. Eger EI. Isoflurane: a review. *Anesthesiology*. 1981;55:559–576.
6. Lockhart SH, Rampil IJ, Yasuda N, Eger EI, Weiskopf RB. Depression of ventilation by desflurane in humans. *Anesthesiology*. 1991;74:484–488.
7. Doi M, Ikeda K. Respiratory effects of sevoflurane. *Anesth Analg*. 1987;66:241–244.
8. Eger EI, Dolan WM, Stevens WC, Miller RD, Way WL. Surgical stimulation antagonises the respiratory depression produced by Forane. *Anesthesiology*. 1972;36:544–549.
*9. Pandit JJ. The variable effect of low-dose volatile anaesthetics on the acute ventilatory response to hypoxia in humans: a quantitative review. *Anaesthesia*. 2002;57:632–643.

*10. Dahan A, Teppema LJ. Influence of anaesthesia and analgesia on the control of breathing. *Br J Anaesth*. 2003;91:40–49.
11. Gordh T. Postural circulatory and respiratory changes during ether and intravenous anesthesia. *Acta Chir Scand*. 1945;92(Suppl 102):26.
12. Duffin J, Triscott A, Whitwam JG. The effect of halothane and thiopentone on ventilatory responses mediated by the peripheral chemoreceptors in man. *Br J Anaesth*. 1976;48:975–981.
13. Knill RL, Gelb AW. Ventilatory responses to hypoxia and hypercapnia during halothane sedation and anesthesia in man. *Anesthesiology*. 1978;49:244–251.
14. Nagyova B, Dorrington KL, Gill EW, Robbins PA. Comparison of the effects of sub-hypnotic concentrations of propofol and halothane on the acute ventilatory response to hypoxia. *Br J Anaesth*. 1995;75:713–718.
15. Temp JA, Henson LC, Ward DS. Does a subanaesthetic concentration of isoflurane blunt the ventilatory response to hypoxia. *Anesthesiology*. 1992;77:1116–1124.
16. van den Elsen MJLJ, Dahan A, Berkenbosch A, DeGoede J, van Kleef JW, Olievier ICW. Does subanesthetic isoflurane affect the ventilatory response to acute isocapnic hypoxia in healthy volunteers. *Anesthesiology*. 1994;81:860–867.

17. Young CH, Drummond GB, Warren PM. Effect of a sub-anaesthetic concentration of halothane on the ventilatory response to sustained hypoxia in healthy humans. *Br J Anaesth*. 1993;71:642–647.
18. Knill RL, Kieraszewicz HT, Dodgson BG, Clement JL. Chemical regulation of ventilation during isoflurane sedation and anaesthesia in humans. *Can Anaes Soc J*. 1983;30:607–614.
19. Temp JA, Henson LC, Ward DS. Effect of a subanesthetic minimum alveolar concentration of isoflurane on two tests of the hypoxic ventilatory response. *Anesthesiology*. 1994;80:739–750.
20. Nagyova B, Dorrington KL, Poulin MJ, Robbins PA. Influence of 0.2 minimum alveolar concentration of enflurane on the ventilatory response to sustained hypoxia in humans. *Br J Anaesth*. 1997;78:707–713.
21. Sjögren D, Sollevi A, Ebberyd A, Lindahl SGE. Isoflurane anesthesia (0.6 MAC) and hypoxic ventilatory response in humans. *Acta Anaesthesiol Scand*. 1995;39:17–22.
22. van den Elsen M, Sarton E, Teppema L, Berkenbosch A, Dahan A. Influence of 0.1 minimum alveolar concentration of sevoflurane, desflurane and isoflurane on dynamic ventilatory response to hypercapnia in humans. *Br J Anaesth*. 1998;80:174–182.
23. Robotham JL. Do low dose inhalational anesthetic agents alter

ventilatory control. *Anesthesiology*. 1994;80:723–726.

24. Nandi PR, Charlesworth CH, Taylor SJ, Nunn JF, Dorè CJ. Effect of general anaesthesia on the pharynx. *Br J Anaesth*. 1991;66:157–162.

25. Mathru M, Esch O, Lang J, et al. Magnetic resonance imaging of the upper airway. Effects of propofol anesthesia and nasal continuous positive airway pressure in humans. *Anesthesiology*. 1996;84:273–279.

26. Ochiai R, Guthrie RD, Motoyama EK. Effects of varying concentrations of halothane on the activity of the genioglossus, intercostals, and diaphragm in cats: an electromyographic study. *Anesthesiology*. 1989;70:812–816.

27. Drummond GB. Influence of thiopentone on upper airway muscles. *Br J Anaesth*. 1989;63:12–21.

28. Boidin MP. Airway patency in the unconscious patient. *Br J Anaesth*. 1985;57:306–310.

29. Morikawa S, Safar P, DeCarlo J. Influence of the head-jaw position upon upper airway patency. *Anesthesiology*. 1961;22:265–270.

30. Heiberg J. A new expedient in administering chloroform. Medical Times and Gazette; 10 Jan 1874, p36

31. Marsh AM, Nunn JF, Taylor SJ, Charlesworth CH. Airway obstruction associated with the use of the Guedel airway. *Br J Anaesth*. 1991;67:517–523.

32. Brain AIJ. The laryngeal mask: a new concept in airway management. *Br J Anaesth*. 1983;55:801–805.

33. Miller AH. Ascending respiratory paralysis under general anaesthesia. *JAMA*. 1925;84:201–202.

34. Jones JG, Faithfull D, Jordan C, Minty B. Rib cage movement during halothane anaesthesia in man. *Br J Anaesth*. 1979;51:399–407.

35. Warner DO, Warner MA, Ritman EL. Human chest wall function while awake and during halothane anesthesia: I Quiet breathing. *Anesthesiology*. 1995;82:6–19.

36. Warner DO, Warner MA, Joyner MJ, Ritman EL. The effect of nitrous oxide on chest wall function in humans and \ dogs. *Anesth Analg*. 1998;86:1058–1064.

37. Lumb AB, Petros AJ, Nunn JF. Rib cage contribution to resting and carbon dioxide stimulated ventilation during 1 MAC isoflurane anaesthesia. *Br J Anaesth*. 1991;67:712–721.

38. Mankikian B, Cantineau JP, Sartene R, Clergue F, Viars P. Ventilatory pattern and chest wall mechanics during ketamine anesthesia in humans. *Anesthesiology*. 1986;65:492–499.

39. Morton CPJ, Drummond GB. Change in chest wall dimensions on induction of anaesthesia: a reappraisal. *Br J Anaesth*. 1994;73:135–139.

40. Reigner J, Ameur MB, Ecoffey C. Spontaneous ventilation with halothane in children: A comparative study between endotracheal tube and laryngeal mask airway. *Anesthesiology*. 1995;83:674–678.

41. Drummond GB. The abdominal muscles in anaesthesia and after surgery. *Br J Anaesth*. 2003;91:73–80.

42. Kaul SU, Heath JR, Nunn JF. Factors influencing the development of expiratory muscle activity during anaesthesia. *Br J Anaesth*. 1973;45:1013–1018.

43. Hewlett AM, Hulands GH, Nunn JF, Heath JR. Functional residual capacity. II: Spontaneous respiration. *Br J Anaesth*. 1974;46:486–494.

44. Fourcade HE, Larson CP, Hickey RF, Bahlman SH, Eger EI. Effects of time on ventilation during halothane and cyclopropane anesthesia. *Anesthesiology*. 1972;36:83–88.

45. Bergman NA. Distribution of inspired gas during anesthesia and artificial ventilation. *J Appl Physiol*. 1963;18:1085–1089.

46. Rutherford JS, Logan MR, Drummond GB. Changes in end-expiratory lung volume on induction of anaesthesia with thiopentone or propofol. *Br J Anaesth*. 1994;73:579–582.

47. Warner DO, Warner MA, Ritman EL. Atelectasis and chest wall shape during halothane anesthesia. *Anesthesiology*. 1996;85:49–59.

*48. Duggan M, Kavanagh BP. Pulmonary atelectasis. A pathogenic perioperative entity. *Anesthesiology*. 2005;102:838–854.

49. Gunnarsson L, Tokics L, Gustavsson H, Hedenstierna G. Influence of age on atelectasis formation and gas exchange impairment during general anaesthesia. *Br J Anaesth*. 1991;66:423–432.

50. Hedenstierna G, Strandberg A, Brismar B, Lundquist H, Svensson L, Tokics L. Functional residual capacity, thoracoabdominal dimensions and central blood volume during general anesthesia with muscle paralysis and mechanical ventilation. *Anesthesiology*. 1985;62:247–254.

51. Muller N, Volgyesi G, Becker L, Bryan MH, Bryan AC. Diaphragmatic muscle tone. *J Appl Physiol*. 1979;47:279–284.

52. Froese AB, Bryan AC. Effects of anesthesia and paralysis on diaphragmatic mechanics in man. *Anesthesiology*. 1974;41:242–255.

53. Reber A, Nylund U, Hedenstierna G. Position and shape of the diaphragm: implications for atelectasis formation. *Anaesthesia*. 1998;53:1054–1061.

54. Krayer S, Rehder K, Beck KC, Cameron PD, Didier EP, Hoffman EA. Quantification of thoracic volumes by three-dimensional imaging. *J Appl Physiol*. 1987;62:591–598.

55. Hedenstierna G, Lundquist H, Undh B, et al. Pulmonary densities during anaesthesia. *Eur Respir J.* 1989;2:528–532.

56. Bendixen HH, Hedley-Whyte J, Laver MB. Impaired oxygenation in surgical patients during general anesthesia with controlled ventilation. *N Engl J Med.* 1963;269:991–996.

57. Hedenstierna G, Tokics L, Strandberg A, Lundquist H, Brismar B. Correlation of gas exchange impairment to development of atelectasis during anaesthesia and muscle paralysis. *Acta Anaesthesiol Scand.* 1986;30:183–191.

58. Lundquist H, Hedenstierna G, Strandberg A, Tokics L, Brismar B. CT-Assessment of dependent lung densities in man during general anaesthesia. *Acta Radiol.* 1995;36:626–632.

59. Serafini G, Cornara G, Cavalloro F, et al. Pulmonary atelectasis during paediatric anaesthesia: CT evaluation and effect of positive end-expiratory pressure (PEEP). *Paediatr Anaesth.* 1999;9:225–228.

60. Hedenstierna G. Invited editorial on "Kinetics of absorption atelectasis during anaesthesia: a mathematical model". *J Appl Physiol.* 1999;86:1114–1115.

61. Nunn JF, Williams IP, Jones JG, Hewlett AM, Hulands GH, Minty BD. Detection and reversal of pulmonary absorption collapse. *Br J Anaesth.* 1978;50:91–100.

62. Rothen HU, Sporre B, Engberg G, Wegenius G, Hedenstierna G. Airway closure, atelectasis and gas exchange during general anaesthesia. *Br J Anaesth.* 1998;81:681–686.

63. Nunn JF. Measurement of closing volume. *Acta Anaesthiol Scand Supp.* 1978;70:154–160.

64. Hedenstierna G, McCarthy G, Bergström M. Airway closure during mechanical ventilation. *Anesthesiology.* 1976;44:114–123.

65. Juno P, Marsh M, Knopp TJ, Rehder K. Closing capacity in awake and anesthetized-paralyzed man. *J Appl Physiol.* 1978;44:238–244.

66. Bergman NA, Tien YK. Contribution of the closure of pulmonary units to impaired oxygenation during anesthesia. *Anesthesiology.* 1983;59:395–401.

67. Joyce CJ, Baker AB. What is the role of absorption atelectasis in the genesis of perioperative pulmonary collapse? *Anaesth Intensive Care.* 1995;23:691–696.

68. Magnusson L, Spahn DR. New concepts of atelectasis during general anaesthesia. *Br J Anaesth.* 2003;91:61–72.

69. Rothen HU, Sporre B, Engberg G, Wegenius G, Reber A, Hedenstierna G. Prevention of atelectasis during general anaesthesia. *Lancet.* 1996;345:1387–1391.

70. Reber A, Engberg G, Wegenius G, Hedenstierna G. Lung aeration: The effect of pre-oxygenation and hyperoxygenation during total intravenous anaesthesia. *Anaesthesia.* 1996;51:733–737.

71. Edmark L, Kostova-Aherdan K, Enlund M, Hedenstierna G. Optimal oxygen concentration during induction of general anesthesia. *Anesthesiology.* 2003;98:28–33.

72. Rothen HU, Sporre B, Engberg G, Wegenius G, Högman M, Hedenstierna G. Influence of gas composition on recurrence of atelectasis after a reexpansion maneuvre during general anesthesia. *Anesthesiology.* 1995;82:832–842.

73. Rothen HU, Sporre HU, Engberg G, Wegenius G, Hedenstierna G. Reexpansion of atelectasis during general anaesthesia may have a prolonged effect. *Acta Anaesthesiol Scand.* 1995;39:118–125.

74. Akça O, Podolsky A, Eisenhuber E, et al. Comparable postoperative pulmonary atelectasis in patients given 30% or 80% oxygen during and 2 hours after colon resection. *Anesthesiology.* 1999;91:991–998.

*75. Benoit Z, Wicky S, Fischer J-F, et al. The effect of increased FIo$_2$ before tracheal extubation on postoperative atelectasis. *Anesth Analg.* 2002;95:1777–1781.

76. Lindahl SGE, Mure M. Dosing oxygen: A tricky matter or a piece of cake? *Anesth Analg.* 2002;95:1472–1473.

77. Lumb AB. Just a little oxygen to breathe as you go off to sleep … is it always a good idea? *Br J Anaesth.* 2007;99:769–771.

78. Joyce CJ, Williams AB. Kinetics of absorption atelectasis during anaesthesia: a mathematical model. *J Appl Physiol.* 1999;86:1116–1125.

79. Agarwal A, Singh PK, Dhiraj S, Pandey CM, Singh U. Oxygen in air (FIo$_2$ 0.4) improves gas exchange in young healthy patients during general anesthesia. *Can J Anesth.* 2002;49:1040–1043.

80. Gunnarson L, Strandberg Å, Brismar B, Tokics L, Lundquist H, Hedenstierna G. Atelectasis and gas exchange impairment during enflurane/nitrous oxide anaesthesia. *Acta Anaesthesiol Scand.* 1989;33:629–637.

81. Rusca M, Proietti S, Schnyder P, et al. Prevention of atelectasis formation during induction of general anesthesia. *Anesth Analg.* 2003;97:1835–1839.

82. Herriger A, Frascarolo P, Spahn DR, Magnusson L. The effect of positive airway pressure during pre-oxygenation and induction of anaesthesia upon duration of non-hypoxic apnoea. *Anaesthesia.* 2004;59:243–247.

83. Neumann P, Rothen HU, Berglund JE, Valtysson J, Magnusson A, Hedenstierna G. Positive end-expiratory pressure prevents atelectasis during general anaesthesia even in the presence of a high inspired oxygen concentration. *Acta Anaesthesiol Scand.* 1999;43:295–301.

84. Rothen HU, Sporre B, Engberg G, Wegenius G, Hedenstierna G. Re-expansion of atelectasis during general anaesthesia: a computed tomography study. *Br J Anaesth*. 1993;71:788–795.

85. Tusman G, Böhm SH, Vazquez de Anda GF, do Campo JL, Lachmann B. 'Alveolar recruitment strategy' improves arterial oxygenation during general anaesthesia. *Br J Anaesth*. 1999;82:8–13.

*86. Rothen HU, Neumann P, Berglund JE, Valtysson J, Magnusson A, Hedenstierna G. Dynamics of re-expansion of atelectasis during general anaesthesia. *Br J Anaesth*. 1999;82:551–556.

87. Hedenstierna G, Tokics L, Lundquist H, Andersson T, Strandberg A, Brismar B. Phrenic nerve stimulation during halothane anaesthesia. Effects on atelectasis. *Anesthesiology*. 1994;80:751–760.

88. Milic-Emili J, Robatto FM, Bates JHT. Respiratory mechanics in anaesthesia. *Br J Anaesth*. 1990;65:4–12.

89. Hirshman CA, Bergman NA. Factors influencing intrapulmonary airway calibre during anaesthesia. *Br J Anaesth*. 1990;65:30–42.

90. Joyner MJ, Warner DO, Rehder K. Halothane changes the relationships between lung resistances and lung volume. *Anesthesiology*. 1992;76:229–235.

91. Pelosi P, Croci M, Calappi E, et al. The prone position during general anesthesia minimally affects respiratory mechanics while improving functional residual capacity and increasing oxygen tension. *Anesth Analg*. 1995;80:955–960.

92. D'Angelo E, Robatto FM, Calderini E, et al. Pulmonary and chest wall mechanics in anesthetized paralyzed humans. *J Appl Physiol*. 1991;70:2602–2610.

93. Yamakage M. Effects of anaesthetic agents on airway smooth muscle. *Br J Anaesth*. 2002;88:624–627.

94. Korenaga S, Takeda K, Ito Y. Differential effects of halothane on airway nerves and muscle. *Anesthesiology*. 1984;60:309–318.

95. Bhatt SB, Kendall AP, Lin ES, Oh TE. Resistance and additional inspiratory work imposed by the laryngeal mask airway: a comparison with tracheal tubes. *Anaesthesia*. 1992;47:343–347.

96. Westbrook PR, Stubbs SE, Sessler AD, Rehder K, Hyatt RE. Effects of anesthesia and muscle paralysis on respiratory mechanics in normal man. *J Appl Physiol*. 1973;34:81–86.

97. Scheidt M, Hyatt RE, Rehder K. Effects of rib cage or abdominal restriction on lung mechanics. *J Appl Physiol*. 1981;51:1115–1121.

98. Campbell EJM, Nunn JF, Peckett BW. A comparison of artificial ventilation and spontaneous respiration with particular reference to ventilation-blood-flow relationships. *Br J Anaesth*. 1958;30:166–175.

99. Nunn JF, Hill DW. Respiratory dead space and arterial to end-tidal CO_2 tension difference in anesthetized man. *J Appl Physiol*. 1960;15:383–389.

100. Casati A, Fanelli G, Torri G. Physiological dead space/tidal volume ratio during face mask, laryngeal mask, and cuffed oropharyngeal airway spontaneous ventilation. *J Clin Anesth*. 1998;10:652–655.

101. Kain ML, Panday J, Nunn JF. The effect of intubation on the dead space during halothane anaesthesia. *Br J Anaesth*. 1969;41:94–102.

102. Tokics L, Hedenstierna G, Svensson L, et al. $\dot{V}/\dot{Q}$ distribution and correlation to atelectasis in anesthetized paralyzed humans. *J Appl Physiol*. 1996;81:1822–1833.

103. Hedenstierna G. Contribution of the multiple inert gas elimination technique to pulmonary medicine 6: Ventilation-perfusion relationships during anaesthesia. *Thorax*. 1995;50:85–91.

104. Rehder K, Knopp TJ, Sessler AD, Didier EP. Ventilation-perfusion relationship in young healthy awake and anesthetized-paralyzed man. *J Appl Physiol*. 1979;47:745–753.

105. Nunn JF. Oxygen – friend and foe. *J R Soc Med*. 1985;78:618–622.

106. Bindslev L, Hedenstierna G, Santesson J, Gottlieb I, Carvallhas A. Ventilation-perfusion distribution during inhalation anaesthesia. *Acta Anaesthesiol Scand*. 1981;25:360–371.

107. Dueck R, Young I, Clausen J, Wagner PD. Altered distribution of pulmonary ventilation and blood flow following induction of inhalational anesthesia. *Anesthesiology*. 1980;52:113–125.

108. Nunn JF, Bergman NA, Coleman AJ. Factors influencing the arterial oxygen tension during anaesthesia with artificial ventilation. *Br J Anaesth*. 1965;37:898–914.

109. Anjou-Lindskog E, Broman L, Broman M, Holmgren A, Settergren G, Öhqvist G. Effects of intravenous anesthesia on VA/Q distribution: a study performed during ventilation with air and with 50% oxygen, supine and in the lateral position. *Anesthesiology*. 1985;62:485–492.

110. Nunn JF, Ezi-Ashi TI. The respiratory effects of resistance to breathing in anesthetized man. *Anesthesiology*. 1961;22:174–185.

111. Moote CA, Knill RL, Clement J. Ventilatory compensation for continuous inspiratory resistive and elastic loads during halothane anesthesia in humans. *Anesthesiology*. 1986;64:582–589.

112. Drummond GB, Cullen JP. Detection of inspiratory resistive

loads after anaesthesia for minor surgery. *Br J Anaesth*. 1997;78:308–310.

113. Isono S, Nishino T, Sugimori K, Misuguchi T. Respiratory effects of expiratory flow-resistive loading in conscious and anesthetized humans. *Anesth Analg*. 1990;70:594–599.

114. Marshall BE, Marshall C. Anesthesia and the pulmonary circulation. In: Covino BG, Fozzard HA, Rehder K, Strichartz G, eds. *Effects of Anesthesia*. Bethesda, Md: American Physiological Society; 1985.

115. Eisenkraft JB. Effects of anaesthetics on the pulmonary circulation. *Br J Anaesth*. 1990;65:63–78.

116. Pelosi P, Croci M, Ravagnan I, et al. The effects of body mass on lung volumes, respiratory mechanics, and gas exchange during anesthesia. *Anesth Analg*. 1998;87:654–660.

117. Pelosi P, Ravagnan I, Giurati G, et al. Positive end-expiratory pressure improves respiratory function in obese but not in normal subjects during anaesthesia and paralysis. *Anesthesiol*. 1999;91:1221–1231.

118. Yoshino J, Akata T, Takahashi S. Intraoperative changes in arterial oxygenation during volume-controlled mechanical ventilation in modestly obese patients undergoing laparotomies with general anesthesia. *Acta Anaesthesiol Scand*. 2003;47:742–750.

119. Klingstedt C, Hedenstierna G, Baehrendtz S, et al. Ventilation-perfusion relationships and atelectasis formation in the supine and lateral positions during conventional mechanical and differential ventilation. *Acta Anaesthesiol Scand*. 1990;34:421–429.

120. Krayer S, Rehder K, Vettermann J, Didier P, Ritman EL. Position and motion of the human diaphragm during anesthesia-paralysis. *Anesthesiology*. 1989; 70:891–898.

121. Cardiopulmonary physiology and pathophysiology as a consequence of laparoscopic surgery. *Chest* 1996; 110: 810–15.

122. O'Malley C, Cunningham AJ. Physiologic changes during laparoscopy. *Anesthesiol Clin North America*. 2001;19:1–19.

123. Sprung J, Whalley DG, Falcone T, Warner DO, Hubmayr RD, Hammel J. The impact of morbid obesity, pneumoperitoneum, and posture on respiratory system mechanics and oxygenation during laparoscopy. *Anesth Analg*. 2002;94:1345–1350.

124. Andersson L, Lagerstrand L, Thörne A, Sollevi A, Brodin L-Å, Odeberg-Wernerman S. Effect of CO_2 pneumoperitoneum on ventilation-perfusion relationships during laparoscopic cholecystectomy. *Acta Anaesthesiol Scand*. 2002;46:552–560.

125. Kazama T, Ikeda K, Kato T, Kikura M. Carbon dioxide output in laparoscopic cholecystectomy. *Br J Anaesth*. 1996;76:530–535.

126. Veering BT, Cousins MJ. Cardiovascular and pulmonary effects of epidural anaesthesia. *Anesth Int Care*. 2000;28:620–635.

127. Sakura S, Saito Y, Kosaka Y. The effects of epidural anesthesia on ventilatory response to hypercapnia and hypoxia in elderly patients. *Anesth Analg*. 1996;82:306–311.

128. Sakura S, Saito Y, Kosaka Y. Effect of extradural anaesthesia on the ventilatory response to hypoxaemia. *Anaesthesia*. 1993;48:205–209.

129. Sakura S, Saito Y, Kosaka Y. Effect of lumbar epidural anesthesia on ventilatory response to hypercapnia in young and elderly patients. *J Clin Anesth*. 1993;5:109–113.

130. Labaille T, Clergue F, Samii K, Ecoffey C, Berdeaux A.

Ventilatory response to CO_2 following intravenous and epidural lidocaine. *Anesthesiology*. 1985;63:179–185.

131. Warner DO, Warner MA, Ritman EL. Human chest wall function during epidural anesthesia. *Anesthesiology*. 1996;85: 761–773.

132. Moir DD. Ventilatory function during epidural analgesia. *Br J Anaesth*. 1963;35:3–7.

133. Kelly MC, Fitzpatrick KTJ, Hill DA. Respiratory effects of spinal anaesthesia for Caesarean section. *Anaesthesia*. 1996;51:1120–1122.

134. Gamil M. Serial peak expiratory flow rates in mothers during caesarean section under extradural anaesthesia. *Br J Anaesth*. 1989;62:415–418.

135. Yun E, Topulos GP, Body SC, Datta S, Bader AM. Pulmonary function changes during epidural anesthesia for Cesarean delivery. *Anesth Analg*. 1996;82:750–753.

136. Reber A, Bein T, Högman M, Khan ZP, Nilsson S, Hedenstierna G. Lung aeration and pulmonary gas exchange during lumbar epidural anaesthesia and in the lithotomy position in elderly patients. *Anaesthesia*. 1998;53:854–861.

137. Jones JG, Sapsford DJ, Wheatley RG. Postoperative hypoxaemia: mechanisms and time course. *Anaesthesia*. 1990;45:566–573.

138. Moller JT, Johannessen NW, Berg H, Espersen K, Larsen LE. Hypoxaemia during anaesthesia – an observer study. *Br J Anaesth*. 1991;66:437–444.

139. Liu S, Carpenter RL, Neal JM. Epidural anesthesia and analgesia: their role in postoperative outcome. *Anesthesiology*. 1995;82: 1474–1506.

140. McKeague H, Cunningham AJ. Postoperative respiratory dysfunction: is the site of surgery crucial? *Br J Anaesth*. 1997;79:415–416.

141. Couture JD, Chartrand D, Gagner M, Bellemare F. Diaphragmatic and abdominal muscle activity after endoscopic cholecystectomy. *Anesth Analg*. 1994;78:733–739.

142. Strandberg A, Tokics L, Brismar B, Lundquist H, Hedenstierna G. Atelectasis during anaesthesia and in the postoperative period. *Acta Anaesthesiol Scand*. 1986;30:154–158.

143. Drummond GB. Diaphragmatic dysfunction: an outmoded concept. *Br J Anaesth*. 1998;80:277–280.

144. Nimmo AF, Drummond GB. Respiratory mechanics after abdominal surgery measured with continuous analysis of pressure, flow and volume signals. *Br J Anaesth*. 1996;77:317–326.

145. Keller C, Brimacombe J. Bronchial mucus transport velocity in paralyzed anesthetized patients: a comparison of the laryngeal mask airway and cuffed tracheal tube. *Anesth Analg*. 1998;86:1280–1282.

Chapter 23

Changes in the carbon dioxide partial pressure

- Hypocapnia occurs when alveolar ventilation is excessive relative to carbon dioxide production and usually results from hyperventilation due to hypoxia, acidosis or lung disease.
- Hypercapnia most commonly occurs because of inadequate alveolar ventilation from a multitude of causes, or more rarely from increased carbon dioxide production.
- Arterial $P\text{CO}_2$ affects the cerebral circulation – hypocapnia may cause potentially harmful vasoconstriction whilst vasodilatation from hypercapnia may increase intracranial pressure.
- Hypercapnia, and the resulting acidosis, both have depressant effects on the cardiovascular system, but these are opposed by the stimulant effects of catecholamine release.

Routine monitoring of end-expiratory and arterial $P\text{CO}_2$ means it should now be possible to avoid both hypo- and hypercapnia under almost all clinical circumstances. However, interest in hypercapnia has continued over recent years for two reasons. First, changes in the approach to artificial ventilation in severe lung injury have led to the use of 'permissive hypercapnia' (page 457). In order to minimise pulmonary damage, minute volume of ventilation is maintained deliberately low, and the arterial $P\text{CO}_2$ is allowed to increase. Secondly, a massive expansion of laparoscopic surgical techniques, mostly using carbon dioxide for abdominal insufflation, has led to the anaesthetist having to control arterial $P\text{CO}_2$ under conditions of significantly increased pulmonary carbon dioxide output (page 347).

Before describing the effects of carbon dioxide on various physiological systems, this chapter will briefly outline the causes of changes in arterial $P\text{CO}_2$.

CAUSES OF HYPOCAPNIA[1]

Hypocapnia can result only from an alveolar ventilation that is excessive in relation to carbon dioxide production. Low values of arterial $P\text{CO}_2$ are commonly found, resulting from artificial ventilation with an excessive minute volume or from voluntary hyperventilation due to psychological disturbance such as hysteria. A low arterial $P\text{CO}_2$ may also result simply from hyperventilation during arterial puncture. Persistently low values may be due to an excessive respiratory drive resulting from one or more of the following causes.

Hypoxaemia is a common cause of hypocapnia, occurring in congenital heart disease with right-to-left shunting, residence at high altitude, pulmonary pathology or any other condition that reduces the arterial $P\text{O}_2$ below about 8 kPa (60 mmHg). Hypocapnia secondary to hypoxaemia opposes the ventilatory response to the hypoxaemia (page 73).

Metabolic acidosis produces a compensatory hyperventilation (air hunger), which minimises the fall in pH that would otherwise occur. This is a pronounced feature of diabetic ketoacidosis; arterial $P\text{CO}_2$ values below 3 kPa (22.5 mmHg) are not uncommon in severe metabolic acidosis. This is a vital compensatory mechanism. Failure to maintain the required hyperventilation, either from fatigue or inadequate artificial ventilation leads to a rapid life-threatening decrease in arterial pH.

Mechanical abnormalities of the lung may drive respiration through the vagus, resulting in moderate reduction of the P_{CO_2}. Thus conditions such as pulmonary fibrosis, pulmonary oedema and asthma are usually associated with a low to normal P_{CO_2} until the patient passes into type 2 respiratory failure (page 393).

Neurological disorders may result in hyperventilation and hypocapnia. This is most commonly seen in those conditions that lead to the presence of blood in the cerebrospinal fluid, such as occurs following head injury or subarachnoid haemorrhage.

CAUSES OF HYPERCAPNIA

It is uncommon to encounter an arterial P_{CO_2} above the normal range in a healthy subject. Any value of more than 6.1 kPa (46 mmHg) should be considered abnormal, but values up to 6.7 kPa (50 mmHg) may be attained by breath holding. It is difficult for the healthy subject to exceed this level by any respiratory manoeuvre other than by breathing mixtures of carbon dioxide in oxygen.

When a patient is hypercapnic, there are only four possible causes:

Increased concentration of carbon dioxide in the inspired gas. This iatrogenic cause of hypercapnia is uncommon but it is dangerous and differs fundamentally from the other causes listed below. It should therefore be excluded at the outset in any patient unexpectedly found to be hypercapnic when breathing via any external equipment. The carbon dioxide may be endogenous from rebreathing or exogenous from carbon dioxide added to the inhaled gases. The latter is now very rare as a supply of carbon dioxide is not provided on modern anaesthetic machines. Hypercapnia from rebreathing is more common, but fortunately its severity is limited by the rate at which the P_{CO_2} can increase. If all the carbon dioxide produced by metabolism is retained and distributed in the body stores, arterial P_{CO_2} can increase no faster than about 0.4–0.8 kPa.min^{-1} (3–6 mmHg.min^{-1}).

Increased carbon dioxide production. If the pulmonary minute volume is fixed by artificial ventilation and carbon dioxide production is increased by, for example, malignant hyperpyrexia, hypercapnia is inevitable. Like the previous category, this is a rare but dangerous cause of hypercapnia during anaesthesia. A less dramatic, but very common, reason for increased carbon dioxide production is sepsis leading to pyrexia, which often results in hypercapnia in artificially ventilated patients.

Though not strictly an increase in production, absorption of carbon dioxide from the peritoneum during laparoscopic surgery has the same respiratory effects and is described on page 347.

Hypoventilation. An inadequate pulmonary minute volume is by far the commonest cause of hypercapnia. Pathological causes of hypoventilation are numerous and considered in Chapter 27 and Figure 27.2. In respiratory medicine, the commonest cause of long standing hypercapnia is chronic obstructive pulmonary disease (COPD).

Increased dead space. This rare cause of hypercapnia is usually diagnosed by a process of exclusion when a patient has a high P_{CO_2}, with a normal minute volume and no evidence of a hypermetabolic state or inhaled carbon dioxide. The cause may be incorrectly configured breathing apparatus, or an excessively large alveolar dead space (page 130). This might be due to pulmonary embolism or a cyst communicating with the tracheobronchial tree and receiving preferential ventilation.

EFFECTS OF CARBON DIOXIDE ON THE NERVOUS SYSTEM

A number of special difficulties hinder an understanding of the effects of changes in P_{CO_2} on any physiological system. First, there is the problem of species difference, which is a formidable obstacle to the interpretation of animal studies in this field. The second difficulty arises from the fact that carbon dioxide can exert its effect either directly, or in consequence of (respiratory) acidosis. The third difficulty arises from the fact that carbon dioxide acts at many different sites in the body, sometimes producing opposite effects on a particular function, such as blood pressure (see below).

Carbon dioxide has at least five major effects on the brain:

- It is a major factor governing cerebral blood flow.
- It influences the intracerebral pressure through changes in cerebral blood flow.
- It is the main factor influencing the intracellular pH, which is known to have important effects on the metabolism, and therefore function, of the cell.

- It may be presumed to exert the inert gas narcotic effect in accord with its physical properties, which are similar to those of nitrous oxide.
- It influences the excitability of certain neurones, particularly relevant in the case of the reticuloactivating system.

The interplay of these effects is difficult to understand, although the gross changes produced are well established.

EFFECTS ON CONSCIOUSNESS

Carbon dioxide has long been known to cause unconsciousness in dogs entering the Grotto del Cane in Italy, where carbon dioxide issuing from a fumarole forms a layer near the ground. It has been widely used as an anaesthetic for short procedures in small laboratory animals. Inhalation of 30% carbon dioxide is sufficient for the production of anaesthesia in humans, but is complicated by the frequent occurrence of convulsions.[2] In patients with ventilatory failure, carbon dioxide narcosis occurs when the P_{CO_2} rises above 12–16 kPa (90–120 mmHg).[3]

Narcosis by carbon dioxide is probably not due primarily to its inert gas narcotic effects, because its oil solubility predicts a very much weaker narcotic than it seems to be. It is likely that the major effect on the central nervous system is by alteration of the intracellular pH, with consequent derangements of metabolic processes. In animals the narcotic effect correlates better with cerebrospinal fluid pH than with arterial P_{CO_2}.[4]

The effects of inhaling low concentrations of carbon dioxide for a prolonged period of time are described on page 305.

CEREBRAL BLOOD FLOW[5]

Cerebral blood flow (CBF) increases with arterial P_{CO_2} at a rate of about 7–15 ml.100g^{-1}.min^{-1} for each kPa increase in P_{CO_2} (1–2 ml.100g^{-1}.min^{-1} per mmHg) within the approximate range 3–10 kPa (20–80 mmHg). The full response curve is S-shaped (Figure 23.1). The response at very low P_{CO_2} is probably limited by the vasodilator effect of tissue hypoxia, and the response above 16 kPa (120 mmHg) seems to represent maximal vasodilatation. The changes shown in Figure 23.1 represent the brain as a whole and it is not possible to generalise about regional changes.

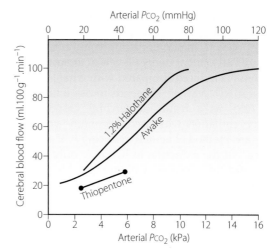

Fig. 23.1 Relationship of cerebral blood flow to arterial P_{CO_2} in awake and anaesthetised patients.

Mechanisms. In the intact animal, CBF is increased in response to P_{CO_2} by a combination of vasodilatation of cerebral blood vessels and an increase in blood pressure (see below). Changes in P_{CO_2} lead to a complex series of events that bring about vasodilation of cerebral blood vessels.[5] In adults, the effect is initiated by changes in the extracellular pH in the region of the arterioles, which alters intracellular calcium levels both directly and indirectly via nitric oxide production and the formation of cyclic GMP. With prolonged hypocapnia, and to a lesser extent hypercapnia, changes in cerebral blood flow return towards baseline after a few hours,[5,6] an effect thought to result from changes in cerebrospinal fluid pH correcting the extracellular acidosis. Sensitivity of the cerebral circulation to carbon dioxide may be lost in a variety of pathological circumstances such as cerebral tumour, infarction or trauma. There is commonly a fixed vasodilatation in damaged areas of brain, which if widespread may cause dangerous increases in intracranial pressure.

Anaesthesia. Inhalational anaesthetics have a direct cerebral vasodilator effect and increase normocapnic CBF considerably.[7,8] They also accentuate the response to both hypocapnia and hypercapnia; that is, they increase the slope of the relationship between P_{CO_2} and CBF (Figure 23.1). In spite of the increased slope during hypocapnia, global CBF during anaesthesia with hyperventilation is normally still greater than when awake.[5] Intravenous anaesthetics such as thiopentone and propofol[9] reduce

CBF at normal P_{CO_2} in accordance with the reduced cerebral oxygen consumption. Vasoconstriction in response to hyperventilation continues to occur (Figure 23.1), but at deeper levels of anaesthesia the response is reduced compared with when awake.[5]

Intracranial pressure (ICP) tends to rise with increasing P_{CO_2} as a result of cerebral vasodilatation. Hyperventilation was used for many years as a standard method of acutely reducing ICP after head injury, but the reduction in ICP may only be short-lived and the effects on CBF are variable. The possibility of *increased* CBF as a result of lowered ICP must be offset against *reduced* CBF from hypocapnic vasoconstriction. It is therefore preferable to monitor ICP, an invasive technique only available in specialised units dealing with head-injured patients. Recent recommendations on the management of head injury therefore advise that hyperventilation should only be used to reduce intracranial pressure when other therapeutic approaches have failed.[10]

EFFECTS ON THE AUTONOMIC AND ENDOCRINE SYSTEMS

Survival in severe hypercapnia is, to a large extent, dependent on the autonomic response. A great many of the effects of carbon dioxide on other systems are due wholly or in part to the autonomic response to carbon dioxide.

Animal studies[11] have clearly shown an increase in plasma levels of both adrenaline and noradrenaline in response to an elevation of P_{CO_2} during apnoeic mass-movement oxygenation (Figure 23.2). In moderate hypercapnia there is a proportionate rise of adrenaline and noradrenaline, but in gross hypercapnia (P_{CO_2} more than 27 kPa or 200 mmHg) there is an abrupt rise of adrenaline. Similar, though variable, changes have been obtained over a lower range of P_{CO_2} in human volunteers inhaling carbon dioxide mixtures.[12,13] Animal studies indicate that the increase in catecholamine release is mediated by direct stimulation of ventrolateral medullary neurones, which respond to elevated P_{CO_2} by increasing sympathetic nerve discharge.[14]

The effect of an increased level of circulating catecholamines is, to a certain extent, offset by a decreased sensitivity of target organs when the pH is reduced. This is additional to the general depressant direct effect of carbon dioxide on target organs. Finally, acetylcholine hydrolysis is reduced at low pH and therefore certain parasympathetic effects may be enhanced during hypercapnia.

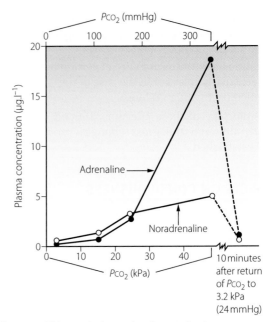

Fig. 23.2 This graph shows the changes in plasma catecholamine levels in the dog during the rise of P_{CO_2} from 2.9 to 45 kPa (22 to 338 mmHg) in the course of 1 hour of apnoeic oxygenation. After 10 minutes of ventilation with oxygen, P_{CO_2} returned to 3.2 kPa (24 mmHg), following which catecholamines were almost back to control values. (Data from reference 11.)

EFFECTS ON OTHER PHYSIOLOGICAL SYSTEMS

RESPIRATORY SYSTEM

Chapter 5 describes the role of carbon dioxide in the control of breathing, and this is not discussed further here.

Pulmonary circulation. An elevated P_{CO_2} causes vasoconstriction in the pulmonary circulation (page 110) but the effect is less marked than that of hypoxia.[15] Nevertheless, in healthy subjects an end-expiratory P_{CO_2} of 7 kPa (52 mmHg) increased pulmonary vascular resistance by 32%, which, along with elevated cardiac output, led to a 60% increase in mean pulmonary arterial pressure.[16] Though regional variations in blood flow have not been demonstrated, this effect is believed to act in a similar fashion to hypoxic pulmonary vasoconstriction (HPV, page 108), tending to divert blood away from underventilated alveoli. Hypocapnia significantly attenuates HPV in animals, though this has not been described in humans. There is evidence from both animal[17] and human[18] studies that pH is the factor responsible for CO_2-mediated changes in the pulmonary vasculature, rather than Pco$_2$ per se.

Oxygenation of the blood. Quite apart from its effect on ventilation, carbon dioxide exerts three other important effects that influence the oxygenation of the blood. First, if the concentration of nitrogen (or other 'inert' gas) remains constant, the concentration of carbon dioxide in the alveolar gas can increase only at the expense of oxygen, which must be displaced. Secondly, an increase in Pco$_2$ causes a displacement of the oxygen dissociation curve to the right (page 192). Finally, in animals, changes in Pco$_2$ are known to affect the distribution of ventilation/perfusion ratios as measured by the multiple inert gas elimination technique (page 126). This results from changes in pH influencing pulmonary vessels as described in the previous paragraph, as well as causing changes in the size of small diameter bronchi.[17]

CARDIOVASCULAR SYSTEM[19]

The effects of carbon dioxide on the circulation are complicated by the alternative modes of action on different components of the system. In general, both hypercapnia and acidosis have direct depressant effects on cardiac myocytes and vascular smooth muscle cells, effects that are normally opposed by the increase in catecholamines caused by elevated Pco$_2$. Under different circumstances these opposing effects make the overall effect of carbon dioxide on the cardiovascular system unpredictable. Despite this problem, moderate degrees of hypercapnia have been proposed to have therapeutic potential in treating septic shock when its effects can mimic the commonly used inotrope dobutamine.[20]

Myocardial contractility and heart rate. Both contractility and heart rate are diminished by elevated Pco$_2$ in the isolated preparation, probably as a result of change in pH. However, in the intact subject the direct depressant effect of carbon dioxide is overshadowed by the stimulant effect mediated through the sympathetic system. In artificially ventilated humans, increased Pco$_2$ raises cardiac output and slightly reduces total peripheral resistance,[13] and blood pressure therefore tends to be increased. Awake healthy subjects studied with non-invasive Doppler echocardiography show similar changes.[16] With an end-expiratory Pco$_2$ of 7 kPa (52 mmHg) cardiac output was increased by about 1 l.min^{-1} as a result of increases in both heart rate and stroke

volume, and accompanied by a small rise in blood pressure. Measurements of left ventricular systolic and diastolic function were unchanged, confirming the dominance of catecholamine stimulation compared with direct depressant effects on the heart. The response of cardiac output to hypercapnia is diminished by most anaesthetics.[13]

Arrhythmias have been reported in awake humans during acute hypercapnia, but seldom seem to be of serious import. One study of normal subjects with modest degrees of hypercapnia did, however, demonstrate an increase in QT dispersion of the electrocardiogram during hypercapnia.[16] This finding reflects regional repolarisation abnormalities of the ventricles and under other circumstances, such as ischaemic heart disease, indicates a propensity to develop life-threatening arrhythmias.

Blood pressure. As described above, an elevated Pco$_2$ usually causes a small increase in blood pressure, an effect seen in both conscious and anaesthetised patients. However, the response is variable and certainly cannot be relied upon as an infallible diagnostic sign of hypercapnia. Hypotension accompanies an elevation of Pco$_2$ if there is blockade of the sympathetic system by, for example, spinal anaesthesia. There is general agreement that hypotension follows a sudden fall of an elevated Pco$_2$.

EFFECT ON THE KIDNEY

Renal blood flow and glomerular filtration rate are little influenced by minor changes of Pco$_2$. However, at high levels of Pco$_2$ there is constriction of the glomerular afferent arterioles, leading to anuria. Long-term hypercapnia results in increased resorption of bicarbonate by the kidneys, further raising the plasma bicarbonate level, and constituting a secondary or compensatory metabolic alkalosis. Long-term hypocapnia decreases renal bicarbonate resorption, resulting in a further fall of plasma bicarbonate and producing a secondary or compensatory metabolic acidosis. In each case the arterial pH returns towards the normal value but the bicarbonate ion concentration departs even further from normality.

EFFECT ON BLOOD ELECTROLYTE LEVELS

The acidosis that accompanies hypercapnia causes leakage of potassium ions from the cells into the plasma. Because it takes an appreciable time for the potassium ions to be transported back into the intracellular compartment, repeated bouts of hypercapnia at short intervals result in a stepwise rise in plasma potassium.

A reduction in the ionised fraction of the total calcium has, in the past, been thought to be the cause of the tetany that accompanies severe hypocapnia. However, the changes that occur are too small to account for tetany, which occurs in parathyroid disease only when there has been a fairly gross reduction of ionised calcium.[21] Hyperexcitability affects all nerves, and spontaneous activity ultimately occurs. The muscle spasms probably result from activity in proprioceptive fibres causing reflex muscle contraction.

The effects of long-term small elevations in inspired carbon dioxide are described on page 305.

HYPERCAPNIA IN CLINICAL PRACTICE

CLINICAL SIGNS

Hyperventilation is the cardinal sign of hypercapnia due to an increased concentration of carbon dioxide in the inspired gas, whether it be endogenous or exogenous. However, this sign will be absent in the paralysed patient and also in those in whom hypercapnia is the result of hypoventilation. Such patients, including those with COPD, constitute the great majority of those with hypercapnia.

Dyspnoea may or may not be present. In patients with central failure of respiratory drive, dyspnoea may be entirely absent. On the other hand, when hypoventilation results from mechanical failure in the respiratory system (airway obstruction, pneumothorax, pulmonary fibrosis, etc.), dyspnoea is usually obvious.

In patients with COPD hypercapnia is usually associated with a flushed skin and a full and bounding pulse with occasional extrasystoles. The blood pressure is often raised but this is not a reliable sign. Muscle twitchings and a characteristic flap of the hands may be observed when coma is imminent. Convulsions may occur. The patient will become comatose when the $P\text{co}_2$ is in the range 12–16 kPa (90–120 mmHg) (see above). Hypercapnia should always be considered in cases of unexplained coma.

Hypercapnia cannot be reliably diagnosed on clinical examination. This is particularly true when there is a neurological basis for hypoventilation. Now that it has become so simple to measure the arterial $P\text{co}_2$, an arterial sample should be taken in all cases of doubt.

Gross hypercapnia. Relatively, few cases of gross hypercapnia are documented, but there are sufficient to indicate that complete recovery from gross hypercapnia without hypoxia is possible and may even be the rule.[22] One report from 1990[23] detailed five instances of hypercapnia without hypoxia in children with arterial $P\text{co}_2$ values in the range 21–36 kPa (155–269 mmHg). All were comatose or stuperose but recovered. A single case report of massive grain aspiration reported survival following a $P\text{co}_2$ of 66.8 kPa (501 mmHg).[24] These cases indicate that, *of the reported cases*, full recovery seems to be the usual outcome. Hypoxia seems to be much more dangerous than hypercapnia.

References

1. Laffey JG, Kavanagh BP. Hypocapnia. *N Engl J Med.* 2002;347:43–53.

2. Leake CD, Waters RM. The anesthetic properties of carbon dioxide. *J Pharmacol Exp Ther.* 928;33:280–281.

3. Refsum HE. Relationship between state of consciousness and arterial hypoxaemia and hypercapnia in patients with pulmonary insufficiency, breathing air. *Clin Sci.* 1963;25:361–367.

4. Eisele JH, Eger EI, Muallem M. Narcotic properties of carbon dioxide in the dog. *Anesthesiology.* 1967;28:856–865.

*5. Brian JE. Carbon dioxide and the cerebral circulation. *Anesthesiology.* 1998;88:1365–1386.

6. Raichle ME, Posner JB, Plum F. Cerebral blood flow during and after hyperventilation. *Arch Neurol.* 1970;23:394–403.

7. Ornstein E, Young WL, Fleischer LH, Ostapkovich N. Desflurane and isoflurane have similar effects on cerebral blood flow in patients with intracranial mass lesions. *Anesthesiology.* 1993;79: 498–502.

8. Cho S, Kujigaki T, Uchiyama Y, Fukusai M, Shibata O, Somikawa K. Effects of sevoflurane with and without nitrous oxide on human cerebral circulation. *Anesthesiology.* 1996;85:755–760.

9. Eng C, Lam AM, Mayberg TS, Lee C, Mathisen T. The influence of propofol with and without nitrous oxide on cerebral blood flow velocity and CO_2 reactivity in humans. *Anesthesiology.* 1992;77:872–879.

10. Yundt KD, Diringer MN. The use of hyperventilation and its impact on cerebral ischaemia in the treatment of traumatic brain injury. *Crit Care Clin.* 1997;13:163–184.

11. Millar RA. Plasma adrenaline and noradrenaline during diffusion respiration. *J Physiol*. 1960;150:79–90.

12. Sechzer PH, Egbert LD, Linde HW, Cooper DY, Dripps RD, Price HL. Effect of CO_2 inhalation on arterial pressure ECG and plasma catecholamines and 17-OH corticosteroids in normal man. *J Appl Physiol*. 1960;15:454–458.

13. Cullen DJ, Eger EI. Cardiovascular effects of carbon dioxide in man. *Anesthesiology*. 1974;41:345–349.

14. Toney GM. Sympathetic activation by the central chemoreceptor 'reflex': new evidence that RVLM vasomotor neurons are involved … but are they enough? *J Physiol*. 2006;577:3.

15. Barer GR, Howard P, McCurrie JR. The effect of carbon dioxide and changes in blood pH on pulmonary vascular resistance in cats. *Clin Sci*. 1967;32:361–376.

16. Kiely DG, Cargill RI, Lipworth BJ. Effects of hypercapnia on hemodynamic, inotropic, lusitropic, and electrophysiological indices in humans. *Chest*. 1996;109:1215–1221.

17. Domino KB, Swenson ER, Hlastala MP. Hypocapnia-induced ventilation/perfusion mismatch: a direct CO_2 or pH-mediated effect. *Am J Respir Crit Care Med*. 1995;152:1534–1539.

18. Loeppky JA, Scotto P, Riedel CE, Roach RC, Chick TW. Effects of acid-base status on acute hypoxic pulmonary vasoconstriction and gas exchange. *J Appl Physiol*. 1992;72:1787–1797.

19. Fox P. Effects of carbon dioxide on the systemic circulation. In: Prys-Roberts C, ed. *The Circulation in Anaesthesia*. Oxford: Blackwell Scientific; 1980.

*20. Wang Z, Su F, Bruhn A, Yang X, Vincent J-L. Acute hypercapnia improves indices of tissue oxygenation more than dobutamine in septic shock. *Am J Respir Crit Care Med*. 2008;177:178–183.

21. Tenney SM, Lamb TW. Physiological consequences of hypoventilation and hyperventilation. *Handbk Physiol Sect 3*. 1965;2:979.

22. Potkin RT, Swenson ER. Resuscitation from severe acute hypercapnia. Determinants of tolerance and survival. *Chest*. 1992;102:1742–1745.

23. Goldstein B, Shannon DC, Todres ID. Supercarbia in children: clinical course and outcome. *Crit Care Med*. 1990;18:166–168.

24. Slinger P, Blundell PE, Metcalf IR. Management of massive grain aspiration. *Anesthesiology*. 1997;87:993–995.

Chapter 24

Hypoxia

KEY POINTS

- Intracellular acidosis from anaerobic metabolism occurs soon after the onset of cellular hypoxia, and is worse when there is a plentiful supply of glucose to the cell.

- Lack of high energy substrates such as ATP and direct effects of hypoxia both inhibit the activity of ion channels, decreasing the transmembrane potential of the cell, leading to increased intracellular calcium levels.

- In nervous tissue the uncontrolled release of excitatory amino acids exacerbates the hypoxic damage.

- Hypoxia also causes the activation of a transcription protein HIF-1, which induces the production of several proteins with diverse functions biological functions.

Chapter 1 explained how all but the simplest forms of life have evolved to exploit the immense advantages of oxidative metabolism. The price they have paid is to become dependent on oxygen for their survival. The essential feature of hypoxia is the cessation of oxidative phosphorylation (page 199) when the mitochondrial Po_2 falls below a critical level. Anaerobic pathways, in particular the glycolytic pathway (see Figure 11.13), then come into play. These trigger a complex series of cellular changes leading first to reduced cellular function and ultimately to cell death.

BIOCHEMICAL CHANGES IN HYPOXIA

DEPLETION OF HIGH-ENERGY COMPOUNDS

Anaerobic metabolism produces only one-nineteenth of the yield of the high-energy phosphate compound

adenosine triphosphate (ATP) per mole of glucose, when compared with aerobic metabolism (page 200). In organs with a high metabolic rate such as the brain, it is impossible to increase glucose transport sufficiently to maintain the normal level of ATP production. Therefore, during hypoxia, the ATP/ADP ratio falls and there is a rapid decline in the level of all high energy compounds (Figure 24.1). Very similar changes occur in response to arterial hypotension. These changes will rapidly block cerebral function, but organs with a lower energy requirement will continue to function for a longer time and are thus more resistant to hypoxia (see below).

Under hypoxic conditions, there are two ways in which reductions in ATP levels may be minimised, both of which are effective for only a short time. First, the high energy phosphate bond in phosphocreatine may be used to create ATP,[2] and initially this slows the rate of reduction of ATP (Figure 24.1). Secondly, two molecules of ADP may combine to form one of ATP and one of AMP (the adenylate kinase reaction). This reaction is driven forward by the removal of AMP (adenosine monophosphate), which is converted to adenosine (a potent vasodilator) and thence to inosine, hypoxanthine, xanthine and uric acid, with irreversible loss of adenine nucleotides. The implications for production of reactive oxygen species are discussed on page 383.

END-PRODUCTS OF METABOLISM

The end-products of aerobic metabolism are carbon dioxide and water, both of which are easily diffusible and lost from the body. The main anaerobic pathway produces hydrogen and lactate ions

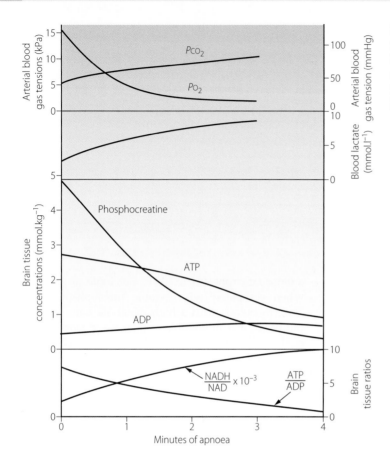

Fig. 24.1 Biochemical changes during 4 minutes of respiratory arrest in rats previously breathing 30% oxygen. Recovery of all values, except blood lactate, was complete within 5 minutes of restarting pulmonary ventilation. (Data from reference 1.)

which, from most of the body, escape into the circulation, where they may be conveniently quantified in terms of the base deficit, excess lactate or lactate/pyruvate ratio. However, the blood–brain barrier is relatively impermeable to charged ions, and therefore hydrogen and lactate ions are retained within the neurones of the hypoxic brain. Lactacidosis can only occur when circulation is maintained to provide the large quantities of glucose required for conversion to lactic acid.

In severe cerebral hypoxia, a major part of the dysfunction and damage is due to intracellular acidosis rather than simply depletion of high energy compounds (see below). Gross hypoperfusion is more damaging than total ischaemia, because the latter limits glucose supply and therefore the formation of lactic acid. Similarly, patients who have an episode of cerebral ischaemia whilst hyperglycaemic (e.g. a stroke) have been found to have more severe brain injury than those with normal or low blood glucose levels at the time of the hypoxic event.[3]

INITIATION OF GLYCOLYSIS[4]

The enzyme 6-phosphofructokinase (PFK) is the rate-limiting step of the glycolytic pathway (see Figure 11.13). Activity of PFK is enhanced by the presence of ADP, AMP and phosphate, which will rapidly accumulate during hypoxia, thus accelerating glycolysis. PFK is, however, inhibited by acidosis, which will therefore quickly limit the formation of ATP from glucose. The intracellular production of phosphate from ATP breakdown also promotes the activity of glycogen phosphorylase, which cleaves glycogen molecules to produce fructose-1,6-diphosphate. This enters the glycolytic pathway below the rate-limiting PFK reaction, and also avoids the expenditure of two molecules of ATP in its derivation from glucose. Therefore four molecules of ATP are produced from one of fructose-1,6-diphosphate in comparison with two from one molecule of glucose. There is no subsequent stage in the glycolytic pathway that is significantly rate-limited by acidosis. Provided glycogen is available within the cell, this second pathway therefore provides a valuable reserve for the production of ATP.

MECHANISMS OF HYPOXIC CELL DAMAGE

Many mechanisms contribute to cell damage or death from hypoxia. The precise role of each is unclear, but there is general agreement that different tissues respond to hypoxia in quite varied ways. Also, the nature of the hypoxic insult has a large effect with differing speed of onset, degree of hypoxia, blood flow, blood glucose concentration and tissue metabolic activity all influencing the resulting tissue dysfunction.

IMMEDIATE CELLULAR RESPONSES TO HYPOXIA[5]

Because of the dramatic clinical consequences of nervous system damage, neuronal cells are the most widely studied and therefore form the basis for the mechanisms described in this section.[2] Changes in the transmembrane potential of a hypoxic neurone are shown in Figure 24.2, along with the major physiological changes that occur. At the onset of anoxia, CNS cells immediately become either slightly hyperpolarised (as shown in Figure 24.2) or depolarised, depending on the cell type. This is followed by a gradual reduction in membrane potential until a 'threshold' value is reached, when a spontaneous rapid depolarisation occurs. At this stage there are gross abnormalities in ion channel function and the normal intracellular and extracellular ionic gradients are abolished, leading to cell death.

Potassium and sodium flux. Hypoxia has a direct effect on potassium channels (page 71), increasing transmembrane K^+ conductance and causing the immediate hyperpolarisation. Potassium begins to leak out from the cell, increasing the extracellular K^+ concentration thus tending to depolarise the cell membrane. Potassium leakage, along with sodium influx, are accelerated when falling ATP levels cause failure of the Na/K ATPase pump. Following rapid depolarisation, sodium and potassium channels probably simply remain open, allowing free

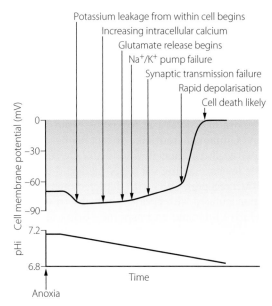

Fig. 24.2 Changes in transmembrane potential and intracellular pH (pHi) in a neuronal cell following the sudden onset of anoxia. Significant physiological events in the course of the hypoxic insult are shown. Once membrane potential reaches zero, cell death is almost inevitable (see text for details). The time between anoxia and rapid depolarisation is highly variable, between about 4 minutes with complete ischaemia to almost an hour with hypoxia and preserved blood flow. (After reference 2.)

passage of ions across the cell membrane leading to cellular destruction.

Calcium. Intracellular calcium concentration increases shortly after the onset of hypoxia. Voltage gated calcium channels open in response to the falling transmembrane potential and the increasing intracellular sodium concentration causes the membrane-bound Na/Ca exchanger to reverse its activity. An altered transmembrane potential is detected within the cell by ryonidine receptors on intracellular organelles leading to release of calcium from the endoplasmic reticulum and mitochondria.[6] This increase in intracellular calcium is generally harmful, causing the activation of ATPase enzymes just when ATP may be critically low, the activation of proteases to damage sarcolemma and the cytoskeleton, and the uncontrolled release of neurotransmitters (see below). At this stage, the cell has probably not been irretrievably damaged by spontaneous depolarisation, but derangement of calcium channel function effectively prevents normal synaptic transmission and therefore cellular function.

Extracellular adenosine, formed from the degradation of AMP, is also believed to play a role in blocking calcium channels during anoxia.[2]

Excitatory amino acid release.[7] The excitatory amino acids glutamate and aspartate are released from many neurones at concentrations of 2–5× normal early in the course of a hypoxic insult, followed by further dramatic increases following rapid depolarisation. Glutamate reuptake mechanisms also fail, and extracellular concentrations quickly reach neurotoxic levels,[7,8] acting via the N-methyl-d-aspartate (NMDA) receptor. Cells with depleted energy stores are particularly susceptible, but the mechanism by which glutamate and aspartate bring about cell damage is unknown.

DELAYED CELLULAR RESPONSES TO HYPOXIA

Following brain injury in humans, cerebral oedema often continues to develop for some hours after the initial insult. There are several possible explanations for this delayed neuronal damage with activation of many different cellular systems being implicated. However, it is a quite different clinical problem that has recently focussed attention on cellular adaptations to hypoxia. The core of many solid malignant tumours has a poor blood supply, caused by the failure of angiogenesis to keep up with the rapid tumour growth. Tumour hypoxia is associated with highly malignant, aggressive tumours, which often respond poorly to treatment. For this reason, much recent research has focussed on understanding the cellular effects of hypoxia, with a view to developing new therapeutic approaches.

Table 24.1 shows the numerous genes that may be induced by hypoxia. Most of the systems activated by hypoxia assist the cell in overcoming the hypoxic conditions, for example erythropoietin to increase haemoglobin concentration, or glycolytic enzymes to increase anaerobic ATP formation. Some activated genes may accelerate cell proliferation and therefore increase tumour malignancy, while other genes are activated that encourage apoptosis and impair tumour growth.[9]

Hypoxia inducible factor 1 (HIF-1).[10–12] Many of these cellular adaptations to hypoxia are mediated by a transcription regulating protein called HIF-1. Under normal conditions cytoplasmic HIF-1 is ubiquitous, but a prolyl-hydroxylase protein (PHD-1) rapidly hydroxylates HIF-1 rendering it inactive. Oxygen is required as a cosubstrate for this reaction such that when cellular hypoxia occurs hydroxylation by PHD-1 fails and HIF-1 remains stable for long enough to initiate transcription of some of the hypoxia induced genes shown in Table 24.1. The HIF-1 system is now seen as a major potential target for therapeutic agents to treat malignancies prone to tumour hypoxia.

ISCHAEMIC PRECONDITIONING[13,14]

Prior exposure of a tissue to a series of short periods of hypoxia, interspersed with normal oxygen levels, has been found to influence the tissue's subsequent response to a prolonged ischaemic insult, a phenomenon known as ischaemic preconditioning. Though mostly studied in heart muscle, ischaemic preconditioning has been demonstrated in other tissues.

Table 24.1 Genes induced by hypoxia and their effects

FUNCTION	GENE	BIOLOGICAL ACTION
Oxygen transport	Erythropoietin	Stimulation of red cell production
	Transferrin	Iron transport
Increased blood flow	VEGF	Angiogenesis
	NO synthase	Vasodilatation
ATP production	Glucose transporter-1	Transfer of glucose into cell
	Hexokinase	
	Aldolase	Glycolysis (see Figure 11.13)
	Pyruvate kinase	
	Lactate dehydrogenase	
pH correction	Carbonic anhydrase	Buffering of metabolic acidosis
Inflammation	Interleukin-6, -8	Activation of inflammatory cells

VEGF, Vascular endothelial growth factor; NO, nitric oxide.

Early protection. Reduction in the damage occurring from an ischaemic period begins immediately after the preconditioning has occurred, and lasts for 2–3 hours. Activation of sarcolemmal and mitochondrial ATP-dependent K channels (K_{ATP}) is believed to be the main mechanism by which protection from ischaemia occurs. After preconditioning, the enhanced activity of K_{ATP} channels helps to maintain the transmembrane potential nearer to normal values, and so slows the rate of progression of the immediate cellular responses to hypoxia described above. During prolonged hypoxia, fluid and electrolyte imbalances also occur across the mitochondrial membrane impairing the ability of the cell to make the best use of any oxygen remaining in the cell. Activated mitochondrial K_{ATP} channels will again reduce the rate at which these changes occur. Extracellular triggers that bring about preconditioning include adenosine, purines, bradykinin or catecholamines, all acting via G-proteins and protein kinase C to cause activation of the K_{ATP} channels.

Late protection. This describes the protection from ischaemia seen about 12 hours after the preconditioning and is less effective than early protection. It is again mediated by activation of K_{ATP} channels, this time brought about by gene transcription of proteins such as inducible nitric oxide synthase, superoxide dismutase (page 385) or cyclo-oxygenase (page 224).

Agents used for preconditioning. Several drugs, but particularly inhalational anaesthetics, can precondition cardiac muscle in a manner similar to brief ischaemic episodes.[13,15] The mechanism is also similar, with most of the effective drugs somehow enhancing K_{ATP} channel activity. Similar responses occur to the noble gases helium and xenon, possibly mediated by modulation of nitric oxide.[16] Unfortunately, impressive laboratory studies of ischaemic preconditioning have so far failed to translate into clinically useful benefits, possibly because of an inability of diseased cardiac muscle to show the same response to preconditioning as that of normal myocardium.[17]

Po_2 LEVELS AT WHICH HYPOXIA OCCURS

CELLULAR Po_2

'Critical Po_2' refers to the oxygen tension below which oxidative cellular metabolism fails. For isolated mitochondria, this is known to be below 0.13 kPa (1 mmHg), and possibly as low as 0.01 kPa (0.1 mmHg) in muscle cells[4] despite their large oxygen consumption. Venous Po_2 approximates to end-capillary Po_2, and though highly variable this is usually in excess of 3 kPa ($\approx$20 mmHg) even in maximally working skeletal muscle. Thus with the minimal Po_2 in the nearby capillary being approximately 200 times greater than that required by the mitochondria, it is difficult to envisage how cellular hypoxia can occur in all but the most extreme situations. There are reasons why this is not the case in vivo.

Measurement of intracellular Po_2 is difficult. The most widely used technique is applicable only to muscle cells and involves measurement of myoglobin saturation, from which Po_2 may be determined. These studies have indicated that intracellular Po_2 is in the range 0.5–2 kPa (3–15 mmHg) depending on cell activity.[4] Many studies have also indicated a minimal difference between the Po_2 in extracellular fluid and within cells.[17] This would indicate a possibly substantial barrier to oxygen diffusion between the capillary and extracellular fluid. Finally, diffusion of oxygen within cells is believed to be slow because of the proteinaceous nature of the cytoplasm, and therefore large variations in intracellular Po_2 are likely to exist. Thus in intact cells, as opposed to isolated mitochondria, critical Po_2 is more likely to be of the order of 0.5–1.3 kPa (3–10 mmHg), much closer to the end-capillary value.[18]

CRITICAL ARTERIAL Po_2 FOR CEREBRAL FUNCTION

The minimal safe level of arterial Po_2 is that which will maintain a safe tissue Po_2. This will depend on many factors besides arterial Po_2, including haemoglobin concentration, tissue perfusion and tissue oxygen consumption. These factors accord with Barcroft's classification of 'anoxia' into anoxic, anaemic and stagnant (page 203), which has previously been shown as a Venn diagram (see Figure 11.16).

This argument may be extended to consider in which circumstances the venous Po_2 (and by implication tissue Po_2) may fall below its critical level corresponding, in normal blood, to 32% saturation and oxygen content of 6.4 ml.dl^{-1}. If the brain has a mean oxygen consumption of 46 ml.min^{-1} and a blood flow of 620 ml.min^{-1}, the arterial/venous oxygen content difference will be 7.4 ml.dl^{-1}. Therefore, *with normal cerebral perfusion, haemoglobin concentration, pH, etc.,* this would correspond to a critical arterial oxygen content of $13.8\,ml.dl^{-1}$, saturation 68% and Po_2 4.8 kPa (36 mmHg). This calculation and others under various different conditions are set out in Table 24.2.

However, the other factors in italics (above) will probably not be normal. They may be unfavourable as a result of multiple pathologies in the patient (e.g. anaemia or a decreased cerebral blood flow). Alternatively, there may be favourable factors, such as polycythaemia in chronic arterial hypoxaemia, or reduced cerebral oxygen requirements during hypothermia or anaesthesia. The possible combinations of circumstances are so great that it is not feasible to consider every possible situation. Instead, certain important examples have been selected which illustrate the fundamentals of the problem, and these are shown in Table 24.2.

Uncompensated ischaemia is dangerous and, with a 45% reduction in cerebral blood flow, any reduction of arterial Po_2 exposes the brain to risk of hypoxia. Uncompensated anaemia is almost equally dangerous, although an increase in cerebral blood flow restores a satisfactory safety margin. In the example in Table 24.2, a 40% reduction of blood oxygen carrying capacity and a 40% increase of cerebral blood flow permits the arterial Po_2 to fall to 5.3 kPa (40 mmHg) without the cerebral venous Po_2 falling below 2.7 kPa (20 mmHg). The last line in Table 24.2 shows the very dangerous combination of anaemia (haemoglobin concentration $11\,g.dl^{-1}$) and cerebral blood flow three-quarters of normal. Neither abnormality is very serious considered separately, but in combination the arterial Po_2 cannot be reduced below its normal value without the risk of cerebral hypoxia.

Table 24.2 is not to be taken too literally, because there are many minor factors that have not been considered. However, it is a general rule that maximal cerebral vasodilatation may be expected to occur in any condition (other than cerebral ischaemia) that threatens cerebral oxygenation. Also, there are circumstances in which the critical organ is not the brain but the heart, liver or kidney.

The most important message of this discussion is that there is no simple answer to the question 'What is the safe lower limit of arterial Po_2?'. Acclimatised mountaineers have remained conscious at high altitude with arterial Po_2 values as low as 3.28 kPa (25 mmHg) (Chapter 17). Patients presenting with severe respiratory disease tend to remain conscious down to similar levels of arterial Po_2. However, both acclimatised mountaineers

and patients with chronic respiratory disease have compensatory polycythaemia and maximal cerebral vasodilatation. Uncompensated subjects who are acutely exposed to hypoxia are unlikely to remain conscious at such low values for arterial Po_2, but considerable individual variation must be expected.

EFFECTS OF HYPOXIA

Hypoxia presents a serious threat to the body, and compensatory mechanisms usually take priority over other changes. Thus, for example, in hypoxia with concomitant hypocapnia, hyperventilation and an increase in cerebral blood flow occur in spite of the decreased Pco_2. Certain compensatory mechanisms will come into play whatever the reason for the hypoxia, although their effectiveness will depend to a large extent on the cause. For example, hyperventilation will be largely ineffective in stagnant or anaemic hypoxia because hyperventilation while breathing air can do little to increase the oxygen content of arterial blood, and usually nothing to increase perfusion.

Hyperventilation results from a decreased arterial Po_2 but the response is non-linear (see Figure 5.7). There is little effect until arterial Po_2 is reduced to about 7 kPa (52.5 mmHg): maximal response is at 4 kPa (30 mmHg). The interrelationship between hypoxia and other factors in the control of breathing is discussed in Chapter 5.

Pulmonary distribution of blood flow is improved by hypoxia as a result of hypoxic pulmonary vasoconstriction (page 108).

The sympathetic system is concerned in many of the responses to hypoxia, particularly the increase in organ perfusion. The immediate response is reflex and is initiated by chemoreceptor stimulation: it occurs before there is any measurable increase in circulating catecholamines, although this does occur in due course. Reduction of cerebral and probably myocardial vascular resistance is not dependent on the autonomic system but depends on local responses in the vicinity of the vessels themselves. With the exception of pulmonary vessels, hypoxia causes vasodilatation of blood vessels almost everywhere in the body. This results mainly from a direct effect of adenosine and other metabolites generated by hypoxia.

Cardiac output is increased by hypoxia, together with the regional blood flow to almost every major organ, particularly the brain.

Table 24.2 Lowest arterial oxygen levels compatible with a cerebral venous Po_2 of 2.7 kPa (20 mmHg) under various conditions

| | BLOOD O$_2$ CAPACITY | BRAIN O$_2$ CONSUMPTION | CEREBRAL BLOOD FLOW | CEREBRAL VENOUS BLOOD | | | | ART./VEN. O$_2$ CONTENT DIFFERENCE | ARTERIAL BLOOD | | | |
| | | | | Po_2 | | SAT. | O$_2$ CONTENT | | O$_2$ CONTENT | SAT. | Po_2 | |
	ml.dl^{-1}	ml.min^{-1}	ml.min^{-1}	kPa	mmHg	%	ml.dl^{-1}	ml.dl^{-1}	ml.dl^{-1}	%	kPa	mmHg
Normal values	20	46	620	4.4	33	63	12.6	7.4	20.0	98	13	100
Uncompensated arterial hypoxaemia	20	46	620	2.7	20	32	6.4	7.4	13.8	68	4.8	36
Arterial hypoxaemia with increased cerebral blood flow	20	46	1240	2.7	20	32	6.4	3.7	10.1	50	3.6	27
Arterial hypoxaemia with polycythaemia	25	46	620	2.7	20	32	8.0	7.4	15.4	61	4.3	32
Arterial hypoxaemia with alkalosis*	20	46	620	2.7	20	46	9.2	7.4	16.6	82	4.9	37
Arterial hypoxaemia with hypothermia†	20	23	620	2.7	20	57	11.4	3.7	15.1	75	3.6	27
Uncompensated cerebral ischaemia	20	46	340	2.7	20	32	6.4	13.5	19.9	98	15	112
Uncompensated anaemia	12	46	620	2.7	20	32	3.8	7.4	11.2	93	8.9	67
Anaemia with increased cerebral blood flow	12	46	870	2.7	20	32	3.8	5.3	9.1	75	5.3	40
Combined anaemia and ischaemia	15	46	460	2.7	20	32	4.8	10.0	14.8	97	12	92

*pH 7.6.
†Temperature 30°C; cerebral O$_2$ consumption reduced to half normal.

Haemoglobin concentration is not increased in acute hypoxia in humans but it is increased in chronic hypoxia due to residence at altitude or respiratory disease.

The oxyhaemoglobin dissociation curve is displaced to the right by an increase in 2,3-DPG and by acidosis which may also be present. This tends to increase tissue Po_2 (see Figure 11.10).

Anaerobic metabolism is increased in severe hypoxia in an attempt to maintain the level of ATP (see above).

References

1. Kaasik AE, Nilsson L, Siesjö BK. The effect of asphyxia upon the lactate, pyruvate and bicarbonate concentrations of brain tissue and cisternal CSF, and upon the tissue concentrations of phosphocreatine and adenine nucleotides in anesthetized rats. *Acta Physiol Scand*. 1970;78:433–437.

2. Martin RL, Lloyd HGE, Cowan AI. The early events of oxygen and glucose deprivation: setting the scene for neuronal death? *Trends Neurosci*. 1994;17:251–256.

3. Candelise L, Landi G, Orazio EN, Boccardi E. Prognostic significance of hyperglycaemia in acute stroke. *Arch Neurol*. 1985;42:661–663.

4. Connett RJ, Honig CR, Gayeski TEJ, Brooks GA. Defining hypoxia: a systems view of $\dot{V}o_2$, glycolysis, energetics, and intracellular Po_2. *J Appl Physiol*. 1990;68:833–842.

*5. Ransom BR, Brown AM. Intracellular Ca^{2+} release and ischemic axon injury: the Trojan horse is back. *Neuron*. 2003;40:2–4.

6. Katchman AN, Hershkowitz N. Early anoxia-induced vesicular glutamate release results from mobilization of calcium from intracellular stores. *J Neurophysiol*. 1993;70:1–7.

7. Choi DW. Cerebral hypoxia: some new approaches and unanswered questions. *J Neurosci*. 1990;10:2493–2501.

8. Ohmori T, Hirashima Y, Kurimoto M, Endo S, Takaku A. In vitro hypoxia of cortical and hippocampal CA1 neurons: glutamate, nitric oxide, and platelet activating factor participate in the mechanism of selective neural death in CA1 neurons. *Brain Res*. 1996;743:109–115.

9. Harris AL. Hypoxia – A key regulatory factor in tumour growth. *Nat Rev Cancer*. 2002;2:38–46.

10. Höpfl G, Ogunshola O, Gassman M. HIFs and tumors – causes and consequences. *Am J Physiol Regul Integr Comp Physiol*. 2004;286:R608–R623.

*11. Semenza GL. HIF-1: mediator of physiological and pathophysiological responses to hypoxia. *J Appl Physiol*. 2000;88:1474–1480.

*12. Berchner-Pfannschmidt U, Frede S, Wotzlaw C, Fandrey J. Imaging of the hypoxia-inducible factor pathway: insights into oxygen sensing. *Eur Respir J*. 2008;32:210–217.

13. Zaugg M, Lucchinetti E, Uecker M, Pasch T, Schaub MC. Anaesthetics and cardiac preconditioning. Part I. Signalling and cytoprotective mechanisms. *Br J Anaesth*. 2003;91:551–565.

14. Zaugg M, Lucchinetti E, Garcia C, Pasch T, Spahn DR, Schaub MC. Anaesthetics and cardiac preconditioning. Part II. Clinical implications. *Br J Anaesth*. 2003;91:566–576.

15. Tanaka K, Ludwig LM, Kersten JR, Pagel PS, Warltier DC. Mechanisms of cardioprotection by volatile anaesthetics. *Anesthesiology*. 2004;100:707–721.

16. Pagel PS, Krolikowski JG, Pratt PF, et al. The mechanism of helium-induced preconditioning: a direct role for nitric oxide in rabbits. *Anesth Analg*. 2008;107:762–768.

17. Rumsey WL, Wilson DF. Tissue capacity for mitochondrial oxidative phosphorylation and its adaptation to stress. In: Fregly MJ, Blatteis CM, eds *Handbook of Physiology, Section 4: Environmental Physiology*. New York & Oxford: Oxford University Press; 1996:1095–1114.

18. Epstein FH, Agmon Y, Brezis M. Physiology of renal hypoxia. *Ann N Y Acad Sci*. 1995;718:72–81.

Chapter 25

Anaemia

KEY POINTS

- Anaemia has little effect on pulmonary gas exchange but decreases oxygen carriage in the arterial blood in direct proportion to the reduction in haemoglobin concentration.
- Mechanisms that compensate for the reduced oxygen delivery include increased cardiac output, increased tissue oxygen extraction and a right shift of the oxyhaemoglobin dissociation curve.
- Older patients or those with poor cardiac reserve compensate less well when anaemic.

Anaemia is a widespread pathophysiological disorder that interferes with oxygen transport to the tissues. In developed countries it has a varied aetiology, including iron deficiency, chronic haemorrhage, end-stage renal failure or depletion of vitamin B_{12}. However, in the Third World it is endemic, major factors including malnutrition and infestation with various parasites such as hookworm and bilharzia. In many countries, haemoglobin concentrations within the range $6-10\,\text{g.dl}^{-1}$ are regarded as normal.

Anaemia per se has no major direct effects on pulmonary function. Arterial P_{O_2} and saturation should remain within the normal range in uncomplicated anaemia, and the crucial effect is on the arterial oxygen content and therefore oxygen delivery. Important compensatory changes are increases in cardiac output, greater oxygen extraction from the arterial blood and to a lesser extent the small rightward displacement of the oxyhaemoglobin dissociation curve. However, there are limits to these

adaptations, which define the minimal tolerable haemoglobin concentration, and also the exercise limits attainable at various levels of severity of anaemia.

Physiological aspects of blood transfusion and blood substitutes are discussed on page 197.

PULMONARY FUNCTION

GAS EXCHANGE

Alveolar P_{O_2} is determined by dry barometric pressure, inspired oxygen concentration and the ratio of oxygen consumption to alveolar ventilation (page 139). Assuming that the first two are unchanged, and there being good evidence that the latter two factors are unaffected in the resting state by anaemia down to a haemoglobin concentration of at least $5\,\text{g.dl}^{-1}$ (see below), then there is no reason why alveolar P_{O_2} or P_{CO_2} should be affected by uncomplicated anaemia down to this degree of severity.

The increased cardiac output (see below) will cause a small reduction in pulmonary capillary transit time which, together with the reduced mass of haemoglobin in the pulmonary capillaries, causes a modest decrease in diffusing capacity (page 152). However, such is the reserve in the capacity of pulmonary capillary blood to reach equilibrium with the alveolar gas (see Figure 9.2) that it is highly unlikely that this would have any measurable effect on the alveolar/end-pulmonary capillary P_{O_2} gradient, which in the normal subject is believed to be of the order of only $10^{-6}\,\text{mmHg}$. Thus pulmonary end-capillary P_{O_2} should also be normal in anaemia.

DOI: 10.1016/B978-0-7020-2996-7.00025-8

Continuing down the cascade of oxygen partial pressures from ambient air to the site of use in the tissues, the next step is the gradient in P_{O_2} between pulmonary end-capillary blood and mixed arterial blood. The P_{O_2} gradient at this stage is caused by shunting and the perfusion of relatively underventilated alveoli. There is no evidence that these factors are altered in anaemia, and arterial P_{O_2} should therefore be normal. Because the peripheral chemoreceptors are stimulated by reduction in arterial P_{O_2} and not arterial oxygen content (page 71), then there should be no stimulation of respiration unless the degree of hypoxia is sufficient to cause anaerobic metabolism and lactacidosis.

THE HAEMOGLOBIN DISSOCIATION CURVE

It is well established that red blood cell 2,3-diphosphoglycerate levels are increased in anaemia (page 194), typical changes being from a normal value of 5 mmol.l^{-1} to 7 mmol.l^{-1} at a haemoglobin concentration of 6 g.dl^{-1}.[1] This results in an increase in P_{50} from 3.6 to 4.0 kPa (27 to 30 mmHg). This rightward shift of the dissociation curve would have a negligible effect on arterial saturation, which has indeed been reported to be normal in anaemia. The rightward shift will, however, increase the P_{O_2} at which oxygen is unloaded in the tissues, mitigating to a small extent the effects of reduction in oxygen delivery so far as tissue P_{O_2} is concerned.

ARTERIAL OXYGEN CONTENT

Although the arterial oxygen saturation usually remains normal in anaemia, the oxygen content of the arterial blood will be reduced in approximate proportion to the decrease in haemoglobin concentration. Arterial oxygen content can be expressed as follows:

$$Ca_{O_2} = ([Hb] \times Sa_{O_2} \times 1.39) + 0.3$$
$$\text{ml.dl}^{-1} \quad \text{g.dl}^{-1} \quad \%/100 \quad \text{ml.g}^{-1} \quad \text{ml.dl}^{-1}$$
$$\text{e.g. } 20 = (14.7 \times 0.97 \times 1.39) + 0.3 \quad (1)$$

where Ca_{O_2} is arterial oxygen content, [Hb] is haemoglobin concentration, Sa_{O_2} is arterial oxygen saturation, 1.39 is the combining power of haemoglobin with oxygen (page 189) and 0.3 is dissolved oxygen at normal arterial P_{O_2}.

OXYGEN DELIVERY

The important concept of oxygen delivery ($\dot{D}_{O_2}$) is considered in detail on page 202. It is defined as the product of cardiac output ($\dot{Q}$) and Ca_{O_2}.

$$\dot{D}_{O_2} = \dot{Q} \times Ca_{O_2}$$
$$\text{ml.min}^{-1} \quad \text{1.min}^{-1} \quad \text{ml.dl}^{-1}$$
$$\text{e.g. } 1050 = 5.25 \times 20 \quad (2)$$

(the right-hand side is multiplied by a scaling factor of 10 to account for the differing units of volume).

Combining equations (1) and (2):

$$\dot{D}_{O_2} = \dot{Q} \times \{([Hb]) \times Sa_{O_2} \times 1.39) + 0.3\}$$
$$\text{ml.min}^{-1} \quad \text{1.min}^{-1} \quad \text{g.dl}^{-1} \quad \%/100 \quad \text{ml.g}^{-1} \quad \text{ml.dl}^{-1}$$
$$\text{e.g. } 1050 = 5.25 \times \{(14.7 \times 0.97 \times 1.39) + 0.3\}$$
$$(3)$$

(the right-hand side is again multiplied by a scaling factor of 10).

Normal values give an oxygen delivery of approximately 1000 ml.min^{-1}, which is about four times the normal resting oxygen consumption of 250 ml.min^{-1}. Extraction of oxygen from the arterial blood is thus 25% and this accords with an arterial saturation of 97% and mixed venous saturation of 72%.

If the small quantity of dissolved oxygen (0.3 ml.dl^{-1}) is ignored, then oxygen delivery is seen to be proportional to the product of cardiac output, haemoglobin concentration and arterial oxygen saturation. There is, of course, negligible scope for any compensatory increase in saturation in a patient with uncomplicated anaemia at sea level.

EFFECT OF ANAEMIA ON CARDIAC OUTPUT

Equation (3) shows that, if other factors remain the same, a reduction in haemoglobin concentration will result in a proportionate reduction in oxygen delivery. Thus a haemoglobin concentration of 7.5 g.dl^{-1}, with unchanged cardiac output, would halve delivery to give a resting value of 500 ml.min^{-1}, which would be approaching the likely critical value. However, patients with quite severe anaemia usually show little evidence of hypoxia at rest and, furthermore, achieve surprisingly good levels of exercise. Because arterial saturation cannot be

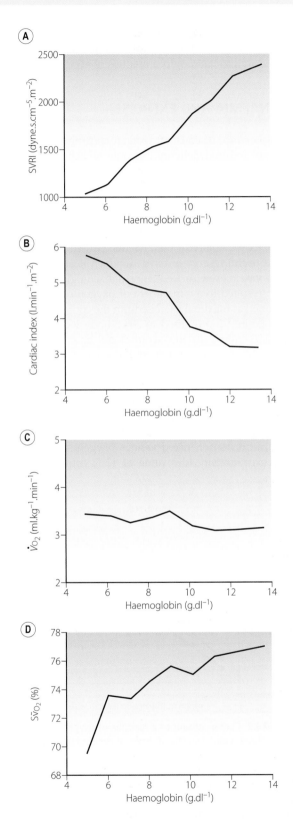

increased, full compensation can be achieved only by a reciprocal relationship between cardiac output and haemoglobin concentration. Thus, if haemoglobin concentration is halved, maintenance of normal delivery will require a doubling of cardiac output. Full compensation may not occur, but fortunately a reduction in haemoglobin concentration is usually accompanied by some increase in cardiac output.

Acute anaemia. Early studies of cardiac output and anaemia involved measurement of cardiovascular parameters in patients before and after treatment for uncomplicated anaemia.[2] Cardiac output was significantly greater before the patients' haemoglobin concentration increased from 5.9 to $10.9 \, g.dl^{-1}$. There was, however, a negative correlation between age and cardiac index in the anaemic state, reflecting the relative inability of the older patient to compensate. More recent studies have involved deliberately reducing the haemoglobin concentration isovolaemically in volunteers and patients.[3-6] One of these studies reduced the haemoglobin concentration from 13.1 to $5.0 \, g.dl^{-1}$, and the effects of this on the cardiovascular system are shown in Figure 25.1.[4] In these healthy volunteers the predictable linear relationship between cardiac index and haemoglobin concentration can easily be seen (Figure 25.1B). The increase in cardiac output seen in response to acute anaemia is much less in anaesthetised patients.[5]

The mechanism underlying the increase in cardiac output is not clear, but is due to increases in both stroke volume and heart rate.[4] Likely explanations for these changes include reduced cardiac afterload due to lowered blood viscosity (Figure 25.1A), and increased preload due to greater venous return secondary to increased tone in capacitance vessels.[7]

Chronic anaemia. In one study of isovolaemic reduction of haemoglobin concentration, down to a mean value of $10 \, g.dl^{-1}$, the anaemia was then maintained at the same level for 14 days.[3] Immediately after induction of anaemia there was a marked increase in

Fig. 25.1 Cardiovascular changes in response to acute isovolaemic reduction of mean haemoglobin concentration from 13.1 to $5.0 \, g.dl^{-1}$. (A) Systemic vascular resistance index (SVRI) falls in direct proportion to Hb concentration as blood viscosity decreases; (B) Cardiac index doubles when Hb has fallen to $5.0 \, g.dl^{-1}$ in these healthy volunteers; (C) Oxygen delivery ($\dot{V}_{O_2}$) remains constant due to the increase in cardiac output exactly matching the decrease in arterial oxygen content; (D) Mixed venous oxygen saturation ($S\bar{v}_{O_2}$) falls as the tissues extract more oxygen. (After reference 4.)

cardiac output (55%), but this decreased to only 14% above control levels after 14 days.

THE INFLUENCE OF CARDIAC OUTPUT ON OXYGEN DELIVERY

Following the acute reduction of haemoglobin concentration in healthy subjects,[3,4] cardiac output increased sufficiently to maintain normal or near-normal oxygen delivery (Figure 25.1C). However, in sustained anaemia, the increase in cardiac output (only 14%) is insufficient to maintain oxygen delivery, which decreases to 25% below control values. Similarly, in a study of anaemic patients,[2] oxygen delivery was reduced in proportion to the degree of anaemia.

Without an increase in cardiac output, it is likely that a haemoglobin concentration of 6–8 g.dl^{-1} would be the minimal level compatible with life. It is clear that the ability of the cardiovascular system to respond to anaemia with an increase in cardiac output is an essential aspect of accommodation to anaemia, and this is less effective in anaesthetised patients, the elderly or other subjects with reduced cardiac reserve.

Relationship between oxygen delivery and consumption. The relationship between oxygen delivery and consumption has been considered on page 202 et seq. When oxygen delivery is reduced, for whatever reason, oxygen consumption is at first maintained at its normal value, but with increasing oxygen extraction and therefore decreasing mixed venous saturation (Figure 25.1D). Below a 'critical' value for oxygen delivery, oxygen consumption decreases as a function of delivery, and is usually accompanied by evidence of hypoxia, such as increased lactate in peripheral blood. Values for critical oxygen delivery depend upon the pathophysiological state of the patient and vary from one condition to another.

It has not been clearly established what is the critical level of oxygen delivery in uncomplicated anaemia in humans. Studies of acutely induced anaemia have found no evidence of tissue hypoxia, though in one study, at a haemoglobin concentration of 5 g.dl^{-1}, oxygen consumption was reduced in spite of oxygen delivery being well maintained. In volunteers maintained at a haemoglobin concentration of 10 g.dl^{-1} for 14 days, oxygen delivery decreased from about 1200 to 900 ml.min^{-1} while oxygen consumption remained virtually unchanged.[3] Similarly, a study of treated anaemic patients found no increase in oxygen consumption when haemoglobin concentration was increased from mean value of 6 to 11 g.dl^{-1}.[2] Thus these patients with long-term anaemia seemed to have all remained above the critical value for oxygen delivery down to haemoglobin values of about 6 g.dl^{-1}.

ANAEMIA AND EXERCISE

Maintenance of constant oxygen consumption in the face of reduced delivery can only be achieved at the expense of a reduction in mixed venous saturation, as a result of increased extraction of oxygen from the arterial blood. This has been clearly demonstrated in both acute (Figure 25.1D) and sustained anaemia.[3] A reduction in the oxygen content of mixed venous blood curtails the ability of the anaemic patient to encroach on a useful reserve of oxygen, which is an important response to exercise. Reduction of haemoglobin to 10 g.dl^{-1} resulted in a curtailment of oxygen consumption attained at maximal exercise from the control values of 3.01 l.min^{-1} (normalised to 70 kg body weight) down to 2.53 l.min^{-1} in the acute stage, and 2.15 l.min^{-1} after 14 days of sustained anaemia (Figure 25.2).[3] The increase in cardiac output required for the same increase in oxygen consumption was greater in the anaemic state, and cardiac output at maximal oxygen consumption was slightly less than under control conditions. Maximal exercise in the anaemic state resulted in a reduction of mixed venous oxygen saturation to the exceptionally low value of 12%, compared with

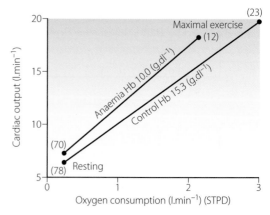

Fig. 25.2 Cardiac output as a function of oxygen consumption during rest and maximal exercise under control and isovolaemic anaemic conditions. Numbers in parentheses indicate mean mixed venous oxygen saturation. (Redrawn from reference 3 on the assumption that mean weight of the subjects was 70 kg, by permission of the author, and the Editors and publishers of Journal of Applied Physiology.)

control values of 23% during maximal exercise with a normal haemoglobin concentration.

Brisk walking on level ground normally requires an oxygen consumption of about $1 \, l.min^{-1}$ and a cardiac output of about $10 \, l.min^{-1}$. At a haemoglobin level of $5 \, g.dl^{-1}$, this would require a cardiac output of about $20 \, l.min^{-1}$ to permit an oxygen consumption of $1 \, l.min^{-1}$ with a satisfactory residual level of mixed venous oxygen saturation. It will be clear that, at this degree of anaemia, cardiac function is a critical factor determining the mobility of a patient.

Exercise tolerance may be limited by either respiratory or circulatory capacity. In uncomplicated anaemia, there is no reason to implicate respiratory limitation, and exercise tolerance is therefore, to a first approximation, governed by the remaining factors in the oxygen delivery equation (3) (above). On the assumption that the maximal sustainable cardiac output is only marginally affected by anaemia, it is to be expected that exercise tolerance will be reduced in direct proportion to the haemoglobin concentration. Available evidence supports this hypothesis (Figure 25.3).

Using haemoglobin to enhance athletic performance. The corollary of the preceding description is the question of improving athletic performance by increasing haemoglobin concentration above the normal range. This used to be achieved by removal of blood for replacement of red cells after a few weeks when the subject has already partially restored his haemoglobin concentration, a procedure known as blood doping. The same effect is now much more conveniently achieved by the administration of erythropoietin. Studies of trained athletes in this area are notoriously difficult, and it is easy to confuse the effects of changes in blood volume and haemoglobin concentration. Furthermore, blood doping involves the subject continuing his training after removal of blood while he is anaemic. This may well make his training more effective, as is the case when training is undertaken at altitude. In the pioneer study of Ekblom et al in 1972,[9] it was reported that, following reinfusion of blood (resulting in an increase in haemoglobin concentration from 13.2 to $14.9 \, g.dl^{-1}$), maximal oxygen consumption was increased from 4.40 to $4.79 \, l.min^{-1}$, and time to exhaustion during uphill treadmill running was extended from 5.43 to 6.67 minutes. These findings were challenged in subsequent studies, but confirmed in a well-controlled study of highly trained runners,[10] in which a mean haemoglobin concentration of $16.7 \, g.dl^{-1}$ was attained with significant increases in maximal oxygen uptake from 4.85 to $5.10 \, l.min^{-1}$. Differences of this magnitude are critically important in the arena of modern athletic competition.

WHAT IS THE OPTIMAL HAEMOGLOBIN CONCENTRATION IN THE CLINICAL SETTING?[11]

Evolution has resulted in a haemoglobin concentration of $13–16 \, g.dl^{-1}$ presumably for sound biological reasons, and this value must represent the best compromise between oxygen carriage, cardiac output and blood viscosity. However, blood transfusion has always been, and currently remains, a hazardous procedure and a haemoglobin concentration of over $10 \, g.dl^{-1}$ was for many years regarded as acceptable. At this level, cardiac output increases are modest and though exercise tolerance may be reduced this is unlikely to trouble the patient. There is evidence that lower values will be acceptable in some circumstances. Jehovah's Witnesses, whose religious beliefs prevent them from consenting to blood transfusion, frequently undergo major surgery and survival is reported following haemoglobin values of less than $3 \, g.dl^{-1}$, albeit with substantial cardiovascular and respiratory support. Studies of these patients[12] indicate that perioperative death is uncommon if haemoglobin concentration remains above $5 \, g.dl^{-1}$. There is also a suggestion that low haemoglobin values may actually be beneficial, with lowered blood viscosity improving blood flow through diseased vessels and

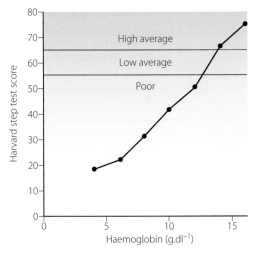

Fig. 25.3 Relationship between capacity for exercise and haemoglobin concentration. (After reference 8 by permission of the authors, and the Editor and publishers of Clinics in Haematology.)

so increasing tissue oxygenation, though evidence for a clinically relevant effect is lacking. A target haemoglobin concentration of $10\,g.dl^{-1}$ may therefore be too conservative in fit healthy patients, or those with chronic anaemia,[13] and a haemoglobin level of $7\,g.dl^{-1}$ is probably acceptable in these groups.[11] This view was confirmed in a randomised controlled study of intensive care patients in whom haemoglobin values of $7–9\,g.dl^{-1}$ were associated with improved outcome compared with those in whom haemoglobin was maintained at over $10\,g.dl^{-1}$.[14]

The organ that limits the acceptable degree of anaemia is the heart, where oxygen extraction is normally in excess of 50%. Increased oxygen extraction as a compensatory mechanism is therefore limited and coronary blood flow must increase to facilitate the greater oxygen requirement of a raised cardiac output. Thus any patient with ischaemic heart disease will be considerably less tolerant of anaemia than those with normal coronary arteries, as shown in the study of intensive care patients already described.[14] For these patients, particularly in the postoperative period when cardiac output is elevated to the same extent as during moderate exercise, the optimal haemoglobin may be as high as $12.8\,g.dl^{-1}$.[15]

Chronic renal failure leads to a lack of renal erythropoietin release and severe symptomatic anaemia results, with patients commonly having haemoglobin levels of less than $8\,g.dl^{-1}$. The availability of recombinant human erythropoietin has allowed partial correction of anaemia in many patients, leading to a substantial improvement in quality of life for most. There is, however, debate about the optimal target haemoglobin concentration to aim for.[16] There is good evidence that the chronic severe anaemia associated with renal disease commonly leads to cardiac complications.[17] Unfortunately, there is also some evidence that correction of haemoglobin to normal values is associated with increased cardiac complications in these patients, and a value of around $12\,g.dl^{-1}$ seems to be the safest compromise.[16]

References

1. Torrance J, Jacobs P, Restrepo A, Eschbach J, Lenfant C, Finch CA. Intraerythrocytic adaptation to anemia. *N Engl J Med*. 1970;283:165–169.

2. Duke M, Abelmann WH. The hemodynamic response to chronic anemia. *Circulation*. 1969;39:503–515.

3. Woodson RD, Wills RE, Lenfant C. Effect of acute and established anemia on O_2 transport at rest, submaximal and maximal work. *J Appl Physiol*. 1978;44:36–43.

4. Weiskopf RB, Viele MK, Feiner J, et al. Human cardiovascular and metabolic response to acute, severe isovolemic anemia. *JAMA*. 1998;279:217–221.

*5. Ickx BE, Rigolet M, Van der Linden PJ. Cardiovascular and metabolic response to acute normovolemic anemia. *Anesthesiology*. 2000;93:1011–1016.

6. Leung J, Weiskopf R, Feiner J, et al. Electrocardiographic ST-segment changes during acute, severe isovolemic hemodilution in humans. *Anesthesiology*. 2000;93:1004–1010.

7. Chapler CK, Cain SM. The physiologic reserve in oxygen carrying capacity: studies in experimental haemodilution. *Can J Physiol Pharmacol*. 1986;64:7–12.

8. Viteri FE, Torun B. Anaemia and physical work capacity. *Clin Hematol*. 1974;3:609–626.

9. Ekblom B, Goldbarg AN, Gullbring B. Response to exercise after blood loss and reinfusion. *J Appl Physiol*. 1972;33:175–180.

10. Buick FJ, Gledhill N, Froese AB, Spriet L, Meyers EC. Effect of induced erythrocythemia on aerobic work capacity. *J Appl Physiol*. 1980;48:636–642.

11. Wedgwood JJ, Thomas JG. Perioperative haemoglobin: an overview of current opinion regarding the acceptable level of haemoglobin in the peri-operative period. *Eur J Anaesthesiol*. 1996;13:316–324.

12. Viele MK, Weiskopf RB. What can we learn about the need for transfusion from patients who refuse blood? The experience with Jehovah's Witnesses. *Transfusion*. 1994;34:396–401.

13. Welch HG, Meehan KR, Goodnough LT. Prudent strategies for elective red blood cell transfusion. *Ann Intern Med*. 1992;116:393–402.

*14. Hébert PC, Wells G, Blajchman MA, et al. A multicenter, randomized, controlled clinical trial of transfusion requirements in critical care. *N Engl J Med*. 1999;340:409–417.

15. Kettler D. 'Permissive anaemia' compared with blood transfusion in patients with cardiac disease: another point of view. *Curr Opin Anaesthesiol*. 1994;7:908–918.

16. Phrommintikul A, Haas SJ, Elsik M, Krum H. Mortality and target haemoglobin concentrations in anaemic patients with chronic kidney disease treated with erythropoietin: a meta-analysis. *Lancet*. 2007;369:381–388.

17. Schunkert H, Hense H-W. A heart price to pay for anaemia. *Nephrol Dial Transplant*. 2001;16:445–448.

Chapter 26

Hyperoxia and oxygen toxicity

KEY POINTS

- Breathing oxygen at increased atmospheric pressure achieves very high arterial Po_2 values but venous Po_2, and therefore minimum tissue Po_2, only increases at three atmospheres absolute pressure.
- Hyperbaric oxygen is used to treat a variety of conditions such as tissue infections, carbon monoxide poisoning and sports injuries, but its use remains controversial.
- Normal metabolic processes, particularly in the mitochondria, produce a range of powerful oxidising derivatives of oxygen, collectively referred to as reactive oxygen species.
- The harmful effects of reactive oxygen species are countered by a combination of ubiquitous enzymes that inactivate reactive oxygen species and endogenous antioxidant molecules.
- The lungs are susceptible to oxygen toxicity, the first measurable signs occurring in healthy subjects after breathing 100% oxygen for approximately 24 hours.

Chapter 24 described the disastrous consequences of lack of oxygen for life forms that depend on it, but for most organisms hypoxia is an infrequent event. However, oxygen itself also has toxic effects at the cellular level, which organisms have had to oppose by the development of complex antioxidant systems. The activity of toxic oxygen derivatives and antioxidant systems is perfectly balanced for most of the time. Nevertheless, there is a strengthening opinion that over many years oxidative mechanisms predominate, and may be responsible for the generalised deterioration in function associated with ageing.[1] In a variety of diseases, or when exposed to extra oxygen, the balance is radically disturbed and oxidative tissue damage results.

HYPEROXIA

Hyperventilation, while breathing air, can raise the arterial Po_2 to about 16 kPa (120 mmHg). Higher levels can be obtained only by oxygen enrichment of the inspired gas and/or by elevation of the ambient pressure. Although the arterial Po_2 can be raised to very high levels, the increase in arterial oxygen content is usually relatively small (Table 26.1). The arterial oxygen saturation is normally close to 95% and, apart from raising saturation to 100%, additional oxygen can be carried only in physical solution. Provided that the arterial/mixed venous oxygen content difference remains constant, it follows that venous oxygen content will rise by the same value as the arterial oxygen content. The consequences in terms of venous Po_2 (Table 26.1) are important because minimum tissue Po_2 approximates more closely to venous than to arterial Po_2. The rise in venous Po_2 is trivial when breathing 100% oxygen at normal barometric pressure, and it is necessary to breathe oxygen at 3 atmospheres absolute (ATA) pressure before there is a large increase in venous and therefore tissue Po_2. This is because most of the body requirement can then be met by dissolved oxygen, and the saturation of capillary and venous blood remains close to 100%.

It is convenient to consider two degrees of hyperoxia. The first applies to the inhalation of oxygen-enriched gas at normal pressure, while the second involves inhaling oxygen at raised pressure and is termed hyperbaric oxygenation.

DOI: 10.1016/B978-0-7020-2996-7.00026-X

Table 26.1 Oxygen levels attained in the normal subject by changes in the oxygen tension of the inspired gas

| | AT NORMAL BAROMETRIC PRESSURE | | AT 2 ATA | AT 3 ATA |
	AIR	OXYGEN	OXYGEN	OXYGEN
Inspired gas P_{O_2} (humidified)				
(kPa)	20	96	190	285
(mmHg)	150	713	1425	2138
Arterial P_{O_2}*				
(kPa)	13	80	175	270
(mmHg)	98	600	1313	2025
Arterial oxygen content[†]				
(ml.dl^{-1})	19.3	21.3	23.4	25.5
Arterial/venous oxygen content difference				
(ml.dl^{-1})	5.0	5.0	5.0	5.0
Venous oxygen content				
(ml.dl^{-1})	14.3	16.3	18.4	20.5
Venous P_{O_2}				
(kPa)	5.2	6.4	9.1	48.0
(mmHg)	39	48	68	360

Oxygen-induced vasoconstriction means tissue perfusion may be reduced by elevation of P_{O_2}. This tends to increase the arterial/venous oxygen content difference, which will limit the rise in venous P_{O_2}. The increases in venous P_{O_2} shown in this table are therefore likely to be greater than in vivo.
*Reasonable values have been assumed for P_{CO_2} and alveolar/arterial P_{O_2} difference.
[†]Normal values assumed for Hb, pH etc.

HYPEROXIA AT NORMAL ATMOSPHERIC PRESSURE

The commonest indications for oxygen enrichment of the inspired gas are the prevention of arterial hypoxaemia ('anoxic anoxia') caused either by hypoventilation (page 399) or by venous admixture (page 133). Oxygen enrichment of the inspired gas may also be used to mitigate the effects of hypoperfusion ('stagnant hypoxia'). The data in Table 26.1 show that there will be only marginal improvement in oxygen delivery (page 202), but it may be critical in certain situations. 'Anaemic anoxia' will be only partially relieved by oxygen therapy but, because the combined oxygen is less than in a subject with normal haemoglobin concentration, the effect of additional oxygen carried in solution will be relatively more important.

Clearance of gas loculi in the body may be greatly accelerated by the inhalation of oxygen, which greatly reduces the *total* tension of the dissolved gases in the venous blood (Table 26.2). This results in the capillary blood having additional capacity to carry away gas dissolved from the loculi.

Table 26.2 Normal arterial and mixed venous blood gas tensions

| | kPa | | mmHg | |
	ARTERIAL BLOOD	VENOUS BLOOD	ARTERIAL BLOOD	VENOUS BLOOD
Breathing air				
P_{O_2}	13.3	5.2	98	39
P_{CO_2}	5.3	6.1	40	46
P_{N_2}	76.0	76.0	570	570
Total gas tension	94.6	87.3	708	655
Breathing oxygen				
P_{O_2}	80.0	6.4	600	48
P_{CO_2}	5.3	6.1	40	46
P_{N_2}	0	0	0	0
Total gas tension	85.3	12.5	640	94

Total gas tensions in venous blood are always slightly less than atmospheric, and this is of critical importance in preventing the accumulation of air in potential spaces such as the pleural cavity, where the pressure is subatmospheric. Oxygen is therefore useful in the treatment of air embolism (page 426) and pneumothorax (page 446).

HYPERBARIC OXYGENATION

MECHANISMS OF BENEFIT

Effect on P_{O_2}. Hyperbaric oxygenation is the only means by which arterial P_{O_2} values in excess of 90 kPa (675 mmHg) may be obtained. However, it is easy to be deluded into thinking that the tissues will be exposed to a similar P_{O_2} as found in the chamber. Terms such as 'drenching the tissues with oxygen' have been used but are meaningless. In fact, the simple calculations shown in Table 26.1, supported by experimental observations, show that large increases in venous and presumably therefore minimum tissue P_{O_2} do not occur until the P_{O_2} of the arterial blood is of the order of 270 kPa (2025 mmHg), when the whole of the tissue oxygen requirements can be met from the dissolved oxygen. However, the relationship between arterial and tissue P_{O_2} is highly variable (page 155), and hyperoxia-induced vasoconstriction in the brain and other tissues limits the rise in venous and tissue P_{O_2}. Direct access of ambient oxygen will increase P_{O_2} in superficial tissues, particularly when the skin is breached.

Effect on P_{CO_2}. An increased haemoglobin saturation of venous blood reduces its buffering power and carbamino carriage of carbon dioxide, possibly resulting in carbon dioxide retention. In fact, the increase in tissue P_{CO_2} from this cause is unlikely to exceed 1 kPa (7.5 mmHg). However, in the brain this might result in a significant increase in cerebral blood flow, causing a secondary rise in tissue P_{O_2}.

Vasoconstriction. An increase in P_{O_2} causes vasoconstriction, which may be valuable for reduction of oedema in the reperfusion of ischaemic limbs and in burns (see below).

Angiogenesis. The growth of new blood vessels is improved when oxygen is increased to more than 1 ATA pressure.[2] There seems to be no effect with 100% oxygen at 1 ATA,[3] and the mechanism by which angiogenesis is promoted is uncertain. When normoxia follows a period of hypoxia, reactive oxygen species (see below) are produced, and these are known to stimulate the production of a variety of growth factors that initiate angiogenesis.[4] The same mechanism may occur during hyperbaric oxygenation.[5]

Anti-bacterial effect. For many years oxygen was believed to play a role in bacterial killing by the formation of reactive oxygen species, particularly in polymorphs and macrophages, though this has recently been refuted (see below). However, oxygen will still have a direct toxic effect on micro-organisms, particularly on anaerobic bacteria, and relief of hypoxia improves the performance of polymorphs.[6]

Boyle's Law effect. The volume of gas spaces within the body is reduced inversely to the absolute pressure according to Boyle's Law (page 515). This effect is additional to that resulting from reduction of the total tension of gases in venous blood (see above).

CLINICAL APPLICATIONS OF HYPERBARIC OXYGENATION[7]

In practice, hyperbaric oxygen therapy means placing a patient into a chamber at 2–3 ATA and providing apparatus to allow them to breathe 100% oxygen, normally a tight fitting facemask. Treatment is usually for about 1–2 hours, and repeated daily for up to 30 days. Since its first use in 1960 enthusiasm for hyperbaric oxygenation has waxed and waned, but its use is still confined to relatively few centres. Clear indications of its therapeutic value have been slow to emerge from controlled trials, which are admittedly very difficult to conduct in the conditions for which benefit is claimed. In particular, a proper 'control' group of patients must undergo a sham treatment in a hyperbaric chamber, which has been used in very few trials. The most commonly accepted indications are as follows.

Infection is the most enduring field of application of hyperbaric oxygenation, particularly anaerobic bacterial infections. High partial pressures of oxygen increase the production of reactive oxygen species, which are cidal not only to anaerobes but also to aerobes. The strongest indications are for clostridial myonecrosis (gas gangrene), refractory osteomyelitis and necrotising soft tissue infections, including cutaneous ulcers.

Gas embolus and decompression sickness are unequivocal indications for hyperbaric therapy and the rationale of treatment is considered above and in Chapter 18.

Carbon monoxide poisoning. In spite of the exploitation of natural gas, there remains a high incidence of carbon monoxide poisoning from automobile exhausts, fires and defective domestic heating appliances. Indications for hyperbaric oxygenation following carbon monoxide poisoning include age over 36 years, loss of consciousness or carboxyhaemoglobin (COHb) levels of more than 25%,[8] and it is now accepted that therapy improves delayed neurological sequelae.[7,9,10]

The rationale of therapy – increased rate of dissociation of COHb – seems simple when the half-life of COHb is approximately 4–5 hours whilst breathing air and only 20 minutes with hyperbaric oxygen. However, breathing 100% oxygen at normal pressure reduces the half life of COHb to just 40 minutes, and therefore in many cases, by the time transport to a hyperbaric chamber is achieved, COHb levels will already be considerably reduced. Other potential benefits of hyperbaric oxygen are believed to derive from minimising the effects of carbon monoxide on cytochrome-*c* oxidase and reducing lipid peroxidation and neutrophil adherence.[9]

Wound healing is improved by hyperbaric oxygenation, even when used intermittently. It is particularly useful when ischaemia contributes to the ineffective healing – for example, in diabetes mellitus or peripheral vascular disease. The mechanisms are similar to those for burns, and, in both cases, improved tissue oxygen levels probably result from direct diffusion of oxygen into the affected superficial tissues and increased release of growth factors.[5]

Sports injuries. Hyperbaric oxygen is believed to expedite recovery from soft-tissue injuries and fractures incurred during competitive sports.[11] Early treatment (within 8 hours) is most effective indicating a probable effect on neutrophil activity at the site of injury.[12]

Multiple sclerosis. In the early 1980s there was great interest in the therapeutic value of hyperbaric oxygenation in multiple sclerosis. A small study reported a favourable response in a double-blind controlled trial in which the treated group received 2 ATA oxygen, while the placebo group inhaled 10% oxygen in nitrogen, also at 2 atmospheres.[13] Unfortunately, these findings were not confirmed in subsequent studies, and a review of 14 controlled trials concluded that hyperbaric oxygen cannot be recommended for the treatment of multiple sclerosis.[14]

OXYGEN TOXICITY

THE OXYGEN MOLECULE AND REACTIVE OXYGEN SPECIES (ROS)[15,16]

Although ground state oxygen (dioxygen) is a powerful oxidising agent, the molecule is stable and has an indefinite half-life. However, the oxygen molecule can be transformed into a range of ROS and other highly toxic substances, most of which are far more reactive than oxygen itself.

The dioxygen molecule (Figure 26.1) is unusual in having two unpaired electrons in the outer (2P) shell. Thus dioxygen itself qualifies as a 'double' free radical, but stability is conferred by the fact that the orbits of the two unpaired electrons are parallel. The two unpaired electrons also confer the property of paramagnetism, which has been exploited as a method of gas analysis that is almost specific for oxygen (page 208).

Singlet oxygen. Internal rearrangements of the unpaired electrons of dioxygen result in the formation of two highly reactive species, both known as singlet oxygen ($1O_2$). In $1\Delta gO_2$ one unpaired electron is transferred to the orbit of the other (Figure 26.1), imparting an energy level 22.4 $kcal.mol^{-1}$ above the ground state. There being no remaining unpaired electron, $1\Delta gO_2$ is not a ROS. In $1\Sigma g^+$, the rotation of one unpaired electron is reversed, which imparts an energy level 37.5 $kcal.mol^{-1}$ above the ground state and this molecule is a ROS. $1\Sigma g^+$ is extremely reactive, and rapidly decays to the $1\Delta gO_2$ form, which is particularly relevant in biological systems and especially to lipid peroxidation.

Superoxide anion. Under a wide range of circumstances, considered below, the oxygen molecule may be partially reduced by receiving a single electron, which pairs with one of the unpaired electrons forming the superoxide anion ($O_2^{\bullet-}$ in Figure 26.1), which is both an anion and a ROS. It is the first and crucial stage in the production of a series of toxic oxygen-derived ROS and other compounds. The superoxide anion is relatively stable in aqueous solution at body pH, but has a rapid biological decay due to the ubiquitous presence of superoxide dismutase (see below). Being charged, superoxide anion does not readily cross cell membranes.

Hydroperoxyl radical. Superoxide anion may acquire a hydrogen ion to form the hydroperoxyl radical thus:

$$O_2^{\bullet-} + H^+ = HO_2^{\bullet}$$

The reaction is pH dependent with a pK of 4.8, so the equilibrium is far to the left in biological systems.

Hydrogen peroxide. Superoxide dismutase (SOD) catalyses the transfer of an electron from one molecule of the superoxide anion to another. The donor molecule becomes dioxygen while the recipient rapidly combines with two hydrogen ions to form hydrogen peroxide (Figure 26.1). Although hydrogen peroxide is not a ROS, it is a powerful and

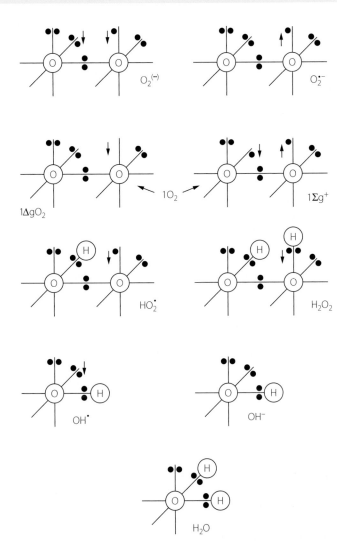

Fig. 26.1 Outer orbital ring of electrons in (from the top left): ground state oxygen or dioxygen (O_2); superoxide anion ($O_2^{\bullet-}$); two forms of singlet oxygen ($1O_2$); hydroperoxyl radical ($HO_2^{\bullet}$); hydrogen peroxide (H_2O_2); hydroxyl radical ($OH^{\bullet}$); hydroxyl ion (OH^-); and water. The arrows indicate the direction of rotation of unpaired electrons. See text for properties and interrelationships.

toxic oxidising agent that plays an important role in oxygen toxicity. The overall reaction is as follows:

$$2O_2^{\bullet-} + 2H^+ \rightarrow H_2O_2 + O_2$$

Hydrogen peroxide is continuously generated in the body. Two enzymes ensure its rapid removal. Catalase is a highly specific enzyme active against only hydrogen, methyl and ethyl peroxides. Hydrogen peroxide is reduced to water thus:

$$2H_2O_2 \rightarrow 2H_2O + O_2$$

Glutathione peroxidase acts against a much wider range of peroxides (R-OOH), which react with glutathione (G-SH) thus:

$$R\text{-}OOH + 2G\text{-}SH \rightarrow R\text{-}OH + G\text{-}S\text{-}S\text{-}G + H_2O$$

Catalase and glutathione peroxidase are discussed further below. Obligatory anaerobic bacteria are normally without catalase.

Three stage reduction of oxygen. Figure 26.2 summarises the three-stage reduction of oxygen to water, which is the fully reduced and stable state. This contrasts with the more familiar single-stage reduction of oxygen to water that occurs in the terminal cytochrome (page 200). Unlike the single-stage reduction of oxygen, the three-stage reaction shown in Figure 26.2 is not inhibited by cyanide.

SECONDARY DERIVATIVES OF THE PRODUCTS OF DIOXYGEN REDUCTION

The Fenton reaction. Although both the superoxide anion and hydrogen peroxide have direct toxic

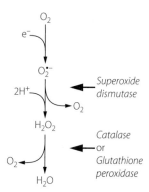

Fig. 26.2 Three-stage reduction of oxygen to water. The first reaction is a single electron reduction to form the superoxide anion reactive oxygen species. In the second stage the first products of the dismutation reaction are dioxygen and a short-lived intermediate, which then receives two protons to form hydrogen peroxide. The final stage forms water, the fully reduced form of oxygen.

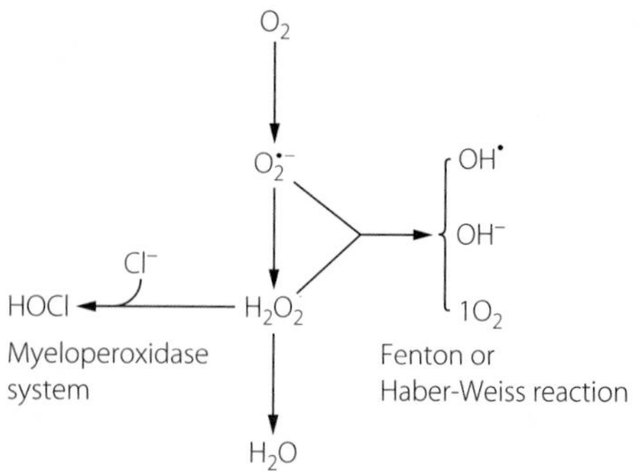

Fig. 26.3 Interaction of superoxide anion and hydrogen peroxide in the Fenton or Haber-Weiss reaction to form hydroxyl free radical, hydroxyl ion and singlet oxygen. Hypochlorous acid is formed from hydrogen peroxide by the myeloperoxidase system. (After reference 17 by courtesy of the Editor of the Journal of the Royal Society of Medicine.)

effects, they interact to produce even more dangerous species. To the right of Figure 26.3 is shown the Fenton or Haber-Weiss reaction, which results in the formation of the harmless hydroxyl ion together with two extremely reactive species, the hydroxyl free radical (OH$^\bullet$) and singlet oxygen (1O$_2$).

$$O_2^{\bullet -} + H_2O_2 \rightarrow OH^- + OH^\bullet + 1O_2$$

The hydroxyl free radical is much the most dangerous ROS derived from oxygen.

The myeloperoxidase reaction.[18] To the left of Figure 26.3 is shown the reaction of hydrogen peroxide with chloride ion to form hypochlorous acid. This occurs in the phagocytic vesicle of the neutrophil and plays a role in bacterial killing. The reaction is accelerated by the enzyme myeloperoxidase, which comprises some 7% of the dried weight of a neutrophil. The myeloperoxidase reaction also occurs immediately after fertilisation of the ovum, and hypochlorous acid so formed causes polymerisation of proteins to form the membrane that prevents the further entry of spermatozoa.

Relationship to ionising radiation. The changes described above have many features in common with those caused by ionising radiation, the hydroxyl radical (OH$^\bullet$) being the most dangerous product in both cases. It is, therefore, hardly surprising that the effect of radiation is increased by high partial pressures of oxygen. As tissue P_{O_2} is reduced below about 2 kPa (15 mmHg), there is progressively increased resistance to radiation

damage until, at zero P_{O_2}, resistance is increased three-fold. This unfortunate effect promotes resistance to radiotherapy of malignant cells in hypoxic areas of tumours (page 444).

Nitric oxide may behave as a ROS by reacting with the superoxide anion to produce peroxynitrite (ONOO$^-$).[15] This molecule can either rearrange itself into relatively harmless nitrite or nitrate (page 194), or give rise to derivatives with similar biological activity to the hydroxyl radical. Conversely, nitric oxide may act as an antioxidant, binding to ferrous iron molecules and preventing them from contributing to the formation of superoxide anion (see below) or the Fenton reaction. The in vivo role of nitric oxide as a ROS or antioxidant therefore remains unclear.[19]

SOURCES OF ELECTRONS FOR THE REDUCTION OF OXYGEN TO SUPEROXIDE ANION

Figure 26.3 shows the superoxide anion as the starting point for the production of many other ROS. The first stage reduction of dioxygen to the superoxide anion is therefore critically important in oxygen toxicity.

Mitochondrial enzymes. NADH dehydrogenase and a variety of other mitochondrial enzymes may 'leak' electrons to molecular oxygen and so produce superoxide anions during normal oxidative respiration.[15,20] Animal studies indicate that this may account for almost 8% of total oxygen consumption, indicating the importance of the highly efficient mitochondrial form of SOD (see below).

The NADPH oxidase system is the major electron donor in neutrophils and macrophages. The electron is donated from NADPH by the enzyme NADPH oxidase, which is located within the membrane of the phagocytic vesicle. This mechanism is activated during phagocytosis and is accompanied by a transient increase in the oxygen consumption of the cells, a process known to be cyanide resistant. This is the so-called respiratory burst, and occurs in all phagocytic cells in response to a wide range of stimuli including bacterial endotoxin, immunoglobulins and interleukins. Superoxide anion is released into the phagocytic vesicle, where it is reduced to hydrogen peroxide which then reacts with chloride ions to form hypochlorous acid in the myeloperoxidase reaction (Figure 26.3). For many years the release of ROS into the phagocyte was believed to be the main way in which bacteria were killed by phagocytes. Recent work on pulmonary neutrophils in mice with pneumococcal infection has refuted this claim, finding no evidence of bacterial killing by neutrophil-generated ROS, though ROS were involved in neutrophil regulation.[21] Powerful protease enzymes released into the phagosome by the neutrophil may be the most important bactericidal mechanism.

Although the NADPH oxidase system has extremely important biological functions, there seems little doubt that its inappropriate activation in marginated neutrophils can damage the endothelium of the lung, and it may well play a part in the production of acute lung injury (Chapter 31).

Xanthine oxidoreductase (XOR) and reperfusion injury.[22] The enzyme XOR is responsible for the conversion of hypoxanthine and xanthine to uric acid (Figure 26.4). XOR is a large (300 kDa) protein involving two separate substrate binding sites, one including flavine adenine dinucleotide cofactor and the other a molybdenum molecule. In vivo, XOR exists in two interchangeable forms, with about 80% existing as xanthine dehydrogenase and the remainder as xanthine oxidase. In both forms XOR catalyses the conversion of both hypoxanthine to xanthine and of xanthine to uric acid, and under normal conditions uses NADH as a cofactor. In ischaemic or hypoxic tissue large quantities of hypoxanthine accumulate (page 363), the availability of NADH declines, and the ratio of the oxidase and dehydrogenase forms of XOR may be reversed. As a result of these changes, when oxygen is restored to the cell, the XOR catalysis of xanthine and hypoxanthine is altered with NAD^+ and dioxygen now being used as cofactors,

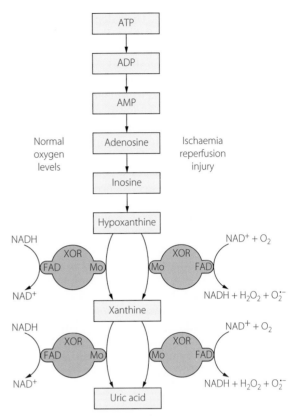

Fig. 26.4 Generation of superoxide anion from oxygen by the activity of xanthine oxidoreductase (XOR). With normal cellular oxygen levels (left side) NADH is the cofactor, binding at the flavine adenine dinucleotide (FAD) site whilst the substrate reacts with the molybdenum binding site at the opposite side of the XOR molecule. Following a period of ischaemia (right side), reperfusion causes NAD^+ and oxygen rather than NADH to react at the FAD binding site of XOR, resulting in the production of hydrogen peroxide or superoxide anion.

resulting in the production of hydrogen peroxide and superoxide anions (Figure 26.4). Thus during reperfusion there may be extensive production of oxygen-derived free radicals. It seems probable that, under certain circumstances, this mechanism may play a role in reperfusion tissue damage or postischaemic shock.[23]

Ferrous iron (Fe^{2+}) loses an electron during conversion to the ferric (Fe^{3+}) state. This is an important component of the toxicity of ferrous iron. A similar reaction also occurs during the spontaneous oxidation of haemoglobin to methaemoglobin (page 196). It is for this reason that large quantities of SOD, catalase and other protective agents are present in the young red blood cell. Their depletion may well determine the lifespan of the cell. Apart from ferrous iron acting as an electron donor, it is a catalyst in the Fenton reaction (see above).

High Po2. Whatever other factors may apply, the production of ROS is increased at high levels of Po_2 by the law of mass action. It would seem that the normal tissue defences against ROS (discussed below) are usually effective only up to a tissue Po_2 of about 60 kPa (450 mmHg). This accords with the development of clinical oxygen toxicity as discussed below. There is also evidence that generation of ROS is increased when normal oxygen usage is increased, for example during exercise.[24]

Exogenous compounds. Various drugs and toxic substances can act as an analogue of NADPH oxidase and transfer an electron from NADPH to molecular oxygen. The best example of this is paraquat which can, in effect, insert itself into an electron transport chain, alternating between its singly and doubly ionised form. This process is accelerated at high levels of Po_2 and so there is a synergistic effect between paraquat and oxygen. Paraquat is concentrated in the alveolar epithelial type II cell where the Po_2 is as high as anywhere in the body. Due to the very short half-life of the oxygen-derived free radicals, damage is confined to the lung. Bleomycin and some antibiotics (e.g. nitrofurantoin) can act in a similar manner. Reactions usually occur at high dose levels, are again potentiated by increased oxygen levels or radiation, and eventually lead to pulmonary fibrosis.

BIOLOGICAL EFFECTS OF ROS

Their use in the regulation of phagocytes, and possibly in the killing of microorganisms is a beneficial role for ROS. Elsewhere within cells, the balance between the detrimental effects of ROS and the antioxidants that counter these (see below) is described as the redox state of the cell. Cellular redox state is believed to be part of an essential, and poorly understood, cell signalling system,[25,26] being involved, for example, in the sensing of oxygen levels in the carotid body. Otherwise, most effects of ROS on biological systems are harmful, and alterations in redox state are linked to a diverse range of diseases.

The three main biochemical targets for ROS damage are deoxyribonucleic acid (DNA), lipids and sulphydryl-containing proteins. All three are also sensitive to ionising radiation. The mechanisms of both forms of damage have much in common and synergism occurs.

DNA. Breakage of chromosomes in cultures of animal lung fibroblasts by high concentrations of oxygen was first demonstrated in 1978[27] (Figure 26.5). In-vivo studies of therapeutic hyperbaric oxygen in humans have also shown DNA damage. However, adverse clinical outcomes from hyperbaric oxygen have not been demonstrated, though susceptible subgroups, who have less effective cellular antioxidant or DNA repair systems, may exist.[28]

Lipids. There is little doubt that lipid peroxidation is a major mechanism of tissue damage by ROS. The interaction of a ROS with an unsaturated fatty acid not only disrupts that particular lipid molecule but also generates another ROS so that a chain reaction ensues until stopped by an antioxidant.[16] Lipid peroxidation disrupts cell membranes and accounts for the loss of integrity of the alveolar/capillary barrier in pulmonary oxygen toxicity.

Proteins. Damage to sulphydryl-containing proteins results in formation of disulphide bridges, which inactivates a range of proteins.

Interference with these fundamental cellular molecules has widespread physiological implications. Superoxide anion, and the peroxynitrite formed from nitric oxide, initiate a wide range of pathological processes, including the inactivation of neurotransmitters, inhibition of proteins, release of cytokines and direct cytotoxic effects (Figure 26.6).[29] Inevitably,

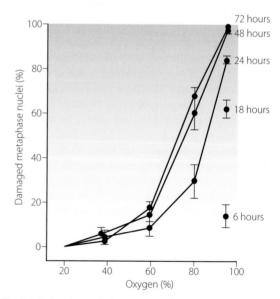

Fig. 26.5 Breakage of chromosomes in a culture of Chinese hamster lung fibroblasts by oxygen at various concentrations and for varying durations of exposure. (Reproduced from reference 27 by courtesy of the Editors of Mutation Research.)

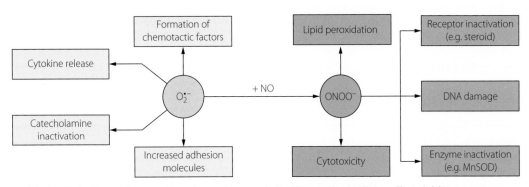

Fig. 26.6 Biochemical effects of superoxide anion and peroxynitrite. These potent cellular effects initiate numerous pathological processes including inflammation, malignancy or cell death. MnSOD, manganese superoxide dismutase. (After reference 29 with permission of the authors.)

cell dysfunction will rapidly occur, followed over the long term by the occurrence of inflammation, malignancy or cell death. Over an animal's lifetime, ROS-induced damage is now closely linked with cardiovascular[30] and neurological disease, cancer[31] and the degenerative changes of ageing.[1]

DEFENCES AGAINST REACTIVE OXYGEN SPECIES

Life in an oxidising environment is possible only because of powerful anti-oxidant defences, which all aerobes have developed (Chapter 1). The defensive systems are freely duplicated and operate in depth.

ANTIOXIDANT ENZYMES

These enzymes are widely distributed in different organs and different species but are deficient in most obligatory anaerobic bacteria. Young animals normally have increased levels of SOD and catalase, which confers greater resistance to oxygen toxicity. The reactions catalysed by antioxidant enzymes have been described above.

Superoxide dismutase.[32,33] Three types of SOD exist, each derived from a separate gene; extracellular SOD, cytoplasmic SOD containing manganese (MnSOD) and mitochondrial SOD containing both copper and zinc (CuZnSOD). Extra production of SOD may be induced by several mechanisms, of which hyperoxia is the most notable, but inflammatory cytokines such as interferon, TNF, interleukins and lipopolysaccharide are important stimulants of SOD production in the intact animal.

Animal studies have consistently shown that induction of SOD confers some protection against the toxic effects of oxygen,[15] and, by implication, enhanced SOD activity may be protective against the wide range of pathological processes described above. There are difficulties in the therapeutic use of SOD because the most important forms are intracellular or mitochondrial enzymes which have very short half-lives in plasma. There is therefore little scope for their use by direct intravenous injection. It is possible for SOD to enter cells if it is administered in liposomes, and extracellular SOD has been used by direct instillation into the lungs.[34] Recent attempts to enhance SOD activity for therapeutic purposes have switched to the development of SOD mimetics.[29] A number of small polycyclic compounds, mostly containing a central manganese molecule, have been found to catalyse the same reactions as SOD, but because of their small size and non-peptide nature they can freely enter the intracellular environment. SOD mimetics have yet to begin clinical trials, but their therapeutic potential for the future looks promising.

Catalase has a cellular and extracellular distribution similar to SOD, with which it is closely linked in disposing of superoxide anion (Figure 26.2). Although studied less extensively, catalase production is believed to be induced by the same factors as SOD. Similarly, trials of exogenous antioxidant enzymes have usually given better results when both SOD and catalase are administered.

Glutathione peroxidase system scavenges not only the ROS themselves but also reactive species formed during lipid peroxidation. Two molecules of the tripeptide (glycine-cysteine-glutamic acid) glutathione (GSH) are oxidised to one molecule of reduced glutathione (GSSG) by the formation of a disulphide bridge linking the cysteine residues. GSH is reformed from GSSG by the enzyme glutathione reductase, protons being supplied by NADPH.

ENDOGENOUS ANTIOXIDANTS

Ascorbic acid is a small molecule with significant antioxidant properties, being particularly important for removal of the hydroxyl free radical. Humans, along with guinea-pigs and bats, lack the enzyme required for the production of ascorbate, and so must ingest sufficient vitamin C to compensate. In these mammals, SOD activity is markedly higher than in those able to produce endogenous ascorbate.[35]

Vitamin E (α-tocopherol) is a highly fat-soluble compound and is therefore found in high concentrations in cell membranes. Predictably, its main antioxidant role is in the prevention of lipid peroxidation chain reactions described above.

Glutathione is found in high concentrations in the airway lining fluid as part of the glutathione peroxidase system described above. Widespread use of paracetamol, which at high doses can reduce glutathione levels in the lung, may attenuate the antioxidant activity provided by glutathione so increasing oxidative stress and possibly contributing to the increasing incidences of asthma and COPD (Chapter 28).[36]

Surfactant may act as an antioxidant in the lung. Animal studies have shown that administration of exogenous surfactant prolongs the duration of oxygen exposure required to cause lung damage.[37]

EXOGENOUS ANTIOXIDANTS

Allopurinol. Because XOR plays a pivotal role in the reactions shown in Figure 26.4 it seemed logical to explore the use of allopurinol, which inhibits a range of enzymes including XOR. As may be expected, benefit was seen mainly following ischaemia-reperfusion injury, but under these conditions allopurinol has multiple effects on purine metabolism and may not be acting as a XOR inhibitor at all.[22]

Iron-chelating agents. Since ferrous iron is both a potent source of electrons for conversion of oxygen to the superoxide anion and a catalyst in the Fenton reaction, desferrioxamine has antioxidant properties in vitro.[38]

These compounds, along with other in vitro antioxidants such as *n*-acetyl cysteine, β-carotene and dimethylsulphoxide have generally failed to live up to their expectations in human disease. There are three possible explanations. First, studies of ROS production and antioxidants in human cells are relatively rare, and there is known to be considerable species variability.[15] Secondly, penetration of the exogenous antioxidant to the site of ROS generation (e.g. mitochondria) or damage (e.g. nuclear DNA) is likely to be poor. Finally, ROS involvement in physiological systems such as neutrophil regulation is crucial, so any non-specific antioxidant activity may be detrimental. Their therapeutic role in oxygen toxicity or diseases known to involve ROS is therefore far from fully clarified.

CLINICAL OXYGEN TOXICITY

The most important clinical conditions in which oxygen has been identified as the sole precipitating cause are oxygen convulsions, pulmonary oxygen toxicity and retrolental fibroplasia.

OXYGEN CONVULSIONS (THE PAUL BERT EFFECT)

It is well established that exposure to oxygen at a partial pressure in excess of 2 atmospheres absolute (2 ATA) may result in convulsions, usually preceded by a variety of non-specific neurological symptoms such as headache, and visual disturbances.[39] This limits the depth to which closed-circuit oxygen apparatus can be used. It is interesting that the threshold for oxygen convulsions is close to that at which brain tissue Po_2 is likely to be sharply increased (Table 26.1). The relationship to cerebral tissue Po_2 is supported by the observation that an elevation of Pco_2 lowers the threshold for convulsions. High Pco_2 increases cerebral blood flow and therefore raises the tissue Po_2 relative to the arterial Po_2. Hyperventilation and anaesthesia each provide limited protection.

Convulsions result from poorly understood changes in cellular interactions between gamma-aminobutyric acid (GABA) and nitric oxide. GABA concentrations decrease in the brain prior to convulsion and the change correlates with the severity of the convulsion.[40] As GABA is an inhibitory neurotransmitter, it is not unreasonable to suggest that a reduced level might result in convulsions. Nitric oxide is known to sensitise neurones to the toxic effects of GABA in hypoxia, and is also involved in hyperoxic convulsions. Nitric oxide inhibitors delay the onset of convulsions in hyperoxia,[41] but paradoxically, the same effect is seen with some

NO donors.[42] Whatever the role of NO, the final common pathway seems to be mediated by disturbed calcium fluxes and increased cyclic-GMP concentration.[41]

Incidence. Hyperbaric oxygen used therapeutically as described above – that is, intermittent exposure to less than 3 ATA – carries little risk of oxygen convulsions. At 2 ATA, a large series reported no convulsions in over 12 000 treatments.[43] Treatment for CO poisoning is associated with a greater incidence of convulsions because of the higher pressures used (normally 2.8–3.0 ATA) and the toxic effects of CO on the brain itself. In this case, 1–2% of patients experience convulsions.[44]

PULMONARY OXYGEN TOXICITY

Pulmonary tissue Po_2 is the highest in the body. In addition, a whole range of other oxidising substances may be inhaled, including common air pollutants and the constituents of cigarette smoke (Chapter 21). The lung is therefore the organ most vulnerable to oxygen toxicity and a range of defence mechanisms have developed. Overall antioxidant activity from both enzymes and other endogenous antioxidants is very high in the fluid lining the respiratory tract. Extracellular SOD is abundant in pulmonary airway tissues, and abnormalities in its regulation may contribute to some lung diseases.[45] Type II alveolar epithelial cells, which produce surfactant (page 23), are believed to also incorporate vitamin E into the surfactant lipids.[46]

Pulmonary oxygen toxicity is unequivocal and lethal in laboratory animals such as the rat. Humans seem to be far less sensitive, but there are formidable obstacles to investigation of both human volunteers and patients. Study of oxygen toxicity in the clinical environment is complicated by the presence of the pulmonary pathology that necessitated the use of oxygen.

Symptoms.[47] High concentrations of oxygen cause irritation of the tracheobronchial tree, which gives rise initially to a sensation of retrosternal tightness. Continued exposure leads to chest pain, cough, and an urge to take deep breaths. Reduced vital capacity is the first measurable change in lung function, occurring after about 24 hours of normobaric 100% oxygen. Oxygen exposure beyond this point leads to the widespread structural changes described below, which ultimately give rise to acute lung injury and possibly irreversible changes in lung function.

Cellular changes.[48] Electron microscopy has shown that, in rats exposed to 1 atmosphere of oxygen, the primary change is in the capillary endothelium, which becomes vacuolated and thin. Permeability is increased and fluid accumulates in the interstitial space. At a later stage, in monkeys, the epithelial lining is lost over large areas of the alveoli. This process affects the type I cell (page 22) and is accompanied by proliferation of the type II cell, which is relatively resistant to oxygen. The alveolar/capillary membrane is greatly thickened, partly because of the substitution of type II for type I cells and partly because of interstitial accumulation of fluid.

Limits of survival. Pulmonary effects of oxygen vary greatly between different species, probably because of different levels of provision of defences against free radicals. Most strains of rat will not survive for much more than 3 days in 1 atmosphere of oxygen. Monkeys generally survive oxygen breathing for about 2 weeks, and humans are probably even more resistant. Oxygen tolerance in humans has been investigated,[49] but these studies are based on reduction in vital capacity etc., which is a very early stage of oxygen toxicity. There is an approximately inverse relationship between Po_2 and duration of tolerable exposure. Thus 20 hours of 1 atmosphere had a similar effect to 10 hours of 2 atmospheres or 5 hours of 4 atmospheres.

Pulmonary oxygen toxicity seems to be related to Po_2 rather than inspired concentration. Early American astronauts breathed 100% oxygen at a pressure of about one-third of an atmosphere for many days (Table 19.1) with no apparent ill effects. There is abundant evidence that prolonged exposure to this environment does not result in demonstrable pulmonary oxygen toxicity, thus establishing a Po_2 of 34 kPa (255 mmHg) as a safe level. It also confirms that the significant factor is partial pressure and not concentration. In contrast, the concentration of oxygen rather than its partial pressure is the important factor in absorption collapse of the lung (see below).

Clinical studies. Some limited information on human pulmonary oxygen toxicity has been obtained from patients in the course of therapeutic administration of oxygen. A study in 1967 of patients who died after prolonged artificial ventilation found more structural pulmonary abnormalities (fibrin membranes, oedema and fibrosis) in those who had received 100% oxygen.[50] However, the higher concentrations of oxygen would probably have been used in the patients with more severe defects in gas exchange, and it is therefore difficult to distinguish between the effects of oxygen itself and the conditions which required its use. A similar group of patients ventilated for long periods with high concentrations of oxygen were reviewed in 1980,[51] and these authors concluded that adverse effects of oxygen on the alveolar epithelium were rarely of practical importance in hypoxaemic patients. An attempt to avoid the complicating factor of pre-existing pulmonary disease was made in 1970[52] by ventilating a group of patients with 100% oxygen for 24 hours after cardiac surgery. Various indices of pulmonary function (V_D/V_T ratio, shunt and compliance) were not significantly different from a control group receiving less than 42% oxygen.

In contrast to these essentially negative findings, a study in 1987 obtained positive findings in a randomised trial involving patients ventilated after cardiac surgery.[53] Venous admixture was significantly greater and arterial P_{O_2} less in patients receiving 50% oxygen compared with the group receiving less than 30%. There are many possible causes for these changes but the authors concluded that unnecessary elevation of inspired oxygen concentration should be avoided, a view from which few would dissent at present.

Pulmonary absorption collapse. Whatever the uncertainties about the susceptibility of humans to pulmonary oxygen toxicity, there is no doubt that high concentrations of oxygen in zones of the lung with low ventilation/perfusion ratios will result in collapse. This occurs routinely during anaesthesia (page 334), and may be demonstrated in the healthy volunteers. A few minutes of breathing oxygen at residual lung volume results in radiological evidence of collapse, a reduced arterial P_{O_2} and substernal pain on attempting a maximal inspiration.[54]

Balancing the risks. Prevention of dangerous hypoxia is always the first priority and must be treated in spite of the various hazards associated with the use of oxygen. Recent guidelines have suggested that emergency oxygen therapy should always by targeted at a pre-determined oxygen saturation, suggested values being 94–98% in most acutely ill patients or 88–92% for those at risk of hypercapnia.[55] When these targets are not achievable by increasing inspired oxygen alone, it is important to remember that oxygen delivery can also be increased by improving cardiac output and haemoglobin levels.

The cornerstone of avoiding the potentially harmful effects of oxygen in the clinical environment is prevention. Although, brief periods of exposure to 100% oxygen appear safe, inspired oxygen concentrations should be titrated against arterial P_{O_2}. This is particularly important in patients exposed to paraquat or bleomycin.

RETROLENTAL FIBROPLASIA (RLF)[56]

Shortly after RLF was first described in 1942, it became established that hyperoxia was the major aetiological factor and led to the use of oxygen being strictly curtailed in the management of neonates. This resulted in an increase in morbidity and mortality attributable to hypoxia and thereafter oxygen was carefully monitored and titrated in the hope of steering the narrow course between the Scylla of hypoxia and the Charybdis of RLF. This policy has not eradicated the condition, and there is some evidence that RLF may occur in infants who have never received additional oxygen. Vitamin E has been used in the attempt to prevent RLF but it is currently believed that hyperoxia is but one of a variety of factors that may cause RLF by changes in the retinal oxygen supply. RLF is increasingly likely to occur with greater degrees of prematurity, and there is a well-established inverse relationship between birth weight and its incidence.

References

1. Ershler WB. A gripping reality: oxidative stress, inflammation, and the pathway to frailty. *J Appl Physiol.* 2007;103:3–5.

2. Thom SR. Hyperbaric oxygen therapy. *Intensive Care Med.* 1989;4:58–63.

3. Marx RE, Ehler WJ, Tayapongsak P, Pierce LW. Relationship of oxygen dose to angiogenesis induction in irradiated tissue. *Am J Surg.* 1990;160:519–524.

4. Maulik N, Das DK. Redox signalling in vascular angiogenesis. *Free Radic Biol Med.* 2002;33:1047–1060.

5. Thom SR. Oxidative stress is fundamental to hyperbaric oxygen therapy. *J Appl Physiol.* 2009;106:988–995.

6. Mandell G. Bactericidal activity of aerobic and anaerobic polymorphonuclear neutrophils. *Infect Immun.* 1974;9:337–341.

7. Tibbles PM, Edelsberg JS. Hyperbaric-oxygen therapy. *N Engl J Med.* 1996;334:1642–1648.

8. Weaver LK, Valentine KJ, Hopkins RO. Carbon monoxide poisoning. Risk factors for cognitive sequelae

and the role of hyperbaric oxygen. *Am J Respir Crit Care Med.* 2007;176:491–497.

*9. Stoller KP. Hyperbaric oxygen and carbon monoxide poisoning: a critical review. *Neurol Res.* 2007;29:146–155.

10. Thom SR. Hyperbaric-oxygen therapy for acute carbon monoxide poisoning. *N Engl J Med.* 2002;347:1105–1106.

11. Babul S, Rhodes EC. The role of hyperbaric oxygen therapy in sports medicine. *Sports Med.* 2000;30:395–403.

12. Staples J, Clement D. Hyperbaric oxygen chambers and the treatment of sports injuries. *Sports Med.* 1996;22:219–227.

13. Fischer BH, Marks M, Reich T. Hyperbaric-oxygen treatment of multiple sclerosis. A randomized, placebo controlled, double blind study. *N Engl J Med.* 1983;308:181–184.

14. Kleijnen J, Knipschild P. Hyperbaric oxygen for multiple sclerosis. Review of controlled trials. *Acta Neurol Scand.* 1995;91:330–334.

15. Kinnula VL, Crapo JD, Raivio KO. Generation and disposal of reactive oxygen metabolites in the lung. *Lab Invest.* 1995;73:3–19.

16. Webster NR, Nunn JF. Molecular structure of free radicals and their importance in biological reactions. *Br J Anaesth.* 1988;60:98–108.

17. Nunn JF. Oxygen – friend or foe. *J Roy Soc Med.* 1985;78:618–622.

18. Fantone JC, Ward PA. Role of oxygen-derived free radicals and metabolites in leukocyte-dependent inflammatory reactions. *Am J Pathol.* 1982;107:397–418.

*19. Dweik RA. Nitric oxide, hypoxia, and superoxide: the good, the bad, and the ugly! *Thorax.* 2005;60:265–267.

20. Turrens JF. Mitochondrial formation of reactive oxygen species. *J Physiol.* 2003;552:335–344.

21. Marriott HM, Jackson LE, Wilkinson TS, et al. Reactive oxygen species regulate neutrophil recruitment and survival in pneumococcal pneumonia. *Am J Respir Crit Care Med.* 2008;177:887–895.

*22. Harrison R. Structure and function of xanthine oxidoreductase: Where are we now? *Free Radic Biol Med.* 2002;33:774–797.

23. Traystman RJ, Kirsch JR, Koehler RC. Oxygen radical mechanisms of brain injury following ischaemia and reperfusion. *J Appl Physiol.* 1991;71:1185–1195.

24. Kantner M. Free radicals, exercise and antioxidant supplementation. *Proc Nutrit Soc.* 1998;57:9–13.

25. Forman HJ, Torres M. Reactive oxygen species and cell signalling. Respiratory burst in macrophage signaling. *Am J Respir Crit Care Med.* 2002;166:S4–S8.

26. Clanton T. Yet another oxygen paradox. *J Appl Physiol.* 2005;99:1245–1246.

27. Sturrock JE, Nunn JF. Chromosomal damage and mutations after exposure of Chinese hamster cells to high concentrations of oxygen. *Mutat Res.* 1978;57:27–31.

*28. Speit G, Dennog C, Radermacher P, Rothfuss A. Genotoxicity of hyperbaric oxygen. *Mutat Res.* 2002;512:111–119.

29. Salvemini D, Riley DP, Cuzzocrea S. SOD mimetics are coming of age. *Nat Rev Drug Discov.* 2002;1:367–374.

30. Rapola JM. Should we prescribe antioxidants to patients with coronary heart disease. *Eur Heart J.* 1998;19:530–532.

31. Hennekens CH, Buring JE, Manson JE, et al. Lack of effect of long-term supplementation with beta carotene on the incidence of malignant neoplasms and cardiovascular disease. *N Engl J Med.* 1996;334:1145–1149.

32. Zelko IN, Mariani TJ, Folz RJ. Superoxide dismutase multigene family: A comparison of the CuZn-SOD (SOD1), Mn-SOD (SOD2), and EC-SOD (SOD3) gene structures, evolution, and expression. *Free Radic Biol Med.* 2002;33:337–349.

*33. Kinnula VL, Crapo JD. Superoxide dismutases in the lung and human lung diseases. *Am J Respir Crit Care Med.* 2003;167:1600–1619.

34. Barnard ML, Baker RR, Matalon S. Mitigation of oxidant injury to lung microvasculature by intratracheal instillation of antioxidant enzymes. *Am J Physiol.* 1995;265:L340–L367.

35. Nandi A, Mukhopadhyay CK, Ghosh MK, Chattopadhyay DJ, Chatterjee IB. Evolutionary significance of vitamin C biosynthesis in terrestrial vertebrates. *Free Radic Biol Med.* 1997;22:1047–1054.

36. McKeever TM, Lewis SA, Smit HA, Burney P, Britton JR, Cassano PA. The association of acetaminophen, aspirin, and ibuprofen with respiratory disease and lung function. *Am J Respir Crit Care Med.* 2005;171:966–971.

37. Ghio AJ, Fracica PJ, Young SL, Piantadosi CA. Synthetic surfactant scavenges oxidants and protects against hyperoxic lung injury. *J Appl Physiol.* 1994;77:1217–1223.

38. Gutteridge JMC, Rowley DA, Griffiths E, Halliwell B. Low-molecular-weight iron complexes and oxygen radical reactions in idiopathix haemochromatosis. *Clin Sci.* 1985;68:463–467.

39. Arieli R, Arieli Y, Daskalovic Y, Eynan M, Abramovich A. CNS oxygen toxicity in closed circuit diving: signs and symptoms before loss of consciousness. *Aviat Space Environ Med.* 2006;77:1153–1157.

40. Wood JD, Watson WJ. Gamma-aminobutyric acid levels in the brain of rats exposed to oxygen at high pressures. *Can J Biochem Physiol.* 1963;41:1907–1913.

41. Wang WJ, Ho XP, Yan YL, Yan TH, Li CL. Intrasynaptosomal free calcium and nitric oxide metabolism in central nervous system toxicity. *Aviat Space Environ Med*. 1998;69:551–555.

42. Bitterman N, Bitterman H. L-arginine-NO pathway and CNS oxygen toxicity. *J Appl Physiol*. 1998;84:1633–1638.

43. Hill RK. Is more better? A comparison of different clinical hyperbaric treatment pressures – a preliminary report. *Undersea Hyperb Med*. 1993;20(suppl):12.

44. Hampson NB, Simonson SG, Kramer CC, Piantadosi CA. Central nervous system oxygen toxicity during hyperbaric treatment of patients with carbon monoxide poisoning. *Undersea Hyperb Med*. 1996;23:215–219.

45. Bowler RP, Crapo JD. Oxidative stress in airways. Is there a role for extracellular superoxide dismutase. *Am J Respir Crit Care Med*. 2002;166:S38–S43.

46. Kolleck I, Sinha P, Rüstow B. Vitamin E as an antioxidant of the lung. Mechanisms of vitamin E delivery to alveolar Type II cells. *Am J Respir Crit Care Med*. 2002;166:S62–S66.

47. Montgomery AB, Luce JM, Murray JF. Retrosternal pain is an early indicator of oxygen toxicity. *Am Rev Respir Dis*. 1989;139:1548–1550.

48. Weibel ER. Oxygen effect on lung cells. *Arch Intern Med*. 1971;128:54–56.

49. Clark JM, Lambertsen CJ, Gelfand R, et al. Effects of prolonged oxygen exposure at 1.5, 2.0, or 2.5 ATA on pulmonary function in men (Predictive studies V). *J Appl Physiol*. 1999;86:243–259.

50. Nash G, Blennerhassett JB, Pontoppidan H. Pulmonary lesions associated with oxygen therapy and artificial ventilation. *N Engl J Med*. 1967;276:368–374.

51. Gilbe CE, Salt JC, Branthwaite MA. Pulmonary function after prolonged mechanical ventilation with high concentrations of oxygen. *Thorax*. 1980;35:907–911.

52. Singer MM, Wright F, Stanley LK, Roe BB, Hamilton WK. Oxygen toxicity in man. A prospective study in patients after open-heart surgery. *N Engl J Med*. 1970;283:1473–1478.

53. Register SD, Downs JB, Stock MC, Kirby RR. Is 50% oxygen harmful? *Crit Care Med*. 1987;15:598–601.

54. Nunn JF, Williams IP, Jones JG, Hewlett AM, Hulands GH, Minty BD. Detection and reversal of pulmonary absorption collapse. *Br J Anaesth*. 1978;50:91–100.

55. O'Driscoll BR, Howard LS, Davison AG. BTS guideline for emergency oxygen use in adult patients. *Thorax*. 2008;63(suppl VI):1–68.

56. Lucey JF, Dangman B. A reexamination of the role of oxygen in retrolental fibroplasia. *Pediatrics*. 1984;73:82–96.

PART 3

Physiology of pulmonary disease

Chapter 27

Ventilatory failure

KEY POINTS

■ Ventilatory failure occurs when alveolar ventilation becomes too low to maintain normal arterial blood gas partial pressures.

■ There are many causes, involving the respiratory centre, the respiratory muscles or their nerve supply and abnormalities of the chest wall, lung or airways.

■ Modest increases in the inspired oxygen concentration will correct hypoxia due to ventilatory failure, but may worsen hypercapnia.

DEFINITIONS

Respiratory failure is defined as a failure of maintenance of normal arterial blood gas partial pressures. Hypoxia as a result of cardiac and other extrapulmonary forms of shunting are excluded from this definition. Respiratory failure may be subdivided according to whether the arterial Pco_2 is normal or low (type 1) or elevated (type 2). Mean of the normal arterial Pco_2 is 5.1 kPa (38.3 mmHg) with 95% limits (2 s.d.) of ±1.0 kPa (7.5 mmHg). The normal arterial Po_2 is more difficult to define because it decreases with age (page 194), and is strongly influenced by the concentration of oxygen in the inspired gas. Mechanisms that contribute to respiratory failure include ventilatory failure (reduced alveolar ventilation) and venous admixture as a result of either pure intrapulmonary shunt or ventilation perfusion mismatch (Chapter 8).

Ventilatory failure is defined as a pathological reduction of the alveolar ventilation below the level required for the maintenance of normal alveolar gas partial pressures. Because arterial Po_2 (unlike arterial Pco_2) is so strongly influenced by shunting, the adequacy of ventilation is conveniently defined by the arterial Pco_2, although it is also reflected in end-expiratory Pco_2 and Po_2. This chapter is concerned mainly with pure ventilatory failure; other causes of respiratory failure are described in the next four chapters.

PATTERN OF CHANGES IN ARTERIAL BLOOD GAS TENSIONS

Figure 27.1 shows, on a Po_2/Pco_2 diagram, the typical patterns of deterioration of arterial blood gases in respiratory failure. The shaded area indicates the normal range of values with increasing age corresponding to a leftward shift. Pure ventilatory failure in a young person with otherwise normal lungs would result in changes along the broken line. Chronic obstructive pulmonary disease (COPD), the most common cause of predominantly ventilatory failure, occurs in older people, and the observed pattern of change is shown within the upper arrow in Figure 27.1. The limit of survival, while breathing air, is reached at a Po_2 of about 2.7 kPa (20 mmHg) and Pco_2 of 11 kPa (83 mmHg). The limiting factor is not Pco_2 but Po_2. This prevents the rise of Pco_2 to higher levels except when the patient's inspired oxygen concentration is increased. It may also be raised above 11 kPa by the inhalation of carbon dioxide. In either event, a Pco_2 in excess of 11 kPa may be considered an iatrogenic disorder. Figure 27.1 also shows the pattern of blood gas changes caused by shunting or pulmonary venous admixture (Chapter 8).

In general, the arterial Po_2 indicates the severity of respiratory failure (assuming that the patient is breathing air), while the Pco_2 indicates the differential

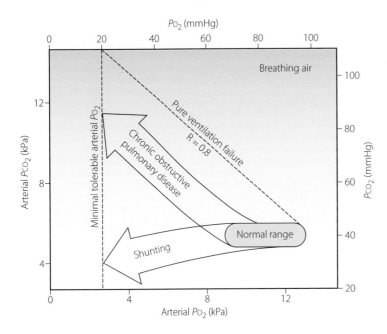

Fig. 27.1 Pattern of deterioration of arterial blood gases in chronic obstructive pulmonary disease and pulmonary shunting. The shaded area indicates the normal range of arterial blood gas partial pressures from 20 to 80 years of age. The oblique broken line shows the theoretical changes in alveolar P_{O_2} and P_{CO_2} resulting from pure ventilatory failure. In chronic obstructive pulmonary disease, the arterial P_{O_2} is always less than the value that would be expected in pure ventilatory failure at the same P_{CO_2} value. Discussion of shunting is to be found in Chapter 8 and further discussion of chronic obstructive pulmonary disease in Chapter 28.

diagnosis between ventilatory failure and shunting as shown in Figure 27.1. In respiratory disease it is, of course, common for ventilatory failure and shunting to coexist in the same patient, and the relative contribution of each mechanism will determine whether type 1 or 2 respiratory failure develops.

TIME COURSE OF CHANGES IN BLOOD GAS TENSIONS IN ACUTE VENTILATORY FAILURE

Although the upper arrow in Figure 27.1 shows the effect of established ventilatory failure on arterial blood gas tensions, short-term deviations from this pattern occur in acute ventilatory failure. This is because the time courses of changes of P_{O_2} and P_{CO_2} in response to acute changes in ventilation are quite different.

Body stores of oxygen are small, amounting to about 1550 ml while breathing air. Therefore, following a step change in the level of alveolar ventilation, the alveolar and arterial P_{O_2} rapidly reach the new value and the half-time for the change is only 30 seconds (see page 205 and Figure 11.19). In contrast, the body stores of carbon dioxide are very large: of the order of 120 litres. Therefore, following a step change in the level of alveolar ventilation, the alveolar and arterial P_{CO_2} only slowly attain the value determined by the new alveolar ventilation. Furthermore, the time course is slower following a reduction of ventilation than an

increase (Figure 10.11) and the half-time of rise of P_{CO_2} following a step reduction of ventilation is of the order of 16 minutes.

The practical point is that, during the early phase of acute hypoventilation, there may be a low P_{O_2} while the P_{CO_2} is increasing but is still within the normal range. Thus the pulse oximeter may, under certain circumstances such as when breathing air, give an earlier warning of hypoventilation than the capnograph. This breaks the rule that the P_{CO_2} is the essential index of alveolar ventilation, and it may be erroneously believed that the diagnosis is shunting rather than hypoventilation.

CAUSES OF VENTILATORY FAILURE[1,2]

The causes of ventilatory failure may be conveniently considered under the headings of the anatomical sites where they arise. These sites are indicated in Figure 27.2. Lesions or malfunctions at sites A to E result in a reduction of input to the respiratory muscles. Dyspnoea may not be apparent and the diagnosis of ventilatory failure may be overlooked on superficial inspection of the patient. Lesions or malfunctions at sites G to J result in evident dyspnoea and no one is likely to miss the diagnosis of hypoventilation. The various sites will now be considered individually.

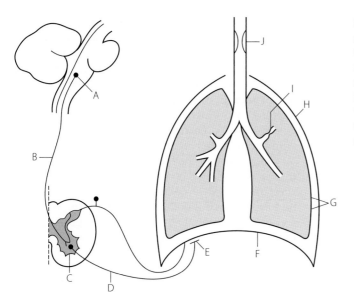

Fig. 27.2 Summary of sites at which lesions, drug action or malfunction may result in ventilatory failure. (A) Respiratory centre. (B) Upper motor neuron. (C) Anterior horn cell. (D) Lower motor neuron. (E) Neuromuscular junction. (F) Respiratory muscles. (G) Altered elasticity of lungs or chest wall. (H) Loss of structural integrity of chest wall and pleural cavity. (I) Increased resistance of small airways. (J) Upper airway obstruction.

A. The respiratory neurones of the medulla are depressed by hypoxia and also by very high levels of $P\text{co}_2$, probably of the order of 40 kPa (300 mmHg) in the healthy unanaesthetised subject, but at a lower $P\text{co}_2$ in the presence of some drugs (see below). Reduction of $P\text{co}_2$ below the apnoeic threshold results in apnoea in the unconscious subject but usually not in the conscious subject. Loss of respiratory sensitivity to carbon dioxide occurs in various types of long-term ventilatory failure, particularly COPD, and this is discussed further on page 412.

A wide variety of drugs may cause central apnoea or respiratory depression (page 77) and these include opioids, barbiturates and most anaesthetic agents, whether intravenous or inhalational. The respiratory neurones may also be affected by a variety of neurological conditions such as raised intracranial pressure, stroke, trauma or neoplasm.

B. The upper motoneurones serving the respiratory muscles are most likely to be interrupted by trauma. Only complete lesions above the third or fourth cervical vertebrae will affect the phrenic nerve and result in total apnoea. However, fracture dislocations of the lower cervical vertebrae are relatively common and result in loss of action of the intercostal and expiratory muscles while sparing the diaphragm. Upper motoneurones may be involved in various disease processes, including tumours, demyelination and, occasionally, in syringomyelia.

C. The anterior horn cell may be affected by various disease processes, of which the most important is poliomyelitis. Fortunately, this condition is now rare in the developed world but it can produce any degree of respiratory involvement up to total paralysis of all respiratory muscles.

D. Lower motoneurones supplying the respiratory muscles are prone to normal traumatic risks and, in former times, the phrenic nerves were surgically interrupted for the treatment of pulmonary tuberculosis. The later stages of motoneurone disease may cause ventilatory failure at this level. Idiopathic polyneuritis (Guillain–Barré syndrome) remains a relatively common neurological cause of ventilatory failure. The syndrome results from an immune-mediated aetiology and is characterised by a rapidly ascending motor nerve paralysis, which in one-third of patients progresses to quadriplegia and total respiratory muscle paralysis.[3] With modern ventilatory support death is fortunately rare, and 85% of sufferers make a complete neurological recovery.

E. The neuromuscular junction is affected by several causes including botulism, neuromuscular blocking drugs used in anaesthesia, organophosphorus compounds and nerve gases. However, myasthenia gravis is by far the most common cause of ventilatory failure at this site, marked respiratory muscle weakness occurring in seemingly mild cases.[4] Myasthenia gravis is an auto-immune disease in which the acetylcholine receptors on the neuromuscular junction are destroyed, leading to progressive weakness. Administration of an anticholinesterase drug such as edrophonium increases acetylcholine concentration at the neuromuscular junction and causes an immediate improvement in symptoms. Immunosuppression or thymectomy are effective current therapies.

F. The respiratory muscles themselves are rarely entirely responsible for ventilatory failure, but they often contribute to reduced alveolar ventilation in a variety of respiratory diseases. For example, the efficiency of contraction of the respiratory muscles is severely impaired by the hyperinflation that normally accompanies COPD. In these patients, although the curvature of the diaphragm may remain normal, the zone of apposition is reduced (see Figures 6.1 and 6.2), and the resultant shortening of diaphragmatic muscle fibres significantly impairs their function.[2] The respiratory muscles may also become fatigued as a result of working against excessive impedance, but this is not thought to occur until very late in the course of most acute respiratory problems.[5] Patients who require critical care commonly develop a polyneuropathy and myopathy of the respiratory muscles, particularly if sepsis is the underlying cause of their multiorgan failure. Activation of cytokines and malnutrition are believed to be contributing mechanisms.[2] Furthermore, following a long period of artificial ventilation, respiratory muscles develop 'disuse atrophy'. These factors all make weaning from ventilation difficult (page 474).

Cardiac failure may result in respiratory muscle weakness due to reduced blood supply,[6] often coupled with low compliance lungs due to pulmonary oedema (Chapter 29).

Assessment of respiratory muscle strength is described on page 97.

G. Loss of elasticity of the lungs or chest wall is a potent cause of ventilatory failure. It may arise within the lungs (e.g. pulmonary fibrosis or acute lung injury), in the pleura (e.g. chronic empyema with fibrinous covering of the pleura), in the chest wall (e.g. kyphoscoliosis) or in the skin (e.g. contracted burn scars in children). It is frequently forgotten that seemingly mild pressures applied to the outside of the chest may seriously embarrass the breathing and even result in total apnoea. A sustained pressure of only 6 kPa (45 mmHg or a depth of 2 feet of water) is sufficient to prevent breathing. This can occur when crowds get out of control and people fall on top of one another, or when either children or adults become accidentally buried under sand or other heavy materials.

H. Loss of structural integrity of the chest wall may result in ventilatory failure, for example from multiple fractured ribs. A condition known as flail chest arises when multiple ribs are broken in two places, allowing the middle, 'flail', rib section to move independently of the anterior and posterior 'fixed' sections. Movement of the flail segment is then determined by changes in intrathoracic pressure; with spontaneous breathing, a paradoxical respiratory movement of the flail segment develops, which if large enough will compromise tidal volume. Flail chest may need to be treated by artificial ventilation with intermittent positive pressure, although conservative treatment with good analgesia, sometimes assisted by rib fixation, is becoming more common.

Closed pneumothorax causes interference with ventilation in proportion to the quantity of air in the chest, and is described on page 445.

I. Small airway resistance remains the commonest and most important cause of ventilatory failure. The physiology of diseases affecting airway resistance is described in Chapter 28 and will not be further discussed here. However, the relationship between airway resistance and ventilatory failure is a complex subject, which is considered below. In the clinical field, airway resistance is less frequently measured but is most often inferred from measurement of ventilatory capacity.

J. Upper airway obstruction occurs in a wide range of conditions such as airway and pharyngeal tumours, upper respiratory tract infections, inhaled foreign bodies and tumour or bleeding in the neck causing external compression of the airway. Stridor is common, and should quickly alert the clinician to the cause of respiratory distress. A smaller airway diameter in babies and children makes them more susceptible than adults to upper airway obstruction, as airway oedema from infections such as croup or epiglottitis quickly causes dramatic stridor. The excellent ability of the respiratory system to overcome increased airway resistance (page 54) is such that ventilatory failure is normally a late development.

INCREASED DEAD SPACE

Very rarely, a large increase in the respiratory dead space may cause ventilatory failure. Minute volume may be increased but the alveolar ventilation is reduced and the patient presents with a high P_{CO_2}

accompanied by a high minute volume. An increase in the arterial/end-expiratory Pco_2 gradient (more than 2 kPa or 15 mmHg) indicates an increase in the alveolar dead space. This condition may be caused by ventilation of large unperfused areas of lung (e.g. an air cyst communicating with the bronchus), pulmonary emboli or pulmonary hypotension. External or apparatus dead space also tends to reduce alveolar ventilation and may be added either intentionally or accidentally.

RELATIONSHIP BETWEEN VENTILATORY CAPACITY AND VENTILATORY FAILURE

Tests for the measurement of ventilatory capacity are described on pages 96 et seq. However, a severe reduction in ventilatory capacity does not necessarily mean that a patient will be in ventilatory failure. Figure 27.3 shows the lack of correlation between FEV_1 and arterial Pco_2 in the grossly abnormal range of FEV_1 0.3–1 litre from a series of patients with COPD.[7]

It should again be stressed that the usual tests of ventilatory capacity depend on the expiratory muscles while the work of breathing is normally achieved by the action of inspiratory muscles.

METABOLIC DEMAND AND VENTILATORY FAILURE

In renal failure, protein intake is a major factor in the onset of uraemia. Similarly, in ventilatory failure, the onset of hypoxia and hypercapnia is directly related to the metabolic demand. Just as patients with renal failure benefit from a low protein diet, so patients with a severe reduction of ventilatory capacity protect themselves by limiting the exercise they take.

As COPD progresses, the ventilatory capacity decreases and the minute volume of breathing required for a particular level of activity increases. The increased ventilatory requirement is because both the dead space and the oxygen cost of breathing increase. The patient is thus trapped in a pincer movement of decreasing ventilatory capacity and increasing ventilatory requirement. As the jaws of the pincer close, there is first a limitation on heavy exercise, then on moderate exercise and so on until the patient is dyspnoeic at rest. At any time his work capacity is limited by the fraction of his ventilatory capacity that he is able to maintain for a given level of oxygen uptake.

The complex interaction between these factors is demonstrated in Figure 27.4, where the upper part shows the normal state. Assuming that an untrained subject can comfortably maintain a minute volume equal to about 30% of his maximal breathing capacity (MBC) without dyspnoea, he has a reserve of ventilatory capacity that is adequate for rest and a power output of 100 watts. However, a power output of 200 watts requires a minute volume that exceeds a third of his MBC and he becomes aware of his breathing at this level of exercise.

Figure 27.4B shows moderately severe COPD with the following changes:

1. MBC reduced from 150 to 60 l.min^{-1}.
2. Dead space/tidal volume ratio increased from 30% to 40%.
3. Oxygen cost of breathing increased by 10% for each level of activity.

Factors 2 and 3 together result in an increased minute volume for each level of activity.

Again, on the assumption that dyspnoea will not be apparent until the minute volume is 30% of MBC, the reserve of ventilation is now sufficient for rest, but 100 watts of power output will result in dyspnoea.

Finally, in Figure 27.4C, the changes have progressed to the point where resting minute volume exceeds 30% of MBC and the patient is dyspnoeic at rest.

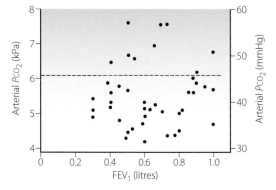

Fig. 27.3 Lack of correlation between arterial Pco_2 and forced expiratory volume in one second (FEV_1) in 44 patients with chronic obstructive pulmonary disease. The broken line indicates the upper limit of normal for Pco_2. (Data from reference 7.)

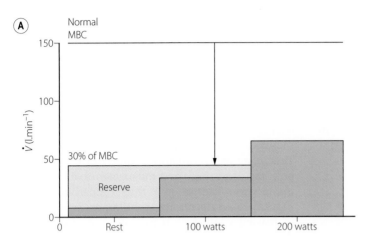

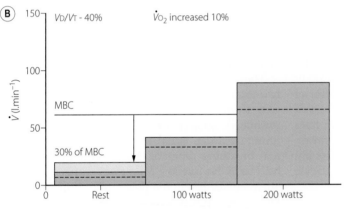

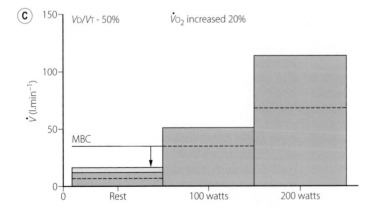

Fig. 27.4 Relationship between maximal breathing capacity (MBC) and ventilatory requirements at rest and work at 100 and 200 watts. The tips of the arrows indicate 30% of MBC, which can usually be maintained without dyspnoea. Ventilatory reserve is between this level and the various ventilatory requirements. (A) Normal. (B) Moderate loss of ventilatory capacity with some increase in oxygen cost of breathing. (C) Severe loss of ventilatory capacity with considerable increase in the oxygen cost of breathing.

BREATHLESSNESS[8]

Breathlessness or dyspnoea has been defined as 'undue awareness of breathing or awareness of difficulty in breathing'.[9] This definition applies to both the awareness of breathing during severe exercise in the healthy subject and the dyspnoea of a patient with respiratory failure or heart failure. In the first case the sensation is normal and to be expected. However, in the latter, it is pathological and should be considered as a symptom.

THE ORIGIN OF THE SENSATION

Hypoxia and hypercapnia may force the patient to breathe more deeply but they are not per se responsible for the sensation of dyspnoea, which arises from the ventilatory response rather than the stimulus itself. Patients with respiratory paralysis caused by poliomyelitis did not usually complain of dyspnoea in spite of abnormal blood gas tensions. Campbell & Guz[9] advanced their reasons for believing that dyspnoea is not akin to pain, though recent studies are now supporting this analogy. Like pain, dyspnoea includes a distressing perception usually referred to as 'air-hunger', which seems to result more from hypercapnia than from the work of breathing.[10] Some patients have dyspnoea at relatively low levels of work of breathing, whereas others show no dyspnoea at high levels of work. Functional imaging of the brain also shows that the cortical areas activated by dyspnoea are close to regions activated by pain.[11] Finally, as for pain, there is undoubtedly a psychological component to the sensation of breathlessness.[12] Dyspnoea arising from respiratory disease, particularly acutely, is often associated with anxiety and panic, which exacerbate the symptom. Conversely, many patients with primary psychological complaints such as panic disorder present with dyspnoea in the absence of any respiratory disease.

In 1963 it was suggested that a major factor in the origin of dyspnoea was an 'inappropriateness' between the tension generated in the respiratory muscles and the resultant shortening of the muscle fibres.[13] This sensory input from muscle spindles would indicate to the brain that breathing was in some way hindered. The theory has since been widened to include other sensory receptors in the respiratory system, again suggesting that dyspnoea results from a mismatch between motor output and sensory input in the respiratory centre.[2] These theories seem to fit observations made during breath holding (pages 76 et seq.), which provide some insight into the origin of the sensation of breathlessness. Blood gas tensions are by no means the only factor limiting breath-holding time, although Po_2 is more important than Pco_2. The sensation that terminates breath holding can be relieved by ventilation without change of blood gas tensions, by bilateral vagal block and by curarisation. Diaphragmatic afferents appear to be more important than those from the intercostals.

It cannot be said that the problem of breathlessness is completely understood at the present time.[2]

The origin seems to be multifactorial and the mechanisms of its generation are clearly complex.

Treatment of breathlessness. Optimal treatment of the underlying disease process that is causing the dyspnoea is clearly the first approach to managing the symptom. However, in the later stages of many respiratory diseases, and in almost all patients with malignancy, breathlessness becomes an intractable and distressing problem. Palliation of breathlessness is now recognised as a valuable form of therapy, and offers further insight into the multifactorial nature of the symptom.[8,14] Simple measures such as a fan blowing on the face are effective, and breathing oxygen relieves dyspnoea in many patients, even some who are not hypoxic.[14] Opioids are effective, whether exogenous or endogenous as a result of exercising.[15] Whether this opioid effect is mediated by reducing the respiratory drive or by simply altering the patient's perception of their breathlessness is unknown.[16]

PRINCIPLES OF THERAPY FOR VENTILATORY FAILURE

Many patients lead normal lives with arterial Pco_2 levels as high as 8 kPa (60 mmHg). Higher levels are associated with increasing disability, largely due to the accompanying hypoxaemia when the patient is breathing air (see Figure 27.1). Treatment may be divided into symptomatic relief of hypoxaemia and attempts to improve the alveolar ventilation.

TREATMENT OF HYPOXAEMIA DUE TO HYPOVENTILATION BY ADMINISTRATION OF OXYGEN

Hypoxia must be treated as the first priority, and administration of oxygen is the fastest and most effective method.

The relationship between alveolar Po_2 and alveolar ventilation is explained on pages 180 et seq. and illustrated in Figure 11.2. If other factors remain constant, an increase in inspired gas Po_2 will result in an equal increase in alveolar gas Po_2. Therefore only small increases in inspired oxygen concentration are required for the relief of hypoxia *due to hypoventilation*. Figure 27.5 shows the rectangular hyperbola relating Pco_2 and alveolar ventilation (as in Figure 10.9), but superimposed are the concentrations of inspired oxygen required to restore a normal alveolar Po_2 for different degrees of alveolar hypoventilation.

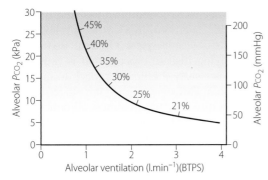

Fig. 27.5 Alveolar P_{CO_2} as a function of alveolar ventilation at rest. The percentages indicate the inspired oxygen concentration that is then required to restore normal alveolar P_{O_2}.

It will be seen that 30% is sufficient for the degree of alveolar hypoventilation that will result in an alveolar P_{CO_2} of 13 kPa (almost 100 mmHg). Clearly this is an unacceptable P_{CO_2}, and therefore 30% can be regarded as the upper limit of inspired oxygen concentration to be used in the palliative relief of hypoxia due to ventilatory failure, without attempting to improve the alveolar ventilation.

The use of very high concentrations of inspired oxygen will prevent hypoxia even in gross alveolar hypoventilation, which carries the risk of dangerous hypercapnia. Although this is itself a strong contraindication to the use of high concentrations of oxygen under these circumstances, the effect may be even worse in patients who have lost their ventilatory sensitivity to carbon dioxide and rely upon their hypoxic drive to maintain ventilation (page 412). Recognition of this potential problem unfortunately resulted in a tendency to withhold oxygen for fear of causing hypercapnia. The rule is that hypoxia must be treated first, because hypoxia kills quickly while hypercapnia kills slowly. However, it must always be remembered that administration of oxygen to a patient with ventilatory failure will do nothing to improve the P_{CO_2} and may make it worse. The arterial P_{CO_2} must be measured if there is any doubt.

IMPROVEMENT OF ALVEOLAR VENTILATION

The only way to reduce the arterial P_{CO_2} is to improve the alveolar ventilation. The first line of therapy is to improve ventilatory capacity by treatment of the underlying cause while simultaneously providing carefully controlled oxygen therapy and avoiding the use of drugs that depress breathing.

The second line is chemical stimulation of breathing. Doxapram stimulates breathing via an action on the peripheral chemoreceptors (page 78) and is effective in treating exacerbations of COPD, but only for the first few hours after admission to hospital.[17]

The third line of treatment is by tracheal intubation or tracheostomy, which may improve alveolar ventilation by reducing dead space and facilitating the control of secretions.

The fourth line of therapy is the institution of artificial ventilation (considered in detail in Chapter 32). It is difficult to give firm guidelines for the institution of artificial ventilation and the arterial P_{CO_2} should not be considered in isolation. Nevertheless, a P_{CO_2} in excess of 10 kPa (75 mmHg) that cannot be reduced by other means in a patient who is deemed recoverable is generally considered as a firm indication. However, artificial ventilation may be required at much lower levels of P_{CO_2} if there is actual or impending respiratory fatigue as a result of increased work of breathing. This may be difficult to diagnose or predict. Although it is now recognised that intense activity by the respiratory muscles results in fatigue, as in the case of other skeletal muscles under similar conditions, it is also thought that ventilatory failure from this cause occurs only very late in the course of most respiratory diseases.

References

1. Roussos C, Koutsoukou A. Respiratory failure. *Eur Respir J*. 2003;22(Supp 47):3S–14S.

*2. Laghi F, Tobin MJ. Disorders of the respiratory muscles. *Am J Respir Crit Care Med*. 2003;168:10–48.

3. Sharsar T, Chevret S, Bourdain F, Raphael JC. Early predictors of mechanical ventilation in Guillain–Barré syndrome. *Crit Care Med*. 2003;31: 278–283.

4. Mier A, Brophy C, Green M. Respiratory muscle function in myasthenia gravis. *Am Rev Respir Dis*. 1988;138:867–874.

5. Roussos C, Zakynthinos S. Fatigue of the respiratory muscles. *Intensive Care Med*. 1996;22:134–155.

6. Hammond MD, Bauer KA, Sharp JT, Rocha RD. Respiratory muscle strength in congestive heart failure. *Chest*. 1990;98:1091–1094.

7. Nunn JF, Milledge JS, Chen D, Doré C. Respiratory criteria of fitness for surgery and anaesthesia. *Anaesthesia*. 1988;43:543–551.

*8. Meek PM, Schwartzstein RM, Adams L, et al. Dyspnea. mechanisms, assessment, and management: A consensus statement. *Am J Respir Crit Care Med*. 1999;159:321–340.

9. Campbell EJM, Guz A. Breathlessness. In: Hornbein TF, ed. *Regulation of breathing, Part II*. New York: Marcel Dekker; 1981.

10. Banzett RB, Pedersen SH, Schwartzstein RM, Lansing RW. The affective dimension of laboratory dyspnea: air hunger is more unpleasant than work/ effort. *Am J Respir Crit Care Med*. 2008;177:1384–1390.

11. von Leupoldt A, Dahme B. Cortical substrates for the perception of dyspnea. *Chest*. 2005;128:345–354.

12. Smoller JW, Pollack MH, Otto MW, Rosenbaum JF, Kradin RL. Panic anxiety, dyspnea, and respiratory disease – Theoretical and clinical considerations. *Am J Respir Crit Care Med*. 1996;154:6–17.

13. Campbell EJM, Howell JBL. The sensation of breathlessness. *Br Med Bull*. 1963;19:36–40.

14. Booth S, Wade R. Oxygen or air for palliation of breathlessness in advanced cancer. *J R Soc Med*. 2002;96:215–218.

15. Mahler DA, Murray JA, Waterman LA, et al. Endogenous opioids modify dyspnoea during treadmill exercise in patients with COPD. *Eur Respir J*. 2009;33:771–777.

16. Jennings A-L, Davies AN, Higgins JPT, Gibbs JSR, Broadley KE. A systematic review of the use of opioids in the management of dyspnoea. *Thorax*. 2002;57: 939–944.

17. Greenstone M, Lasserson TJ. Doxapram for ventilatory failure due to exacerbations of chronic obstructive pulmonary disease. *Cochrane Database Syst Rev*. 2003;1:CD000223.

Chapter 28

Airways disease

KEY POINTS

- Whatever the cause, airway narrowing leads to expiratory flow limitation, gas trapping, and hyperinflation of the lung, which manifests itself as breathlessness.
- Asthma involves intermittent, reversible, airway obstruction caused by airway inflammation and bronchial smooth muscle contraction, both as a result of mediators released from mast cells and eosinophils.
- Chronic obstructive pulmonary disease is progressive and poorly reversible airway narrowing caused by airway inflammation and loss of lung tissue elasticity, mostly as a result of smoking-induced activation of airway neutrophils.
- Cystic fibrosis is an inherited disease in which abnormal chloride transport in the airway impairs the normal pulmonary defence mechanisms, leading to chronic and destructive pulmonary infections.

This chapter considers the physiological changes seen in the three most common diseases of the pulmonary airways: asthma, chronic obstructive pulmonary disease (COPD) and cystic fibrosis. The first two of these have many clinical and physiological features in common, and together constitute the vast majority of respiratory disease seen in clinical practice.

ASTHMA

Lung diseases resulting from air pollution and infection have decreased dramatically in recent decades, but have been almost entirely replaced by asthma. It is estimated that 300 million people have asthma worldwide, with a prevalence that has increased by approximately 50% per decade. In developed countries the increasing prevalence is believed to have now levelled off at 10–15% of the population, but asthma may be continuing to become more common in the developing world (see below).[1–3] In contrast to many respiratory diseases, the onset of asthma is usually in early childhood or in young adulthood. The prevalence of asthma amongst children in the developed world increased 2–3-fold in the last 50 years, though this has also now stopped increasing.[4] Although the prevalence is no longer increasing, hospital admissions for asthma worldwide continue to rise, though fortunately deaths attributable to asthma have been falling consistently since the 1980s.[1,5]

CLINICAL FEATURES

Asthma causes recurrent episodes of chest 'tightness', wheezing, breathlessness and coughing as a result of airway narrowing from a combination of inflammation of the small airways and contraction of bronchial smooth muscle in the lower airway. The term 'asthma' includes a wide spectrum of illnesses, varying from a wheezy 6-month-old baby with a viral infection to a young adult with multiple allergies manifested as wheeze or an older patient with chronic lung disease. In the last case, clinical features of asthma merge with those of COPD, and differentiation between the two is difficult. Whatever the clinical presentation, there are three closely related phases of an episode of asthma, as follows.

Bronchoconstriction occurs early in an asthma 'attack'. This is particularly prominent in allergic asthma when, within minutes of exposure to an allergen, wheezing develops. Narrowing of small airways occurs due to contraction of airway smooth muscle in response to the cellular mechanisms described below. Bronchoconstriction in different regions of lung is not uniform, and positron emission tomography (PET) studies have shown that ventilation becomes patchy with clusters of poorly ventilated lung regions.[6,7] This might be expected to cause maldistribution of ventilation and perfusion, but another study using PET showed that blood flow to the poorly ventilated areas is also reduced,[8] presumably illustrating the efficiency of hypoxic pulmonary vasoconstriction (page 108). Heterogeneity of bronchoconstriction has significant implications for inhaled therapy, as these studies infer that most of an inhaled drug will be deposited in the better ventilated regions rather than where it is most needed.[6]

With more severe bronchoconstriction airway closure begins to occur during expiration, gas trapping occurs, and the lungs become hyperinflated.[9] Eventually, the patient is attempting to breath in when the lungs are almost at total lung capacity, and a sensation of inspiratory dyspnoea results, even though the defect is with expiration. Physiological effects of hyperinflation are described on page 411.

Bronchoconstriction may quickly subside, either spontaneously or with treatment, but more commonly progresses to a late phase reaction.

Late-phase reactions are characterised by inflammation of the airway and develop a few hours after the acute bronchoconstriction. Airway obstruction continues, and cough with sputum production develops. Asthma precipitated by respiratory tract infection may 'bypass' the acute bronchoconstriction phase and the onset of symptoms is then more gradual.

Airway hyper-responsiveness (AHR) describes the observation that asthmatic subjects become wheezy in response to a whole range of stimuli that have little effect on normal individuals. Stimuli include such things as cold air, exercise, pollution (page 322) or inhaled drugs and occur via the neural pathways present in normal lungs (page 50). Methacholine or histamine can be used to measure AHR accurately by determining the inhaled concentration that gives rise to a 20% reduction in forced expiratory volume in one second (FEV_1).[10] Inhaled adenosine also causes airway narrowing, but unlike histamine and methacholine it does not act directly on bronchial smooth muscle.[11] Bronchoconstriction in response to adenosine involves release of mediators from inflammatory cells, so the response is sensitive to the inflammatory state of the airway. For this reason, it is hoped that adenosine provocation may prove useful for monitoring the effectiveness of anti-inflammatory treatment of asthma patients, or even for differentiating between asthma and COPD.[11]

The degree of AHR seen in patients with asthma is highly variable. Severe asthma is associated with continuous AHR, whilst in mild asthma, the patient's response will be normal between wheezy episodes.

CELLULAR MECHANISMS OF ASTHMA[12-14]

Many cell types are involved in the pathophysiology of asthma. A summary of the interactions between these cells is shown in Figure 28.1, which also shows the principal cytokines that facilitate communication between the cells.

Mast cells are plentiful in the walls of airways and alveoli and also lie free in the lumen of the airways where they may be recovered by bronchial lavage. Mast cell activation is the main cause of the immediate bronchospasm seen in allergen-provoked asthma. The surface of the mast cell contains a large number of binding sites for the immunoglobulin IgE. Activation of the cell results from antigen bridging of only a small number of these receptors, and may also be initiated by complement fractions C3a, C4a and C5a, substance P, physical stimulation and many drugs and other organic molecules.

The triggering mechanism of the mast cell is thus extremely sensitive, and is mediated by an increase in inositol triphosphate and intracellular calcium ions. Within 30 seconds of activation, there is degranulation with discharge of a range of preformed mediators listed in Table 28.1. Histamine acts directly on H_1 receptors in the bronchial smooth muscle fibres to cause contraction, on other H_1 receptors to increase vascular permeability, and on H_2 receptors to increase mucus secretion. The granules also contain proteases, mainly tryptase, which can detach epithelial cells from the basement membrane resulting in desquamation and possibly activating neuronal reflexes causing further bronchospasm.

The second major event after mast cell activation is the initiation of synthesis of arachidonic acid derivatives (see Figure 12.3). The most important derivative of the cyclo-oxygenase pathway is prostaglandin PGD_2, which is a bronchoconstrictor, although its clinical significance is still not clear. The lipoxygenase pathway results in the formation of leukotriene (LT) C_4, from which two further peptide leukotrienes, LTD_4 and LTE_4, are formed (see Figure 4.9).

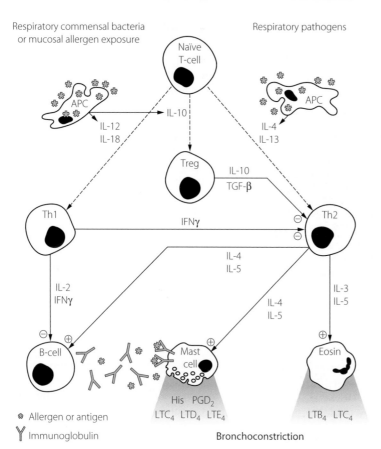

Respiratory commensal bacteria or mucosal allergen exposure

Respiratory pathogens

Naïve T-cell

APC

IL-12
IL-18

IL-10

APC

IL-4
IL-13

Treg

IL-10
TGF-β

Th1

IFNγ

⊖
⊖

Th2

IL-4
IL-5

IL-2
IFNγ

IL-4
IL-5

IL-3
IL-5

⊖ ⊕
B-cell

⊕
Mast cell

⊕
Eosin

Allergen or antigen

Immunoglobulin

His PGD₂
LTC₄ LTD₄ LTE₄

LTB₄ LTC₄

Bronchoconstriction

Fig. 28.1 Inflammatory cells involved in the pathogenesis of asthma, and the cytokines by which they communicate with each other. For details see text. The immunological pathways shown are based on a combination of animal and human studies. Eosin, eosinophil; Th2 and Th1, sub-types of T-lymphocyte 'helper' cells; Treg, regulatory lymphocyte; B-cell, B-lymphoctye; APC, antigen presenting cell; IL, interleukin; IFN, interferon; TGF, transforming growth factor.

Table 28.1 Mediators released from mast cells when activated by IgE

PREFORMED MEDIATORS	NEWLY GENERATED MEDIATORS	CYTOKINES
Histamine	Prostaglandin D₂	Interleukins 3, 4, 5, 6
Heparin	Thromboxane A₂	and 13
Serotonin	Leukotrienes C₄,	Granulocyte/
Lysosomal	D₄ and E₄	macrophage-colony
enzymes:		stimulating factor
Tryptase		Tumour necrosis
Chymase		factor
β-Galactosidase		Platelet activating
β-Glucuronidase		factor
Hexosaminidase		

Finally, mast cells also release a variety of cytokines, some of which are contained within the granules whilst others are generated de novo on activation of the cell. Interleukin-5 (IL-5) and granulocyte/macrophage colony stimulating factor (GM-CSF) are chemotactic for eosinophils whilst IL-4 stimulates IgE production by B-lymphocytes and so amplifies the activation of mast cells.

Eosinophils are freely distributed alongside mast cells in the submucosa, and are believed to be the principal cell involved in the late-phase reaction of asthma. In particular, they release LTB_4 and LTC_4, which are potent bronchoconstrictors with a prolonged action. They are attracted to the area by GM-CSF, which is released by many inflammatory cells, before being activated by IL-5 and IL-3 originating from mast cells and lymphocytes.

Lymphocytes have an important role in the control of mast cell and eosinophil activation.[14] Activated B-lymphocytes are responsible for production of the antigen specific IgE needed to cause mast cell degranulation. B-cells are in turn controlled by two subsets of T 'Helper' lymphocytes, known as Th1 and Th2 cells.

Th2 cells are important pro-inflammatory cells in asthma, promoting both bronchospasm and inflammation by stimulation of mast cells, eosinophils and B-lymphocytes with IL-3, IL-4 and IL-5. The Th2 cell is non-specific in its response, and relies on stimulation by IL-4 and IL-13 from antigen presenting cells (APC) both for its generation from naïve T-cells and its subsequent activation to produce its own pro-inflammatory cytokines. It is not clear from where APCs originate, but they are probably located in the airway mucosa. Once activated by their specific antigen, the APC migrates to lymphoid tissue in the lungs to control the division of naïve lymphocytes into their various sub-types. In the case of Th2 stimulation, the APC is responding to a range of lung pathogens and this is the immunological pathway involved in normal pulmonary defences against infection.

Th1 cells are also generated from naïve T-cells in lymphoid tissue in response to cytokines released by activated APCs, but for Th1 generation the cytokines concerned are IL-12 and IL-18. Th1 cells normally act as anti-inflammatory cells by producing interferon and IL-2, which inhibit the activity of Th2 and B-cells.

The relative activity of the opposing effects of Th1 and Th2 lymphocytes was, until recently, believed to play an important role in the development and severity of asthma. However, this convenient explanation, based mainly on studies in animals, is now thought to be an over-simplification of the situation in humans, particularly with respect to the generation of Th1 cells.[15]

A third sub-type of T-lymphocyte is now thought to be involved in immune regulation of the lung.[14,15,16] Regulatory T-cells (Treg) are again generated from naïve T-cells, this time in response to IL-10 released by activated APCs. Activation of the APCs to produce the anti-inflammatory cytokines IL-10, IL-12 and IL-18 is believed to occur in response to antigens from respiratory tract commensal bacteria or from exposure to high levels of allergens.[14] Treg cells exert an anti-inflammatory effect by secretion of IL-10 and transforming growth factor β (TGF-β), which modify the activities of both Th1 and Th2 cells.

Nitric oxide (NO) is detectable in small concentrations in the expired air of normal subjects.[17] It is produced from the mucosa of the whole respiratory tract, including the nose and nasal sinuses. Nitric oxide acts as the neurotransmitter for the non-cholinergic parasympathetic bronchodilator pathway in normal lungs (page 51), is involved in control of vascular tone in all tissues and is present in blood. In asthmatic patients with active disease, NO concentration in expired air is two to ten times greater than non-asthmatics (page 414).[18] In this situation, the extra NO is derived from inducible NO-synthase (iNOS, page 107) in the airway mucosa. Cytokines produced by the inflammatory cells already described are believed to result in increased production of iNOS.[19]

CAUSES OF AIRWAY OBSTRUCTION IN ASTHMA[20]

Airway smooth muscle (ASM). Stimulation of bronchial smooth muscle by the substances shown in Figure 28.1 and Table 28.1 explains some of the airway narrowing seen in asthma, particularly during the acute and early stages. During deliberately induced bronchoconstriction ASM cells in asthmatic subjects also respond differently to stretching (by taking a deep inspiration) compared with in non-asthmatic subjects. In the normal lung deep inspiration causes ASM relaxation which ameliorates the bronchoconstriction, whilst in asthmatic subjects the ASM fails to respond or even contracts, exacerbating the bronchoconstriction.[21] This is a poorly understood aspect of ASM physiology.[22]

Inflammation. Airway narrowing during the late phase response, or in severe asthma, results from inflammation of the airway. Many cytokines released during asthma have effects on blood vessel permeability and therefore cause oedema of the epithelium and basement membrane.[23] Protease enzymes break down normal epithelial architecture generating defects in the epithelial barrier, leading to further inflammation and eventually detachment of the epithelium from the basement membrane. Finally, hypersecretion of mucus and impaired mucociliary clearance are both recognised features of asthma, and this correlates with the flow limitation seen in individual patients. These changes in the thickness of the airway lining translate into a significant reduction in airway cross-sectional area, and thus a large increase in resistance (page 44). Mucus, inflammatory cells and epithelial debris cause obstruction of small airways, compounded by flow limitation preventing an effective cough.

Airway remodelling.[13,24,25] Repeated activation of inflammatory pathways inevitably leads to attempts by the body to repair the tissue concerned. In the lung, this results in morphological changes to both the airway smooth muscle and the respiratory epithelium. Hyperplasia of smooth muscle cells causes thickening of the airway wall even when the muscle is relaxed, and exacerbates the airway narrowing that occurs with muscle contraction because a lesser degree of muscle shortening now causes a greater reduction in the airway lumen. Goblet cell hyperplasia occurs, worsening the hypersecretion of mucus seen with airway inflammation. Finally, in asthmatic patients, there is thickening of the lamina reticularis of the epithelial basement membrane and changes to the extracellular matrix, thought to be mediated by Th2 secreted cytokines, and ultimately resulting in collagen deposition and long term loss of lung function. The clinical significance of airway remodelling in asthma is unknown, but remodelling is believed to be responsible for the long-term decline in lung function seen in some asthma patients. Airway remodelling may begin before asthma becomes severe, or is even diagnosed at all,[26] and though reducing airway inflammation with steroids may delay remodelling, drugs to reverse the structural changes are as yet undiscovered.[27]

AETIOLOGY OF ASTHMA[2]

Genetics.[28] Asthma, along with other allergic diseases, has a substantial genetic component with several genomic regions known to be linked with developing the disease.[29] Environmental factors invariably contribute to the development of clinical disease, but genetic susceptibility to asthma is strong. Two reasons explain this observation. First, the genes for most of the cytokines involved in asthma are found close together on chromosome 5, and asthmatic patients may have increased expression of these, so encouraging formation of an allergic phenotype.[12] Secondly, human lymphocyte antigens (HLA), which are involved in sensitisation of APCs to specific antigens, are part of the major histocompatibility complex allowing immunological 'self recognition', and so are inherited. It is possible that some HLA types are particularly active in the processing of common allergens and thus the stimulation of Th2 cells or the suppression of Treg cells.

A genome-wide scan of patients with asthma identified a specific gene that is strongly associated with bronchial hyperresponsiveness.[29,30] The gene codes for a protein named ADAM33, part of a large family of proteins with diverse functions, including the control of cell–cell and cell–matrix interactions. In lung tissue ADAM33 protein is found in smooth muscle and fibroblasts, but not epithelial cells, indicating its possible role in airway remodelling in asthma.

Maternal allergic disease is more likely to be passed to offspring than paternal disease, though this may relate to modification of the fetal immune system in utero rather than a true genetic influence. During pregnancy, lymphocyte subsets Th1 and Th2 are closely involved in the prevention of maternal rejection, and abnormalities at this stage may influence the activity of Th1 and Th2 cells in the offspring's immune system, leading to allergic diseases, including asthma, in later life.[31]

Allergy. Changes in living conditions are believed to have contributed to the increase in asthma prevalence. In the developing world, population shifts from rural to urban environments have reduced exposure to parasitic infections and increased exposure to other allergens, and it seems likely that the extensive IgE and mast cell systems that formally inactivated parasites now respond to urban allergens. In the developed world, changes in living conditions have resulted in a dramatic increase in allergen exposure, in particular house dust mite (HDM, *Dermatophagoides pteronyssinus*), domestic animals and fungi. Asthma is more common in affluent families, and correlates with exposure to HDM, which thrives in warm, humid houses with extensive carpeting and bedding. These conditions are ideal for the HDM and its food supply of shed skin flakes. Simply inhaling allergens is only part of the explanation of how allergen exposure causes asthma, and once again pregnancy plays a role. Allergen taken in by the mother is believed to cross the placenta and influence immunological development before birth. Neonatal T-lymphocytes taken from children who subsequently develop asthma already show a reduced production of interferon-γ in response to allergen, indicating an existing immunological susceptibility to asthma.[32]

Infection.[33] Viral respiratory tract infections cause wheezing in many asthmatics and account for over half of acute exacerbations of asthma. In infants, respiratory syncytial or parainfluenza viruses are common, whilst in adults a 'common cold' rhinovirus is the most usual pathogen. Viral infection gives rise to an immune response involving many cells and cytokines, but T-lymphocytes are particularly important and undergo both virus-specific and generalised activation. Inevitably, Th2 activity is increased giving rise to wheeze and airway inflammation by the mechanisms described above (Figure 28.1). In addition, stimulation of allergic mechanisms in susceptible individuals continues for some time after the viral symptoms have subsided. Thus, for example, after a simple rhinovirus infection allergen-induced histamine production and eosinophil-induced late-phase reactions remain increased for 4–6 weeks.[34]

Hygiene hypothesis.[35] This hypothesis to explain the rising incidence of asthma claims that in the clean, hygienic, developed world children are exposed to fewer infections or other environmental antigens than only a few decades ago. It is known that some infections may have a protective role in preventing the initiation of asthma in early childhood.[33] Children who are exposed to more infections in early life, such as those with older siblings or children living on farms, are less likely to develop allergic disease. This led to a suggestion that lower infection rates in the population at large and effective immunisation programmes may have contributed to the rising incidence of asthma. Measles virus, *Mycobacterium tuberculosis*, respiratory and gastro-intestinal commensal bacteria, some respiratory viral infections and hepatitis A virus all have the potential to reduce asthma development by modification of the lymphocyte sub-types shown in Figure 28.1. Other micro-organisms to which the modern human is now less commonly exposed, termed 'old friends' by the authors,[36] include lactobacilli from untreated dairy products, saprophytic mycobacteria found in mud, and helminths (worms). All three are known to promote activity of Treg cells and so potentially protect against the development of asthma (Figure 28.1). For many of these micro-organisms exposure to the entire microbe is not required and beneficial immune responses may be gained from exposure to antigens found in the dust and dirt of the environment.

Pollution. Trends in air pollution have not generally followed trends in asthma prevalence over recent decades, the levels of many pollutants declining whilst asthma becomes more common. Laboratory evidence described on page 322 describes how, in comparison with normal subjects, asthmatics develop wheeze when exposed to lower inhaled concentrations of nitrogen dioxide and sulphur dioxide. The levels required to cause wheezing are still higher than commonly encountered in the atmosphere, and though there is some evidence linking air pollution episodes to respiratory problems the effect is believed to be small.

A role for air pollution in the initiation of asthma has also remained elusive, though there is now some evidence that exposure to traffic pollution may increase asthma incidence in children (page 321). Animal experiments indicate that common air pollutants can sensitise the airway to allergens, probably by disturbance of mucociliary clearance.

Gastric reflux.[37] Gastro-oesophageal reflux symptoms are common in asthmatics, and are believed to be involved in the production of cough or wheeze in many patients. Acid in the distal oesophagus may, via a vagally mediated reflex, provoke either broncho-constriction itself or airway hypersensitivity to allergen. In more severe cases, oesophageal reflux leading to aspiration of small amounts of acid into the airway can provoke severe bronchospasm. In patients with asthma who are resistant to treatment or have mainly nocturnal symptoms, reflux should be considered as a cause, though treatment of the reflux has an inconsistent effect on the asthma symptoms.[38]

Paracetamol. Depletion of glutathione in the lung (page 385) and oxidative stress are potential mechanisms to explain a link between asthma and paracetamol.[39] In a cohort study of over 121 000 adults, frequent use of paracetamol was associated with the development of asthma.[40] A recent study of over 200 000 children aged 6–7 years has also found an association between use of paracetamol in the first year of life and developing childhood asthma.[41] Other explanations may explain this association apart from the paracetamol, for example, children who have frequent infections may be given paracetamol more often. However, given that the increasing use of paracetamol in children has followed a similar timescale to the rising incidence in childhood asthma, further research may soon reveal a relatively simple explanation for the current childhood asthma epidemic.

ASPIRIN–INDUCED ASTHMA (AIA)[42,43]

The involvement of arachidonic acid derivatives in the normal control of bronchial smooth muscle (see Table 4.2 and page 53) predicts that drugs blocking these pathways may influence the airways of asthma patients. This is indeed the case, with aspirin, and the closely related non-steroidal anti-inflammatory drugs, sometimes causing bronchospasm in asthma patients. Based on patient history alone only 2.7% of asthma patients report wheezing in response to aspirin, but when provocation with oral aspirin is carried out 21% of patients develop a reduction in FEV_1.[44] Many asthmatic patients who are sensitive to aspirin have a characteristic clinical presentation. Typically, AIA develops in patients at around 30 years of age, preceded for a few years by rhinitis and nasal polyps, and occurs in more female than male patients.

Mechanism of aspirin sensitivity. Inhibitors of the cyclo-oxygenase (COX) pathway in the airway will reduce synthesis of the bronchodilator prostaglandin PGE_2. Reduced synthesis of PGE_2 cannot alone account for AIA; patients with AIA also have increased production of LTE_4, a potent broncho-constrictor.[42] This effect on the lipo-oxygenase pathway is not mediated by aspirin itself, and possibly results from loss of inhibition of lipo-oxygenase by PGE_2. Genetic polymorphisms for the enzymes involved in leukotriene production may explain why some patients are aspirin sensitive.[45] Multiple isoforms of COX exist (page 224) and COX-1 seems to be responsible for most cases of AIA. Coxibs, a group of drugs that specifically inhibit COX-2, seem to be safe for use in AIA patients.[42] The analgesic effects of paracetamol (acetaminophen) may be mediated by inhibition of COX-3,[46] and a small subset of patients with AIA develop bronchospasm in response to paracetamol.[44] This sensitivity to paracetamol usually involves only a mild reaction in response to high doses of the drug, and occurs in less than 2% of asthmatic patients.

PRINCIPLES OF THERAPY[47]

Detailed guidelines on the treatment of asthma are published for both the UK[48] and the USA,[49] and are beyond the scope of this book. Except in mild asthma treatment has now moved away from the traditional bronchodilator inhaler 'when needed' approach of the past. The emphasis is now on continuous treatment with drugs and other strategies aimed at preventing exacerbations and suppressing airway inflammation. Therapeutic approaches include the following.

Bronchodilators remain a common treatment for relief of acute bronchospasm. The β_2-adreno-ceptor agonists (page 51) are widely used, and recent developments include wider use of longer acting drugs,[50] though concerns remain about the mortality for patients using these drugs in the long-term.[51] Other bronchodilator drugs include inhibitors of leukotriene receptors on bronchial smooth muscle (page 53), blocking the effects of LTC_4, LTD_4 and LTE_4. They are effective in treating asthma, including the bronchospasm seen in the late-phase reaction, and may be particularly useful in patients with exercise-induced or aspirin-induced asthma.[52]

Steroids,[53,54] either inhaled or oral, are an invaluable method of prophylaxis and treatment in asthma. The anti-inflammatory effect of steroids is complex and incompletely elucidated. Steroids act on a glucocorticoid receptor found in the cytoplasm of cells, following which, the receptor–drug complex can enter the nucleus and regulate the transcription of numerous genes.[53] By a combination of direct and indirect effects on transcription, steroids inhibit the synthesis of a wide range of inflammatory proteins including cytokines, adhesion molecules and inflammatory receptors.

Allergen-avoidance is an attractive strategy for the prevention of asthma in patients with known allergies. Low humidity is very effective in reducing HDM, and therefore at high altitude (above 1500 m or 5000 ft) HDM allergen is non-existent. Several studies have used this to compare asthma severity in normal and HDM-free high altitude environments, and have found improvements in both clinical and cellular measures of asthma severity.[55] However, the rather drastic intervention of moving to high altitude is clearly not practical, and reduction of allergen load in the home is considerably less effective. Measures include removing carpets, reducing temperature and humidity, application of acaricides to kill HDM and encasing mattresses in allergen-impermeable membranes. Some studies have reported clinical benefits, but a meta-analysis did not support this approach.[56]

CHRONIC OBSTRUCTIVE PULMONARY DISEASE

Clinical features of COPD are similar to those of asthma with wheeze, cough and dyspnoea, but the airflow limitation is poorly reversible with bronchodilators. Much older patients are affected by COPD than asthma, and the progressive nature of the process leads to more serious interruption of normal activities and eventually respiratory failure (page 393). COPD accounts for between 3.8% and 4.9% of deaths worldwide, rates which are similar in high, middle and low-income countries and believed to still be increasing.[57,58,59]

Unlike asthma, where airway obstruction is usually intermittent, COPD is characterised by progressive chronic airflow limitation along with intermittent exacerbations, particularly in winter.[60] These exacerbations vary from a slight worsening of symptoms to a life-threatening deterioration, and are usually caused by either viral or bacterial infections,[61] possibly exacerbated by air pollution.

AETIOLOGY OF COPD[62]

Smoking is the major aetiological factor in COPD. The accelerated decline in FEV_1 seen with smoking is shown in Figure 21.1, and the 15–20% of smokers who develop COPD probably represent an extreme response to this effect of tobacco smoke. Attempts to identify the genes responsible for this susceptibility to COPD in smokers are at an early stage (page 318).[63,64]

Both asthma and COPD are characterised pathologically by airway narrowing and inflammation, but the causes and clinical course of the two diseases are quite different. Improved understanding of the pathology of COPD and asthma has uncovered a variety of major differences between the two, and these are shown in Figure 28.2. It is believed that around 10% of patients have a mixture of the two disease processes.[65]

The cellular mechanisms underlying airway inflammation in COPD relate to the disease's strong association with smoking, with activation of neutrophils and macrophages (page 320) rather than the eosinophils and mast cells seen in asthma.

Neutrophil activation causes the release of several protease enzymes, including neutrophil elastase, which degrades pulmonary elastin leading to the loss of lung tissue elasticity that is a characteristic feature of COPD. Smoking also induces oxidative stress in the airways, again potentially leading to irreversible tissue damage (page 320).

Three pathophysiological changes give rise to COPD – emphysema, mucous hypersecretion of larger airways, and small airway obstruction.

Emphysema may be defined as permanent enlargement of airspaces distal to the terminal bronchiole accompanied by destruction of alveolar walls.[66] The process begins by enlargement of normal interalveolar holes, followed by destruction of the entire alveolar septum. Both ventilation and perfusion of the emphysematous area are therefore reduced, and, though some mismatch of ventilation and perfusion may occur in widespread emphysema, localised areas, as usually seen in COPD, have little effect. The loss of elastic tissue contained within the alveolar septa is, however, important, and reduces the elastic recoil of the pulmonary tissue so contributing to closure of small airways, particularly during expiration.

Current views on the cellular defect responsible for emphysema involve the relationship between protease and antiprotease activity in the lung.[66–68] These enzymes are normally released following

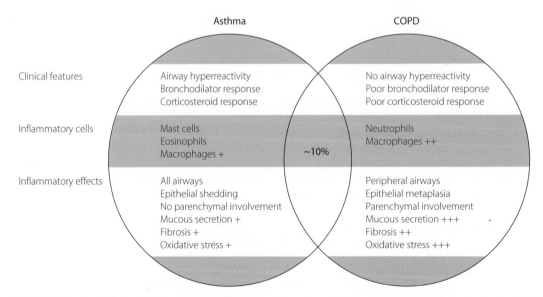

Fig. 28.2 Clinical and pathological differences between chronic obstructive pulmonary disease and asthma. Approximately 10% of patients have features characteristic of both diseases and may be described as having 'wheezy bronchitis'. (After reference 65 by permission of the author and publishers of Chest.)

activation of neutrophils (e.g. neutrophil elastase) or macrophages in response to tobacco smoke or infection. A deficiency of the most well known antiprotease, α_1-antitrypsin, is a significant risk factor for early development of emphysema (page 221). Disturbances of less well understood protease–antiprotease systems, such as the matrix metalloproteases group of enzymes,[68] are now also believed to be involved in the generation of emphysema, as these proteases are normally involved in remodelling of the extracellular lung matrix.[66] Proteases with activity against elastin are likely to be responsible for generating emphysema. Elastin deposition in the lung occurs early in life, and is minimal beyond late adolescence. Later, any pulmonary elastin lost through disease is likely to be replaced with collagen so reducing lung elasticity, and probably explaining the general decline in lung recoil throughout life.

Small airway obstruction plays a major role in COPD, but its aetiology is controversial.[62,69] Part of the expiratory airflow limitation results from emphysema as described above. It is also likely that changes in the airway wall itself contribute. Inflammatory changes in small airways are ubiquitous in COPD, and may lead to mucosal thickening, hypertrophy of bronchial smooth muscle and ultimately to deposition of collagen in the outer airway wall.[62]

Large airway disease consists of goblet cell hyperplasia, mucosal oedema and production of excessive amounts of mucus. Recurrent respiratory tract infections and smoking undoubtedly contribute, and a chronic productive cough is the result. This feature of COPD is not always present, and its contribution to overall airway obstruction is variable. In some patients, extensive and long-standing inflammation of the large airways gives rise to permanent thickening of the airway wall within the cartilaginous airways, and so causes clinically important degrees of obstruction.[69]

Hyperinflation. Airflow limitation in small airways results from a combination of airway narrowing and loss of elastic recoil of lung tissue. The latter is of major importance in maintaining the patency of airways less than 1 mm in diameter (page 18), which lack supporting cartilage in their walls. Expiratory flow limitation leads to prolonged expiratory time constants in affected lung units, and incomplete expiration (gas trapping).[70] Lung volume is therefore forced to increase and the patient becomes dyspnoeic, particularly during any situation that requires a greater minute volume

such as exercise. Hyperinflation of the lung will, in theory, tend to oppose expiratory airway closure (see Figure 4.5), but it also causes a significant reduction in the efficiency of the respiratory muscles. In particular, the diaphragm becomes displaced caudally and, in severe disease, flattened, reducing the zone of apposition (see Figure 6.1) and causing much of the muscle activity to either oppose the opposite side of the diaphragm or pull the lower ribcage inwards rather outwards (see Figure 6.2). In time, lung hyperinflation becomes permanent with expansion of the chest wall (barrel chest) and irreversible flattening of the diaphragm.

When a patient with COPD develops an acute exacerbation airway obstruction worsens acutely and dynamic hyperinflation occurs. This is the same concept as seen during artificial ventilation (page 476), when the expiratory time becomes so long that expiration is incomplete, and end-expiratory lung volume increases acutely. Apart from the inevitable severe dyspnoea, the respiratory muscles also become even less efficient, ventilation/perfusion mismatching worsens, and gas exchange deteriorates.[71]

Respiratory muscles in COPD. The diaphragm, and to a lesser extent the intercostal muscles, are abnormal in patients with COPD. The fibre type shifts towards fatigue-resistant Type 1 fibres (page 91), and the contractile mechanisms of the fibres becomes less efficient.[61,72] Whether these changes result from the chronic stretching of the diaphragm caused by hyperinflation or from systemic inflammation as a result of the COPD is unknown, but the effect is to further impair the ventilatory capacity.

PRINCIPLES OF THERAPY[73,74]

As for asthma, detailed guidelines for the treatment of COPD have been published.[75] Surgical procedures used to treat COPD are described on page 496.

Smoking cessation is central to all forms of treatment for COPD. The rate of the progressive decline in lung function returns to that of a non-smoker (see Figure 21.1) and symptoms improve. Patients with COPD have often been heavy smokers for a considerable number of years, and smoking cessation may therefore need great determination. Patients usually only become permanent non-smokers after multiple attempts at quitting, though nicotine replacement and other drug therapies may improve this poor success rate.

Medical treatment.[76] Inhaled bronchodilators may be used. Their efficacy depends on the reversibility of the airways disease in each patient. Both β_2-agonists and anticholinergic drugs (page 51) are used, and long-acting drugs becoming more widely used though concerns continue about the mortality of COPD patients using long-acting β_2-agonists.[77] Corticosteroids are not as effective for treating COPD as they are for asthma.[78] The inflammatory cells involved are different (Figure 28.2), and may be less susceptible to steroid suppression. Oxidative stress present in COPD airways from neutrophil activation and smoking may inhibit one of the transcription enzymes normally stimulated by steroid drugs.[79]

Medical treatment also involves active management of exacerbations. Management of the underlying disease with antibiotics and oxygen is required. Artificial ventilation is commonly required, and non-invasive ventilation (page 464) is now accepted as the best initial option for these patients.[80]

Supplemental oxygen[81] at low inspired concentrations for 15–24 hours a day improves survival in patients with severe COPD associated with hypoxia. There may also be some benefit of oxygen therapy for COPD patients who desaturate on exercise, both in terms of preventing the desaturation and improving their exercise capacity.

OXYGEN THERAPY IN COPD[82]

The previous classification of patients with advanced COPD into 'pink puffers' and 'blue bloaters' has now been replaced with Type 1 and Type 2 respiratory failure respectively (page 393). Which pattern occurs in an individual patient depends on the relative contributions of airway disease, emphysema and loss of lung elasticity, along with their central chemoreceptor sensitivity to carbon dioxide. Whatever the type of their respiratory failure, administration of oxygen to patients with severe COPD can lead to hypercapnia. Two main mechanisms are believed to be responsible.

Ventilatory depression by oxygen.[82] Patients with type 2 respiratory failure may be relying on their hypoxic drive to maintain ventilation. If this is abolished, as, for example, by the achievement of a high arterial Po_2, hypoventilation or even apnoea may result. However, studies investigating oxygen-induced hypercapnia in COPD have failed to find consistent changes in minute ventilation during either periods of stable respiratory symptoms[83] or acute exacerbations.[84] Reduction in minute ventilation in response to oxygen was either too small to explain adequately the changes in Pco_2, or only transient,

returning towards baseline ventilation after a few minutes. Nevertheless, in one of these reports,[84] of 22 subjects studied, two developed severe respiratory depression leading to dangerous hypercapnia after just 15 minutes of breathing 100% oxygen. A small proportion of patients with COPD therefore seem to be susceptible to oxygen induced respiratory depression.

Altered ventilation perfusion relationships with oxygen have been proposed to explain hypercapnia seen in COPD patients in whom minute ventilation remains essentially unchanged.[83,84,85] Alveolar Po_2 is known to contribute to hypoxic pulmonary vasoconstriction (page 108) and so help to minimise $\dot{V}/\dot{Q}$ mismatch. Administration of oxygen may therefore abolish hypoxic pulmonary vasoconstriction in poorly ventilated areas, increasing blood flow to these areas, and so reducing blood flow to other lung regions with normal or high ventilation to perfusion ratios.[83] These areas will then contribute further to alveolar dead space and so cause an increase in arterial Pco_2 (page 130).

Which of these mechanisms predominates in an individual patient is currently difficult to predict. Administration of oxygen to patients with COPD must therefore be undertaken with great care, and accompanied by suitable monitoring of both oxygenation and arterial Pco_2.

CYSTIC FIBROSIS[86]

Cystic fibrosis (CF) is an autosomal recessive genetic disorder affecting Caucasian individuals of whom 1 in 25 carry the gene. The disease affects approximately 1 in 2500 births and abnormal CF genes can be identified prenatally. Prediction of phenotype from genetic screening is complex because there is a wide spectrum of clinical disease,[87] the severity of which is determined by environmental factors (e.g. smoking) and genetic modifiers of the abnormal CF gene.[88] Mortality from CF remains high, but has been improving dramatically for some years, and the anticipated life expectancy for a person born with CF in the year 2000 is now 50 years.[89] Thus, although the number of CF births is constant, improved survival means that the prevalence of CF is increasing steadily.

Cystic fibrosis affects epithelial cell function in many body systems, but gastrointestinal and respiratory functions are the most important; this chapter discusses only the latter. Abnormalities of pulmonary airway defence mechanisms lead to lifelong colonisation of the CF lung with bacteria. Recurrent airway infection produces hypersecretion of mucus, cough and over many years, destruction of normal lung architecture including bronchiectasis.

AETIOLOGY OF CF

Biochemical abnormality

The molecular mechanisms of CF have been the focus of extensive research for many years, which has led to CF being one of the most completely understood of inherited diseases. As long ago as 1989 the gene responsible for CF was identified.[90] It is located on chromosome 7, and codes for a protein named cystic fibrosis transmembrane regulator (CFTR) found in epithelial cells. The CFTR protein functions as a membrane-bound active chloride channel, and plays a major role in controlling salt concentration in epithelial secretions. Sweat production is influenced by CFTR function, allowing measurement of the sodium concentration in sweat to remain a relatively simple investigation for diagnosis, being over twice normal in CF patients.

The CFTR comprises three types of protein subunit.[91] A ring of membrane spanning domains form a channel through the lipid bilayer of the cell wall (Figure 28.3). Attached to the intracellular aspect of these are two nucleotide-binding domains (NBDs) that use ATP when the channel is activated. Finally, a single regulatory domain (R) protein is loosely attached to the NBDs and can move away from the NBDs to 'open' the channel and allow chloride to pass into or out of the cell (Figure 28.3). Intracellular protein kinase A activates the channel by binding to the regulatory domain of CFTR, whilst ATP provides the energy and is dephosphorylated by the NBDs. Over 1000 different mutations of the CF gene have been identified, and can result in no CFTR being formed, failure of the different protein domains to align correctly or failure of the CFTR to become incorporated into the cell membrane. In normal subjects the CFTR protein also acts by inhibiting nearby epithelial sodium channels, a link which is believed to be defective in CF further impairing the regulation of airway lining fluid (page 219).[92]

Causes of lung disease

The sequence of events by which abnormal CFTR function leads to pulmonary pathology remains

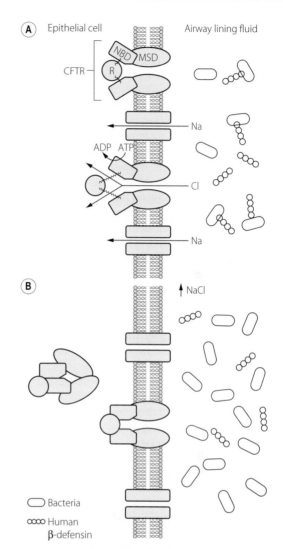

Fig. 28.3 Sodium and chloride transport across the pulmonary epithelial cell wall in cystic fibrosis. (A) Normal lung. Cystic fibrosis transmembrane regulator (CFTR) chloride channel in the closed (upper) and open (lower) positions showing movement of the regulator domain (R). Sodium transport follows chloride via passive Na channels due to altered transmembrane potentials. Bacteria in the airway lining fluid may be inactivated by human β-defensin. (B) Cystic fibrosis. The CFTR proteins are defective so do not locate in the membrane, or are non-functional when they do. Sodium and chloride concentration is therefore abnormally high in the airway, which may inactivate human β-defensin or alter airway lining fluid function and so allow bacterial proliferation. MSD, membrane spanning domain; NBD, nucleotide binding domain.

controversial. Abnormalities of the airway lining fluid and mucus result in poor defences against inhaled pathogens. Bacterial colonisation occurs early in the disease process, and CF patients have an exaggerated inflammatory response to a variety of airway pathogens. A cycle becomes established in which bacterial infection leads to airway inflammation, mucus production and more infection, associated with progressive lung tissue damage. Abnormal CFTR function may adversely affect the ability of the airway to remove inhaled pathogens by a variety of mechanisms, as follows.

Salt-defensin hypothesis. The human lung produces a variety of endogenous antibiotics, of which the most-studied is human β-defensin (HBD), which may play an important role in preventing pulmonary infection. Consisting of a 64 amino acid peptide, HBD has been shown to be inactivated by increased sodium chloride concentrations, so allowing proliferation of bacteria in CF lungs (Figure 28.3).[93]

Inflammation first hypothesis. This proposes that airway inflammation is the primary event in CF lungs, possibly caused by abnormal cytokine production. Inflammatory changes in the airways then lead to excessive and abnormal mucus production and colonisation with pathogens.

Cell-receptor hypothesis. In normal lung, the CFTR found on epithelial cells, along with a range of cell surface glycoproteins, binds many bacterial pathogens as part of the normal process for killing inhaled microorganisms. Abnormal pH around epithelial cells from CF lung inhibits the binding of lung pathogens found in CF.

Depleted airway surface liquid hypothesis. Despite the altered sodium and chloride transport in the CF lung epithelial cells, the 'sol', or periciliary layer of the airway surface liquid (page 219) is believed to be isotonic.[87] However, the volume of periciliary fluid is reduced, and this disturbs the physical linkage between the cilia and the periciliary and mucous layers of ASL, effectively preventing the normal clearance of the ASL. The mucous layer becomes abnormally deep and viscous, which inhibits the function of endogenous antimicrobial systems such as HBD, lactoferrin and lysozyme, and also creates a layer of hypoxic mucus in which anaerobic bacteria can thrive.[94]

PRINCIPLES OF THERAPY

Conventional treatment[95,96] involves assisting the clearance of airway secretions by physiotherapy, postural drainage and exercise. The viscous mucous layer of ASL results in part from degradation of the numerous inflammatory cells found in infected airways, and it is DNA from these cells that can aggregate and further increase viscosity. Treatment with inhaled recombinant human DNAase reduces the viscosity of sputum, and is a useful adjunct to physical methods of mucus clearance. Antibiotic therapy, for both infective exacerbations and maintenance therapy, is now used for all patients and is believed to be the main reason for improved survival in CF.

Lung transplantation is now a recognised treatment for CF, and is described in Chapter 33.

Gene therapy has held great potential for therapy ever since the CF gene was identified, but unfortunately this potential has not been realised.[97,98] A normal CFTR gene can be produced, but the problem arises in incorporating the gene into the airway cells and stimulating its expression into functioning CFTR in vivo. Gene delivery either in liposomes or viral vectors has been attempted, but the functional effect is poor with only transient or small changes in CFTR expression. A more promising approach is to incorporate the normal gene into the fetus, which bypasses immunological reactions and should provide a permanent correction of the defective gene. This has been achieved in mice,[99] but studies of this type in humans are currently prohibited by international ethical convention.

ASSESSMENT OF AIRWAY DISEASE BY EXHALED BREATH ANALYSIS

Exhaled nitric oxide. Nitric oxide is detectable in small concentrations in the expired air of normal subjects.[17] It is produced from the mucosa of the whole respiratory tract, including the nose and nasal sinuses. Nitric oxide acts as the neurotransmitter for the non-cholinergic parasympathetic bronchodilator pathway in normal lungs (page 51), is involved in control of vascular tone in all tissues and is present in blood. By varying the size of breath and expiratory flow rates it may be possible to measure NO released from different areas of the respiratory system.[100] When inflammation is present in the airways, extra NO is produced by inducible NO-synthase (iNOS, page 107) in the airway mucosa, and the exhaled NO level increases. For example in asthmatic patients with active disease, NO concentration in expired air is two to ten times greater than non-asthmatics.[18] Exhaled NO levels may be used as a non-specific marker of airway inflammation in asthma, including in children,[101] and this technique is now beginning to be advocated for use in clinical practice though its exact role remains unclear.[102,103]

Exhaled breath condensate (EBC).[104] This technique is at an earlier stage of development than exhaled NO, but has enormous potential. Liquid condensate from the lungs is analysed for a range of substances that reflect lung pathology. The concentrations of the biomarkers are very low, often close to the detection limits of the analysers, giving rise to a significant variability in results. Nevertheless, EBC has been used to assess the oxidative stress of the lungs by measuring hydrogen peroxide or lung inflammation using condensate pH or prostaglandin levels.[104,105] In future, by analysing DNA obtained from EBC, a non-invasive test for lung cancer is a possibility, which would be a major advance considering that a majority of lung cancers have spread beyond the primary tumour when diagnosed.[106]

References

1. Braman SS. The global burden of asthma. *Chest.* 2006;130:4S–12S.
*2. Eder W, Ege MJ, von Mutius E. The asthma epidemic. *N Engl J Med.* 2006;355:2226–2235.
3. Holgate ST. The epidemic of asthma and allergy. *J R Soc Med.* 2004;97:103–110.
4. Anderson HR, Gupta R, Strachan DP, Limb ES. 50 years of asthma: UK trends from 1955 to 2004. *Thorax.* 2007;62:85–90.
5. Wijesinghe M, Weatherall M, Perrin K, Crane J, Beasley R. International trends in asthma mortality rates in the 5- to 34-year age group. A call for closer surveillance. *Chest.* 2009;135:1045–1049.
*6. Venegas JG, Winkler T, Musch G, et al. Self-organised patchiness in asthma as a prelude to catastrophic shifts. *Nature.* 2005;434:777–782.
7. Venegas J. Linking ventilation heterogeneity and airway hyper-responsiveness in asthma. *Thorax.* 2007;62:653–654.
8. Harris RS, Winkler T, Tgavalekos N, et al. Regional pulmonary perfusion, inflation, and ventilation defects in bronchoconstricted patients with asthma. *Am J Respir Crit Care Med.* 2006;174:245–253.
9. Cormier Y, Lecours R, Legris C. Mechanisms of hyperinflation in asthma. *Eur Respir J.* 1990;3:619–624.
10. Lötvall J, Inman M, O'Byrne P. Measurement of airway hyper-responsiveness: new considerations. *Thorax.* 1998;53:419–424.
11. Polosa R, Rorke S, Holgate ST. Evolving concepts on the value of adenosine hyper-responsiveness in asthma and chronic obstructive pulmonary disease. *Thorax.* 2002;57:649–654.
12. Lee TH. Cytokine networks in the pathogenesis of bronchial asthma: implications for therapy. *J R Coll Phys Lond.* 1998;32:56–64.
13. Bousquet J, Jeffery PK, Busse WW, Johnson M, Vignola AM. Asthma: from bronchoconstriction to airways inflammation and remodeling. *Am J Respir Crit Care Med.* 2000;161:1720–1745.
*14. Umetsu DT, McIntyre J, Akbari O, Macaubas C, DeKruyff RH. Asthma: an epidemic of dysregulated immunity. *Nat Immunol.* 2002;3:715–720.
15. van Oosterhout AJM, Motta AC. Th1/Th2 paradigm: not seeing the forest for the trees? *Eur Respir J.* 2005;25:591–593.
16. Larché M. Regulatory T cells in allergy and asthma. *Chest.* 2007;132:1007–1014.
17. DuBois AB, Kelley PM, Douglas JS, Mohsenin V. Nitric oxide production and absorption in trachea, bronchi, bronchioles, and respiratory bronchioles of humans. *J Appl Physiol.* 1999;86:159–167.
18. Frank TL, Adisesh A, Pickering AC, et al. Relationship between exhaled nitric oxide and childhood asthma. *Am J Respir Crit Care Med.* 1998;158:1032–1036.
19. Hamid Q, Springall DR, Riveros-Moreno V, et al. Induction of nitric oxide synthase in asthma. *Lancet.* 1993;342:1510–1513.
20. Nadel JA, Busse WW. Asthma. *Am J Respir Crit Care Med.* 1998;157:S130–S138.
21. Berend N, Salome C. Can a deep breath blow away the fog surrounding airway hyper-responsiveness? *Am J Respir Crit Care Med.* 2007;176:109–111.
22. Bates JHT. How should airway smooth muscle be punished for causing asthma? *J Appl Physiol.* 2008;104:575–576.
23. Jeffery PK, Godfrey RW, Ädelroth E, Nelson F, Rogers A, Johansson S-A. Effects of treatment on airway inflammation and thickening of basement membrane reticular collagen in asthma. *Am Rev Respir Dis.* 1992;145:890–899.
24. McParland BE, Macklem PT, Paré PD. Airway wall remodelling: friend or foe. *J Appl Physiol.* 2003;95:426–434.
25. Fixman ED, Stewart A, Martin JG. Basic mechanisms of

development of airway structural changes in asthma. *Eur Respir J.* 2007;29:379–389.

26. Pohunek P, Roche WR, Tarzikova J, Kurdmann J, Warner JO. Eosinophilic inflammation in the bronchial mucosa in children with bronchial asthma. *Eur Respir J.* 2000;11(Supp 25):160S.

27. Boulet L-P, Sterk PJ. Airway remodelling: the future. *Eur Respir J.* 2007;30:831–834.

*28. Martinez FD. Genes, environments, development and asthma: a reappraisal. *Eur Respir J.* 2007;29:179–184.

29. Van Eerdewegh P, Little RD, Dupuis J, et al. Association of the ADAM33 gene with asthma and bronchial hyper-responsiveness. *Nature.* 2002;418:426–430.

30. Holgate ST, Holloway JW. Is big beautiful? The continuing story of ADAM33 and asthma. *Thorax.* 2005;60:263–264.

31. Warner JA, Jones AC, Miles EA, Colwell BM, Warner JO. Maternofetal interaction and allergy. *Allergy.* 1996;51:447–451.

32. Tang MLK, Kemp AS, Thorburn J, Hill DJ. Reduced interferon-γ secretion in neonates and subsequent atopy. *Lancet.* 1994;344:983–985.

33. Folkerts G, Busse WW, Nijkamp FP, Sorkness R, Gern JE. Virus-induced airway hyper-responsiveness and asthma. *Am J Respir Crit Care Med.* 1998;157:1708–1720.

34. Calhoun WJ, Dick EC, Schwartz LB, Busse WW. A common cold virus, rhinovirus 16, potentiates airway inflammation after segmental antigen bronchoprovocation in allergic subjects. *J Clin Invest.* 1994;94:2200–2208.

35. Cullinan P. Childhood allergies, birth order and family size. *Thorax.* 2006;61:3–5.

36. Rook GAW, Adams V, Hunt J, Palmer R, Martinelli R, Brunet LR. Mycobacteria and other environmental organisms as immunomodulators for immunoregulatory disorders. *Springer Semin Immunopathol.* 2004;25:237–255.

37. Harding SM, Richter JE. The role of gastroesophageal reflux in chronic cough and asthma. *Chest.* 1997;111:1389–1402.

38. Jain S. Proton-pump inhibitor therapy for gastroesophageal reflux disease. Does it treat the asthma? *Chest.* 2005;127:1097–1098.

39. Eneli I, Sadri K, Camargo C, Barr RG. Acetaminophen and the risk of asthma. The epidemiologic and pathophysiologic evidence. *Chest.* 2005;127:604–612.

40. Barr RG, Wentowski CC, Curhan GC, et al. Prospective study of acetaminophen use and newly diagnosed asthma among women. *Am J Respir Crit Care Med.* 2004;169:836–841.

41. Beasley R, Clayton T, Crane J, et al. Association between paracetamol use in infancy and childhood, and risk of asthma, rhinoconjunctivitis, and eczema in children aged 6–7 years: analysis from phase three of the ISAAC programme. *Lancet.* 2008;372:1039–1048.

42. Farooque S, Lee TH. Aspirin sensitivity and eicosanoids. *Thorax.* 2008;63:2–4.

43. Farooque SP, Lee TH. Aspirin-sensitive respiratory disease. *Annu Rev Physiol.* 2009;71:465–487.

44. Jenkins C, Costello J, Hodge L. Systematic review of prevalence of aspirin induced asthma and its implications for clinical practice. *BMJ.* 2004;328:434–437.

45. Szczeklik A, Sanak M. Genetic mechanisms in aspirin-induced asthma. *Am J Respir Crit Care Med.* 2000;161:S142–S146.

46. Schwab JM, Schluesener HJ, Laufer S. COX-3: just another COX or the solitary elusive target of paracetamol? *Lancet.* 2003;361:981–982.

47. Fanta CH. Asthma. *N Engl J Med.* 2009;360:1002–1014.

48. British Thoracic Society, Scottish Intercollegiate Guidelines Network. British guideline on the management of asthma. *Thorax.* 2008;63:iv1–iv121.

49. National Heart, Lung, and Blood Institute. *National Asthma Education and Prevention Program, Expert Panel.* Bethesda, MD: National Institutes of Health; 2007. Report 3: guidelines for the diagnosis and management of asthma. Publication No. 07-4051.

50. Tattersfield AE, Harrison TW. β-adrenoceptor polymorphisms: focus moves to long-acting β-agonists. *Am J Respir Crit Care Med.* 2006;173:473–474.

51. Beasley R, Martinez FD, Hackshaw A, Rabe KF, Sterke PJ, Djukanovic R. Safety of long-acting β-agonists: urgent need to clear the air remains. *Eur Respir J.* 2009;33:3–5.

52. Busse W, Kraft M. Cysteinyl leukotrienes in allergic inflammation: strategic target for therapy. *Chest.* 2005;127:1312–1326.

53. Barnes PJ. Molecular mechanisms of corticosteroids in allergic disease. *Allergy.* 2001;56:928–936.

54. Adcock IM, Barnes PJ. Molecular mechanisms of corticosteroid resistance. *Chest.* 2008;134:394–401.

55. Custovic A, Simpson A, Chapman MD, Woodcock A. Allergen avoidance in the treatment of asthma and atopic disorders. *Thorax.* 1998;53:63–72.

56. Gotzsche PC, Hammarquist C, Burr M. House dust mite control measures in the management of asthma: meta-analysis. *BMJ.* 1998;317:1105–1110.

57. Calverley PMA, Walker P. Chronic obstructive pulmonary disease. *Lancet.* 2003;362:1053–1061.

*58. Viegi G, Pistelli F, Sherrill DL, Maio S, Baldacci S, Carrozzi L. Definition, epidemiology and natural history of COPD. *Eur Respir J*. 2007;30:993–1013.

59. Mannino DM, Buist AS. Global burden of COPD: risk factors, prevalence, and future trends. *Lancet*. 2007;370:765–773.

60. Aaron SD. COPD exacerbations. Predicting the future from the recent past. *Am J Respir Crit Care Med*. 2009;179:335–336.

61. Ottenheijm CAC, Heunks LMA, Sieck GC, et al. Diaphragm dysfunction in chronic obstructive pulmonary disease. *Am J Respir Crit Care Med*. 2005;172:200–205.

*62. Barnes PJ, Shapiro SD, Pauwels RA. Chronic obstructive pulmonary disease: molecular and cellular mechanisms. *Eur Respir J*. 2003;22:672–688.

63. Sandford AJ, Silverman EK. Chronic obstructive pulmonary disease 1: Susceptibility factors for COPD – the genotype–environment interaction. *Thorax*. 2002;57:736–741.

64. Anthonisen NR. 'Susceptible' smokers? *Thorax*. 2006;61: 924–925.

65. Barnes PJ. Mechanisms in COPD. Differences from asthma. *Chest*. 2000;117:10S–14S.

66. Hogg JC, Senior RM. Chronic obstructive pulmonary disease 2: Pathology and biochemistry of emphysema. *Thorax*. 2002;57:830–834.

67. Turino GM. Emphysema in COPD: consequences and causes. *Thorax*. 2006;61:1031–1032.

68. Turino GM. Proteases in COPD. A critical pathway to injury. *Chest*. 2007;132:1724–1725.

69. Tiddens HAWM, Paré PD, Hogg JC, Hop WCJ, Lambert R, De Jongste JC. Cartilaginous airway dimensions and airflow obstruction in human lungs. *Am J Respir Crit Care Med*. 1995;152:260–266.

70. Man SFP, McAlister FA, Anthonisen NR, Sin DD. Contemporary management of chronic obstructive pulmonary disease. Clinical applications. *JAMA*. 2003;290:2313–2316.

71. O'Donnell DE, Parker CM. COPD exacerbations. 3: Pathophysiology. *Thorax*. 2006;61:354–361.

72. McKenzie D. To breathe or not to breathe: the respiratory muscles and COPD. *J Appl Physiol*. 2006;101:1279–1280.

73. Celli BR. Update on the management of COPD. *Chest*. 2008;133:1451–1462.

*74. Sutherland ER, Cherniak RM. Management of chronic obstructive pulmonary disease. *N Engl J Med*. 2004;350: 2689–2697.

75. Pauwels RA, Buist AS, Calverley PMA, Jenkins CR, Hurd SS. Global strategy for the diagnosis, management, and prevention of chronic obstructive pulmonary disease. NHLBI/WHO Global Initiative for Chronic Obstructive Lung Disease (GOLD) Workshop summary. *Am J Respir Crit Care Med*. 2001;163:1256–1276.

76. Barnes PJ. Emerging pharmacotherapies for COPD. *Chest*. 2008;134:1278–1286.

77. Sears MR. Long-acting bronchodilators in COPD. *Chest*. 2008;133:1057–1058.

78. Niewoehner DE, Wilt TJ. Inhaled corticosteroids for chronic obstructive pulmonary disease. *Am J Respir Crit Care Med*. 2007;175:103–104.

79. Barnes PJ, Ito K, Adcock IM. Corticosteroid resistance in chronic obstructive pulmonary disease: inactivation of histone deacetylase. *Lancet*. 2004;363:731–733.

80. Plant PK, Elliott MW. Chronic obstructive pulmonary disease 9: Management of ventilatory failure in COPD. *Thorax*. 2003;58:537–542.

81. Drummond MB, Wise RA. Oxygen therapy in COPD: what do we know?. *Am J Respir Crit Care Med*. 2007;176:321–326.

*82. O'Driscoll BR, Howard LS, Davison AG, on behalf of the British Thoracic Society. BTS guideline for emergency oxygen use in adult patients. *Thorax*. 2008;63:vi1–vi68.

83. Sassoon CSH, Hassell KT, Mahutte CK. Hyperoxic-induced hypercapnia in stable chronic obstructive pulmonary disease. *Am Rev Respir Dis*. 1987;135:907–911.

84. Aubier M, Murciano D, Milic-Emili J, et al. Effects of the administration of O_2 on ventilation and blood gases in patients with chronic obstructive pulmonary disease during acute respiratory failure. *Am Rev Respir Dis*. 1980;122:747–754.

85. Crossley DJ, McGuire GP, Barrow PM, Houston PL. Influence of inspired oxygen concentration on deadspace, respiratory drive, and $Paco_2$ in intubated patients with chronic obstructive pulmonary disease. *Crit Care Med*. 1997;25:1522–1526.

86. O'Sullivan BP, Freedman SD. Cystic fibrosis. *Lancet*. 2009;373:1891–1904.

*87. Boucher RC. New concepts of the pathogenesis of cystic fibrosis lung disease. *Eur Respir J*. 2004;23:146–158.

88. Vanscoy LL, Blackman SM, Collaco JM, et al. Heritability of lung disease severity in cystic fibrosis. *Am J Respir Crit Care Med*. 2007;175:1036–1043.

89. Dodge JA, Lewis PA, Stanton M, Wilsher J. Cystic fibrosis mortality and survival in the UK: 1947–2003. *Eur Respir J*. 2007;29:522–526.

90. Kerem B, Rommens JM, Buchanan JA, et al. Identification of the cystic fibrosis gene: genetic analysis. *Science*. 1989;245:1073–1080.

91. Stern M, Geddes D. Cystic fibrosis: basic chemical and cellular mechanisms. *Br J Hosp Med*. 1996;55:237–240.

92. Donaldson SH, Boucher RC. Sodium channels and cystic fibrosis. *Chest*. 2007;132:1631–1636.

93. Goldman MJ, Anderson GM, Stolzenberg ED, Kari UP, Zasloff M, Wilson J. Human β-defensin-1 is a salt-sensitive antibiotic in lung that is inactivated in cystic fibrosis. *Cell*. 1997;88:553–560.

94. Tunney MM, Field TR, Moriarty TF, et al. Detection of anaerobic bacteria in high numbers in sputum from patients with cystic fibrosis. *Am J Respir Crit Care Med*. 2008;177:995–1001.

95. Yankaskas JR, Marshall BC, Sufian B, Simon RH, Rodman D. Cystic fibrosis adult care: consensus conference report. *Chest*. 2004;125(suppl 1):1S–39S.

96. Flume PA, O'Sullivan BP, Robinson KA, et al. Cystic fibrosis pulmonary guidelines. Chronic medications for maintenance of lung health. *Am J Respir Crit Care Med*. 2007;176:957–969.

97. Kolb M, Martin G, Medina M, Ask K, Gauldie J. Gene therapy for pulmonary diseases. *Chest*. 2006;130:879–884.

98. Driskell RA, Engelhardt JF. Current status of gene therapy for inherited lung diseases. *Annu Rev Physiol*. 2003;65:585–612.

99. Larson JE, Morrow SL, Happel L, Sharp JF, Cohen JC. Reversal of cystic fibrosis phenotype in mice by gene therapy in utero. *Lancet*. 1997;349:619–620.

100. George SC. How accurately should we estimate the anatomical source of exhaled nitric oxide?. *J Appl Physiol*. 2008;104:909–911.

101. Brussee JE, Smit HA, Kerkhof M, et al. Exhaled nitric oxide in 4-year-old children: relationship with asthma and atopy. *Eur Respir J*. 2005;25:455–461.

102. Grob NM, Dweik RA. Exhaled nitric oxide in asthma from diagnosis, to monitoring, to screening: are we there yet? *Chest*. 2008;133:837–839.

103. Pedersen S, O'Byrne PM. Exhaled nitric oxide in guideline-based asthma management. *Lancet*. 2008;372:1015–1017.

*104. Barnes PJ, Chowdhury B, Kharitonov SA, et al. Pulmonary biomarkers in chronic obstructive pulmonary disease. *Am J Respir Crit Care Med*. 2006;174:6–14.

105. Holz O. Catching breath: monitoring airway inflammation using exhaled breath condensate. *Eur Respir J*. 2005;26:371–372.

106. Powell CA. Waiting to exhale. *Am J Respir Crit Care Med*. 2008;177:246–247.

Chapter 29

Pulmonary vascular disease

DOI: 10.1016/B978-0-7020-2996-7.00029-5

KEY POINTS

- Pulmonary oedema occurs when increases in pulmonary capillary pressure or the permeability of the alveolar/capillary membrane cause fluid to accumulate in the interstitium and alveoli.
- Pulmonary embolism, with either thrombus or air, partially occludes the pulmonary circulation causing an increase in alveolar dead space and pulmonary arterial hypertension.
- Pulmonary hypertension most commonly results from long-term hypoxia or elevated left atrial pressure, and involves reduced nitric oxide production and remodelling of the pulmonary blood vessels.

PULMONARY OEDEMA

Pulmonary oedema is defined as an increase in pulmonary extravascular water, which occurs when transudation or exudation exceeds the capacity of the lymphatic drainage. In its more severe forms there is free fluid in the alveoli.

ANATOMICAL FACTORS

The pulmonary capillary endothelial cells abut against one another at fairly loose junctions which are of the order of 5 nm wide.[1] These junctions permit the passage of quite large molecules and the pulmonary lymph contains albumin at about half the concentration in plasma. Alveolar epithelial cells are connected by tight junctions at their alveolar surface with a gap of only about 1 nm. Under normal circumstances the tightness of these junctions prevents the escape of large molecules, such as albumin, from the interstitial fluid into the alveoli. However, the proteins that make up the tight junction are not simply passive structural units, and can, for example in response to nitric oxide, be modified and allow an increase in permeability across the tight junction.[2,3]

The lung has a well-developed lymphatic system draining the interstitial tissue through a network of channels around the bronchi and pulmonary vessels towards the hilum. Lymphatic vessels are seen in the juxtaseptal alveolar region (see below) and are commonly found in association with bronchioles. Down to airway generation 11 (see Table 2.1), the lymphatics lie in a potential space around the air passages and vessels, separating them from the lung parenchyma. In the hilum of the lung, the lymphatic drainage passes through several groups of tracheobronchial lymph glands, where they receive tributaries from the superficial subpleural plexus. Most of the lymph from the left lung usually enters the thoracic duct where it can be conveniently sampled in animals. The right side drains into the right lymphatic duct.

The normal lymphatic drainage from human lungs is astonishingly small – only about 10 ml per hour. However, lymphatic flow can increase up to ten times this value when transudation into the interstitial spaces is increased.[4] This presumably occurs when pulmonary oedema is threatened but it cannot be conveniently measured in man.

PULMONARY FLUID DYNAMICS

For intravascular fluid to enter the alveoli it must traverse three barriers. First, it must move from the microcirculation into the interstitial space (across

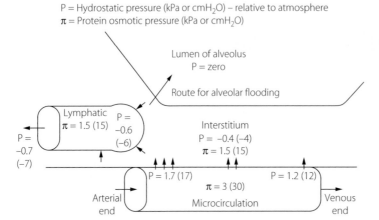

P = Hydrostatic pressure (kPa or cmH$_2$O) – relative to atmosphere
π = Protein osmotic pressure (kPa or cmH$_2$O)

Lumen of alveolus
P = zero

Route for alveolar flooding

Lymphatic
π = 1.5 (15) P = –0.6 (–6)

P = –0.7 (–7)

Interstitium
P = –0.4 (–4)
π = 1.5 (15)

P = 1.7 (17)   P = 1.2 (12)
π = 3 (30)

Arterial end   Microcirculation   Venous end

Fig. 29.1 Normal values for hydrostatic and plasma protein osmotic pressures in the pulmonary microcirculation and interstitium. (Values taken from reference 5.)

the endothelium), secondly through the interstitium and finally from the interstitial space into the alveoli (across the epithelium) (Figure 29.1).

Fluid exchange across the endothelium. This is promoted by the hydrostatic pressure difference between capillary and interstitium but counteracted by the osmotic pressure of the plasma proteins. The balance of pressures is normally sufficient to prevent any appreciable transudation but it may be upset in a wide variety of pathological circumstances.

It is customary to display the relationship between fluid flow and the balance of pressures in the form of the Starling equation. For the endothelial barrier this is as follows:

$$\dot{Q} = K[(Pcap - Pint) - \Sigma(\Pi cap - \Pi int)]$$

$\dot{Q}$ is the flow rate of transudated fluid which, in equilibrium, will be equal to the lymphatic drainage.

K is the hydraulic conductance (i.e. flow rate of fluid per unit pressure gradient across the endothelium).

$Pcap$ is the hydrostatic pressure in the pulmonary capillary.

$Pint$ is the hydrostatic pressure in the interstitium.

Σ is the reflection coefficient, in this case applying to albumin. It is an expression of the permeability of the endothelium to the solute (albumin). A value of unity indicates total reflection corresponding to zero concentration of the solute in the interstitial fluid. A value of zero indicates free passage

of the solute across the membrane and, with equal concentrations on both sides of the membrane, the solute could exert no osmotic pressure across the membrane. This normally applies to the crystalloids in plasma.

Πcap is the osmotic pressure the solute exerts within the pulmonary capillary.

Πint is the osmotic pressure the solute exerts in the interstitium.

Under normal circumstances in humans, the pulmonary lymph flow ($\dot{Q}$) is about 10 ml per hour with a protein content about half that of plasma. The pulmonary microvascular pressure ($Pcap$) is in the range 0–2 kPa (0–15 mmHg), relative to atmosphere, depending on the vertical height in the lung field. Furthermore, there is a progressive decrease in capillary pressure from its arterial to its venous end, since approximately one-half the pulmonary vascular resistance is across the capillary bed (see Figures 7.2 and 29.1). In this context, it is meaningless to think of a single value for the mean pulmonary capillary pressure.

The hydrostatic pressure in the interstitial space ($Pint$) of the lung is not easy to measure. Animal studies using micropuncture techniques obtained subatmospheric pressures of −0.40 to −1.25 kPa (−4 to −12.5 cmH$_2$O).[6] In the excised lung there was no vertical gradient in interstitial pressures such as might have been expected from the effect of gravity, but this was observed when measurements were made with the chest and pleura intact.[6]

The reflection coefficient for albumin (Σ) in the healthy lung is about 0.5. The overall osmotic pressure gradient between blood and interstitial fluid is about 1.5 kPa (11.5 mmHg). Thus there is a fine balance between forces favouring and opposing transudation. There is a considerable safety margin in the upper part of the lung where the capillary hydrostatic pressure is lowest. However, in the dependent part of the lung, where the hydrostatic pressure is highest, the safety margin is slender.

Fluid dynamics within the interstitium. It is now accepted that the interstitium does not simply act as a passive conduit for fluid transfer to the lymphatics.[7,8] Proteoglycan and hyaluron molecules are present in the pulmonary interstitium of animals, and function like a gel to absorb water to minimise increase in interstitial pressure and prevent hydration of other extracellular structures such as collagen.[9] Regional differences in the properties of these molecules are believed to be responsible for the establishment of a pressure gradient between the septal interstitium and the juxtaseptal region where lymphatic channels originate. This gradient may promote, and allow some control of, fluid flow from the endothelium to the lymphatics in the normal lung.[7]

With increased fluid transfer across the endothelium, the interstitial space can accommodate large volumes of water with only small increases in pressure, the interstitial compliance being high. Some 500 ml can be accommodated in the interstitium and lymphatics of the human lungs with a rise of pressure of only about 0.2 kPa (2 cmH$_2$O).[5] Eventually, the capacity of the molecules to absorb water is exceeded, and the proteoglycan structure breaks down, possibly leading to disturbances of nearby collagen molecules and therefore basement membrane function, producing alveolar oedema.[7] Alterations of interstitial proteoglycan structure during lung injury may contribute to the greater likelihood of pulmonary oedema under these circumstances (Chapter 31).

Fluid exchange across the alveolar epithelium. The permeability of this barrier to gases is considered in Chapter 9. It is freely permeable to gases, water and hydrophobic substances but virtually impermeable to albumin.

There is now considerable evidence of active fluid clearance from the alveoli in normal human lungs.[3,10,11] For methodological reasons, most studies of this system have involved Type II alveolar epithelial cells, but the same processes are believed to occur in Type I cells and in clara cells in the distal airways. On the alveolar side of these cells, the cell membrane contains epithelial sodium channels (ENaC)[12] and cystic fibrosis transmembrane conductance regulator (CFTR) channels (page 413), which actively pump

sodium and chloride ions respectively into the cell.[3] On the interstitial border of the cells, chloride moves passively out of the cell and the Na$^+$/K$^+$-ATPase channel actively removes sodium from the cell. Water from the alveolus follows these ion transfers down an osmotic gradient into the interstitium. Aquaporins are found in human alveolar epithelial cells, suggesting that water movement may be facilitated by these water channel proteins, but their role in normal adult lung remains unclear.[3]

A small amount of active clearance of fluid from the alveoli occurs under normal circumstances, but these systems become vital when pulmonary oedema threatens. Active removal of alveolar fluid by alveolar epithelial cells increases within one hour of the onset of oedema.[13] Stimulation of β_2 adrenoceptors by catecholamines increases the affinity of existing Na$^+$/K$^+$-ATPase channels for sodium and causes new channels to be incorporated into the cell membrane from intracellular endosomal stores. After a few hours, a variety of hormones[13] (e.g. thyroxine, aldosterone, glucocorticoids) and cytokines[3,11] (e.g. tumour necrosis factor) induce the transcription of new Na$^+$/K$^+$-ATPase channels and increase fluid clearance. These mechanisms are important both for minimising the severity of pulmonary oedema and clearing oedema fluid once the precipitating cause has resolved.

STAGES OF PULMONARY OEDEMA

There is presumably a prodromal stage in which pulmonary lymphatic drainage is increased, but there is no increase in extravascular water. This may progress to the following stages.

Stage I. Interstitial pulmonary oedema. In its mildest form, there is an increase in interstitial fluid but without passage of oedema fluid into the alveoli. With the light microscope this is first detected as cuffs of distended lymphatics, typically '8'-shaped around the adjacent branches of the bronchi and pulmonary artery (Figure 29.2). Electron microscopy shows fluid accumulation in the alveolar septa but this is characteristically confined to the 'service' side of the pulmonary capillary which contains the stroma, leaving the geometry of the 'active' side unchanged (see page 21 and Figure 2.7). Thus, gas exchange is better preserved than might be expected from the overall increase in lung water. Interstitial swelling is however not without risks, and swelling on the service side will eventually cause narrowing of the capillary lumen, though this does not occur until pulmonary oedema is advanced.

Stage I
Interstitial pulmonary oedema

Stage II
Crescentic filling of alveoli

Stage III
Alveolar flooding

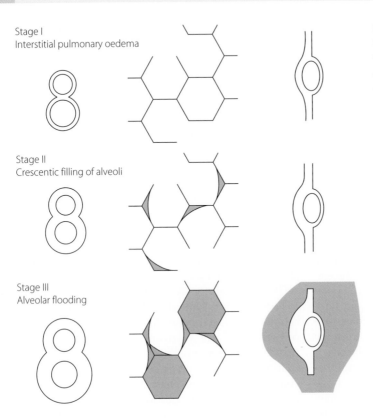

Fig. 29.2 Schematic diagram of the stages in the development of pulmonary oedema. On the left is shown the development of the cuff of distended lymphatics around the branches of the bronchi and pulmonary arteries. In the middle is the appearance of the alveoli by light microscopy (fixed in inflation). On the right is the appearance of the pulmonary capillaries by electron microscopy. The active side of the capillary is to the right. See text for details.

Physical signs are generally minimal in stage I, except perhaps for mild dyspnoea, particularly with exercise. The alveolar/arterial Po_2 gradient is normal or only slightly increased.

Stage II. Crescentic filling of the alveoli. With further increase in extravascular lung water, interstitial oedema of the alveolar septa is increased and fluid begins to pass into some alveolar lumina. It first appears as crescents in the angles between adjacent septa, at least in lungs which have been fixed in inflation (Figure 29.2). The centre of the alveoli and most of the alveolar walls remain clear, and gas exchange is not grossly abnormal, but dyspnoea at rest is likely and the characteristic butterfly shadow may be visible on the chest radiograph.

Stage III. Alveolar flooding. In the third stage, there is quantal alveolar flooding. Some alveoli are totally flooded while others, frequently adjacent, have only the crescentic filling or else no fluid at all in their lumina. It seems that fluid accumulates up to a point at which a critical radius of curvature results in surface tension sharply increasing the transudation pressure gradient. This produces flooding on an all-or-none basis for each individual alveolus. Due to the effect of gravity on pulmonary vascular pressures

(page 123), alveolar flooding tends to occur in the dependent parts of the lungs. Râles can be heard during inspiration and the lung fields show an overall opacity superimposed on the butterfly shadow.

Clearly there can be no effective gas exchange in the capillaries of an alveolar septum which is flooded on both sides, and blood flow through these alveoli constitutes venous admixture or shunt. This results in an increased alveolar/arterial Po_2 gradient and hypoxaemia, which may be life threatening. Blood flow to the oedematous lung regions is slightly reduced by hypoxic pulmonary vasoconstriction (page 108), possibly in conjunction with interstitial swelling causing capillary narrowing (see above), but the shunt commonly remains substantial.

Hypercapnia is not generally a problem. In less severe pulmonary oedema, there is usually an increased respiratory drive, due partly to hypoxaemia and partly to stimulation of J receptors (page 68). As a result the Pco_2 is usually normal or somewhat decreased.

Stage IV. Froth in the air passages. When alveolar flooding is extreme, the air passages become blocked with froth, which moves to and fro with breathing.

This effectively stops all gas exchange and is rapidly fatal unless treated.

AETIOLOGY OF PULMONARY OEDEMA

On the basis of the Starling equation, it is possible to make a rational approach to the aetiology of pulmonary oedema. There are three groups of aetiological factors, classified according to their effect on factors in the Starling equation.

Increased capillary pressure (haemodynamic pulmonary oedema). This group comprises the commonest causes of pulmonary oedema. There is an elevation of the hydrostatic pressure gradient across the pulmonary capillary wall, until it exceeds the osmotic pressure of the plasma proteins. Interstitial fluid accumulates until it overwhelms the ability of the interstitium to absorb fluid and transport it to the lymphatics. Fluid then begins to enter the alveoli and will initially be actively removed by the alveolar epithelial cells until this system is also overwhelmed. The oedema fluid has a protein content which is less than that of normal pulmonary lymph or plasma.[5] Apart from transudation in accord with the Starling equation, severe pulmonary capillary hypertension may result in loss of structural integrity (see below).

Causes of an increase in pulmonary capillary pressure are numerous:

- Absolute hypervolaemia may result from overtransfusion, from excessive and rapid administration of other blood volume expanders or from acute renal failure.
- Relative pulmonary hypervolaemia may result from redistribution of the circulating blood volume into the lungs. Examples of how this may occur include use of the Trendelenburg position or vasopressor drugs that act on the systemic circulation to a greater extent than the pulmonary circulation and so redirect blood into the pulmonary circulation.
- Raised pulmonary capillary pressure will inevitably result from an increase in pulmonary venous pressure.[4,8] This may occur from any form of left heart failure, most commonly left ventricular failure or mitral valve lesions.
- Increased pulmonary blood flow may raise the pulmonary capillary pressure sufficiently to precipitate pulmonary oedema. This may result from a left-to-right cardiac shunt, anaemia or, rarely, as a result of exercise.

Increased permeability of the alveolar/capillary membrane (permeability oedema). This group comprises the next commonest causes of pulmonary oedema. The mechanism is the loss of integrity of the alveolar/capillary membrane, allowing albumin and other macromolecules to enter the alveoli. The osmotic pressure gradient which opposes transudation is then lost. The oedema fluid has a protein content that approaches that of plasma.

The alveolar/capillary membrane can be damaged either directly or indirectly by many agents, which are reviewed in Chapter 31. Apart from the possibility of the condition progressing to acute lung injury, permeability pulmonary oedema is always potentially very dangerous. The presence of protein in the alveoli tends to make the oedema refractory and the protein may become organised into a so-called hyaline membrane.

'Stress failure' of the pulmonary capillaries occurs when the pulmonary capillary pressure is increased in the range 3–5 kPa (30–50 cmH₂O). Discontinuities appear in the capillary endothelium and type I alveolar epithelial cells, while the basement membrane often remains intact.[4,14] This would seem to result in increased permeability and leakage of protein into the alveoli. The gaps tend to occur in the cell body, rather than at the junctions between the cells. High-altitude pulmonary oedema (page 286) is an example of this mechanism.

Decreased osmotic pressure of the plasma proteins. The Starling equation indicates that the osmotic pressure of the plasma proteins is a crucial factor opposing transudation. Although seldom the primary cause of pulmonary oedema, a reduced plasma albumin concentration is very common in the seriously ill patient and it must inevitably decrease the microvascular pressure threshold at which transudation commences.

Neurogenic pulmonary oedema may follow head injuries or other cerebral lesions. Evidence for the existence of pulmonary venous sphincters has provided a possible mechanism for neurogenic pulmonary oedema.[15] Constriction of these sphincters, either due to circulating adrenaline or a neural response, could cause an abrupt increase in pulmonary capillary pressure. A study of neurogenic pulmonary oedema in humans supported this hypothesis by demonstrating that the oedema fluid often has a low protein content suggesting a haemodynamic mechanism (see above).[15]

Re-expansion pulmonary oedema is described on page 445 and pulmonary oedema following lung resection on page 495.

PRINCIPLES OF THERAPY

Immediate treatment aims to restore the arterial Po_2 to normal values. The inspired oxygen concentration should be increased, up to 100% if necessary. Sitting the patient up is a simple way to reduce central blood volume. Treatment of the underlying cause of pulmonary oedema follows directly from the Starling equation and an understanding of the aetiology.

Haemodynamic pulmonary oedema. Treatment aims to reduce left atrial pressure. Depending on the precise aetiology, treatment is directed towards improvement of left ventricular function and/or reduction of blood volume. The latter may be quickly and easily achieved by peripheral vasodilatation. Drugs that predominantly dilate the capacitance (venous) system, such as nitrates or angiotensin-converting enzyme inhibitors, will be most effective. This mechanism is probably also responsible for the beneficial effects of furosemide and diamorphine in the acute situation. Diuretics act more slowly but are useful for long-term treatment. Essentially the patient is titrated to the left along his Frank–Starling curve (Figure 29.3). In addition the curve is moved upwards and to the left, if this is possible, using positive inotropes as an adjunct to correction of left ventricular malfunction, for example from ischaemia. The further the curve can be moved, the greater will be that part of it lying in the safe quadrant between low cardiac output on one hand and pulmonary oedema on the other.

Permeability pulmonary oedema. Treatment should be directed towards restoration of the integrity of the alveolar/capillary membrane. Unfortunately, no particularly successful measures are available towards this end. It is, however, important to minimise left atrial pressure even though this is not the primary cause of the oedema. Attempts may be made to increase the plasma albumin concentration if it is reduced.

Artificial ventilation and positive end-expiratory pressure (PEEP). Severe pulmonary oedema causes degrees of hypoxia that may quickly be lethal. Tracheal intubation and positive pressure ventilation is therefore commonly required, and the results are often spectacular. Froth in the airways may be aspirated, and any areas of atelectasis occurring along with the oedema improved. Artificial ventilation is often combined with PEEP, resulting in further improvements

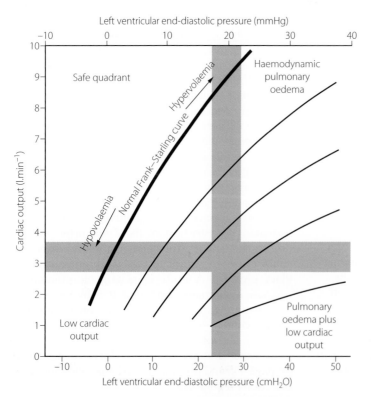

Fig. 29.3 Quadrant diagram relating cardiac output to left ventricular end-diastolic pressure. The thick curve is a typical normal Frank–Starling curve. To the right are shown curves representing progressive left ventricular failure. *Top left* is the safe quadrant, which contains a substantial part of the normal curve, but much less of the curves representing ventricular failure. *Top right* is the quadrant representing normal cardiac output but raised left atrial pressure, attained at the upper end of relatively normal Frank–Starling curves (e.g. hypervolaemia). There is a danger of haemodynamic pulmonary oedema. *Bottom left* is the quadrant representing normal or low left atrial pressure but low cardiac output, attained at the lower end of all curves (e.g. hypovolaemia). The patient is in shock. *Bottom right* is the quadrant representing both low cardiac output and raised left atrial pressure. There is simultaneous danger of pulmonary oedema and shock, and the worst Frank–Starling curves hardly leave this quadrant.

in arterial P_{O_2}. It was originally thought that the positive pressures drove the fluid back into the circulation, but evidence that extravascular lung water is reduced by PEEP is contradictory, with few human studies. Animal studies of pulmonary oedema indicate that by increasing the lung volume, the capacity of the interstitium to hold liquid is increased.[16] Similarly, with haemodynamic pulmonary oedema in dogs, PEEP does not alter the total amount of lung water but a greater proportion is in the extra-alveolar interstitial space,[17] and lymphatic drainage is increased.[18] With haemodynamic pulmonary oedema positive pressure ventilation has beneficial effects on the function of the failing heart (page 480) and it is probably this effect, rather than any effect on the lungs, that causes the clinical benefit in humans.

CLINICAL MEASUREMENT

Pulmonary vascular pressures. As an indication of impending or actual haemodynamic pulmonary oedema, the most physiological measurement is the pulmonary artery occlusion pressure (page 113), which equates to pulmonary venous pressure. In clinical practice the use of this technique is declining, with less invasive estimates of pulmonary vascular pressures being preferred such as echocardiography.

Permeability of the alveolar/capillary membrane. The only practical approach in humans is measurement of the rate of loss of a gamma-emitting tracer molecule from the lung into the circulation. The most sensitive tracer is ^{99m}TcDTPA (metastable technetium-99-labelled diethylene triamine penta-acetate, molecular weight 492 daltons).[19] The half-time of clearance from the lung fields is usually in the range 40–100 minutes in the healthy non-smoker. The half-time is reduced below 40 minutes following a variety of lung insults. However, it is within the range 10–40 minutes in apparently healthy smokers and this limits its scope for the early detection of a damaged alveolar/capillary membrane.

Lung water. Measurement of lung water in the intact subject has proved difficult. A great deal of effort has been devoted to the double indicator method. This uses the techniques for the measurement of pulmonary or central blood volume by dye dilution but with two indicators. One indicator is chosen to remain within the circulation while the other (usually 'coolth' or tritiated water) diffuses into the interstitial fluid. Extravascular lung water is then derived as the difference between the volumes as measured

with the two indicators. These methods are limited because a high level of accuracy is required to demonstrate small changes in lung water, though clinically acceptable results may now be obtained reasonably conveniently.[20]

PULMONARY EMBOLISM

The pulmonary circulation may be occluded by embolism, which may be gas, thrombus, fat, tumour or foreign body. The architecture of the microvasculature is well adapted to minimise the effects of embolism. Large numbers of pulmonary capillaries tend to arise at right angles from metarterioles and there are abundant anastomoses throughout the microcirculation. This tends to preserve circulation distal to the impaction of a small embolus. Nevertheless, a large pulmonary embolus is a serious and potentially lethal condition.

THROMBOEMBOLISM[21,22]

The commonest pulmonary embolus consists of detached venous thromboses from veins in the thigh and the pelvic venous plexuses. Smaller thrombi are filtered in the lungs without causing symptoms but larger emboli may impact in major vessels, typically at a bifurcation forming a saddle embolus. There may be a catastrophic increase in pulmonary vascular resistance with acute right heart failure or cardiac arrest.

Diagnosis of pulmonary thrombo-embolus.[22] Massive pulmonary thrombo-embolus causes rapid cardiac arrest and death, and over half the cases are undiagnosed except at autopsy.[23] Similarly, small pulmonary emboli may be completely asymptomatic, but often precede more significant, or lethal, embolism later. For patients with intermediate-sized emboli, a combination of pleuritic chest pain, dyspnoea and tachypnoea is indicative of pulmonary embolus. Changes in the electrocardiogram following pulmonary embolus reflect disturbed right-sided cardiac function secondary to elevated pulmonary arterial pressure and are generally non-specific and only occur after a large embolism. A variety of imaging techniques are available, with computed tomography (CT) scanning now regarded as the investigation of choice for diagnosis of pulmonary thrombo-embolism (Figure 29.4). Pulmonary radioisotope perfusion or ventilation-perfusion scans may detect smaller emboli not seen with CT scanning, but the technique has low sensitivity,[24] particularly in patients with pre-existing lung disease.

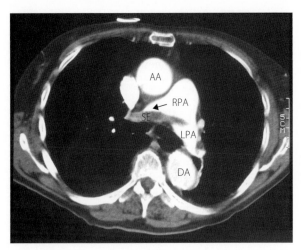

Fig. 29.4 Spiral computed tomographic scan of pulmonary thromboemboli. Intravenous contrast injected immediately before scanning makes the blood vessels appear white. Emboli then appear as darker areas within the blood vessel lumen. Saddle embolus (SE) situated mainly in the right pulmonary artery (RPA). AA, ascending aorta; DA, descending aorta; LPA, left pulmonary artery. (I am indebted to Celia Craven, Superintendent Radiographer, St James's Hospital, Leeds for supplying the scans.)

Pathophysiology.[21,25] Three mechanisms give rise to the physiological changes seen in pulmonary embolism. First is physical occlusion of the pulmonary vascular system. Second, platelet activation within the thrombus leads to release of 5-hydroxytryptamine (5-HT, serotonin) and thromboxane A_2, causing a further increase in pulmonary vascular resistance. Finally, the right ventricle commonly is unable to overcome the raised pulmonary vascular resistance and cardiac output falls, eventually culminating in right heart failure.

The primary respiratory lesion is an increase in alveolar dead space with an increased arterial/end-tidal Pco_2 gradient. Carbon dioxide elimination is therefore reduced and if ventilation remains unchanged arterial Pco_2 slowly climbs, until elimination is restored in spite of the large dead space.[26] However, in awake patients hypercapnia is unusual because hyperventilation is almost always present and arterial Pco_2 is usually below the normal range.[25] The cause of respiratory stimulation is unclear, but may involve stimulation of J-receptors as in air embolism (see below), or hypoxia if present.

Arterial Po_2 is also decreased. This results from derangement of normal ventilation perfusion relationships. Initially, whilst cardiac output remains normal, partial obstruction of the pulmonary circulation results in excessive blood flow to those lung regions that are still perfused, giving a low ventilation/perfusion ratio in these areas. When cardiac output begins to decrease as a result of a failing right ventricle, pulmonary perfusion will fall below normal levels and low mixed venous oxygen content will exacerbate the abnormal ventilation/perfusion relationships (page 134). Elevated right atrial pressures, as a consequence of pulmonary hypertension, may cause right-to-left intracardiac shunting[21] through an unsuspected patent foramen ovale (page 217).

Bronchospasm is a well recognised complication[27] and has been attributed to the 5-HT released from platelets and also to local hypocapnia in the part of the lung without effective pulmonary circulation. Pulmonary compliance may be reduced with large pulmonary emboli, but the mechanism of this change is unknown. Pulmonary infarction, which might be expected to occur, is rarely a problem. The lung can obtain oxygen directly from air within the airways and alveoli, from backflow along pulmonary veins, and from the bronchial circulation. Only when these sources are also impaired does infarction occur, for example when localised pulmonary oedema or pulmonary haemorrhage into the airways occurs in conjunction with embolism.

Principles of therapy.[22] Anticoagulation with intravenous heparin is the mainstay of treatment and prevents further clot from forming, either in lung or elsewhere, and allows endogenous fibrinolysis to proceed. If right ventricular dysfunction occurs, which is relatively easy to assess using echocardiography,[28] or haemodynamic instability is present due to a low cardiac output, thrombolytic therapy may also be used. Surgical embolectomy is now reserved for patients with significant pulmonary embolism who are unable to receive, or unresponsive to, other forms of treatment.

AIR EMBOLISM

An embolus may arise from pneumothorax or pulmonary barotrauma but is most commonly iatrogenic. In neurosurgery, the usual cause of air embolism is the use of the sitting position for posterior fossa surgery. A subatmospheric venous pressure at the operative site allows air to enter dural veins, which are held open by their structure. In open cardiac surgery, it is almost impossible to remove all traces of air from the cardiac chambers before closing the heart. Some small degree of air embolism is almost inevitable in all types of intravenous therapy, but catastrophic air embolism can occur when compression bags are used to accelerate the flow rate of intravenous fluids or blood bags that accidentally already contain air.

Detection of air embolism. Early diagnosis of air embolism is essential in neurosurgery, and there are three principal methods in routine use. Bubbles in circulating blood give a very characteristic sound with a precordial Doppler probe. The method is, if anything, too sensitive, because a shower of very small bubbles produces a particularly large signal. The simplest method is based on the end-expired CO_2 concentration, which is easily measured from capnography. Many factors influence the end-expiratory concentration (page 169) but a sudden decrease is likely to be either cardiac arrest or air embolism. Transoesophageal echocardiography is an efficient method of detecting air embolism[29] and, furthermore, it is the only practicable method of detecting paradoxical air embolism (see below).

Pathophysiology of air embolus. Provided there is no major intracardiac right-to-left shunt, small quantities of air are filtered out by the lungs where they are gradually excreted and little harm results. Alveolar dead space is increased according to the proportion of the pulmonary circulation that is occluded. The resultant increase in arterial/end-expiratory $P\text{co}_2$ gradient is the basis of detection of air embolism by capnography as described above. Pulmonary arterial pressure is increased by a large embolus due to the right ventricle working against an increased pulmonary vascular resistance. Finally, in animal studies, airway resistance is increased following air embolism, an effect mediated by arachidonic acid metabolites, possibly in conjunction with platelet activation and stimulation of pulmonary irritant receptors.[30]

Massive air embolism (probably in excess of 100 ml) may cause cardiac arrest by accumulation in the right ventricle, where compression of the air bubble prevents ventricular ejection of blood. Treatment then requires aspiration of air through a cardiac catheter, which is difficult. In lesser degrees of embolisation during surgery, reduced cardiac output probably also contributes to the sudden reduction in end-expiratory $P\text{co}_2$.

Paradoxical air embolism. Rarely, there may be passage of air emboli from the right to left heart without there being an overt right-to-left shunt. This is important because air then enters the systemic arterial circulation where there may be embolism and infarction, particularly of the brain. It is possible to pass a probe through such a foramen ovale in over 25% of the adult population (page 217), but paradoxical embolism does not usually occur because pressure is slightly higher in the left atrium than the right. However, under many circumstances, such as following pulmonary embolism, right atrial pressure may be elevated to the point that a right-to-left shunt occurs.

FAT EMBOLISM[31]

Fracture of long bones or major orthopaedic surgery may be associated with fat embolism.[32] This term is not strictly correct, as the features of 'fat embolism syndrome' result from release of bone marrow micro-emboli. Some degree of fat embolism occurs in almost all patients having hip and knee replacement surgery, but clinical sequelae occur in less than 1% of these.

Microscopic intravascular bone marrow fragments promote intravascular coagulation and platelet adherence, particularly under the conditions of venous stasis present during surgery, and so develop into larger 'mixed' emboli. There is initially an increase in physiological dead space but this is soon accompanied by an increase in shunt. Release of inflammatory mediators in the lung causes bronchospasm, increases capillary permeability and leads to localised pulmonary oedema.[32]

Lipid seems to pass through the pulmonary circulation to invade the systemic circulation. Surface forces between blood and lipid are much less than between blood and air and so would not offer the same hindrance to passage through the lungs. In the systemic circulation, fat emboli cause characteristic petechiae in the anterior axillary folds and there is often evidence of cerebral involvement.[31]

AMNIOTIC FLUID EMBOLISM[33,34]

Amniotic fluid embolism occurs rarely during delivery, but is fatal in over half of cases. Death normally results from cardiovascular disturbances and haemorrhage secondary to coagulopathy. Pulmonary vascular resistance is increased, but animal studies indicate that pulmonary hypertension is only transient, returning to normal after just a few minutes. The reasons for this effect on the pulmonary circulation remain unclear. Amniotic fluid and fetal cells in the circulation may cause no cardiovascular changes, and either an immune-mediated response, or the release of vasoactive mediators such as endothelin or prostaglandins have been suggested as mechanisms causing the clinical syndrome.

PULMONARY HYPERTENSION

There are many causes of pulmonary hypertension, which are classified as either primary or secondary (Table 29.1). The latter is much more common, and is therefore considered first.

SECONDARY PULMONARY HYPERTENSION

Respiratory disease. Pulmonary vascular resistance is increased by almost any pulmonary disease that results in chronic hypoxia (Table 29.1). Similar changes occur with intermittent hypoxia caused, for example, by sleep apnoea (Chapter 16). The change is initially temporary and reversible but progresses to become permanent. Nitric oxide (NO) production by pulmonary endothelium contributes to the normal low resistance of the pulmonary circulation (page 107). Hypoxia has been shown to reduce this basal NO secretion,[35] and further work has identified reduced production of constitutive nitric oxide synthase as the mechanism.[36]

Cardiac disease. Valvular disease of the left heart leads to an elevation of pressure in the left atrium and pulmonary veins. Increases in pulmonary capillary pressure from this cause tend to be long-term, and lead to remodelling of the pulmonary circulation. Smooth muscle hypertrophy and fibrosis of the pulmonary vasculature cause pulmonary arterial hypertension and, eventually, right heart failure (cor pulmonale).[4,8] A low cardiac output, either from the original valvular heart disease or the resulting right heart failure, results in reduction of mixed venous Po_2, which then causes further increases in pulmonary vascular resistance.

Treatment should first be directed towards improving the underlying condition, particularly if this is causing chronic or intermittent hypoxia. Long-term administration of oxygen, during the day and during sleep, is beneficial and recommended for any patient with hypoxia and pulmonary hypertension.[37] Vasodilator therapy is complicated by the lack of drugs with specific action on the pulmonary circulation, and is discussed below.

PRIMARY PULMONARY HYPERTENSION[38,39]

Pulmonary hypertension occurring in the absence of hypoxia is termed primary pulmonary hypertension (PPH) and has a prevalence of approximately 1300 per million. It is a progressive disease, which normally presents in early adulthood with worsening shortness of breath and eventually right heart failure. There is a familial contribution to PPH, and it may rarely be associated with advanced liver disease or the use of some older appetite suppressant drugs. Prognosis is poor, with most patients dying within three years of diagnosis.

Pathophysiology. The disease is characterised by proliferation of endothelial cells, hypertrophy of pulmonary arterial smooth muscle, and by thrombosis within pulmonary vessels.[40] Abnormal endothelial function is believed to be where the primary defect occurs, and nitric oxide related functions are abnormal. The defect seems to arise in communication between endothelial and smooth muscle cells, though this has yet to be fully characterised.[41]

Treatment.[37,38,42,43] In recent years a variety of drugs have been developed that lower pulmonary arterial pressures (page 111), all of which are now used for treating PPH. Prostacyclin and its analogues are the mainstays of PPH therapy, particularly now that orally active agents are becoming

Table 29.1 Causes of pulmonary hypertension

PRIMARY	SECONDARY		
	RESPIRATORY	CARDIAC	OTHER
Primary pulmonary hypertension	COPD	Left heart failure	Sleep apnoea
Hepato-pulmonary syndrome	Emphysema	Valvular disease	Lupus
	Pulmonary fibrosis	Congenital disease	Scleroderma
	Cystic fibrosis		Rheumatoid arthritis
	Chronic embolism		HIV infection
			Vasculitis

available.[44] Endothelin receptor antagonists are also now in routine use, though the debate continues about whether selective or non-selective drugs are best.[45] PPH remains a common indication for lung transplantation (Chapter 33).

HEPATOPULMONARY SYNDROME (HPS)

This clinical syndrome describes the combination of liver disease, pulmonary vascular dilatation and impaired oxygenation.[46] In this syndrome the pulmonary circulation becomes abnormally dilated. Pulmonary capillary diameter at rest is normally <7 μm, though with physiological increases in cardiac output, for example during exercise, this may increase up to 15 μm. In HPS pulmonary capillaries can be as large as 100 μm in diameter, and pulmonary arteriovenous or portopulmonary shunts may develop. Hypoxia is therefore the result of widespread areas with low ventilation/perfusion ratios, including shunts. With a high cardiac output state, which is common in liver failure, a diffusion barrier also develops when a large blood flow passes through dilated pulmonary capillaries leaving insufficient time for diffusion of oxygen into the blood (Chapter 9).

Pulmonary capillary dilatation in HPS results from excessive nitric oxide production, levels of which are increased in expired breath analysis (page 414). What stimulates the excess NO production is unknown, with contenders including production of endothelin-1 or tumour necrosis factor alpha (TNFα). Excessive production of carbon monoxide by the haemoxygenase system has also been implicated as carboxyhaemoglobin levels are high in patients with HPS.[47]

Treatment of HPS with NO antagonists has shown variable results, though using a TNFα antagonist may be useful for its prevention. Liver transplantation reverses the syndrome, though the time taken for the lung to recover is variable.

References

1. DeFouw DO. Ultrastructural features of alveolar epithelial transport. *Am Rev Respir Dis.* 1983;127(suppl 5):S9–S13.

2. Bhattacharya J. The alveolar water gate. *Am J Physiol Lung Cell Mol Physiol.* 2004;286:L257–L258.

*3. Matthay MA, Folkesson HG, Clerici C. Lung epithelial fluid transport and the resolution of pulmonary edema. *Physiol Rev.* 2002;82:569–600.

4. Gehlbach BK, Geppert E. The pulmonary manifestations of left heart failure. *Chest.* 2004;125:669–682.

5. Staub NA. Pathophysiology of pulmonary oedema. In: Staub NA, Taylor AE, eds. *Edema.* New York: Raven Press; 1984.

6. Miserocchi G, Negrini D, Gonano C. Direct measurement of interstitial pulmonary pressure in in situ lung with intact pleural space. *J Appl Physiol.* 1990;69:2168–2174.

7. Bhattacharya J. The microphysiology of lung liquid clearance. *Adv Exp Med Biol.* 1995;381:95–108.

8. Drake RE, Doursout MF. Pulmonary edema and elevated left atrial pressure: Four hours and beyond. *News Physiol Sci.* 2002;17:223–226.

9. Negrini D, Passi A, De Luca G, Miserocchi G. Pulmonary interstitial pressure and proteoglycans during development of pulmonary oedema. *Am J Physiol.* 1996;270:H2000–H2007.

10. Matthay MA, Clerici C, Saumon G. Active fluid clearance from the distal air spaces of the lung. *J Appl Physiol.* 2002;93:1533–1541.

11. Sznajder JI, Factor P, Ingbar DH. Lung edema clearance: role of Na$^+$-K$^+$-ATPase. *J Appl Physiol.* 2002;93:1860–1866.

12. Eaton DC, Helms MN, Koval M, Bao HF, Jain L. The contribution of epithelial sodium channels to alveolar function in health and disease. *Annu Rev Physiol.* 2009;71:403–423.

13. Crandall ED, Matthay MA. Alveolar epithelial transport. Basic science to clinical medicine. *Am J Respir Crit Care Med.* 2001;162:1021–1029.

14. Tsukimoto K, Mathieu-Costello O, Prediletto R, Elliott AR, West JB. Ultrastructural appearances of pulmonary capillaries at high transmural pressures. *J Appl Physiol.* 1991;71:573–582.

15. Smith WS, Matthay MA. Evidence for a hydrostatic mechanism in human neurogenic pulmonary edema. *Chest.* 1997;111:1326–1333.

16. Gee MH, Williams DO. Effect of lung inflation on perivascular cuff fluid volume in isolated dog lung lobes. *Microvasc Res.* 1979;17:192–196.

17. Paré PD, Warriner B, Baile EM, Hogg JC. Redistribution of pulmonary extravascular water with positive end-expiratory pressure in canine pulmonary edema. *Am Rev Respir Dis.* 1983;127:590–593.

18. Mondéjar EF, Mata GV, Cärdenas A, Mansilla A, Cantalejo F, Rivera R. Ventilation with positive end-expiratory pressure reduces extravascular lung water and increases lymphatic flow in hydrostatic pulmonary oedema. *Crit Care Med*. 1996;24:1562–1567.

19. Jones JG, Royston D, Minty BD. Changes in alveolar-capillary barrier function in animals and humans. *Am Rev Respir Dis*. 1983;127(suppl 5):S51–S59.

20. Godje O, Peyerl M, Seebauer T, Dewald O, Reichart B. Reproducibility of double indicator dilution measurements of intrathoracic blood volume compartments, extravascular lung water, and liver function. *Chest*. 1998;113:1070–1077.

21. Goldhaber SZ, Elliott CG. Acute pulmonary embolism: Part I. Epidemiology, pathophysiology, and diagnosis. *Circulation*. 2003;108:2726–2729.

*22. Tapson VF. Acute pulmonary embolism. *N Engl J Med*. 2008;358:1037–1052.

23. Ryu JH, Olson EJ, Pellikka PA. Clinical recognition of pulmonary embolism: problem of unrecognized and asymptomatic cases. *Mayo Clin Proc*. 1998;73:873–879.

24. PIOPED investigators. Value of the ventilation/perfusion scan in acute pulmonary embolism: results of the Prospective Investigation of Pulmonary Embolism Diagnosis (PIOPED). *JAMA*. 1990;263:2753–2759.

25. Santolicandro A, Prediletto R, Fornai E, et al. Mechanisms of hypoxemia and hypocapnia in pulmonary embolism. *Am J Respir Crit Care Med*. 1995;152:336–347.

26. Breen PH, Mazumdar B, Skinner SC. How does experimental pulmonary embolism decrease CO_2 elimination? *Respir Physiol*. 1996;105:217–224.

27. Windebank WJ, Boyd G, Moran F. Pulmonary thromboembolism presenting as asthma. *BMJ*. 1973;1:90–94.

28. Goldhaber SZ. Assessing the prognosis of acute pulmonary embolism. Tricks of the trade. *Chest*. 2008;133:334–336.

29. Furuya H, Okumura F. Detection of paradoxical air embolism by transesophageal echocardiography. *Anesthesiology*. 1984;60:374–377.

30. Chen HF, Lee BP, Kou YR. Mechanisms underlying stimulation of rapidly adapting receptors during pulmonary air embolism in dogs. *Respir Physiol*. 1997;109:1–13.

31. Mellor A, Soni N. Fat embolism. *Anaesthesia*. 2001;56:145–154.

32. Hofmann S, Huemer G, Salzer M. Pathophysiology and management of the fat embolism syndrome. *Anaesthesia*. 1998;53(suppl 2):35–37.

33. Davies S. Amniotic fluid embolus: a review of the literature. *Can J Anaesth*. 2001;48:88–98.

34. O'Shea A, Eappen S. Amniotic fluid embolism. *Int Anesthesiol Clin*. 2007;45:17–28.

35. Adnot S, Raffestin B. Pulmonary hypertension: NO therapy? *Thorax*. 1996;51:762–764.

36. McQuillan L, Leung G, Marsden P, Kostyk S, Kourembanas S. Hypoxia inhibits expression of NOS via transcriptional and posttranscriptional mechanisms. *Am J Physiol*. 1994;36:H1921–H1927.

37. Badesch DB, Abman SH, Simonneau G, Rubin LJ, McLaughlin VV. Medical therapy for pulmonary arterial hypertension. Updated ACCP evidence-based clinical practice guidelines. *Chest*. 2007;131:1917–1928.

38. Humbert M. Update in pulmonary arterial hypertension 2007. *Am J Respir Crit Care Med*. 2008;177:574–579.

39. Gaine SP, Rubin LJ. Primary pulmonary hypertension. *Lancet*. 1998;352:719–725.

40. Rich S. Clinical insights into the pathogenesis of primary pulmonary hypertension. *Chest*. 1998;114:237S–241S.

*41. Budhiraja R, Tuder RM, Hassoun PM. Endothelial dysfunction in pulmonary hypertension. *Circulation*. 2004;109:159–165.

42. Peacock AJ. Treatment of pulmonary hypertension. *BMJ*. 2003;326:835–836.

43. National Pulmonary Hypertension Centres of the UK and Ireland. Consensus statement on the management of pulmonary hypertension in clinical practice in the UK and Ireland. *Thorax*. 2008;63:ii1–ii41.

44. Gomberg-Maitland M, Olschewski H. Prostacyclin therapies for the treatment of pulmonary arterial hypertension. *Eur Respir J*. 2008;31:891–901.

45. Dupuis J, Hoeper MM. Endothelin receptor antagonists in pulmonary arterial hypertension. *Eur Respir J*. 2008;31:407–415.

46. Rodriguez-Roisin R, Krowka MJ. Hepatopulmonary syndrome – a liver-induced lung vascular disorder. *N Engl J Med*. 2008;358:2378–2387.

47. Arguedas MR, Drake BB, Kapoor A, Fallon MB. Carboxyhemoglobin levels in cirrhotic patients with and without hepatopulmonary syndrome. *Gastroenterology*. 2005;128:328–333.

Chapter 30

Diseases of the lung parenchyma and pleura

KEY POINTS

- Lung collapse occurs either from compression of lung tissue or by absorption of gas from lung units with occluded, or severely narrowed, airways.
- Many forms of interstitial lung disease exist, varying from purely inflammatory conditions (alveolitis), to those involving progressive fibrosis with minimal lung inflammation.
- Lung fibrosis arises from an imbalance between the cellular systems responsible for inflammation and tissue repair.
- Lung cancer is a common malignancy which is difficult to treat effectively, and mostly preventable by avoiding tobacco smoke and radon exposure.
- Pleural effusion, infection and pneumothorax remain common occurrences and can all impair respiratory function in the short or long term.

PULMONARY COLLAPSE

Pulmonary collapse may be defined as an acquired state in which the lungs or part of the lungs become airless. Atelectasis is strictly defined as a state in which the lungs of a newborn have never been expanded, but the term is widely used as a synonym for regional pulmonary collapse.

Collapse may be caused by two different mechanisms. The first of these is loss of the forces opposing the elastic recoil of the lung, which then decreases in volume to the point at which airways are closed and gas is trapped behind the closed airways. The second is obstruction of airways at normal lung volume, which may be due to many different causes. This also results in trapping of gas behind the obstructed airway. Whatever the cause of the airway closure, there is rapid absorption of the trapped gas because the total partial pressure of gases in mixed venous blood is always less than atmospheric (see Table 26.2). This generates a subatmospheric pressure more than sufficient to overcome any force tending to hold the lung expanded.

Pulmonary collapse during anaesthesia is described in Chapter 22.

LOSS OF FORCES OPPOSING RETRACTION OF THE LUNG

The lungs are normally prevented from collapse by the outward elastic recoil of the ribcage and any resting tone of the diaphragm. The pleural cavity normally contains no gas but, if a small bubble of gas is introduced, its pressure is subatmospheric (see Figure 3.5). Pulmonary collapse due to loss of forces opposing lung retraction may be considered under five headings as follows.

Voluntary reduction of lung volume. It seems unlikely that voluntary reduction of lung volume below closing capacity will cause overt collapse of lung in a subject breathing air. However, in older subjects, there is an increase in the alveolar/arterial P_{O_2} gradient, suggesting trapping of alveolar gas (see Figure 22.11).

Excessive external pressure. Ventilatory failure is the more prominent aspect of an external environmental pressure in excess of about 6 kPa (60 cmH$_2$O), which is not communicated to the airways (page 396). However, some degree of pulmonary collapse could also occur and this is a normal consequence of the great depths attained by diving mammals while breath holding. An approximately normal

DOI: 10.1016/B978-0-7020-2996-7.00030-1

lung volume is maintained during conventional diving operations when respired gas is maintained at the surrounding water pressure, though this does not occur with surface diving or snorkelling (page 297).

Loss of integrity of the ribcage. Multiple rib fractures or the old operation of thoracoplasty may impair the elastic recoil of the ribcage to the point at which partial lung collapse results. This depends entirely on the extent of the injury to the ribcage, but multiple adjacent ribs fractured in two places will usually result in collapse. However, extensive trauma to the rib cage also causes interference with the mechanics of breathing which is generally more serious than collapse (page 396).

Intrusion of abdominal contents into the chest. Extensive atelectasis results from a congenital defect of the diaphragm. Abdominal contents may completely fill one-half of the chest with total atelectasis of that lung. In adults, similar changes may occur with a large hiatus hernia, or ascites may push the diaphragm into the thoracic cavity. Paralysis of one side of the diaphragm causes the diaphragm to lie higher in the chest, with a tendency to basal collapse on that side.

Space occupation of the pleural cavity. Air introduced into the pleural cavity (pneumothorax) reduces the forces opposing retraction of the lung and this is a potent cause of collapse. The same effect occurs when the pleural cavity is occupied by an effusion, empyema or haemothorax. Pleural disease is discussed on page 444 et seq.

ABSORPTION OF TRAPPED GAS

Absorption of alveolar gas trapped beyond obstructed airways may be the consequence of reduction in lung volume by the mechanisms described above. However, it is the primary cause of collapse when there is total or partial airway obstruction at normal lung volume. Obstruction is commonly due to secretions, pus, blood or tumour but may be due to intense local bronchospasm or airway oedema.

Gas trapped beyond the point of airway closure is absorbed by the pulmonary blood flow. The total of the partial pressures of the gases in mixed venous blood is always less than atmospheric (see Table 26.2), although pressure gradients for the individual component gases between alveolar gas and mixed venous blood may be quite different.

The effect of respired gases. If the patient has been breathing 100% oxygen prior to obstruction the alveoli will contain only oxygen, carbon dioxide and water vapour. Because the last two together normally amount to less than 13.3 kPa (100 mmHg), the alveolar P_{O_2} will usually be in excess of 88 kPa (660 mmHg). However, the P_{O_2} of the mixed venous blood is unlikely to exceed about 6.7 kPa (50 mmHg), so the alveolar/mixed venous P_{O_2} gradient will be of the order of 80% of an atmosphere. Absorption collapse will thus be rapid and there will be no nitrogen in the alveolar gas to maintain inflation. This has important implications during anaesthesia, when 100% oxygen is commonly administered (page 336).

The situation is much more favourable in a patient who has been breathing air, as most of the alveolar gas is then nitrogen, which is at a tension only about 0.5 kPa (4 mmHg) below that of mixed venous blood.[1] Alveolar nitrogen tension rises above that of mixed venous blood as oxygen is absorbed and eventually the nitrogen will be fully absorbed. Collapse must eventually occur but the process is much slower than in the patient who has been breathing oxygen. Figure 30.1 shows a computer simulation of the time required for collapse with various gas mixtures.[2] Nitrous oxide/oxygen mixtures may be expected to be absorbed almost as rapidly as 100% oxygen. This is partly because nitrous oxide is much more soluble in blood than nitrogen, and partly because the mixed venous tension of nitrous oxide is usually much less than the alveolar tension, except after a long period of inhalation.

When the inspired gas composition is changed *after* obstruction and trapping occur, complex patterns of absorption may ensue. The inhalation of nitrous oxide, after airway occlusion has occurred while breathing air, results in temporary expansion of the trapped volume (Figure 30.1). This is caused by large volumes of the more soluble nitrous oxide passing from blood to alveolus in exchange for smaller volumes of the less soluble nitrogen passing in the reverse direction. This phenomenon also applies to any closed air space in the body, such as closed pneumothorax, gas emboli, bowel, and the middle ear with a blocked pharyngotympanic (Eustachian) tube. It is potentially dangerous and may contraindicate the use of nitrous oxide as an anaesthetic.

Magnitude of the pressure gradients. It needs to be stressed that the forces generated by the absorption of trapped gases are very large. The total partial pressure of gases in mixed venous blood is normally 87.3 kPa (655 mmHg). The corresponding pressure

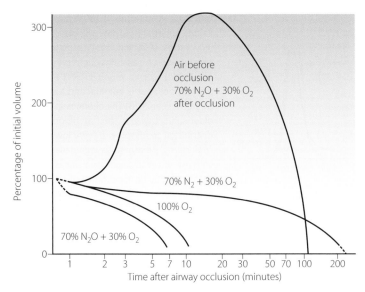

Fig. 30.1 Predicted rates of absorption from alveoli of differing gas mixtures. The lower curves show the rate of absorption of the contents of sections of the lung whose air passages are obstructed, resulting in sequestration of the contents. The upper curve shows the expansion of the sequestered gas when nitrous oxide is breathed by a patient who has recently developed regional airway obstruction whilst breathing air. In all other cases, it is assumed that the inspired gas is not changed after obstruction has occurred. Similar considerations apply to closed gas cavities elsewhere in the body. (Reproduced from reference 2 by permission of the authors and the publishers of Anaesthesia.)

of the alveolar gases is 95.1 kPa (713 mmHg), allowing for water vapour pressure at 37°C. The difference, 7.8 kPa (58 mmHg or 78 cmH$_2$O), is sufficient to overcome any forces opposing recoil of the lung. Absorption collapse after breathing air may therefore result in drawing the diaphragm up into the chest, reducing ribcage volume or displacing the mediastinum. If the patient has been breathing oxygen, the total partial pressure of gases in the mixed venous blood is barely one-tenth of an atmosphere (see Table 26.2) and absorption of trapped alveolar gas generates enormous forces.

Effect of reduced ventilation/perfusion ratio. Absorption collapse may still occur in the absence of total airway obstruction provided that the ventilation/perfusion ($\dot{V}/\dot{Q}$) ratio is sufficiently reduced. Older subjects, as well as those with a pathological increase in scatter of $\dot{V}/\dot{Q}$ ratios, may have substantial perfusion of areas of lung with $\dot{V}/\dot{Q}$ ratios in the range 0.01–0.1. This shows as a characteristic 'shelf' in the plot of perfusion against $\dot{V}/\dot{Q}$ (Figure 30.2). These grossly hypoventilated areas are liable to collapse if the patient breathes oxygen (Figure 30.2B). If the $\dot{V}/\dot{Q}$ ratio is less than 0.05, ventilation even with 100% oxygen cannot supply the oxygen that is removed (assuming the normal arterial/mixed venous oxygen content difference of 0.05 ml.ml^{-1}). As the $\dot{V}/\dot{Q}$ ratio decreases below 0.05, so the critical inspired oxygen concentration necessary for collapse also decreases (Figure 30.2C). The flat part of the curve between $\dot{V}/\dot{Q}$ ratios of 0.001 and 0.004 means that small differences in

inspired oxygen concentration in the range 20–30% may be very important in determining whether collapse occurs or not. There is no difficulty in demonstrating that pulmonary collapse may be induced in healthy middle-aged subjects breathing oxygen close to residual volume.[3,4]

DIAGNOSIS OF PULMONARY COLLAPSE

The diagnosis may be made on physical signs of decreased air entry and chest dullness but reliance is usually placed on chest radiography. Pulmonary opacification is seen, along with indirect signs of thoracic volume loss such as displacement of interlobular fissures, raised diaphragms, and displaced hilar or mediastinal structures.[7] In the upright position, collapse is commonest in the basal segments, often concealed behind the cardiac shadow unless the exposure is appropriate. Areas of atelectasis are clearly seen with computerised tomography (see Figure 22.10).

Collapse results in a reduction in pulmonary compliance, but the value of this in diagnosis is limited by the wide scatter of normal values. A sudden reduction in compliance may give an indication of collapse, provided, of course, that control measurements were available before collapse. Collapse also reduces the functional residual capacity and arterial P_{O_2}. However, in a patient with impaired oxygenation a reduction in arterial P_{O_2} cannot distinguish between the three very common conditions of pulmonary collapse, consolidation and oedema.

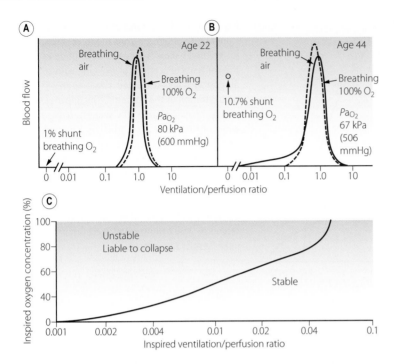

Fig. 30.2 Inspiration of 100% oxygen causes collapse of alveoli with very low $\dot{V}/\dot{Q}$ ratios. (A) The minor change in the distribution of blood flow (in relation to $\dot{V}/\dot{Q}$ ratio) when a young subject breathes oxygen. Collapse is minimal and a shunt of 1% develops. (B) The changes in an older subject with a 'shelf' of blood flow distributed to alveoli with very low $\dot{V}/\dot{Q}$ ratios. Breathing oxygen causes collapse of these alveoli and this is manifested by disappearance of the shelf and development of an intrapulmonary shunt of 10.7%. (C) The inspired oxygen concentration relative to the inspired $\dot{V}/\dot{Q}$ ratio that is critical for absorption collapse. (After reference 5 by permission of the authors and the publishers of the Journal of Clinical Investigation, and from reference 6 by permission of the authors and the publishers of Journal of Applied Physiology.)

PRINCIPLES OF THERAPY

Therapy depends on the physiological abnormality. Factors opposing the elastic recoil of the lung should be removed wherever possible. For example, pneumothorax, pleural effusion and ascites may be corrected. In other cases, particularly impaired integrity of the chest wall, it may be necessary to treat the patient with artificial ventilation. Re-expansion of collapsed lung often requires high pressures to be applied (page 336), but it is usually possible to restore normal lung volume.

When collapse is caused by regional airway obstruction, the most useful methods in both treatment and prevention are by chest physiotherapy, combined when necessary with tracheobronchial toilet, through either a tracheal tube or a bronchoscope. Fibreoptic bronchoscopy alone will often clear an obstructed airway and permit re-expansion, particularly with lobar atelectasis.[8]

Voluntary maximal inspirations are effective in clearing areas of absorption collapse in subjects who had been breathing oxygen near residual volume.[4] This manoeuvre is the basis of the 'incentive spirometer', which is used to prevent postoperative lung collapse.

With artificial ventilation a logical approach is hyperinflation of the chest or an artificial 'sigh'. Some ventilators were designed to provide an intermittent

'sigh' but evidence of its efficacy was never found. Current strategies to prevent pulmonary collapse during artificial ventilation are described in Chapter 32.

PULMONARY CONSOLIDATION (PNEUMONIA)

Inflammation of areas of lung parenchyma, usually due to infection, can lead to the accumulation of exudate within the alveoli and small airways, causing consolidation. Areas of consolidation may be patchy, and referred to as bronchopneumonia, or confined to discrete areas of the lung, forming lobar pneumonia. Pulmonary collapse frequently occurs in conjunction with pneumonia as a result of airway narrowing in surrounding lung areas. Clinical features of pyrexia, cough, sputum production and dyspnoea occur with signs of consolidation such as bronchial breathing, chest dullness and inspiratory crackles, though physical signs may be absent in bronchopneumonia. Diagnosis again relies on chest radiography, where consolidation appears as pulmonary shadowing, sometimes accompanied by an 'air bronchogram'. With resolution of the infection, cough becomes more productive, and the lung returns to normal within a few weeks.

Effects on gas exchange. Patients with pneumonia are commonly hypoxic. Consolidated areas of lung behave in a similar fashion to collapse, forming an intrapulmonary shunt through which mixed venous blood flows. In addition, there is an increase in areas with low $\dot{V}/\dot{Q}$ ratios (<0.1), but the contribution of these areas to impaired oxygenation is believed to be small because of hypoxic pulmonary vasoconstriction. Administration of oxygen to patients with pneumonia causes a further widening of the scatter of $\dot{V}/\dot{Q}$ ratios, implying a reduction in hypoxic pulmonary vasoconstriction,[9] but nevertheless results in a considerable improvement in arterial Po_2. In comparison with collapsed lung, consolidation is commonly associated with a worse pulmonary shunt and therefore more severe hypoxia. Many of the inflammatory mediators released as part of the response to infection act as local pulmonary vasodilators, in effect over-riding hypoxic pulmonary vasoconstriction.

PATHOPHYSIOLOGY[10]

Airway inflammation was described in detail in Chapter 28. Invasion of the lower respiratory tract with viruses and bacteria leads to further inflammatory changes characterised by migration of neutrophils from the circulation into the lung tissue. Depending on the pathogen involved, the stimulus for this migration may originate from the lung epithelial cells or alveolar macrophages. Chemokines released from these cells initiate neutrophil margination, and a range of proinflammatory cytokine pathways begin. Once in the lung tissue and activated, neutrophils are highly effective killers of the invading pathogen (page 455). As part of this process an inflammatory exudate develops that leads to consolidation of the lung tissue. The exudate is a complex mixture or invading organisms, inflammatory cells (dead and alive), immunoglobulins and other immune mediators, fluid transudate from increased capillary permeability, and products resulting from destruction of lung tissue as a result of protease activity.

Margination of neutrophils. Before a neutrophil can contribute to the inflammatory response it must stick to the blood vessel wall (margination), migrate across the endothelium, interstitium and epithelium, and become activated ready to contribute to pathogen removal (see Figure 31.2). These activities are controlled by an extensive series of cytokines in a very similar fashion to airway inflammation (see Figure 28.1). Lymphocytes again play an important role, but in parenchymal inflammation macrophages have an important control function instead of the eosinophils and mast cells involved in airway inflammation.

Neutrophil margination has been extensively studied in the systemic circulation. Selectins expressed on the surface of endothelial cells transiently bind the neutrophil causing it to roll along the blood vessel wall. Eventually, different adhesion molecules on the endothelial cell (e.g. intercellular adhesion molecule-1, ICAM-1) bind to specific receptors on the neutrophil surface (e.g. β_2 integrins CD11/CD18) causing a more firm adhesion to the endothelium. Once 'caught' by the endothelial cell, cytokines are released and neutrophil activation begins. The way in which neutrophils are marginated in the lung differs from elsewhere in the body.[11,12] Adhesion to endothelial cells occurs predominantly in the pulmonary capillary, rather than in venules as in the systemic circulation. Adhesion to the capillary wall can occur by either a CD11/CD18-dependent mechanism, or by another mechanism that seems to be independent of all the adhesion molecules normally required for margination in a systemic capillary.[13] Selectin-induced rolling of neutrophils may not occur. Adhesion is facilitated by a slow transit time for neutrophils across pulmonary capillaries. Human neutrophils are of similar size to red blood cells, but are much less deformable, so neutrophils take up to 120 seconds to traverse a pulmonary capillary compared with less than a second for a red blood cell.[11] Inflammatory mediators may cause changes to the biomechanical properties of neutrophils, in particular, a stiffening of the cell that will further impede its movement through the pulmonary capillary.[14] Once adhered to the pulmonary capillary wall neutrophils may become flattened, leaving some capillary lumen available for blood flow. In this position, emigration into the pulmonary tissue begins and the neutrophil moves through small holes in the capillary basal laminae, being guided by chemokines released from epithelial cells and possibly assisted by fibroblasts in the interstitial space (Figure 30.3).[15]

INTERSTITIAL LUNG DISEASE AND PULMONARY FIBROSIS

Diffuse pulmonary inflammation occurs in a wide variety of conditions, which are summarised in Table 30.1. Pneumonitis may simply resolve, as in pneumonia, leaving no permanent damage, but with long-term inflammation varying degrees of pulmonary fibrosis develop.

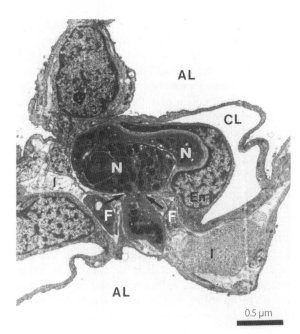

Fig. 30.3 Neutrophil emigration in rabbit lung during streptococcal pneumonia. This electron micrograph shows that the neutrophils (N), which are normally the same diameter as a pulmonary capillary, are elongated so leaving capillary lumen (CL) partly patent. These neutrophils have already emigrated from the capillary lumen across the endothelium (En), and one is now passing into the interstitium (I) through a small hole in the capillary basement membrane (arrows). The pseudopod of the neutrophil is in close contact with fibroblasts (F), which may be guiding the neutrophil through the defect in the basement membrane. AL, alveolar lumen. (Figure kindly provided by Professor DC Walker. Reproduced from reference 15 by permission of the author and publishers of Microvascular Research.)

Clinical features. vary according to the aetiology. Pneumonitis alone (i.e. without fibrosis) may be asymptomatic at first, progressing to a cough and dyspnoea, and in severe cases gives rise to systemic symptoms such as fever. When accompanied by fibrosis, dyspnoea becomes worse, and basal inspiratory crackles are present on examination. Lung function tests show a typical restrictive pattern with similar reductions in both forced vital capacity and forced expiratory volume in one second (page 96). Diffuse reticular shadows develop on chest radiography, and high-resolution CT scanning of the lungs shows either 'ground glass' appearances, which correlate with pneumonitis, or 'honeycombing', which represent more advanced fibrosis.

CAUSES OF PULMONARY FIBROSIS

These have been summarised in Table 30.1.

Drug induced fibrosis may follow lung injury induced by oxygen toxicity (page 387) precipitated by, for example, bleomycin, but the mechanism of this response is poorly understood.

Inorganic dusts.[16] Occupational exposure to asbestos fibres (asbestosis) or silica (silicosis) for many years leads to pulmonary fibrosis. Inhaled dust particles between 1 and 3 μm in diameter reach the alveoli and are ingested by macrophages. Different dust types have variable persistence in the lung, some being rapidly cleared and others persisting within the pulmonary macrophage for many years. In addition, the total (lifetime) fibre burden probably correlates with the degree of resulting fibrosis.

Organic dusts may cause lung inflammation by an immune mechanism, a condition referred to as extrinsic allergic alveolitis. The allergen is normally derived from a fungus to which the patient has occupational exposure, giving rise to a host of disease names such as farmer's lung, malt worker's lung etc. Bird fancier's lung differs in that it is precipitated by exposure to IgA derived from domestic birds. In extrinsic allergic alveolitis, pneumonitis results from activation of T-lymphocytes and IgG mediated inflammation. If caught early enough, and avoidance measures taken, allergic alveolitis resolves completely, but with continued exposure fibrosis develops.

Systemic diseases that lead to fibrosis are numerous and the mechanisms obscure. Many of the diseases associated with lung fibrosis have an immunological basis. For example, sarcoidosis results from T-lymphocyte activation in response to an unknown stimulus, whilst many connective tissue diseases are known to have an autoimmune aetiology. These immune changes are therefore likely to cause activation of the pulmonary inflammatory cells described below.

Radiation lung damage[17] is seen following radiotherapy for tumours in or near the chest. Radiation pneumonitis develops over several weeks following radiotherapy, while fibrosis may take up to 2 years to develop. Cellular radiation damage occurs when cell division occurs, so susceptible cells in the lung are those with the greatest rate of turnover. Thus radiation injury begins with damage to type II pneumocytes and capillary endothelial cells, which results in altered surfactant and interstitial pulmonary oedema (page 423) respectively.

Table 30.1 Causes of interstitial pneumonitis and pulmonary fibrosis

CAUSES	SUBGROUPS	EXAMPLES
Drug induced	Anti-cancer	Bleomycin, busulphan, cyclophosphamide, methotrexate
	Antibiotics	Isoniazid, nitrofurantoin, sulphonamides
	Others	Amiodarone
Dust	Inorganic	Silicosis
		Asbestosis
	Organic	Farmer's lung
Infections	Viral	Viral pneumonia
		HIV
	Other	*Mycoplasma*
		Opportunistic infections
Systemic disease	Connective tissue disease	Rheumatoid arthritis, scleroderma, systemic lupus erythematosus, ankylosing spondylitis
	Others	Sarcoidosis, histiocytosis, uraemia
Miscellaneous	Acute inflammation	Acute lung injury
	Inhalation injury	Smoke, cadmium, sulphur dioxide
	Radiation lung damage	
	Cryptogenic fibrosing alveolitis	

A cascade of inflammatory cell activation will then follow, often proceeding to fibrosis.[18]

Idiopathic pulmonary fibrosis (IPF),[19] synonymous with cryptogenic fibrosing alveolitis, includes all cases of pulmonary fibrosis in which no cause can be found. It is the most common type of pulmonary fibrosis, occurs more commonly in males and is of uncertain aetiology. Patients with CFA have extensive activation of pulmonary inflammatory cells and cytokines as described below. There is also accumulation of neutrophils, and this indicates a role for pulmonary oxidant injury (page 382) in IPF. Whatever the cause, IPF can be rapidly progressive with a median survival from diagnosis of just a few years.

CELLULAR MECHANISMS OF PULMONARY FIBROSIS[20,21]

Lung inflammation has been described earlier in this chapter as well as in Chapters 28 and 31. Progression to pulmonary fibrosis is not inevitable, but predicting which patients, and which underlying diseases, do progress is important clinically. There has been extensive research into the mechanisms of fibrosis, though a useful prognostic test remains a distant prospect.

Inflammation anywhere in the body is naturally succeeded by a cellular healing process that involves the laying down of new collagen. The lung is no exception, and pulmonary fibrosis is a result of excessive deposition of collagen in the lung extracellular matrix.

In pulmonary fibrosis the initial disease process is diverse (Table 30.1) and may cause changes in either type I or type II alveolar epithelial cells, pulmonary macrophages, neutrophils or T-lymphocytes.[22] Interactions between these cells produce numerous cytokines, which amplify the inflammatory response and initiate cellular repair mechanisms. Once these repair mechanisms are established, apoptosis occurs in the inflammatory cells and tissue repair proceeds. Transforming growth factor-β (TGF-β) is believed to be the most important cytokine involved in stimulating tissue repair, and probably acts as the final common pathway for most mechanisms leading to fibrosis.[23] Caveolin-1, which is a structural protein forming caveoli on the plasma membrane of many cells, is believed to be the endogenous regulator of TGF-β activity.[20] Myofibroblasts are the cells responsible for repairing the extracellular matrix in lung tissue, this matrix forming the scaffolding on which new lung tissue is formed. Once myofibroblasts have completed their task, they too undergo apoptosis.

In most causes of pulmonary fibrosis this well-controlled sequence of events is abnormal. The activity of acute inflammatory cells may not subside once the stimulus has been removed, and prolonged stimulation of repair mechanisms will occur. Alternatively, the normal mechanisms that terminate myofibroblast activity may be defective. The combination of inherited differences in the expression of cytokines or their receptors and the range of environmental stimuli described above is believed to result in pulmonary fibrosis. For example, an inherited defect in the expression of caveolin-1 may allow the actions of TGF-β to go unchecked. The intriguing possibility of abnormal apoptosis in lung cells has been suggested to explain pulmonary fibrosis.[24] Type I alveolar epithelial cells may undergo premature apoptosis and so prolong the inflammatory stimulus by continued exposure of underlying tissue. Alternatively, once tissue repair is complete, myofibroblasts may fail to respond to normal apoptotic stimuli and continue to remodel the extracellular matrix.

In a similar fashion to emphysema (page 410), excessive myofibroblast activity leads to a reduction in the amount of elastin present. Synthesis of elastin in normal lung is minimal in adults, and though there is some evidence of increased production in pulmonary fibrosis the elastic fibres formed are abnormal and probably non-functional.[25] Loss of elasticity by this mechanism causes collapse of both alveolar and small airway walls leading to a reduction in compliance and the area available for gas exchange.

PRINCIPLES OF THERAPY[26,27]

Where feasible, removal of the stimulant for lung inflammation or fibrosis is vital. Though this may not halt the development of fibrosis, for example following irradiation, it may limit the degree of pulmonary damage that occurs. Few patients with IPF gain any benefit from treatment with steroids, and predicting who will respond is difficult. Second-line treatment is with cytotoxic drugs such as azathioprine and cyclophosphamide, though with similar poor results. Recent elucidation of the cytokines involved in pulmonary fibrosis has led to optimism about future therapeutic approaches,[23] with many drugs that affect these processes currently under development.[27]

LUNG CANCER[28]

At the start of the 20th century lung cancer was a rare disease, but by the end of the century improved longevity and greater exposure to environmental carcinogens had led to lung cancer becoming one of the most common preventable causes of death in the world.[29,30] Improvements in the success rates for treatment of lung cancer have been less than

for malignancies in other organs, and the overall 5-year survival rate for lung cancer remains poor at only 15.7%.[29] It has been estimated that 1.2 million people worldwide died of lung cancer in 2002.[30]

EPIDEMIOLOGY

Occupational exposure to lung carcinogens such as asbestos was one of the earliest causative factors for lung malignancy to be identified, with several other occupational agents subsequently being linked with lung cancer such as arsenic, cadmium, beryllium and silica. Co-existing lung disease and diet have also been shown to be linked with the development of lung cancer. The role of these factors in causing lung cancer is however now known to be insignificant compared with exposure to environmental radon and the overwhelming role of tobacco smoke.

Tobacco.[30] Tobacco smoking (Chapter 21) is responsible for 90% of lung cancers in countries where smoking is common, and on a population scale lung cancer rates mirror smoking rates with an approximate lag time of 20 years. This is an ominous statistic for many currently developing countries where smoking rates are still increasing. Both the number of cigarettes smoked per day and the duration of being a smoker are positively correlated with the risk of developing lung cancer, though the latter is the more strong association. Quitting smoking has the predictable opposite effect with the risk of developing lung cancer decreasing with every year of continued abstinence, though the risk never falls as low as that for a lifetime non-smoker. Changes to cigarettes over the last 60 years such as the introduction of filtered cigarettes, and low tar and nicotine brands, were all aimed at reducing the health risks of smoking. Although some studies have demonstrated a reduced disease burden of smoking, the overall effect of these changes on lung cancer risk is believed to be negligible.

Smoking prevalence amongst men was at a peak approximately 20 years before the peak for women, so at present the lung cancer incidence in men is declining whilst in women the incidence continues to increase, and lung cancer is now the commonest cause of cancer-related death in women. The greater incidence of lung cancer in women is not caused solely by differences in smoking prevalence, but on a dose-for-dose basis women also seem to be more susceptible to the carcinogens found in cigarette smoke with an odds ratio of between 1.2 and

1.7 compared with men for developing lung cancer with equivalent smoking habits.[31] Studies from several countries have also shown that lung cancer incidence is higher in lower socio-economic groups, an observation which is again not entirely explained by differing smoking habits.

Most of the carcinogens in tobacco smoke are found amongst the 3500 compounds that make up the particulate phase, or 'tar', of cigarette smoke (page 318) and their mechanism of carcinogenesis is described below.

Radon. The second most important cause of lung cancer is environmental exposure to radon gas.[32] Radon is part of the natural decay series of uranium (Figure 30.4) and both elements are ubiquitous in the soil and rocks of the world though in widely varying concentrations. Radon gas is approximately eight times heavier than air and therefore tends to accumulate in the cellars and basements of dwellings, making it an important indoor pollutant.[33] The highest concentrations are found in mines, in particular uranium mines, therefore miners are the group most exposed to radon and an association between these occupations and lung cancer has been described for centuries. Residential exposure to radon may account for 10% of deaths from lung cancer or make an even greater contribution to the relatively rare cases of lung cancer in non-smokers.[32,34]

Radon is an inert gas, so when inhaled into the lung there will be no chemical reaction with other molecules, and with a molecular weight of 222 its diffusion within the alveolus (page 147) and absorption into the blood will both be slow. Most inhaled radon will therefore be exhaled in the same breath, but the most common environmental isotope, [222]radon, has a half life of only 3.8 days so whilst in the airway some of the radon will decay. The decay products are mostly solids which may be deposited in the airways, and also have short half-lives (Figure 30.4). As a result, inhaled radon and its progeny are a source of large quantities of alpha irradiation.

In comparison with beta and gamma radiation the alpha particle, made up of two protons and two neutrons, contains an enormous amount of energy and is therefore more harmful to biological molecules. For a sub-atomic particle, an alpha particle has a large mass and when travelling at around $15\,000\,\text{km.s}^{-1}$ this equates to a large kinetic energy. The strong positive charge of the alpha particle causes the electron shells of nearby atoms to rapidly

slow the particle, dissipating its energy in a much smaller area than other forms of radiation. Alpha particles travel only a few centimetres in air, and probably only 30–50 µm in living tissue. It is unknown whether the alpha particles released in the lung by radon inhalation can penetrate deeply enough into the airway epithelium to damage the rapidly dividing epithelial stem cells, which are far more likely to be a source of a malignancy than superficial, non-dividing, cells. An alternative explanation is that the radioactive progeny of radon are absorbed by other pulmonary cells such as macrophages and carried deeper into lung tissue.

CARCINOGENESIS OF LUNG CANCER[34,35]

Radiation. There are three postulated mechanisms by which an alpha particle may initiate malignancy. Firstly, when individual cells are traversed by a single alpha particle only 20% die, and the molecular damage in the survivors doubles their gene mutation rate.[36] Second, the cells surrounding those hit by the alpha particle are damaged by molecular products released from the directly hit cell, an observation known as the bystander effect. Third, much of the positive charge of an alpha particle is neutralised in tissue by removal of electrons from the abundant and nearby water molecules, initiating the production of a range of reactive oxygen species (Chapter 26).

Tobacco smoke carcinogens. Tobacco smoke contains 44 known human carcinogens, but two groups are of significance to the formation of lung cancer, polycyclic aromatic hydrocarbons (PAHs) and nitrosamines. As for radiation, much of the molecular damage is caused by the carcinogens generating reactive oxygen species. The normal defence mechanisms (page 385) are overwhelmed, and DNA, RNA, lipids and protein molecules are damaged by oxidation reactions. Many tobacco carcinogens also directly react with DNA either by causing methylation of bases within the DNA or simply by forming adducts between themselves and the DNA molecule. These various chemical changes to the DNA molecule will either interfere with transcription immediately, or induce mutations when the DNA replicates during subsequent cell divisions, so explaining why rapidly dividing cells are more susceptible to malignant change.

Molecular mechanisms of carcinogenesis. In order to appreciate how the various molecular injuries bring about malignant change it is useful to review

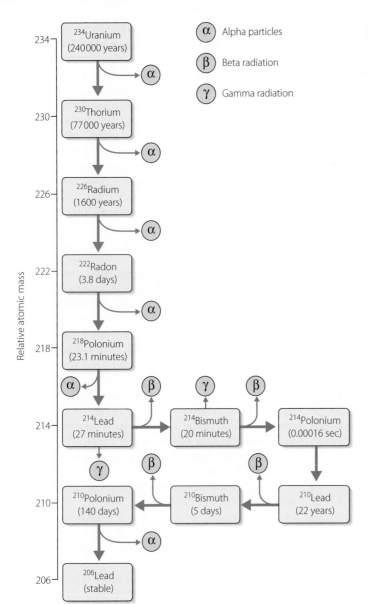

Fig. 30.4 Decay series of ^{234}uranium to stable ^{206}lead. An inhaled ^{222}radon molecule will decay to ^{210}lead within minutes, releasing three alpha and two beta particles in the process.

the normal biochemical systems that produce functioning proteins within a cell from the genes within the cell nucleus, and the normal phases of the cell cycle. Transcription of genes in eukaryotic cells has several complex stages:

1. Exposure of the gene. The human genome is large, and the vast amount of DNA that makes up this genome needs to be highly compacted to fit within the cell nucleus. The double helix of the DNA molecule is wrapped tightly around histone protein complexes, and these nucleosomes are linked together by DNA strands before further histone protein interactions compress the nucleosomes into a compact structure termed chromatin. Most of the genes that may be required are therefore not accessible to transcription proteins, and the nucleosomes must first be rearranged to expose the required gene.

2. Transcription. Numerous proteins, referred to as transcriptional factors, are required to control and initiate transcription from the gene

by binding to the required promoter region. In conjunction with less specific RNA polymerase proteins a single strand of pre-mRNA chain is then produced as the entire complex moves along the gene.

3. Post-transcriptional processing. The pre-mRNA undergoes considerable processing before it is suitable for translation. Methylation of RNA nucleotides near the ends of the chain makes the molecule more stable, varying amounts of redundant RNA are cleaved from the end of the molecule to better delineate the terminal sequence of the RNA, and large sections of redundant RNA (introns) are spliced from the molecule and the sections required for the protein production (exons) joined together and the final mRNA molecule formed.

4. Translation. Eukaryotic ribosomes consist of two subunits which must first dissociate before reforming as an initiation complex with the mRNA molecule, an initial tRNA and a methionine molecule. Elongation of the peptide chain then begins with individual tRNA molecules delivering each amino acid and one GTP molecule providing the energy for each addition. When the end of the translatable RNA sequence is reached a series of release factors are activated which complete the peptide chain and release it from the ribosome before dissociating the mRNA, tRNA and ribosome subunit proteins from each other.

5. Protein modifications. Proteins that ultimately reside in the cytoplasm are produced by free ribosomes, whilst proteins destined either for export from the cell or placement in the cell membrane are produced in the ribosomes bound to endoplasmic reticulum. Many sections of the initial peptide chain include 'signal peptides' that guide the post-transcriptional processing of proteins, for example by facilitating correct folding of the peptide chain or by binding the protein to the correct transporter systems within the cell.

As part of the normal cell cycle, all cells pass through various stages of division:

- G0 – the cell is quiescent, i.e. it is metabolically active, performing its normal functions, and not moving through the cell cycle towards division;
- G1 – the cell is preparing for division by producing the macromolecules required;
- S – synthesis phase when the DNA content of the cell is being replicated;
- G2 – preparation for mitosis when the cell organelles are arranged ready for physical division;
- M – mitosis when the cell divides.

Regulation of progression between these phases, particularly G1 to S and G2 to M, is controlled by a complex group of proteins called cyclin-dependent kinases (CDK). These proteins may, for example, be required to 'hold' the cell in the S phase until all the DNA has been replicated, and failure of this system will lead to premature replication of the cell, producing two progeny each with an abnormal DNA complement. Much of the activity of CDK is post-transcriptional, i.e. new CDK molecules are not being produced. Instead, control of the protein is exerted by phosphorylation and dephosphorylation of the various CDK components, with the degree of phosphorylation affecting the structure, and therefore activity, of the CDK. Alteration of a single base pair in the gene for a CDK will change a single amino acid of the CDK molecule and so fundamentally disturb the regulation of cell division.

A further way in which molecular damage within a cell may promote malignant change is via apoptosis, or programmed physiological cell death. Apoptosis is regulated by many of the same genes as those responsible for control of cell division so abnormalities of these systems may also prolong the life of a cell beyond its normal physiological term, so contributing to tumour growth.

Considering the continuous bombardment with toxic chemicals and radiation that airway cells receive and the myriad steps at which the production and function of a protein could be harmed, and cell division disturbed, it seems surprising that not everybody develops a lung malignancy. Many cells will be killed by the radiation or tobacco constituents, but the resulting tissue damage is quickly repaired, and though in the long term this repeated inflammation and repair cycle may itself damage lung tissue (see Figure 21.1), lung cancer does not result. Even more cells will be damaged, but the body's extensive and incompletely understood cellular repair mechanisms prevent malignancy developing. For a cell to become malignant, the cellular damage must fundamentally alter the cell's passage through the cell cycle or progress towards apoptosis in such a way that tissue growth becomes uncontrolled, which is the fundamental characteristic of a malignant cell.

The immune system has a role in preventing the development of cancer. Cell-mediated immunity involves T-lymphocytes recognising the body's own cells via the major histocompatibility (MHC) antigens present on the surface of all cells. In cancer cells, the damage to DNA and its transcription into proteins may produce abnormal or absent MHC proteins or may cause the cell to display other abnormal peptide molecules that the T-lymphocytes recognise as abnormal. An example is the presence on the cell surface of a malignant cell of peptide chains that are similar enough to those displayed by cells infected with a virus to cause the T-lymphocyte to attack the cell. By this mechanism we are protected against the formation of clinically apparent cancers, and differences in immune responsiveness may explain why some individuals are more vulnerable to developing malignancies. Modulation of the immune response to cancer cells is a potentially very useful future strategy to improve cancer treatment and prevention, for example by immunisation.

Target genes for pulmonary carcinogenesis.[35,37] Abnormal functioning of two groups of genes contribute to causing lung cancer – oncogenes and tumour suppressor genes. Oncogenes involved include:

- *ras* genes, which code for a G-protein involved in signal transduction of growth factor receptors on the cell surface. Mutations of the *ras* gene in lung cancer stimulate excessive cell growth even with normal levels of growth factor.
- *myc* proteins are transcription factors that are involved in controlling the transition of cells from the G0 to G1 phases of cell division, and though the *myc* gene is of normal structure in lung cancer it is over-expressed, amplifying its effect.
- *bcl-2* oncogene is normally involved in controlling cell division in the embryo or in adult stem cells, and it also has a role in controlling the timing of apoptosis. This gene is also over-expressed in some lung cancers, so facilitating cell proliferation and delaying apoptosis.

The physiological function of tumour suppressor genes is to respond to stress signals within a cell. Thus if a cell undergoes a period of hypoxia, oxidative stress, or incurs damage to its DNA, these genes are activated and will either delay progress through the cell cycle to allow time for damage to be repaired, or hasten apoptosis to prevent further cellular dysfunction. Tumour suppressor genes involved in lung cancer include:

- *p53.* Depending on the circumstances, activation of the p53 gene holds the cell in the G1 phase or induces apoptosis. A wide range of p53 mutations occur in lung cancer including deletions and altered splicing of the pre-mRNA.
- *RB* gene, which codes for one of the proteins involved in controlling transition from the G1 to S phase of cell division. Mutation of the RB gene probably produces a protein structure that is only slightly altered, but unable to be phosphorylated as required to hold the cell in the G1 phase so allowing cell division to progress too rapidly.

Better understanding of the genetic basis of lung cancer should lead to improved survival from the disease, though realisation of this ambition has been limited so far. Early detection of lung cancer by identifying abnormal gene expression in bronchial epithelial cells has been hindered by the finding of many abnormalities in histologically normal cells.[37] Many of the genetic abnormalities described above are associated with poor response to treatment, which is of little help to the patient involved, but hopefully will, in future, allow the best form of treatment to be determined.

CLINICAL ASPECTS[38]

Unfortunately, in a majority of patients their lung cancer has already spread beyond the primary tumour by the time symptoms develop. This remains the main reason for the continued poor outcomes for lung cancer treatment compared with many other malignancies. There is therefore a desperate need for a useable screening test for lung cancer, but none has yet emerged, though low-dose CT and various biomarkers[39] from the blood or exhaled gases (page 415) are currently being considered. In the meantime, avoidance of tobacco smoke and radon[32] remain the best options for prevention of lung cancer.

Pathology. Lung cancers can be divided into small cell lung cancer (SCLC) and non-small cell lung cancer (NSCLC), which is further divided into squamous cell carcinoma and adenocarcinoma. Squamous cell carcinomas account for around one-third of lung cancers, and mostly arise from central airways, often growing peri-bronchially to cause airway narrowing without necessarily being visible from within the airway lumen. They tend to be slow growing, metastasise late, and in the periphery of the lung may undergo central necrosis and cavitation. Adenocarcinomas also account for around one-third of lung cancers, but predominantly arise in the periphery of the lung, are faster growing than squamous cell carcinomas, and metastasise early via the blood or lymphatics. Finally, the NSCLC tumours include a range of different pathological malignancies, all of which share highly malignant characteristics including early spread via the lymphatic system.

Clinical features. Cough is the most common symptom of lung cancer, occurring in most patients at some stage of their disease, though cough is such a common complaint in smokers that this remains a very non-specific symptom. A cough arises from the lung cancer normally by direct irritation of the airway wall, either from within the lumen or from the peribronchial tissue, and is typically positional as the tumour presses on the airway in specific postures. Haemoptysis is the second commonest symptom, occurring in half of patients, and varying from staining of expectorated sputum to massive haemoptysis if the tumour erodes into a major thoracic vessel. Wheezing as a result of small airway occlusion by a peripheral lung tumour occurs in around 10% of patients and may be misdiagnosed as adult onset asthma. Narrowing of larger airways causes stridor, though this is only believed to occur when the cross-sectional airway is reduced by more than 75%. Dyspnoea, chest pain and chest infections (usually distal to an airway obstructed by tumour) are other pulmonary symptoms resulting from lung tumours. Invasion of nearby thoracic structures by a lung cancer causes a host of other presentations, such as pleural effusion (page 445), Horner's or Pancoast's syndrome from invasion of the sympathetic chain and brachial plexus nerves respectively, or obstruction of the superior vena cava. Finally, any lung cancer, but particularly NSCLC, may present with the symptoms and signs of distant metastases.

PRINCIPLES OF THERAPY FOR LUNG CANCER

A detailed description of the complex subject of treating lung cancer is beyond the scope of this book, and guidelines are available.[40] There are three main therapeutic options and their use is dependent on many factors, of which the two most important are the type of tumour and the stage at which the disease presents:

1. Surgery. Lung resection is described in Chapter 33. Resection of the tumour, a lobe of lung, or entire lung is normally done for NSCLC tumours that have not spread beyond the lung or local lymph nodes. For SCLC diagnosed at an early stage lung resection may be performed with the intention of curing the patient, but chemotherapy and radiotherapy are also used for the more malignant SCLC tumours as distant spread must be assumed to have occurred at diagnosis.

2. Chemotherapy. All anti-cancer drugs must affect malignant cells in such a way as to induce apoptosis or necrosis. A summary of the drugs used most commonly for treatment of lung cancer, and their mechanism of action and common side effects, is shown in Table 30.2.

Chemotherapy may be used as an adjuvant treatment for patients having surgical management, or may be used as the mainstay of treatment in more advanced NSCLC. Some form of chemotherapy is invariably used for treatment of SCLC. Most chemotherapy regimes involve administering drugs from two or more different groups to maximise the chances of successfully killing the malignant cells. Chemotherapy is normally given in multiple short courses, mostly to allow the patient to recover from the inevitable toxicity (Table 30.2). Also, this pattern of administration may increase the efficacy of the cytotoxic drugs as repeated hits by the drug encourages the malignant cells to all become aligned in the same phase of the cell cycle. Chemotherapy alone is unlikely to ever be curative. A 1-cm lung cancer is estimated to contain 10^9 malignant cells.[35] If a dose of chemotherapy kills 99.9% of those cells, then 10^6 still remain after the treatment, and this number will increase during the recovery period between treatments. Thus many treatments are required, with the associated toxicity, and in theory it is not possible to kill every malignant cell. However, given that the immune system is also known to have significant cytotoxic abilities, chemotherapy can reduce the tumour cell burden to such an extent that T-lymphocytes may completely remove the cancer.

3. Radiotherapy. Treatment with radiotherapy is indicated either as an adjunct to surgery for localised spread of NSCLC, in combination with chemotherapy for advanced NSCLC, or for treatment of SCLC.[40] Considering that radiation is responsible for causing a proportion of lung cancers it may appear surprising that the same form of energy is used in its treatment. For therapeutic use the same molecular mechanisms of radiation damage are utilised to kill malignant cells rather than to subtly

Table 30.2 Examples of chemotherapeutic agents used for treatment of lung cancer

GROUP	MECHANISM OF ACTION	TOXICITY	EXAMPLES
Alkylating agents	Alkylation of DNA, RNA and proteins	Myelosuppression Nausea and vomiting	Cyclophosphamide, ifosfamide
Platinum analogs	Cross-linking of DNA strands	Nausea and vomiting Nephrotoxicity	Cisplatin, carboplatin
Microtubular inhibitors	Inhibition of microtubulin – arrest of mitosis or induction of apoptosis	Neurotoxicity Myelosuppression	Vincristine, vinblastine, paclitaxel, docetaxel
Topoisomerase inhibitors	Inhibits DNA unwinding and breakage-reunion reactions	Myelosuppression Alopecia Myocardial toxicity	Etoposide, doxorubicin, irinotecan, topotecan
Antimetabolites	Analog of cytidine – halts DNA replication	Myelosuppression	Gemcitabine

damage them to induce malignancy as described above. The aim of radiotherapy is to focus the most intense area of radiation energy on the tumour itself whilst minimising radiation exposure to nearby normal tissue, though collateral tissue damage is inevitable and results in considerable toxicity from radiotherapy. There are wide species differences in the ability of cells to withstand radiation, with mammalian cells being very vulnerable, and within mammals different tissues have differing susceptibility to radiation injury, this being indirectly related to the rate of cell division of the tissue. Thus bone marrow, the gastrointestinal tract and skin, with their large populations of rapidly dividing cells, are the tissues most vulnerable to radiation injury.

A major determinant of the sensitivity of a tumour cell to killing by radiation is the Po_2 in the cell when it is irradiated, with most mammalian tumour cells requiring two to three times more radiation to cause cell death when hypoxic. This observation supports the hypothesis that much of the molecular damage induced by radiation is mediated via reactive oxygen species. Animal studies have demonstrated that many solid tumours have hypoxic centres, an observation which is believed to result from an inability of angiogenesis to keep pace with the rapidly growing tumour so leaving some regions with no blood supply. Positron emission tomography may be used to detect hypoxic tissue within tumours, and in a study of patients with NSCLC 48% of the tumour volume was found to be hypoxic, with a majority of tumours containing areas with an estimated Po_2 below 0.27 kPa (2 mmHg), a level at which radiation sensitivity would be poor.[41]

PLEURAL DISEASE

PHYSIOLOGY OF THE PLEURAL SPACE

Two pleural layers exist: the first lines the inside of the thoracic cavity (parietal pleura) including the diaphragm, and the second (visceral pleura) covers the lung from the hilum outwards including the major and minor pulmonary fissures. The opposing elastic forces of lung and chest wall (Chapter 3) cause a pressure of 3–5 cmH$_2$O below atmospheric to exist in the pleural space. The pleural space facilitates mechanical coupling between the chest wall and the lungs and to do this efficiently, that is with minimal loss of energy, there should be minimal friction between the two structures. The visceral and parietal pleura must therefore slide easily against each other, and this is achieved by the presence of a small amount of pleural fluid and a layer of surfactant molecules on the surface of the mesothelial cells lining both pleural membranes.[42]

An average 70 kg human has a total pleural surface area of 4000 cm^2 containing approximately 18 ml of pleural fluid,[43] which is an ultrafiltrate of plasma containing only small amounts of protein (approximately 1 g.dl^{-1}). Pleural fluid production is determined by the same Starling's forces that determine movement of fluid across capillary walls (page 420). In the parietal pleura, which is supplied by the systemic circulation, the negative intrapleural pressure results in an increased hydrostatic pressure gradient, so favouring fluid movement out of the capillary, but the pleural mesothelial cells are less permeable to protein than systemic capillaries so producing an oncotic gradient that opposes fluid movement out of the capillary. The net effect in parietal pleura is a gradient of about 6 cmH$_2$O for fluid to move from the capillary into the pleural space.[38] The blood supply of the visceral pleura derives from the bronchial circulation or the pulmonary circulation, both of which drain to the low pressure pulmonary venous system, and the hydrostatic pressure gradient is therefore much smaller than in parietal pleura, and no fluid movement is believed to occur from the visceral pleura into the pleural space. Another source of pleural fluid, particularly under pathological conditions, is direct flow from the interstitial space of the lung.

Fluid leaves the pleural space via the lymphatic system draining directly through openings, called stomata, between the parietal pleural and lymphatic channels. Stoma are up to 6 μm in diameter so permitting fluid, proteins and cells to pass through, and are probably more numerous in the caudal and diaphragmatic regions of the pleura, where pleural fluid accumulates due to gravity. Under physiological conditions pleural fluid turnover is about 0.01 ml.kg^{-1}.h^{-1} but when excess fluid accumulates in the pleural space drainage can increase by about 28 times.[38]

PLEURAL EFFUSION

Excessive production of pleural fluid will eventually overwhelm the ability of the lymphatic system to drain the pleural space, and fluid accumulates. There are numerous reasons for excessive pleural fluid production, and these are divided into two main groups:[38]

1. *Transudative* effusions contain fluid with a low protein concentration and arise from an increased hydrostatic pressure gradient or a low protein concentration in the blood, both of which will favour fluid transfer out of the capillary into the pleural space. Congestive heart failure, liver cirrhosis and nephrotic syndrome are common examples, and the effusions are commonly bilateral as the same factors affect both pleural cavities.

2. *Exudative* effusions have high protein content, are commonly unilateral, and arise because of increased permeability of the mesothelial cells, usually caused by pathology involving the pleura such as malignancy, infection or following trauma or surgery. Pleural effusions as a result of thoracic malignancy are often caused simply by tumour cells and debris blocking the stomata.

Investigation of pleural effusions requires care to avoid unnecessary drainage of the effusion with the associated possibility of introducing an infection. Provided the patient's serum protein levels are normal then the protein level in the effusion fluid will differentiate between exudates and transudates, and cytology of the cells in the effusion fluid will allow relatively easy diagnosis in 60% of malignant effusions.[44]

Re-expansion of lung following drainage of a pleural effusion can result in pulmonary oedema of the expanded lung, and it is suggested that no more than 1 litre of fluid should be removed at one time. There is some evidence that recently expanded lung tissue has a leaky microvasculature,[45] caused either by physical loss of integrity of the tight junctions between endothelial cells or by the generation of negative interstitial hydrostatic pressures favouring movement of fluid out of the capillary (page 420). It remains unclear whether the likelihood of pulmonary oedema occurring relates to the volume of fluid removed or the amount of negative pressure created by its removal. A recent study of 185 patients found that re-expansion pulmonary oedema only occurred in 2.7% of patients and was unrelated to the volume of fluid removed provided that the intrathoracic pressure was not allowed to fall below −20 cmH$_2$O.[46]

PNEUMOTHORAX

This occurs when air enters the pleural cavity either from the outside across a defect in the chest wall and parietal pleura or from the lung or mediastinum through a defect in the visceral pleura. The many causes of pneumothorax are usually divided into spontaneous and acquired aetiology and are outlined in Table 30.3.

Primary spontaneous pneumothorax is the most common cause (Figure 30.5A) and is postulated to result from rupture of small, thin-walled cysts in the immediate subpleural lung tissue, referred to as blebs if less than 2 cm in diameter or bullae if greater than 2 cm (Figure 30.5B).[47] Blebs or bullae are seen in most patients presenting with a primary spontaneous pneumothorax,[47] but are also present in 6% of the normal healthy population, so their role in causing pneumothorax remains controversial.[48] Whatever the cause, varying degrees of collapse of a lung will inevitably impair gas exchange, and arterial hypoxaemia occurs in three-quarters of patients with a pneumothorax on presentation, with

Table 30.3 Common causes of pneumothorax

SPONTANEOUS		ACQUIRED	
Primary	Rupture of subpleural bleb	Iatrogenic	Central venous access
			Lung biopsy
			Post-laparoscopy
Secondary	Bullous disease (COPD)		Blunt trauma ± rib fracture
	Cystic fibrosis	Traumatic	Penetrating trauma
	Asthma		
	Lung cancer	Barotrauma	Artificial ventilation (Chapter 32)
	Lung metastasis		
	Oesophageal rupture		
	Marfan's syndrome		
	Pneumocystis pneumonia		
	Lung abscess		

COPD, chronic obstructive pulmonary disease.

the hypoxaemia being worse with larger pneumothoraces or underlying lung disease.[49]

Tension pneumothorax. Occasionally, the defect in the lung or chest wall through which air gains entry to the pleura forms a valve mechanism and a tension pneumothorax occurs. During inspiration, air is sucked into the pleural space but cannot leave the pleura during expiration. A large pneumothorax develops and increased respiratory effort reduces intrapleural pressure further, until the pressure in the affected hemithorax remains above atmospheric throughout almost the entire respiratory cycle. Ventilation of the lung on the affected side ceases, the lung collapses and severe hypoxaemia occurs. A more dramatic effect is the shift of the mediastinum away from the pneumothorax, which causes a sudden and catastrophic reduction in venous return and therefore cardiac output. Insertion of a cannula into the affected hemithorax relieves the pressure, creates an open pneumothorax, and invariably saves the patient's life.

Principles of therapy for pneumothorax

Treatment of a pneumothorax depends on its size and the patient's symptoms.[49] If the patient is not breathless and the rim of air between the lung and the inside of chest wall on a chest radiograph is less

than 2 cm wide then no intervention is required. For larger or symptomatic pneumothoraces aspiration of air is performed and the chest radiograph reviewed to confirm lung expansion. If this is unsuccessful, then a chest drain is placed, complete lung re-expansion confirmed (Figure 30.5C), and the drain left in place until there is no further air leak and full lung expansion for 24 hours. If the lung fails to re-expand with a chest drain in situ or an air leak persists for days, then surgery is usually required. During surgery any visible blebs or bullae at the lung apex are resected, and a pleurodesis (page 496) performed, following which the lung is re-expanded under direct vision.

Absorption of air from the pleura. For small asymptomatic pneumothoraces, or following treatment as described above, complete resolution of a closed pneumothorax requires air to be reabsorbed from the pleura. How quickly this occurs depends on the partial pressure gradients of the various gases between the pleura and the circulation, in particular the venous blood where partial pressures are lowest (see Table 26.2). Two phases of gas reabsorption will theoretically occur: phase 1, when gases in the pleura come into equilibrium with the venous blood and phase 2, when the gas is absorbed. For phase 1, the cause of the pneumothorax is important in that the gas entering the pleura may be either air from the outside or alveolar gas from the lung. When ambient air, which is likely to be dry, enters the pleural space the first change to occur is a small increase in volume as water vapour humidifies the gas. Oxygen will be absorbed into the blood and carbon dioxide diffuses into the pleural space, but these two volume changes should be approximately equal and cause little change in volume.

For partial pressures, the loss of oxygen from the pleural air is partially offset by the gain of water vapour and carbon dioxide, but overall the nitrogen partial pressure increases slightly, and some nitrogen will slowly be absorbed into the circulation. When alveolar gas, which is already humidified and contains carbon dioxide, enters the pleural space the only change will be the absorption of a small amount of oxygen and a slight reduction in the volume of the pneumothorax, and therefore lung re-expansion. In patients breathing oxygen at the time of a pneumothorax (originating from the lung) the situation is, in theory, more favourable as the alveolar gas is now almost entirely oxygen and most of the pneumothorax will be quickly absorbed into the blood stream. A similar phenomenon has been observed if the

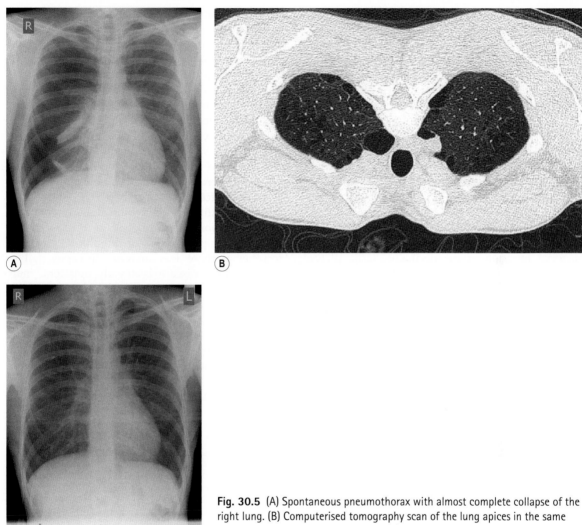

Fig. 30.5 (A) Spontaneous pneumothorax with almost complete collapse of the right lung. (B) Computerised tomography scan of the lung apices in the same patient showing multiple lung blebs. (C) The pneumothorax has been treated by the insertion of a chest drain, with complete re-expansion of the lung.

pneumothorax involves carbon dioxide entering the pleural space during laparoscopic surgery (technically a capnothorax) following which complete resolution occurred within two hours.[50] In both these situations nitrogen from the blood will diffuse into the pleural space, but this process is very slow compared with oxygen or carbon dioxide absorption.

In phase 2 of reabsorption of a pneumothorax the partial pressures of each gas in the pleural space are in equilibrium with the venous blood. Fortunately the subatmospheric total gas partial pressure of venous blood (Table 26.2) maintains small gradients that facilitate slow reabsorption of the pneumothorax. A further theoretical benefit of breathing

oxygen may be obtained during phase 2 of pneumothorax reabsorption. The greater the inspired oxygen concentration the lower is the blood P_{N_2}, so increasing the rate of diffusion of nitrogen from the pleura into the blood. An opposite problem occurs when using nitrous oxide in patients with a closed pneumothorax, when the nitrous oxide in the blood diffuses down its concentration gradient into the pneumothorax, increasing its volume.

These theoretical considerations are harder to demonstrate in practice. Though not investigated for some years, there is agreement that absorption of gas from a pneumothorax is slow, with the most widely quoted estimate being that 1.8% of the hemithorax volume is absorbed per day.[51] This means that a small pneumothorax occupying 15% of hemithorax volume will take approximately 10 days to resolve fully. Animal studies have shown a dose-dependent reduction in the time taken for a pneumothorax to resolve with increasing inspired oxygen fraction, the duration being approximately halved by breathing 50% oxygen compared with air.[52] A small study in humans from 1971 found that during periods breathing an unspecified high oxygen concentration resolution of the pneumothorax was approximately 4 times faster than when breathing air.[53]

EMPYEMA[38]

Empyema thoracis is a condition resulting from bacterial infection of the normally sterile pleural space. Almost two-thirds of patients with pneumonia develop a 'simple', non-infected, pleural effusion by direct movement of interstitial fluid from the infected lung tissue into the pleural space.[54] In around 10% of these effusions bacterial spread from the underlying pneumonia follows, and an empyema develops. Other, less common, causes of empyema include its development as a complication of trauma, thoracic surgery, pneumothorax or diagnostic thoracocentesis. The bacterial infection of the pleural fluid follows the normal stages of inflammation, with influx of white cells eventually causing the formation of pus. In empyema, deposition of fibrin begins early and is aggressive, and within a few weeks a thick layer of collagen (referred to as 'rind' or 'peel') is deposited on both pleural spaces. If left untreated the process continues until pleural fibrosis causes contraction of the chest wall and lung (fibrothorax).

A restrictive pattern of reduced lung function occurs with forced expiratory volume in one second (FEV_1) and forced vital capacity (FVC) values of half predicted normal being typical.[55] Early intervention with antibiotics, fibrinolysis or chest drainage may limit the progression of the fibrotic process.[56] However if these less invasive therapies fail or restrictive lung disease is already apparent, more extensive intervention is required in the form of surgical drainage or decortication, in which the peel formed on the pleura, particularly the parietal layer, is stripped off to allow the underlying lung to re-expand. Decortication is associated with a significant mortality and numerous other serious complications but improves lung function significantly,[55] though return to normal lung volumes rarely occurs.[38]

References

1. Klocke FJ, Rahn H. The arterial-alveolar inert gas ('N_2') difference in normal and emphysematous subjects, as indicated by the analysis of urine. *J Clin Invest.* 1961;40:286–294.

2. Webb SJS, Nunn JF. A comparison between the effect of nitrous oxide and nitrogen on arterial Po_2. *Anaesthesia.* 1967;22:69–81.

3. Nunn JF, Coleman AJ, Sachithanandan T, Bergman NA, Laws JW. Hypoxaemia and atelectasis produced by forced expiration. *Br J Anaesth.* 1965;37:3–12.

4. Nunn JF, Williams IP, Jones JG, Hewlett AM, Hulands GH, Minty BD. Detection and reversal of pulmonary absorption collapse. *Br J Anaesth.* 1978;50:91–100.

5. Wagner PD, Laravuso RB, Uhl RR, West JB. Continuous distributions of ventilation-perfusion ratios in normal subjects breathing air and 100% O_2. *J Clin Invest.* 1974;54:54–68.

6. Dantzker DR, Wagner PD, West JB. Instability of lung units with low VA/Q ratios during O_2 breathing. *J Appl Physiol.* 1975;38:886–895.

7. Ashizawa K, Hayashi K, Aso N, Minami K. Lobar atelectasis: diagnostic pitfalls on chest radiography. *Br J Radiol.* 2001;74:89–97.

8. Kreider ME, Lipson DA. Bronchoscopy for atelectasis in the ICU. *Chest.* 2003;124:344–350.

9. Gea J, Roca J, Torres A, Agusti AGN, Wagner PD, Rodriguez-Roisin R. Mechanisms of abnormal gas exchange in patients with pneumonia. *Anesthesiology.* 1991;75:782–789.

*10. Mizgerd JP. Acute lower respiratory tract infection. *N Engl J Med.* 2008;358:716–727.

11. Hogg JC, Walker BA. Polymorphonuclear leucocyte traffic in lung inflammation. *Thorax.* 1995;50:819–820.

12. D'Ambrosio D, Mariani M, Panina-Bordignon P, Sinigaglia F. Chemokines and their receptors guiding T lymphocyte recruitment in lung inflammation. *Am J Respir Crit Care Med.* 2001;164:1266–1275.

*13. Doerschuk CM, Tasaka S, Wang Q. CD11/CD18-dependent and -independent neutrophil emigration in the lungs. How do neutrophils know which route to take. *Am J Respir Cell Mol Biol.* 2000;23:133–136.

14. Doerschuk CM, Mizgerd JP, Kubo H, Qin L, Kumasaka

T. Adhesion molecules and cellular biomechanical changes in acute lung injury. *Chest.* 1999;116:37S–43S.

15. Walker DC, Behzad AR, Chu F. Neutrophil migration through preexisting holes in the basal laminae of alveolar capillaries and epithelium during streptococcal pneumonia. *Microvasc. Res.* 1995;50:397–416.

16. Mossman BT, Churg A. Mechanisms in the pathogenesis of asbestosis and silicosis. *Am J Respir Crit Care Med.* 1998;157:1666–1680.

17. Movsas B, Raffin TA, Epstein AH, Link CJ. Pulmonary radiation injury. *Chest.* 1997;111:1061–1076.

18. Rubin P, Johnston CJ, Williams JP, McDonald S, Finkelstein JN. A perpetual cascade of cytokines postirradiation leads to pulmonary fibrosis. *Int J Radiat Oncol Biol Phys.* 1995;33:99–109.

19. Noth I, Martinez FJ. Recent advances in idiopathic pulmonary fibrosis. *Chest.* 2007;132:637–650.

20. Verma S, Slutsky AS. Idiopathic pulmonary fibrosis – new insights. *N Engl J Med.* 2007;356:1371–1372.

*21. Thannickal VJ, Toews GB, White ES, Lynch JP, Martinez FJ. Mechanisms of pulmonary fibrosis. *Annu Rev Med.* 2004;55:395–417.

22. Kumar RK, Lykke AWJ. Messages and handshakes: cellular interactions in pulmonary fibrosis. *Pathology.* 1995;27:18–26.

23. Bartram U, Speer CP. The role of transforming growth factor β in lung development and disease. *Chest.* 2004;125:754–765.

24. Uhal BD. Apoptosis in lung fibrosis and repair. *Chest.* 2002;122:293S–298S.

25. Pierce RA, Mariani TJ, Senior RM. Elastin in lung development and disease. *Ciba Found Symp.* 1995;192:199–214.

26. Gross TJ, Hunninghake GW. Idiopathic pulmonary fibrosis. *N Engl J Med.* 2001;345:517–525.

27. Bouros D, Antoniou KM. Current and future therapeutic approaches in idiopathic pulmonary fibrosis. *Eur Respir J.* 2005;26:693–702.

28. Herbst RS, Heymach JV, Lippman SM. Lung cancer. *N Engl J Med.* 2008;359:1367–1380.

29. Alberg AJ, Ford JG, Samet JM. Epidemiology of lung cancer. *Chest.* 2007;132:29S–55S.

30. Parkin DM, Bray F, Ferlay J, Pisani P. Global cancer statistics, 2002. *CA Cancer J Clin.* 2005;55:74–108.

31. Zang EA, Wynder EL. Differences in lung cancer risk between men and women: Examination of the evidence. *J Natl Cancer Inst.* 1996;88:183–192.

32. Gray A, Read S, McGale P, Darby S. Lung cancer deaths from indoor radon and the cost effectiveness and potential of policies to reduce them. *BMJ.* 2009;338:215–218.

33. Samet J. Residential radon and lung cancer: End of the story?. *J Toxicol Environ Health Part A.* 2006;69:527–531.

34. Alavanja MCR. Biologic damage resulting from exposure to tobacco smoke and from radon: implication for preventive interventions. *Oncogene.* 2002;21:7365–7375.

35. Pass HI, Mitchell JB, Jihnson DH, Turrisi AT, Minna JD, eds. *Lung Cancer, Principles and Practice.* Philadelphia: Lippincott Williams & Wilkins; 2000.

36. Hei TK, Wu L-J, Liu S-X, Vannais D, Waldren CA, Randers-Pehrson G. Mutagenic effects of a single and an exact number of particles in mammalian cells. *Proc Natl Acad Sci.* 1997;94:3765–3770.

37. Sun S, Schiller JH, Spinola M, Minna JD. New molecular targeted therapies for lung cancer. *J Clin Invest.* 2007;117:2740–2750.

38. Shields TW, LoCicero J, Ponn RB, Rusch VW, eds. *General Thoracic Surgery.* 6th ed. Philadelphia: Lippincott Williams & Wilkins; 2005.

39. Hirschowitz EA. Biomarkers for lung cancer screening: interpretation and implications of an early negative advanced validation study. *Am J Respir Crit Care Med.* 2009;179:1–3.

40. Alberts WM. Diagnosis and management of lung cancer. Executive summary: ACCP Evidence-based clinical practice guidelines. *Chest.* 2007;132:1–19.

41. Rasey JS, Koh W, Evans ML, et al. Quantifying regional hypoxia in human tumors with positron emission tomography of [^{18}F] fluoromisonidazole: A pretherapy study of 37 patients. *Int J Radiat Oncol Biol Phys.* 1996;136:417–428.

42. Miserocchi G. Physiology and pathophysiology of pleural fluid turnover. *Eur Respir J.* 1997;10:219–225.

*43. Zocchi L. Physiology and pathophysiology of pleural fluid turnover. *Eur Respir J.* 2002;20:1545–1558.

44. Maskell NA, Butland RJA. BTS guidelines for the investigation of a unilateral pleural effusion in adults. *Thorax.* 2003;58:8–17.

45. Wilkinson PD, Keegan J, Davies SW, Bailey J, Rudd RM. Changes in pulmonary microvascular permeability accompanying re-expansion oedema: evidence from dual isotope scintigraphy. *Thorax.* 1990;45:456–459.

46. Feller-Kopman D, Berkowitz D, Boiselle P, Ernst A. Large-volume thoracentesis and the risk of re-expansion pulmonary edema. *Ann Thorac Surg.* 2007;84:1656–1662.

47. Amjadi K, Alvarez GG, Vanderhelst E, Velkeniers B, Lam M, Noppen M. Prevalence of blebs or bullae among young healthy adults. A thoracoscopic investigation. *Chest.* 2007;132:1140–1150.

48. Baumann MH. To bleb or not to bleb? *Chest.* 2007;132:1110–1112.

49. Henry M, Arnold T, Harvey J. BTS guidelines for the management of spontaneous

pneumothorax. *Thorax.* 2003;58(suppl 1):39–52.

50. Karayiannakis AJ, Anagnostoulis S, Michailidis K, Vogiatzaki T, Polychronidis A, Simopoulos C. Spontaneous resolution of massive right-sided pneumothorax occurring during laparoscopic cholecystectomy. *Surg Laparosc Endosc Percutan Tech.* 2005;15:100–103.

51. Flint K, Al-Hillawi AH, Johnson NMcI. Conservative management of spontaneous pneumothorax. *Lancet.* 1984;323:687–688.

52. England GJ, Hill RC, Timberlake GA, et al. Resolution of experimental pneumothorax in rabbits by graded oxygen therapy. *J Trauma.* 1998;45:333–334.

53. Northfield TC. Oxygen therapy for spontaneous pneumothorax. *BMJ.* 1971;4:86–88.

54. Anon. Managing empyema in adults. *Drug Ther Bull.* 2006;44:17–21.

55. Rzyman W, Skokowski J, Romanowicz G, Lass P, Dziadziuszko R. Decortication in chronic pleural empyema – effect on lung function. *Eur J Cardiothorac Surg.* 2002;21:502–507.

56. Davies CWH, Gleeson FV. Davies RJO. BTS guidelines for the management of pleural infection. *Thorax.* 2003;58(suppl 2):18–28.

Chapter 31

Acute lung injury

KEY POINTS

- Acute lung injury is lung inflammation that develops in response to a variety of both pulmonary and generalised acute diseases.
- The clinical features of acute lung injury vary from mild, self-limiting dyspnoea to rapidly progressive and fatal respiratory failure.
- Widespread pulmonary inflammation causes increased permeability of the alveolar capillary membrane leading to flooding and collapse of alveoli and severely impaired gas exchange.
- Artificial ventilation in severe acute lung injury is challenging, though a 'protective ventilation' strategy using small tidal volumes and moderate levels of positive end-expiratory pressure is beneficial.

Acute lung injury (ALI) describes a characteristic form of parenchymal lung disease, and represents a wide range of severity from short-lived dyspnoea to a rapidly terminal failure of the respiratory system, when the term acute respiratory distress (ARDS) is normally used. The syndrome was first described in 1967 when Ashbaugh et al[1] reported a condition in adults that seemed similar to the respiratory distress syndrome seen in infants. One of the subjects reported in this original paper was aged only 11 years, and in recognition of the fact that respiratory distress syndrome is known to occur in children the term *adult* respiratory distress syndrome should be avoided. There are a great many other synonyms for ALI, including acute respiratory failure, shock lung, respirator lung, pump lung and Da Nang lung.

CLINICAL ASPECTS OF ACUTE LUNG INJURY[2,3,4]

DEFINITION

There is no single diagnostic test, and confusion has arisen in the past from differing diagnostic criteria. This has complicated comparisons of incidence, mortality, aetiology and efficacy of therapy in different centres. To address this problem, European–American consensus conferences produced the following widely accepted definitions.[5]

Acute lung injury diagnosis requires the presence of four criteria:

1. Acute onset (less than 7 days) of impaired oxygenation.
2. Severe hypoxaemia defined as a Pa_{O_2} to $F_{I_{O_2}}$ ratio of ≤ 40 (Pa_{O_2} in kPa) or ≤ 300 (Pa_{O_2} in mmHg).
3. Bilateral diffuse infiltration on the chest radiograph consistent with pulmonary oedema.
4. Absence of left atrial hypertension.

Acute respiratory distress syndrome is defined in almost identical terms except that the impairment of gas exchange is worse with a Pa_{O_2} to $F_{I_{O_2}}$ ratio of ≤ 26.7 (kPa) or ≤ 200 (mmHg).

These definitions are now widely accepted and have been extremely helpful in researching ALI, particularly epidemiological studies. However, there are several provisos to their use in the clinical situation. For example, it is possible for patients with diseases that elevate left atrial pressure to also have ALI, but they would fall outside the strict definition.

DOI: 10.1016/B978-0-7020-2996-7.00031-3

Also, many earlier definitions suggest that one or more of the known predisposing conditions should have been present and that the clinical course has followed the recognised pattern (see below). Finally, it is noted that the histology is usually diagnostic but it is seldom indicated or advisable to take a lung biopsy. There is no reliable laboratory test to confirm the diagnosis (see below).

In part, the diagnosis of ALI depends on exclusion of other conditions. Sometimes it is not easy to separate it from other diseases such as pulmonary embolus, pulmonary oedema, fibrosing alveolitis, or diffuse pneumonia, which may present many similar features.

Scoring systems. Various attempts have been made to derive a single numerical value to assess the severity of ALI. Murray et al[6] proposed an expanded three-part definition comprising distinction between acute and chronic phases, identification of aetiological and associated conditions and a numerical lung injury score, details of which are shown in Table 31.1.

PREDISPOSING CONDITIONS AND RISK FACTORS FOR ALI

Although the clinical and histopathological pictures of ALI are remarkably consistent, they have been described as the sequel to a large range of predisposing conditions (Table 31.2). There are, however, very important differences in the progression of ALI and its response to treatment, depending on the underlying cause and associated pathology. Nevertheless, recognition of the predisposing conditions is crucially important for predicting which patients are at risk and the establishment of early diagnosis.

The conditions listed in Table 31.2 are not equally likely to proceed to ALI. Studies have consistently identified sepsis syndrome (see below) as the condition most likely to result in development of ALI with about 40% of patients being affected.[7] Patients who have aspirated gastric contents, received multiple emergency transfusions or incurred pulmonary contusions have a 17–24% chance of developing ALI. Overall, 25% of patients with a single risk factor develop ARDS but this rises to 42% with two factors and 85% with three. Age and sex do not affect the likelihood of developing ALI.

Sepsis syndrome is defined as a systemic response to proven or presumed infection, with hyper- (or hypo-) thermia, tachycardia, tachypnoea, and one or more organs exhibiting signs of hypoperfusion or

Table 31.1 Lung injury score[6]

Chest X-ray appearance	No alveolar consolidation		0
	Alveolar consolidation confined to 1 quadrant		1
	Alveolar consolidation confined to 2 quadrants		2
	Alveolar consolidation confined to 3 quadrants		3
	Alveolar consolidation in all 4 quadrants		4
Hypoxaemia score $Pa_{O_2}:F_{IO_2}$	Pa_{O_2} in kPa:	Pa_{O_2} in mmHg:	
	≥40	≥300	0
	30–39.9	225–299	1
	23.3–29.9	175–224	2
	13.3–23.2	100–174	3
	<13.3	<100	4
Positive end-expiratory pressure (when ventilated)	kPa	cmH_2O	
	≤0.5	≤5	0
	0.6–0.8	6–8	1
	0.9–1.1	9–11	2
	1.2–1.4	12–14	3
	≥1·5	≥15	4
Respiratory system compliance (when available)	$l.kPa^{-1}$	$ml.cmH_2O^{-1}$	
	≥0.8	≥80	0
	0.6–0.79	60–79	1
	0.4–0.59	40–59	2
	0.2–0.39	20–39	3
	≤0.19	≤19	4

$Pa_{O_2}:F_{IO_2}$ is the ratio of arterial P_{O_2} to the fractional concentration of oxygen in the inspired gas. The final lung injury score is the mean of the individual scores for each of the components which are included in the assessment.

Score	
0	No lung injury
0.1–2.5	Mild to moderate ALI
>2.5	Severe ALI (ARDS)

dysfunction. There is usually altered cerebral function, arterial hypoxaemia, lactacidosis and oliguria. Many cases of ALI represent the pulmonary manifestation of the multi-organ dysfunction syndrome (MODS) that is a feature of this condition, and ALI is frequently associated with circulatory failure (septic shock).

Pulmonary and extrapulmonary ALI. Gattinoni et al[8] proposed that patients with ALI should be considered as two separate groups. Pulmonary ALI results from clinical conditions that cause direct lung injury, whilst extrapulmonary ALI follows indirect lung injury (Table 31.2). These two sub-groups of

Table 31.2 Some predisposing conditions for ALI

DIRECT LUNG INJURY	INDIRECT LUNG INJURY
Common:	*Common:*
Pneumonia	Sepsis
Aspiration of gastric contents	Severe non-thoracic trauma
	Multiple transfusions of
Less common:	blood-products
Lung contusion	
Near drowning	*Less common:*
Inhalation of toxic gases or vapours	Acute pancreatitis
Fat or amniotic fluid embolus	Cardiopulmonary bypass
Reperfusion oedema, e.g. following	Severe burns
lung transplantation	Drug overdose
	Disseminated intravascular
	coagulation

ALI have been shown to differ with respect to pathological mechanisms, appearances on chest radiographs and CT scans, abnormalities of respiratory mechanics and response to ventilatory strategies.[9]

INCIDENCE AND MORTALITY[10]

In the past, the lack of accepted definitions of lung injury led to widely varying estimates of the incidences of ALI and ARDS. Despite more consistent diagnostic criteria in recent years, the estimated incidence of ALI remains variable at 18–79 cases per year per 100 000 population.[11] The reasons for this variation in estimates of the incidence of ALI is unknown.[2] Around 70% of cases of ALI are severe enough to be classified as ARDS.

There is, however, considerable agreement that mortality from ALI is high: two decades ago in excess of 50% of patients died whatever the criteria of diagnosis. Outcome has improved in recent years with current estimates of around a 40% mortality rate, but still with wide variability,[3,12] and only slow progress.[13] There appears to be no difference in the mortality of ALI arising from pulmonary or extrapulmonary causes.[14]

CLINICAL COURSE

Four phases may be recognised in the development of severe ALI. In the first the patient is dyspnoeic and tachypnoeic but there are no other abnormalities. The chest radiograph is normal at this stage, which lasts for about 24 hours. In the second phase there

is hypoxaemia but the arterial P_{CO_2} remains normal or subnormal. There are minor abnormalities of the chest radiograph. This phase may last for 24–48 hours. Diagnosis is easily missed in these prodromal stages and is very dependent on the history of one or more predisposing conditions.

It is only in phase three that the diagnostic criteria of ALI become established. There is significant arterial hypoxaemia due to an increased alveolar/arterial P_{O_2} gradient, and the arterial P_{CO_2} may be slightly elevated. The lungs become stiff and the chest radiograph shows the characteristic bilateral diffuse infiltrates. Ventilatory support is usually instituted at this stage, but many patients escape this intervention and are managed on respiratory wards rather than in intensive care.[15]

The fourth phase is often terminal and comprises massive bilateral consolidation with unremitting hypoxaemia even when ventilated with very high inspired oxygen concentrations. Dead space is substantially increased and the arterial P_{CO_2} is only with difficulty kept in the normal range.

Not every patient passes through all these phases and the condition may resolve at any stage. It is difficult to predict whether the condition will progress and there is currently no useful laboratory test. Serial observations of the chest radiograph, the alveolar/arterial P_{O_2} gradient and the function of other compromised organs are the best guides to progress. The more systems in failure, the worse is the outlook.

PATHOPHYSIOLOGY

Alveolar/capillary permeability is increased substantially throughout the course of ALI.[16] This may be demonstrated by the enhanced transit of various tracer molecules across the alveolar/capillary membrane (page 425).[17]

Maldistribution of ventilation and perfusion.[18] Computerised tomography (CT) of patients with ARDS shows that opacities representing collapsed areas are distributed throughout the lungs in a heterogeneous manner but predominantly in the dependent regions.[19] Following a change in posture, the opacities move to the newly dependent zones within a few minutes.[20] The most conspicuous functional disability is the shunt (Figure 31.1), which is usually so large (often more than 40%) that increasing the inspired oxygen concentration cannot produce a normal arterial P_{O_2} (see the isoshunt chart, Figure 8.11). CT scans of patients with ALI also demonstrate

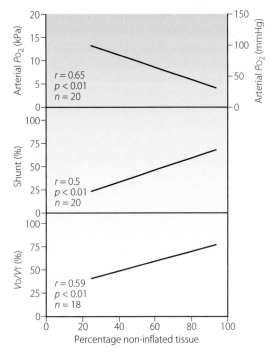

Fig. 31.1 Relationship of arterial P_{O_2}, shunt and physiological dead space (V_D/V_T) to the percentage of non-inflated lung tissue seen by computed tomography in patients with acute respiratory distress syndrome, artificially ventilated with positive end-expiratory pressure of 0.5 kPa (5 cmH$_2$O). (After reference 19.)

substantial areas of lung overdistension.[21] These areas contribute to the increased dead space, which may exceed 70% of tidal volume and requires a large increase in minute volume to attempt to preserve a normal arterial P_{CO_2}. Both shunt and dead space correlate strongly with the non-inflated lung tissue seen with CT (Figure 31.1).

Lung mechanics. In established ARDS, lung compliance is greatly reduced and the static compliance of the respiratory system (lungs + chest wall) is of the order of 300 ml.kPa^{-1} (30 ml.cmH$_2$O^{-1}).[22] Patients with pulmonary and extrapulmonary forms of ARDS (see above) have different abnormalities of respiratory system mechanics.[8] Respiratory system compliance is reduced to a similar extent in both groups, but the abnormality is mostly with lung compliance when lung disease is the cause, and chest wall compliance with extrapulmonary causation.

Functional residual capacity is reduced by collapse and increased elastic recoil.

Mean total resistance to airflow was found to be 1.5–2 kPa.l^{-1}.s (15–20 cmH$_2$O.l^{-1}.s),[22] or about three times that of anaesthetised patients with normal lungs, measured by the same technique. Using the model shown in Figure 4.4, some two-thirds of the total resistance in patients with ARDS could be assigned to visco-elastic resistance of tissue, although the airway resistance was still about twice normal.

Oxygen consumption by the lung. Pulmonary oxygen consumption (page 212) can be very high in patients with severe ALI. It is possible that some of this represents reactive oxygen species formation (see Chapter 26), but the increase in pulmonary oxygen consumption does not seem to correlate with various markers of pulmonary inflammation at the time the measurement is made.[23]

MECHANISMS OF ACUTE LUNG INJURY

HISTOPATHOLOGY

Although of diverse aetiology, the histological appearances of ARDS are remarkably consistent and this lends support for ARDS being considered a discrete clinical entity. Histological changes at autopsy may be divided into two stages, as follows.[24]

Acute stage. The acute stage is characterised by damaged integrity of the blood–gas barrier. The changes are primarily in the inter-alveolar septa and cannot be satisfactorily seen with light microscopy. Electron microscopy shows extensive damage to the type I alveolar epithelial cells (page 22), which may be totally destroyed. Meanwhile the basement membrane is usually preserved and the endothelial cells still tend to form a continuous layer with apparently intact cell junctions. Endothelial permeability is nevertheless increased and interstitial oedema is found, predominantly on the 'service' side of the capillary as seen in other forms of pulmonary oedema (page 421). Protein-containing fluid leaks into the alveoli, which also contain red blood cells, leukocytes and strands of fibrin. Intravascular coagulation is common,[25] and, in patients with septicaemia, capillaries may be completely plugged with leukocytes, and the underlying endothelium damaged.

Chronic or fibroproliferative stage. Attempted repair and proliferation predominate in the chronic stage of ARDS. Within a few days of the onset of the condition, there is a thickening of endothelium, epithelium and the interstitial space. The type I epithelial cells are destroyed and replaced by type II cells, which proliferate but do not differentiate into type I cells as usual. They remain cuboidal and about ten times the thickness of the type I cells they have replaced. This appears to be a non-specific response to damaged type I cells, and is similar to that which results from exposure to high concentrations of oxygen (page 387).

The interstitial space is greatly expanded by oedema fluid, fibres and a variety of proliferating cells. In the same way as for other causes of pulmonary fibrosis, extracellular matrix remodelling begins (page 437). Fibrosis commences after the first week and ultimately fibrocytes predominate: extensive fibrosis is seen in resolving cases. These fibroproliferative changes may occur earlier in pulmonary, compared with extrapulmonary, causes of ARDS.[26]

CELLULAR MECHANISMS[27]

The diversity of predisposing conditions suggests that there may be several possible mechanisms, at least in the early stages of development of ALI, but the end-result is remarkably similar. In all cases, lung injury seems to begin with damage to the alveolar/capillary membrane. This is followed by progressive inflammation leading to alveolar epithelial cell injury, alveolar transudation, pulmonary vasoconstriction and capillary obstruction.

Cells that are capable of damaging the alveolar capillary membrane include neutrophils, basophils, macrophages and platelets. Damage may be inflicted by a large number of substances, including bacterial endotoxin, reactive oxygen species, proteases, thrombin, fibrin, fibrin degradation products, arachidonic acid metabolites and innumerable pro-inflammatory cytokines. It seems improbable that any one mechanism is responsible for all cases of ALI. It is more likely that different mechanisms operate in different predisposing conditions and in different animal models of ALI.

Neutrophils have a key role in human ALI.[28] Although ALI can still be induced in neutrophil depleted animals, patients with ARDS have large numbers of neutrophils and associated cytokines in bronchoalveolar lavage (BAL) fluid samples. Neutrophil activation may occur in response to a large number of substances, some of which are illustrated in Figure 31.2. Which of these are important in ALI is unknown, but likely to depend on the predisposing condition; for example, complement component C5a is known to be involved in sepsis-related ALI. Margination of neutrophils from the pulmonary capillary into the lung parenchyma is the first stage

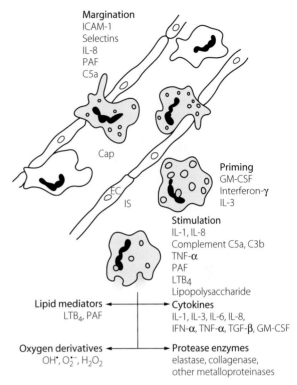

Fig. 31.2 Neutrophil activation and the main cytokines and mediators involved. This takes place in three stages. *Margination*, when neutrophils adhere to the capillary (Cap) wall and migrate between endothelial cells (EC) into the interstitial space (IS); *priming*, when the cells generate preformed mediators and lysozomal contents; and *stimulation*, when neutrophils release the various mediators shown. The scheme shown is based on studies of both systemic and pulmonary inflammation. Neutrophil margination may occur by different mechanisms in pulmonary capillaries (see page 435). For explanation of abbreviations see text.

of neutrophil activation and has been described on page 435. During margination and once in the interstitium, the neutrophil is 'primed' – that is, stimulated to produce preformed mediators ready for release, and to establish the bactericidal contents of their lysosomes. Finally, stimulation results from a whole host of cytokines, some derived from other inflammatory cells (macrophages, lymphocytes or endothelial cells) and some from other neutrophils, so amplifying the process. Stimulation causes release of a whole host of inflammatory mediators (Figure 31.2), and is also associated with inappropriate release of lysosomal contents. Instead of being released into phagocytic vesicles containing bacteria, they come into direct contact with the endothelium, which is thereby damaged.

Four groups of substances released from neutrophils (Figure 31.2) are considered to contribute to lung damage, as follows.

1. Cytokines.[27,29] Neutrophils are capable of producing numerous cytokines, most of which are pro-inflammatory. Tumour necrosis factor (TNF)-α and interleukin (IL)-1β have widespread pro-inflammatory effects including activation of endothelial cells to upregulate the adhesion molecules ICAM-1 (intercellular adhesion molecule) and selectins, which facilitate margination of further inflammatory cells (page 435). Complement component C5a, platelet activating factor (PAF) and IL-8 accelerate margination. Granulocyte macrophage colony stimulating factor (GM-CSF) and IL-3 contribute to priming of further neutrophils along with interferon-γ released from other inflammatory cells. Finally, IL-1, IL-8 and TNF-α all exert positive feedback on neutrophils, causing further stimulation. Transforming growth factor-β (TGF-β) is the principal anti-inflammatory cytokine produced by neutrophils, and is responsible for fibroblast stimulation and the development of pulmonary fibrosis (page 437).

2. Protease enzymes lead to extensive tissue damage in the lung. The most damaging is elastase which, unlike its name suggests, is very non-specific, with proteolytic activity against collagen, fibrinogen and many other proteins as well as elastin. Matrix metalloproteinases are more specific for individual substrates such as collagen.

3. Reactive oxygen species and related compounds (see Chapter 26) are powerful and important bactericidal agents, which also have the capacity to damage the endothelium by lipid peroxidation and other means. In addition, they inactivate α_1-antitrypsin, an important anti-protease enzyme (page 221).

4. Lipid derived mediators include prostaglandins, thromboxanes and leukotrienes (LT), but LTB$_4$ and PAF are the most important in ALI. These two act in the same way as other cytokines to amplify neutrophil activation, and in addition, PAF damages endothelial cells directly and promotes intravascular coagulation.[25]

Macrophages and basophils. Macrophages are already present in the normal alveolus (page 23) but their numbers increase greatly in ALI. They produce a wide range of bactericidal agents and cytokines similar to those of the neutrophil. Lung macrophages produce IL-10, which suppresses gene expression of many cytokines, and so acts as one of the very few anti-inflammatory cytokines so far identified in ALI.[29]

Platelets are present in the pulmonary capillaries in large number in ARDS. Aggregation in the capillary is associated with increased capillary hydrostatic pressure, possibly due to release of arachidonic acid metabolites.

Besides giving rise to pulmonary oedema, many of the mediators released by these inflammatory cells have other effects that contribute to the pulmonary changes seen in ALI. For example, arachidonic acid metabolites cause pulmonary venoconstriction, which will raise pulmonary capillary pressure and compound the effect of increased permeability. Accumulation of platelets and neutrophils along with intravascular coagulation will occlude pulmonary vessels, producing pulmonary hypertension and unperfused lung units. It has also been noted that many proteins, including albumin, but particularly fibrin monomer, can antagonise the action of surfactant so fundamentally altering lung mechanics.[30]

The potential contribution to ALI of lung damage secondary to artificial ventilation is described on page 481.

PRINCIPLES OF THERAPY[31,32]

Aggressive treatment of the underlying cause in conjunction with supportive therapy remains the mainstay of current management. Optimal management of the cardiovascular system and fluid balance[10] is a vital component of ALI treatment as any increase in pulmonary capillary pressure (e.g. from fluid overload) may lead to catastrophic pulmonary oedema. Respiratory support requires artificial ventilation in all but the most minor degrees of ALI.

ARTIFICIAL VENTILATION IN ALI[33,34,35]

General principles of artificial ventilation and the resulting physiological effects are described in detail in the next chapter. In this section, only the problems associated with ventilation of patients with ALI are described.

The lungs of patients with severe ALI may be conveniently divided into three hypothetical sections.[36]

First, there will be some 'normal' areas, usually in the non-dependent region. Second, there will be areas of lung, usually in dependent regions, with such severe collapse and alveolar flooding that ventilation of these areas will be impossible. Finally, there will be an intermediate area with poorly ventilated or collapsed alveoli that are capable of being 'recruited' by appropriate artificial ventilation, with a resultant improvement in gas exchange. Though the relative amounts of each section will vary greatly according to the severity of the ALI, there will always be *some* lung in the final area, and so capable of recruitment.

Tidal volume. The recognition that positive pressure ventilation can lead to lung damage (page 481) has led to a change in ventilatory technique used in patients with ALI. Overdistension of alveoli by application of large tidal volumes is a significant factor in lung damage. In particular, because of the extensive areas of pulmonary collapse a typical patient with ALI may only have approximately one-third of the lung being ventilated. Thus use of a normal tidal volume ($10–12\,ml.kg^{-1}$) will, for the few alveoli being ventilated, equate to a tidal volume of three times usual for normal healthy lungs, which equates to over 2 litres in a 70 kg subject.

Pressure-controlled ventilation (page 465) is now the preferred technique in most centres to avoid the problems outlined in the previous paragraph. However, with pressure-controlled ventilation in lungs with low compliance, such as ALI, the delivery of an adequate minute volume may be difficult. Two techniques are advocated to deal with this problem. First, inverse I/E ratios may be used, in which expiratory time is shorter than inspiratory time, allowing the delivery of a larger tidal volume. Second, the hypercapnia that results from the inadequate minute volume may be partially ignored. Known as permissive hypercapnia,[37] arterial P_{CO_2} is allowed to increase until such time as the respiratory acidosis is deemed detrimental, though the impact of this strategy remains controversial.[38]

Positive end expiratory pressure (PEEP). In patients with ALI PEEP reduces the amount of non-inflated lung tissue seen at CT scan,[19] particularly in dependent lung regions.[39] Shunt fraction and therefore the arterial P_{O_2} (Figure 31.3) also improve. Reduced pulmonary compliance means that cardiac output is better maintained than might be expected (page 48), with a reduction of about 20% with PEEP of 1.5 kPa (15 cm H_2O) (Figure 31.3).

The ideal PEEP value to use has been controversial for decades. Differing end-points (shown here in parentheses) have given rise to numerous terms such as 'optimal' PEEP (lowest physiological shunt fraction), 'best' PEEP (optimal static lung compliance), 'preferred' PEEP (best oxygen delivery), and 'least' PEEP (acceptable values for arterial P_{O_2}, inspired oxygen and cardiac output). High levels of PEEP should result in increased alveolar recruitment and improved oxygenation, but normal alveoli can only enlarge in response to PEEP to a certain extent, above which dramatic increases in alveolar pressure, and possible damage, occur (pages 482 et seq.). Identifying this point has vexed intensivists for some time. It has been suggested that PEEP be increased until the lower inflection of the patient's respiratory system static compliance curve is reached (point A in Figure 31.4), which is normally between 10–15 cmH_2O.[40] The pressure seen at the lower point of inflection is believed to represent the pressure at which most recruitable alveoli have been opened, while the upper inflection point (B in Figure 31.4) designates the point above which overdistension of alveoli may occur.[33] A pressure-volume curve in ARDS patients has also been compared to chest CT scans, and may prove useful in ascertaining which patients have significant potentially recruitable regions of lung.[41]

In clinical practice using higher levels of PEEP (13.2 cmH_2O) versus lower levels (8.3 cmH_2O) has been shown to improve oxygenation, but this did not result in any difference in survival.[42] Possible reasons for this lack of outcome benefit include adverse effects of the higher PEEP on the lungs or cardiovascular system, or that some patients with ALI may have very little 'recruitable' volume of lung.[43]

Protective ventilation strategy.[44] In ALI, the ventilatory strategy used must balance the conflicting requirements of maintaining adequate gas exchange in severely diseased lungs while simultaneously avoiding damaging the lungs by the use of large tidal volumes, high airway pressures or harmful levels of inspired oxygen. Protective ventilation describes a widely advocated ventilatory strategy that may achieve the best compromise, and involves using small tidal volumes to prevent alveolar overdistension and moderate levels of PEEP to maintain alveolar recruitment. Initial tidal volumes used for ventilation should be between $6–8\,ml.kg^{-1}$ using pressure controlled ventilation. PEEP is set using a pressure–volume curve or increased until arterial P_{O_2} is adequate or cardiovascular depression occurs. If plateau airway pressure exceeds 35 cmH_2O, or the inspired oxygen level required to obtain acceptable

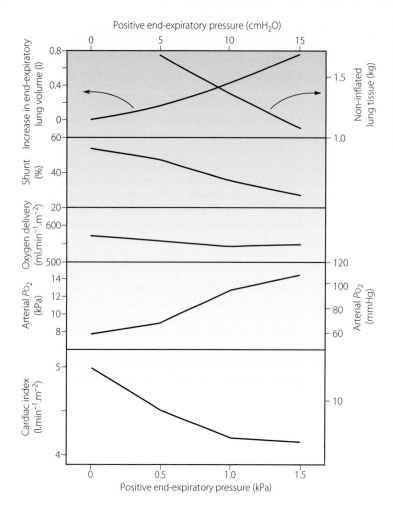

Fig. 31.3 Effect of positive end-expiratory pressure on various factors influencing oxygen delivery in patients with acute respiratory distress syndrome. Although arterial P_{O_2} is increased, cardiac output is decreased and there is no significant change in oxygen transport. (Data on non-inflated lung tissue are from reference 19; remaining data from reference 39.)

arterial P_{O_2} exceeds 0.65, then an alternative ventilatory strategy should be considered.[33] Protective ventilation is the only intervention in the management of ALI that has consistently been found to improve mortality.[35,44,45]

Alternative ventilatory strategies.[4,33] Many other techniques have been described as part of respiratory support for patients with ARDS who continue to have unacceptably poor gas exchange despite the use of protective ventilation. None of these have been shown to improve clinical outcome. Possible interventions include:

- recruitment manoeuvres, similar to those described for atelectasis during anaesthesia (page 336), may be used. Transient, self-limiting, bradycardia and/or desaturation is common, but the manoeuvres do improve oxygenation,[46]

though this has not been shown to improve outcomes from severe ALI.

- inverse-ratio ventilation (page 470)
- prone position. In the prone position both ventilation and perfusion become more uniform, and the areas of atelectasis in dependent lung regions change position, re-forming in the anterior (now dependent) regions.[20] About two-thirds of patients demonstrate an improvement in oxygenation on turning prone, though this is normally not sustained and repeated turning of the patient may be required
- inhaled nitric oxide (page 111)[47]
- high frequency ventilation (page 473)[48]
- extrapulmonary gas exchange (page 484)
- partial liquid ventilation.[49]

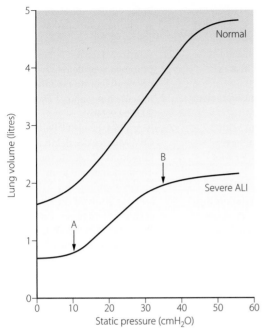

Fig. 31.4 Static pressure versus lung volume curves for patients receiving positive pressure ventilation. Note the severely reduced lung volume and compliance in ALI. Point A indicates the lower inflection of the curve, above which compliance is considerably improved. Application of positive end-expiratory pressure of approximately 12 cmH$_2$O in this patient will therefore improve tidal volume relative to the ventilatory pressure required. Point B indicates the upper inflection point, above which alveolar overdistension may occur, therefore, in this patient, airway pressure should ideally be maintained below 35 cmH$_2$O.

Table 31.3 Summary of pharmacological interventions suggested for the treatment of ALI or ARDS

THERAPY	EXAMPLES	PROPOSED MECHANISM
Pulmonary vasodilators	Prostacyclin	Non-specific pulmonary vasodilator
	Nitric oxide	Regional pulmonary vasodilator (see text)
	Almitrine	Enhancement of hypoxic pulmonary vasoconstriction
Surfactant	Artificial surfactants	Replace depleted alveolar surfactant, may also have anti-inflammatory properties
Anti-inflammatory	Steroids	General anti-inflammatory
	Ketoconazole	Inhibits thromboxane synthesis
	Ibuprofen/ Indomethacin	Inhibits prostaglandin production
	Prostaglandin E$_1$	Inhibits platelet aggregation, vasodilator
	Pentoxifylline	Reduces neutrophil chemotaxis and activation
	Endotoxin/TNF/ IL-1 antagonists	Inhibition of specific aspects of inflammatory response
Anti-oxidants	N-acetylcysteine	Increased glutathione activity (page 385)
	Recombinant human manganese SOD	Replaces epithelial extracellular SOD (page 385)
Anticoagulants	Heparin	Reduce fibrin deposition in alveoli

N.B. All the therapies listed have been shown to have beneficial effects in in-vitro or animal studies of ALI. There is insufficient evidence of improved outcome for any of the therapies listed to be recommended for routine use in human ALI.

SOD, superoxide dismutase (page 385); TNF, tumour necrosis factor; IL-1, interleukin 1.

OTHER THERAPEUTIC OPTIONS

Specific therapy for ALI is the goal of much research, which is directed particularly towards the control of sepsis and the development of antagonists to the various mediators considered above.[31] In most cases it has proved difficult to demonstrate their efficacy in the clinical setting. Detailed description of these, and several other pharmacological approaches to the treatment of ALI, is beyond the scope of this book, but a summary is shown in Table 31.3.

References

1. Ashbaugh DG, Bigelow DB, Petty TL, Levine BE. Acute respiratory distress in adults. *Lancet*. 1967;2:319–323.

2. Ware LB, Matthay MA. The acute respiratory distress syndrome. *N Engl J Med*. 2000;342:1334–1349.

*3. Wheeler AP, Bernard GR. Acute lung injury and the acute respiratory distress syndrome: a clinical review. *Lancet*. 2007;369:1553–1565.

4. Leaver K, Evans TW. Acute respiratory distress syndrome. *BMJ*. 2007;335:389–395.

5. Bernard GR, Artigas A, Brigham KL, et al. The American–European consensus conference on ARDS: definitions, mechanisms, relevant outcomes, and clinical trial coordination. *Am J Respir Crit Care Med*. 1994;149:818–824.

6. Murray JF, Matthay MA, Luce JM, Flick MR. An expanded definition of the adult respiratory distress syndrome. *Am Rev Respir Dis*. 1988;138:720–723.

7. Hudson LD, Millberg JA, Anardi D, Maunder RJ. Clinical risks for development of the acute respiratory distress syndrome. *Am J Respir Crit Care Med*. 1995;151:293–301.

8. Gattinoni L, Pelosi P, Suter PM, Pedoto A, Vercesi P, Lissoni A. Acute respiratory distress syndrome caused by pulmonary and extrapulmonary disease. Different syndromes? *Am J Respir Crit Care Med*. 1998;158:3–11.

*9. Pelosi P, D'Onofrio D, Chiumello D, et al. Pulmonary and extrapulmonary acute respiratory distress syndrome are different. *Eur Respir J*. 2003;22(suppl 42):48S–56S.

10. Rivers EP. Fluid-management strategies in acute lung injury – liberal, conservative, or both? *N Engl J Med*. 2006;354:2598–2600.

11. Milberg JA, Davis DR, Steinberg KP, Hudson LD. Improved survival of patients with acute respiratory distress syndrome (ARDS): 1983–1993. *JAMA*. 1995;273:306–309.

12. Rubenfeld GD, Herridge MS. Epidemiology and outcomes of acute lung injury. *Chest*. 2007;131:554–562.

13. Brochard L, Rouby J-J. Changing mortality in acute respiratory distress syndrome? Yes, we can! *Am J Respir Crit Care Med*. 2009;179:177–178.

14. Agarwal R, Srinivas R, Nath A, Jindal S. Is the mortality higher in the pulmonary vs the extrapulmonary ARDS? A meta-analysis. *Chest*. 2008;133:1463–1473.

15. Quartin AA, Campos MA, Maldonado DA, Ashkin D, Cely CM, Schein RMH. Acute lung injury outside of the ICU. Incidence in respiratory isolation on a general ward. *Chest*. 2009;135:261–268.

16. Sinclair DG, Braude S, Haslam PL, Evans TW. Pulmonary endothelial permeability in patients with severe lung injury: Clinical correlates and natural history. *Chest*. 1994;106:535–539.

17. Rocker GM. Bedside measurement of pulmonary capillary permeability in patients with acute lung injury. What have we learned? *Intensive Care Med*. 1996;22:619–621.

18. Sinclair SE, Albert RK. Altering ventilation-perfusion relationships in ventilated patients with acute lung injury. *Intensive Care Med*. 1997;23:942–950.

19. Gattinoni L, Pesenti A, Bombino M, et al. Relationships between lung computed tomographic density, gas exchange, and PEEP in acute respiratory failure. *Anesthesiology*. 1988;69:824–832.

20. Gattinoni L, Pelosi P, Vitale G, Pesenti A, D'Andrea L, Mascheroni D. Body position changes redistribute lung computed-tomographic density in patients with acute respiratory failure. *Anesthesiology*. 1991;74:15–23.

21. Vieira SRR, Puybasset L, Richecoeur J, et al. A lung computed tomographic assessment of positive end-expiratory pressure-induced lung overdistension. *Am J Respir Crit Care Med*. 1998;158:1571–1577.

22. Tantucci C, Corbeil C, Chasse M, et al. Flow and volume dependence of respiratory system flow resistance in patients with adult respiratory distress syndrome. *Am Rev Respir Dis*. 1992;145:355–360.

23. Jolliet P, Thorens JB, Nicod L, Pichard C, Kyle U, Chevrolet JC. Relationship between pulmonary oxygen consumption, lung inflammation, and calculated venous admixture in patients with acute lung injury. *Intensive Care Med*. 1996;22:277–285.

24. Bachofen M, Weibel ER. Structural alterations and lung parenchyma in the adult respiratory distress syndrome. *Clin Chest Med*. 1982;3:35–43.

25. Schultz MJ, Dixon B, Levi M. The pulmonary protein C system: preventive or therapeutic target in acute lung injury? *Thorax*. 2009;64:95–97.

26. Negri EM, Hoelz C, Barbas CSV, Montes GS, Saldiva PHN, Capelozzi VL. Acute remodeling of parenchyma in pulmonary and extrapulmonary ARDS. An autopsy study of collagen and elastic system fibres. *Pathol Res Pract*. 2002;198:355–361.

*27. Bhatia M, Moochhala S. Role of inflammatory mediators in the pathophysiology of acute respiratory distress syndrome. *J Pathol*. 2004;202:145–156.

*28. Abraham E. Neutrophils and acute lung injury. *Crit Care Med*. 2003;31(supp):S195–S199.

29. Ward PA. Role of complement, chemokines, and regulatory cytokines in acute lung injury. *Ann N Y Acad Sci*. 1996;796:104–112.

30. Seeger W, Stöhr G, Wolf HRD, Neuhof H. Alteration of surfactant function due to protein leakage. *J Appl Physiol*. 1985;58:326–338.

31. Artigas A, Bernard GR, Carlet J, et al. The American–European consensus conference on ARDS, Part 2: Ventilatory, pharmacologic, supportive therapy, study design strategies and issues related to recovery and remodelling. *Intensive Care Med*. 1998;24:378–398.

32. Brower RG, Ware LB, Berthiaume Y, Matthay MA. Treatment of ARDS. *Chest*. 2001;120:1347–1367.

33. Malarkkan N, Snook NJ, Lumb AB. New aspects of ventilation in acute lung injury. *Anaesthesia*. 2003;58:647–667.

*34. Rouby J-J, Constantin J-M, Giradi CrdeA, Zhang M, Lu Q. Mechanical ventilation in patients with acute respiratory distress syndrome. *Anesthesiology*. 2004;101:228–234.

35. Girard TD, Bernard GR. Mechanical ventilation in ARDS. A state-of-the-art review. *Chest*. 2007;131:921–929.

36. Gattinoni L, Pesenti A. ARDS: the non-homogenous lung: facts and hypotheses. *Intensive Crit Care Digest*. 1987;6:1–4.

37. Laffey JG, O'Croinin D, McLoughlin P, Kavanagh BP. Permissive hypercapnia – role in protective lung ventilatory strategies. *Intensive Care Med*. 2004;30:347–356.

38. Kavanagh BP. Therapeutic hypercapnia: careful science, better trials. *Am J Respir Crit Care Med*. 2005;171:96–97.

39. Gattinoni L, D'Andrea L, Pelosi P, Vitale G, Pesenti A, Fumagalli R. Regional effects and mechanism of positive end-expiratory pressure in early adult respiratory distress syndrome. *JAMA*. 1993;269:2122–2127.

40. Rupie E, Dambrosio M, Servillo G, et al. Titration of tidal volume and induced hypercapnia in acute respiratory distress syndrome. *Am J Respir Crit Care Med*. 1995;152:121–128.

41. Rouby J-J, Lu Q, Vieira S. Pressure/volume curves and lung computed tomography in acute respiratory distress syndrome. *Eur Respir J*. 2003;22(suppl 42): 27S–36S.

42. Brower RG, Lanken PN, MacIntyre N, et al. Higher versus lower positive end-expiratory pressures in patients with the acute respiratory distress syndrome. *N Engl J Med*. 2004;351:327–336.

43. Slutsky AS, Hudson LD. PEEP or no PEEP – lung recruitment may be the solution. *N Engl J Med*. 2006;354:1839–1841.

44. Matthay MA, Calfee CS. Therapeutic value of a lung protective ventilation strategy in acute lung injury. *Chest*. 2005;128:3089–3091.

45. Petrucci N, Iacovelli W. Ventilation with lower tidal volumes versus traditional tidal volumes in adults for acute lung injury and acute respiratory distress syndrome. *Cochrane Database Syst Rev*. 2003;3. CD003844.

46. Fan E, Wilcox E, Brower RG, et al. Recruitment maneuvers for acute lung injury: a systematic review. *Am J Respir Crit Care Med*. 2008;178:1156–1163.

47. Adhikari N, Granton JT. Inhaled nitric oxide for acute lung injury. No place for NO? *JAMA*. 2004;291:1629–1631.

48. Chan KPW, Stewart TE, Mehta S. High-frequency oscillatory ventilation for adult patients with ARDS. *Chest*. 2007;131: 1907–1916.

49. Kacmarek RM, Wiedemann HP, Lavin PT, Wedel MK, Tütüncü AS, Slutsky AS. Partial liquid ventilation in adult patients with acute respiratory distress syndrome. *Am J Respir Crit Care Med*. 2006;173:882–889.

Chapter 32

Respiratory support and artificial ventilation

KEY POINTS

- Non-invasive ventilation may be used to increase airway pressure and support a failing respiratory system without the need for tracheal intubation or tracheostomy.
- Intermittent positive pressure ventilation can be delivered by a variety of different techniques, many of which are coordinated with the patient's own respiratory efforts.
- Positive end-expiratory pressure increases the functional residual capacity, reduces airway resistance and may prevent or reverse lung collapse.
- Any increase in mean intra-thoracic pressure, as seen during positive pressure ventilation, impairs venous return, increases pulmonary vascular resistance and so reduces cardiac output.
- Artificial ventilation may damage the lung by exerting excessive pressures or volumes on lung tissue, or by causing repeated opening and closure of small airways with each breath.
- A clinically useful artificial lung remains only a distant possibility, although extracorporeal systems that partially replace pulmonary gas exchange continue to evolve.

The previous five chapters have outlined the numerous ways in which the respiratory system may fail to achieve its primary objective of gas exchange. This chapter describes the various techniques available to replace, either partially or totally, the gas exchange function of the respiratory system.

Respiratory support is required when there is impaired action of the patient's respiratory muscles or a severe dysfunction of the mechanics of breathing.

It may also be used to improve oxygenation of arterial blood even when $P\text{CO}_2$ is within normal limits. Artificial ventilation is defined as the provision of the minute volume of respiration by external forces. For most clinical applications, current practice has moved more towards respiratory 'support' or 'assist' in which the patient's breathing is assisted, but not entirely replaced, by a variety of techniques described throughout this chapter. Provision of the whole minute ventilation by artificial means is now only seen during anaesthesia with paralysis and in the most critically ill patients.

NON-INVASIVE VENTILATION[1,2]

Non-invasive ventilation is defined as respiratory support without establishing a tracheal airway. It may be achieved by either negative pressure ventilation, or positive pressure ventilation via a mask or similar device.

NEGATIVE PRESSURE VENTILATION[3]

This requires the application of subatmospheric pressure to the trunk. It was first reported in 1929[4] and widely used for the following 30 years during polio epidemics. Enthusiasm for the technique has fluctuated since, but there continues to be interest in negative pressure ventilation for a small group of patients.[5]

Animal studies comparing negative and positive pressure ventilation show that lung perfusion is the same with both modes, but that ventilation is more evenly distributed and oxygenation better with negative pressure ventilation.[6] Negative pressure

DOI: 10.1016/B978-0-7020-2996-7.00032-5

ventilation continues to have a place in the management of respiratory failure due to neuromuscular disorders,[3] central apnoeas,[1] or in paediatric intensive care.[5]

Cabinet ventilators, often referred to as an 'iron lung', require the whole body except the head to be encased in a cabinet with an airtight seal around the neck. An intermittent negative pressure is then applied in the tank, causing inspiration, with passive expiration as normal. A superimposed continuous negative pressure may also be applied, which provides the negative pressure equivalent of positive end-expiratory pressure (PEEP). In terms of the airway-to-ambient pressure gradient cabinet ventilators are identical in principle to positive pressure ventilation, with similar effects on cardiovascular and respiratory physiology. Collapse of the extrathoracic upper airway during inspiration may occur, particularly during sleep. Vomiting or regurgitation of gastric contents exposes the patient to the danger of aspiration during the inspiratory phase, and fatalities have occurred under particularly distressing circumstances.

Cuirass and jacket ventilators are a simplified form of cabinet ventilators in which the application of subatmospheric pressure is confined to the trunk or anterior abdominal wall. Function depends on a good airtight seal. They are less efficient than cabinet ventilators and suffer from the same disadvantages. However, they are much more convenient to use and may be useful to supplement inadequate spontaneous breathing.

Hayek oscillator is a form of cuirass that encircles the trunk and allows high frequency ventilation (see below) with a continuous negative pressure.[7] It facilitates a wide range of tidal volumes, and some degree of control of the functional residual capacity (FRC). It may be used during surgery on the airway so avoiding the need for any form of tracheal tube.[8]

NON–INVASIVE POSITIVE PRESSURE VENTILATION[1,2]

Positive pressure ventilation may be delivered using soft masks that fit over the mouth and nose, the nose only, or with a clear plastic helmet over the entire head (sealed around the neck). Most ventilator systems used are pressure generators and so are 'leak tolerant'; that is, flow automatically increases to compensate for a pressure drop due to gas leakage. With nasal ventilation, positive pressure in the nasopharynx normally displaces the soft palate

anteriorly against the tongue, thus preventing escape of gas through the mouth. Adverse effects of nasal ventilation include eye irritation, conjunctivitis and facial skin necrosis. Helmet systems avoid these complications, but have a volume of around 10 litres which inevitably causes some rebreathing making hypercapnia a potential problem. The high volume in the helmet also results in a time delay when changing the pressure in the helmet to support ventilation or when sensing a spontaneous breath with pressure changes (see below).[9]

Techniques of ventilation are similar to invasive artificial ventilation. Ventilator modes that use patient triggering are better tolerated than controlled ventilation, particularly in awake patients, but both techniques are used. Pressure controlled ventilation or pressure support ventilation (PSV, see below) are commonly used, as is continuous positive airway pressure (CPAP). In bilevel positive airway pressure (bilevel PAP) the ventilator pressure steps between two preset values for inspiration and expiration, and, except for the terminology used to describe the pressures, is the same as PSV with CPAP.[1]

Ventilation may be provided continually during acute respiratory problems, or only at night for long-term respiratory disease.[10] The use of nasal CPAP for treating the sleep apnoea hypopnoea syndrome has been described on page 275. In this case, benefit occurs simply be displacing the soft palate away from the posterior pharyngeal wall. Benefit in other respiratory diseases is more difficult to explain, but possible mechanisms include:[2]

- resting fatigued respiratory muscles
- delivery of a higher inspired oxygen concentration by the use of a tight fitting facemask (page 206)
- augmentation of minute ventilation to reduce hypercapnia
- prevention or re-expansion of areas of atelectasis, as seen when using PEEP (see below)
- reduction of cardiac pre-load in patients with heart failure (page 480).

Clinical applications.[2,11] NIV is now advocated for the treatment of acute respiratory failure from numerous causes, though outcome evidence supporting its use is variable as follows:

- Chronic obstructive pulmonary disease (COPD) exacerbations (page 409). NIV is now first line treatment for this situation, and improves survival, reduces the need for invasive ventilation and reduces the length of hospital stay. The case for long-term treatment of COPD remains controversial, with some benefits in some sub-groups only.[12]

- Cardiogenic pulmonary oedema may be successfully treated with NIV, reducing the need for tracheal intubation and improving mortality.[13] The mechanism of this beneficial effect is explained on page 480.
- Acute lung injury (ALI). NIV instituted early in the course of ALI (Chapter 31) may reduce the need for tracheal intubation and improve gas exchange,[14,15] but the evidence for improved survival is currently inconclusive.[11]
- Failure of weaning from invasive ventilation (page 474). NIV may be used to gradually wean patients from invasive ventilation, a strategy that is particularly useful in patients with COPD[16] or obesity.[17]

INTERMITTENT POSITIVE PRESSURE VENTILATION (IPPV)

PHASES OF THE RESPIRATORY CYCLE

Inspiration. During IPPV, the mouth (or airway) pressure is intermittently raised above ambient pressure. The inspired gas then flows into the lungs in accord with the resistance and compliance of the respiratory system. If inspiration is slow, the distribution is governed mainly by regional compliance. If inspiration is fast, there is preferential ventilation of parts of the lungs with short time constants (Figure 3.7). Different temporal patterns of pressure may be applied, as discussed below.

Expiration. During IPPV, expiration results from allowing mouth pressure to fall to ambient. Expiration is then passive, and differs from expiration during spontaneous breathing in which diaphragm muscle tone is gradually reduced (page 63). Expiration may be impeded by the application of PEEP. In the past, expiration was sometimes accelerated by the application of a subatmospheric pressure, termed negative end-expiratory pressure (NEEP), though this technique is no longer used. Expiration to ambient pressure is termed zero end-expiratory pressure (ZEEP).

If the inflating pressure is maintained for several seconds, the resulting tidal volume will be indicated by the following relationship:

$$\text{Tidal volume} = \text{sustained inflation pressure} \times \text{total static compliance}$$

Thus, for example, a sustained inflation pressure of $10 \, cmH_2O$ with a static compliance of $0.5 \, l.kPa^{-1}$ $(50 \, ml.cmH_2O^{-1})$ would result in a lung volume $500 \, ml$ above functional residual capacity (FRC).

TIME COURSE OF INFLATION AND DEFLATION

Equilibration according to the above equation usually takes several seconds. When the airway pressure is raised during inspiration, it is opposed by the two forms of impedance – the elastic resistance of lungs and chest wall (Chapter 3) and resistance to air flow (Chapter 4). At any instant, the inflation pressure equals the sum of the pressures required to overcome these two forms of impedance. The pressure required to overcome elastic resistance equals the lung volume above FRC divided by the total (dynamic) compliance, while the pressure required to overcome air flow resistance equals the air flow resistance multiplied by the instantaneous flow rate.

The effect of applying a constant pressure (or square wave inflation) is shown in Figure 32.1. The two components of the inflation pressure vary during the course of inspiration while their sum remains constant. The component overcoming air flow resistance is maximal at first and declines exponentially with air flow as inflation proceeds. The component overcoming elastic resistance increases with the lung volume. With normal respiratory mechanics in the unconscious patient, the change in lung volume should be 95% complete in about 1.5 seconds, as in Figure 32.1.

The approach of the lung volume to its equilibrium value is according to an exponential function of the wash-in type (see Appendix E). The time constant, which is the time required for inflation to 63% of the equilibrium value, equals the product of resistance and compliance. Normal values for an unconscious patient are as follows:

$$\text{Time constant} = \text{resistance} \times \text{compliance}$$

$$0.5 \text{ second} = 1 \, kPa.l^{-1}.s \times 0.5 \, l.kPa^{-1}$$

or

$$0.5 \text{ second} = 10 \, cmH_2O.l^{-1}.s \times 0.05 \, l.cmH_2O^{-1}$$

The time constant is the time that would be required to reach equilibrium if the initial inspiratory flow rate were maintained. It is sometimes more convenient

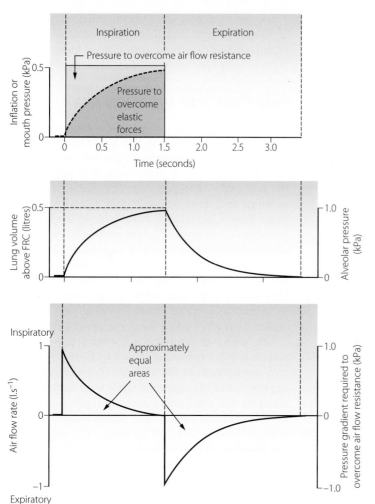

Fig. 32.1 Artificial ventilation by intermittent application of a constant pressure (square wave) followed by passive expiration. Inspiratory and expiratory flow rates are both exponential. Assuming that air flow resistance is constant, it follows that flow rate and pressure gradient required to overcome resistance may be shown on the same graph. Lung volume and alveolar pressure may be shown on the same graph if compliance is constant. Values are typical for an anaesthetised supine paralysed patient: total dynamic compliance, $0.5\,l.kPa^{-1}$ ($50\,ml.cmH_2O^{-1}$); pulmonary resistance $0.3\,kPa.l^{-1}.s$ ($3\,cmH_2O.l^{-1}.s$); apparatus resistance $0.7\,kPa.l^{-1}.s$ ($7\,cmH_2O.l^{-1}.s$); total resistance, $1\,kPa.l^{-1}.s$ ($10\,cmH_2O.l^{-1}.s$); time constant, $0.5\,s$.

to use the half-time, which is 0.69 times the time constant. The inflation curve is shown in full with further mathematical detail in Appendix E.

It is normal practice for the inspiratory phase to be terminated after 1 or 2 seconds at which time the lung volume will still be increasing. Inflation pressure is not then the sole arbiter of tidal volume but must be considered in relation to the duration of the inspiratory phase.

If expiration is passive and mouth pressure remains at ambient, the driving force is the elevation of alveolar pressure above ambient, caused by elastic recoil of lungs and chest wall. This pressure is dissipated in overcoming air flow resistance during expiration. In Figure 32.1, during expiration the alveolar pressure (proportional to the lung volume above FRC) is directly proportional to expiratory flow rate, and all three quantities decline according

to a wash-out exponential function with a time constant which is again equal to the product of compliance and resistance.

THE EFFECT OF CHANGES IN INFLATION PRESSURE, RESISTANCE AND COMPLIANCE

The heavy line in Figure 32.2 shows the inflation curve for the normal parameters of an unconscious paralysed patient as listed in Table 32.1. These are the same values that were considered above. The basic curve is a single exponential approaching a lung volume 0.5 litre above FRC with a time constant of 0.5 seconds.

Changes in inflation pressure do not alter the time constant of inflation, but directly influence the amount of air introduced into the lungs in a given number of time constants. In Figure 32.2, each point

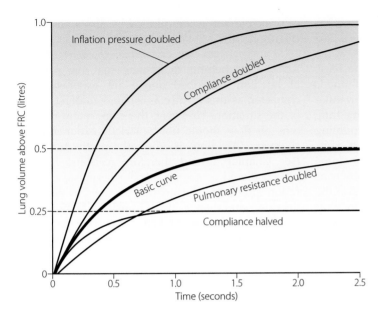

Fig. 32.2 Effect of changes in various factors on the rate of inflation of the lungs. Fixed relationships: final tidal volume achieved = inflation pressure × compliance; time constant = compliance × resistance. (See also Table 32.1.)

Table 32.1 Parameters for inflation curves shown in Figure 32.2

	BASIC CURVE	PULMONARY RESISTANCE DOUBLED	INFLATION PRESSURE DOUBLED	COMPLIANCE DOUBLED	COMPLIANCE HALVED
Inflation pressure					
(kPa)	1	1	2	1	1
(cmH$_2$O)	10	10	20	10	10
Compliance					
(l.kPa^{-1})	0.5	0.5	0.5	1	0.25
(ml.cmH$_2$O^{-1})	50	50	50	100	25
Final tidal volume (l)	0.5	0.5	1	1	0.25
Pulmonary resistance					
(kPa.l^{-1}.s)	1	2	1	1	1
(cmH$_2$O.l^{-1}.s)	10	20	10	10	10
Time constant					
(seconds)	0.5	1	0.5	1	0.25

on the curve labelled 'inflation pressure doubled' is twice the height of the corresponding point on the basic curve for the same time.

Effect of changes in compliance and resistance. If the compliance is doubled, the equilibrium tidal volume is also doubled. However, the time constant (product of compliance and resistance) is also doubled and therefore the equilibrium volume is approached more slowly (Figure 32.2). Conversely, if the compliance is halved, the equilibrium tidal volume is also halved and so is the time constant.

Changes in resistance have a direct effect on the time constant of inflation but do not affect the equilibrium tidal volume. Thus the effect of an increased resistance on tidal volume is through the reduction in inspiratory flow rate. Within limits, this can be counteracted by prolonging inspiration or by increasing the inflation pressure and the degree of overpressure (explained below). The effects, shown in Figure 32.2, apply not only to the whole lung but also to regions that may have different compliances, resistances and time constants (page 121).

Overpressure. Increasing the inflation pressure has a major effect on the time required to achieve a particular lung volume above FRC. In Figure 32.3, the lung characteristics are the same as for the basic curve in Figure 32.2. If the required tidal volume is 475 ml, this is achieved in 1.5 seconds with an inflation pressure of 10 cmH₂O. However, the same lung volume is achieved in only 0.3 seconds by doubling the inflation pressure. The application of a pressure that, if sustained, would give a tidal volume higher than that which is intended, is known as overpressure; it is used extensively to increase the inspiratory flow rate and so to shorten the inspiratory phase. The use of a subatmospheric pressure to increase the rate of passive expiration is similar in principle but is complicated by airway trapping (Figure 32.3B).

Deviations from true exponential character of expiration. It is helpful to assume that the patterns of air flow described above are exponential in character, as this greatly assists our understanding of the situation. However, there are many reasons why air flow should not be strictly exponential in character. Air flow is normally partly turbulent (see Chapter 4) and therefore resistance cannot be considered as a constant. Furthermore, as expiration proceeds, the calibre of the air passages decreases and there is also a transition to more laminar flow as the instantaneous flow rate decreases. Approximation to a single exponential function

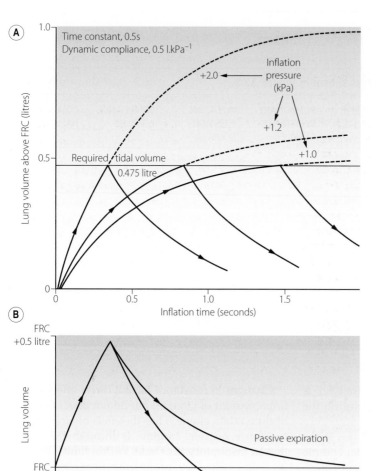

Fig. 32.3 (A) How the duration of inflation may be shortened by the use of overpressure. Inflation curves are shown for +2 kPa (+20 cmH₂O) (equilibrium 1 litre), +1.2 kPa (+12 cmH₂O) (equilibrium 0.6 litre) and +1 kPa (+10 cmH₂O) (equilibrium 0.5 litre). With a required tidal volume of 0.475 litre note the big reduction in duration of inflation needed when the inflation pressure is increased from 1 to 2 kPa (10 to 20 cmH₂O). (B) How expiration is influenced by the use of a subatmospheric pressure or 'negative phase'. Expiration may be terminated at the FRC after 0.6 s, or may be prolonged, in which case the lung volume will fall to 0.2 litre below FRC.

is nevertheless good enough for many practical purposes.

ALTERNATIVE PATTERNS OF APPLICATION OF INFLATION PRESSURE

Constant pressure or square wave inflation has been considered above because it is the easiest for mathematical analysis. There are, however, an almost infinite number of pressure profiles that may be applied for IPPV. There is no very convincing evidence of the superiority of one over the other, except that distribution of inspired gas is improved if there is a prolongation of the period during which the applied pressure is maximal. This permits better

ventilation of the 'slow' alveoli and is not very important in patients with relatively healthy lungs.

Constant flow rate ventilators are extensively used, and Figure 32.4 shows pressure, volume and flow changes in a manner analogous to Figure 32.1.

CONTROL OF DURATION OF INSPIRATION

Three methods are in general use.

1. Time cycling terminates inspiration after a pre-set time. With constant pressure generators and constant flow generators, a separate and variable timing system is used. With constant flow generators, inspiratory time has a direct effect on the tidal volume. With constant pressure generators the

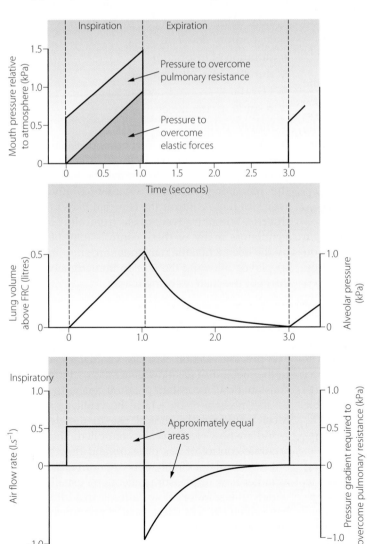

Fig. 32.4 Artificial ventilation by intermittent application of a constant-flow, with passive expiration. Note that inspiratory flow rate is constant. Assuming that pulmonary resistance is constant, it follows that a constant amount of the inflation pressure is required to overcome flow resistance. Lung volume and alveolar pressure may be shown on the same graph if compliance is constant. Values are typical for an anaesthetised supine paralysed patient: total dynamic compliance, $0.5 \, l.kPa^{-1}$ ($50 \, ml.cmH_2O^{-1}$); pulmonary resistance $0.3 \, kPa.l^{-1}.s$ ($3 \, cmH_2O.l^{-1}.s$); apparatus resistance $0.7 \, kPa.l^{-1}.s$ ($7 \, cmH_2O.l^{-1}.s$); total resistance, $1 \, kPa.l^{-1}.s$ ($10 \, cmH_2O.l^{-1}.s$); time constant, $0.5 \, s$.

relationship is more complex, as described above (see Figure 32.3).

2. *Volume cycling* terminates inspiration when a preset volume has been delivered. In the absence of a leak this should guarantee the tidal volume even if the compliance or resistance of the lungs changes within limits. Formerly, volume-cycled ventilators were based on a reciprocating pump of preset tidal volume. Nowadays they are more likely to be flow generators with an inspiratory flow sensor that terminates inspiration when the required volume has been delivered.

3. *Pressure cycling* terminates inspiration when a particular airway pressure is achieved. This in no way guarantees the tidal volume. Increased airway resistance, for example, would limit inspiratory flow rate and cause a more rapid increase in mouth pressure, thus terminating the inspiratory phase. Pressure-cycled ventilators are almost invariably flow generators.

Limitations on inspiratory duration. Whatever the means of cycling, it is possible to add a limitation on inspiratory duration, usually as a safety precaution. For example, a pressure limitation can be added to a time-cycled or a volume-cycled ventilator. This can either function as a pressure relief valve or it can terminate the inspiratory phase.

THE INSPIRATORY TO EXPIRATORY (I:E) RATIO

For a given minute volume of ventilation, it is possible to vary within wide limits the duration of inspiration and expiration and the ratio between the two. A common pattern is about 1 second for inspiration, followed by 2–4 seconds for expiration (I:E ratio 1:2–1:4), giving respiratory frequencies in the range 12–20 breaths per minute. The problem is whether changes from this pattern confer any appreciable benefit in terms of gas exchange. Reduction of the inspiratory time to less than 1 second may cause an increase in dead space, but there is no evidence that the duration of inspiration (in the range 0.5–3 seconds) has any appreciable effect on the alveolar/arterial P_{O_2} gradient. Thus the accepted view seems to be that 1 second is a reasonable minimal time for inspiration.

Inverse I:E ratio ventilation has the effect of increasing the mean lung volume and so may be expected to achieve some of the advantages of PEEP as considered below. It may be achieved either by slowing the inspiratory flow rate (shallow ramp) or by holding the lung volume at the end of inspiration (inspiratory pause), the latter seeming to be more logical. *I:E* ratios as high as 4:1 have been used but 2:1 is generally preferable. The degree of inverse *I:E* ratio used is limited by the cardiovascular disturbances seen with the technique (see below) and the time available for expiration. If the latter is unduly curtailed, FRC will be increased, generating so-called 'intrinsic-PEEP' (see below).

Gas redistribution during an inspiratory hold reduces the dead space (page 130) and so results in a lower P_{CO_2} for the same minute volume. This permits the use of a lower peak inflation pressure.

INTERACTION OF VENTILATOR CONTROLS

The usual controls that are provided on an artificial ventilator are drawn from the following list:

- tidal volume
- inspiratory flow rate
- duration of inspiration
- duration of expiration
- I:E ratio
- respiratory frequency
- minute volume

It will be found that the maximum possible number of independent controls is three. A setting of any three on this list will determine the values for all the remaining variables. Opinion is divided on which of these controls the clinician likes to operate directly. With the advent of electronically controlled ventilators many of these controls may be altered by the user, while the remainder are simultaneously displayed allowing the user to immediately see the effect of the changes being made.

CLINICAL USE OF IPPV

The previous section classifies ventilators according to the method of gas flow generation – for example, constant flow or constant pressure generators – based on the mechanism by which the ventilator worked. Most ventilators in clinical use in the developed world are now electronically controlled. These allow accurate control of gas pressure and flow throughout the ventilator circuit, and can normally perform as either flow or pressure generators, usually with a variety of inspiratory flow patterns. In addition, they have given rise to a whole host of previously impossible ventilatory techniques, a majority of which are dependent on the ventilator responding appropriately to the patient's own respiratory efforts.

INTERACTIONS BETWEEN PATIENT AND VENTILATOR

For many years there have been ventilators in which the inspiratory phase could be triggered with a spontaneous breath, and mechanical ventilators could be modified to facilitate a mandatory minute volume of ventilation, as described below. Electronic ventilators continuously monitor tidal volume, whether generated by the patient (spontaneous breath) or artificially (ventilator breath). With this information available it is a simple task to achieve, by electronic means, a predetermined minute volume, number of breaths, etc. by introducing extra ventilator breaths when necessary. The challenge for ventilator design in recent years has been the speed and sensitivity with which ventilators can sense, and respond to, the patient's own respiratory efforts in order to synchronise ventilator and spontaneous breaths. Without this synchronisation, a patient with any reasonable spontaneous respiratory effort begins to 'fight' against the ventilator[18] leading to discomfort, poor gas exchange and cardiovascular disturbance.

There are two ways by which a ventilator may detect the onset of a spontaneous breath.[19]

Pressure sensing. At the onset of a respiratory effort, the patient will generate a reduction in pressure within the circuit, which may be detected in the ventilator. This pressure wave travels through the circuit at approximately the speed of sound, and so reaches the ventilator within 12 ms, following which the pressure sensor must respond, and flow into the circuit be increased to facilitate inspiration. Overall, these events take approximately 100 ms to occur, which is undetectable by the patient. The pressure drop required to trigger inspiration is now always measured relative to circuit (not atmospheric) pressure, to allow the use of CPAP during ventilation. The time taken to trigger the ventilator increases with decreased sensitivity settings – that is, when a greater pressure drop is required for triggering. Pressure triggering is also affected by the circuit compliance, which is a function of the circuit volume and the stiffness of the tubing.

Flow sensing. Detection of inspiratory flow may trigger a ventilator breath or some type of respiratory assist (see below). Most current intensive care ventilators provide a continuous base flow around the ventilator circuit of 2–20 l.min^{-1}. Any difference between ventilator inflow and outflow represents the patient's respiration. Flow triggering occurs in approximately 80 ms, irrespective of the sensitivity setting. A high base flow provides adequate inspiratory flow for the patient at the start of inspiration and the flow rate is increased when the ventilator is triggered. Flow sensing can also detect the end of inspiration, and is used in pressure support ventilation (see below).

VENTILATORY MODES IN COMMON USE

In addition to control mode ventilation (CMV), there are now a range of ventilation patterns. Many of these are essentially the same but have different nomenclature owing to their development by rival ventilator manufacturers. Those in common use are described below and shown graphically in Figure 32.5.

Mandatory minute volume (MMV). Introduced in the 1970s, this was a simple technique for controlling the volume of artificial ventilation so that the total of spontaneous and artificial ventilation did not fall below a preset value. If the patient was able to achieve the preset level of MMV ventilator breaths did not occur. Achievement of the preset MMV by a rapid, shallow respiratory pattern commonly seen in intensive care patients was a major disadvantage of MMV. Electronic ventilators allow MMV to be used, and can co-ordinate the mandatory breaths with patient respiration to a greater degree than the original mechanical technique, including varying both the inspiratory pressure and timing to suit individual patient requirements.[20]

Assist-control ventilation or synchronised IPPV (Figure 32.5C). This was one of the earlier ventilatory modes that depended on patient triggering of ventilator breaths. It is essentially the same as volume preset IPPV except that breaths are triggered by the patient, normally as a result of reduced circuit pressure. A maximum time delay between breaths is incorporated, following which a breath will be generated by the ventilator if spontaneous triggering has ceased. There is no provision for spontaneous breathing between ventilator breaths.

Airway pressure release ventilation (Figure 32.5D).[21] This ventilation mode differs significantly from all other forms of positive pressure ventilation and is essentially the reverse of IPPV. It consists of maintaining the breathing system at an upper airway pressure level (P$_{high}$), which is intermittently released to a lower airway pressure level (P$_{low}$), causing the patient to *exhale* to FRC. The pattern of the imposed breaths is similar to that of reversed I:E ratio. The patient is able to breathe spontaneously throughout the entire respiratory cycle, but most of the time this will be during P_{high} when inspiration will start from a lung volume greater than FRC. Artificial breaths are thus within the conventional tidal range set by his FRC, while spontaneous inspirations are usually within his inspiratory reserve. More frequent and longer periods at P_{low} lead to a greater minute volume, and so improved elimination of carbon dioxide, and a lower mean airway pressure, but are also associated with greater likelihood of pulmonary collapse in injured lungs and, as a consequence, worsening of oxygenation.

Synchronised intermittent mandatory ventilation (SIMV) (Figure 32.5E). Intermittent mandatory ventilation was introduced in the 1970s, followed a few years later by the ability to synchronise ventilator breaths with the patient's own respiratory effort as described above. The essential feature of SIMV is to allow the patient to take a spontaneous breath between artificial breaths. This confers three major advantages. First, a spontaneous inspiration is not obstructed by a closed inspiratory valve and this helps to prevent the patient fighting the ventilator. The second advantage is the facilitation of weaning, which is considered below.

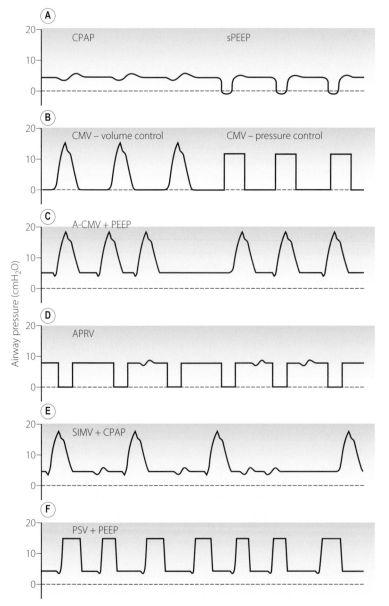

Fig. 32.5 Airway pressure during a variety of commonly used modes of ventilation. (A) CPAP, continuous positive airway pressure and sPEEP, true positive end-expiratory pressure applied during spontaneous breathing. (B) CMV, control mode ventilation showing volume and pressure-controlled inspiration. (C) A-CMV, assist-control mode ventilation where breaths are triggered by a fall in circuit pressure. When apnoea occurs, ventilator breaths occur without triggering. (D) APRV, airway pressure release ventilation with an upper airway pressure (P_{high}) of 8 cmH$_2$O and simultaneous spontaneous breathing. (E) SIMV, synchronised intermittent mandatory ventilation, as for A-CMV except that spontaneous breathing can occur between ventilator breaths. (F) PSV, pressure support ventilation in which pressure-controlled breaths are triggered by the patient, who also controls the duration of each breath. In practice, many ventilators allow combinations of these modes, such as SIMV, PSV and PEEP together.

Thirdly, the patient is able to breathe spontaneously at any time during prolonged ventilation; this may prevent respiratory muscle atrophy and helps to reduce the mean intrathoracic pressure. Most ventilators now provide SIMV as a normal feature with either pressure or volume controlled breaths and it is used extensively, often in conjunction with pressure support ventilation (see below).

Pressure support ventilation (PSV) (Figure 32.5F).[22] In this system a spontaneous inspiration triggers a rapid flow of gas that increases until airway pressure reaches a preselected level. Flow sensing by the ventilator is also then able to detect when the spontaneous inspiration ends, at which point the pressure support ceases, and expiration occurs. The purpose is not to provide a prescribed tidal volume, but to assist the patient in making an inspiration of a pattern that lies largely within his own control. The level of support may be increased until the pressure is sufficient to provide the full tidal volume (maximal pressure support) and may be gradually reduced as the patient's ventilatory capacity improves. The amount of pressure support provided does seem to be inversely related to the work of breathing.

HIGH FREQUENCY VENTILATION[23]

High frequency ventilation may be classified into the following three categories:

1. High frequency positive pressure ventilation (HFPPV) is applied in the frequency range 1–2 Hz (60–120 breaths. min^{-1}) and can be considered as an extension of conventional IPPV techniques. Although many conventional ventilators will operate within this frequency range, specially designed ventilators have been used.

2. High frequency jet ventilation (HFJV) covers the frequency range 1–5 Hz. Inspiration is driven by a high velocity stream of gas from a jet, which may or may not entrain gas from a secondary supply. Humidification with HFJV is technically difficult, and if done properly requires equipment as complex as the ventilator itself. The position of the jet may be proximal to the patient, in the hope of avoiding dead space, or more distal which is safer in terms of mucosal trauma and thermal injury from cooling due to the Joule–Kelvin effect.[23] A unique advantage is the ability to ventilate through a narrow cannula, as for example through the cricothyroid membrane.

3. High frequency oscillatory ventilation (HFOV)[24,25] covers the frequency range 3–10 Hz and the flows are usually generated by an oscillating pump making a fourth connection to a T-piece. At these high frequencies, the respiratory waveform is usually sinusoidal, including active expiration. Tidal volumes are inevitably small and are difficult to measure.

The relationship between tidal volume and dead space during high frequency ventilation is crucial to an understanding of the technique. It is useless to infer values for tidal volume and dead space from measurements made under other circumstances and yet it is very difficult to make direct measurements of these variables under the actual conditions of high frequency ventilation, especially in humans. A study of anaesthetised subjects during HFPPV up to frequencies of 2 Hz, maintained arterial P_{CO_2} approximately constant at about 5 kPa (37.5 mmHg).[26] As frequency increased from conventional ventilation at 15 breaths.min^{-1} to HFPPV at 2 Hz it was necessary to double the minute volume (Table 32.2). The actual volume of the physiological dead space decreased with decreasing tidal volume to reach a minimal value of about 90 ml at 1 Hz. However, the normal proportionality between dead space and tidal volume (page 130) was not maintained. Dead space/tidal volume ratio increased from 37%

Table 32.2 Gas exchange during high frequency ventilation

		RESPIRATORY FREQUENCY		
		15 bpm 0.25 Hz	60 bpm 1 Hz	120 bpm 2 Hz
Arterial P_{CO_2}	kPa	4.8	4.8	4.9
	mmHg	36	36	37
$\dot{V}$	l.min^{-1}	6.8	10.2	14
V_T	ml	454	170	117
V_D (physiol.)	ml	165	96	88
V_D/V_T ratio	%	36	56	75

bpm, breaths per minute. Data from reference 26.

at 15 breaths.min^{-1} to 75% at 2 Hz, which explains the requirement for the increased minute volume. The situation is more complex at higher frequencies. One study found that tidal volumes of at least 100 ml were still required at frequencies of 15 Hz, corresponding to an *applied* minute volume of 90 l.min^{-1}, which would indicate a dead space/tidal volume ratio of over 90%.[27] There are severe technical difficulties in the measurement of the actual delivered tidal volumes which, though undoubtedly less than the pump settings, are probably much larger than the external movements of the thorax would suggest.

End-expiratory pressure is inevitably raised at high frequencies because the duration of expiration will be inadequate for passive exhalation to FRC, the time constant of the normal respiratory system being about 0.5 second (see above). Therefore, the use of respiratory frequencies above about 2 Hz will usually result in 'intrinsic' PEEP, and hence an increased end-expiratory lung volume, which is likely to be a major factor promoting favourable gas exchange.

Gas mixing and streaming is likely to be modified at high frequencies. The sudden reversals of flow direction are likely to set up eddies that blur the boundary between dead space and alveolar gas, thus improving the efficiency of ventilation. It has been suggested that such 'enhanced diffusion' or 'augmented dispersion' plays a major role in gas exchange during HFOV.[25,27] Air passages dilated by intrinsic PEEP may contribute to this effect. Furthermore, cardiac mixing of gases becomes relatively more important at small tidal volumes.[28]

The clinical indications for high frequency ventilation remain unclear. The techniques have been used mainly for weaning from artificial ventilation in adults and for respiratory support in babies.[24] There is also agreement on its special role for patients with bronchopleural fistula and the technique is particularly convenient when there is no airtight junction between ventilator and the tracheobronchial tree, during surgery on the airway for example (page 491). There is no doubt that effective gas exchange is usually possible with high frequency ventilation but clinical advantages over conventional artificial ventilation are less clear. Randomised trials generally failed to demonstrate any significant advantage over conventional methods of ventilation.[29] Although there are enthusiasts, others believe that it is merely a technique in search of an application. Of the various techniques described, HFOV is currently the most popular in intensive care units,

with renewed interest in its use for patients with severe ALI (Chapter 31). Use of HFOV can maintain a reasonably high mean airway pressure to prevent lung collapse whilst still allowing adequate ventilation without high peak airway pressures that may cause overdistension of alveoli.[25]

WEANING[30,31]

Weaning describes the process by which artificial ventilation is gradually withdrawn and the patient returned to normal respiration. In practice it is useful to think of two stages: the withdrawal of respiratory support and the removal of any artificial airway, usually a tracheal tube or tracheostomy. Only the first of these stages is considered here.

Predicting successful weaning. Before weaning can be attempted, the balance between ventilatory load and capacity must be favourable. Extra demands on the respiratory system may originate from increased oxygen consumption, commonly as a result of sepsis, but also occasionally from thyrotoxicosis, convulsions or shivering. Reduced respiratory system compliance or increased airway resistance also impose additional loads on the respiratory system. The capacity of the respiratory system to wean depends on having, first, adequate ventilation perfusion matching and, secondly, low intrapulmonary shunt and respiratory dead space. Finally, good respiratory muscle function must be achieved (page 92), including correction of any metabolic disturbance and provision of adequate blood supply to the muscles; that is, the patient must have reasonable cardiovascular function. Numerous different measurements of lung function have been reported to predict successful weaning from ventilatory support. Some of the more widely accepted ones are shown in Table 32.3.

No single variable is a reliable indicator of success, with most having very low predictive values. This has led to the development of more complex scoring systems, which include the Compliance, Rate, Oxygenation, Pressure (CROP) score, calculated as:

$$\text{CROP} = \text{dynamic Crs} \times PI_{max} \times (Pa_{O_2}/PA_{O_2})/\text{respiratory rate}$$

(Crs, respiratory system compliance; PI_{max} maximum inspiratory pressure).

Rate:volume ratio (RVR) score is respiratory rate (breaths.min^{-1}) divided by tidal volume (litres) measured over one minute without artificial ventilation.

Table 32.3 Measurements of lung function used to assess suitability for weaning from artificial ventilation

MEASUREMENT	VALUE FOR SUCCESSFUL WEANING
Measured on ventilator:	
$Pa_{O_2} : Fi_{O_2}$ ratio	> 20 (Pa_{O_2} in kPa) or 150 (Pa_{O_2} in mmHg)
Resting minute volume	< 10 l.min^{-1}
Negative inspiratory force	-20 to -30 cmH$_2$O
Pl_{max}	-15 to -30 cmH$_2$O
$P_{0.1}/Pl_{max}$	> 0.3
CROP score	≥ 13 ml.breath^{-1}.min
Measured during brief period of spontaneous breathing:	
Respiratory rate	< 30 breaths.min^{-1}
Tidal volume	> 4–6 ml.kg^{-1}
Respiratory rate : tidal volume ratio	> 60 breaths.l^{-1}
RVR score	≤ 105 breaths.min^{-1}.l^{-1}

Pl_{max}, maximal inspiratory pressure; $P_{0.1}$, mouth occlusion pressure 0.1 s after the onset of inspiration; CROP and RVR score, see text for details. (After references 32 and 33.)

A CROP score of ≥ 13 ml.breath^{-1}.min^{-1} or a RVR score ≤ 105 breath.min^{-1}.l^{-1} are both reasonable predictors of successful weaning.[33]

Techniques for weaning. Recent guidelines suggest that once these predictors indicate that discontinuation of ventilation may be possible, a spontaneous breathing trial should be used.[30,31] During this trial, which should last approximately 30 minutes, the patient breathes spontaneously with only minimal respiratory support, and is closely observed to ensure that respiratory pattern, patient comfort, gas exchange and cardiovascular stability are all acceptable. If this trial of spontaneous breathing fails, appropriate degrees of ventilatory support should be recommenced, and a further trial of spontaneous breathing performed at 24-hour intervals if the predictors of successful weaning remain satisfactory.

Ventilation strategies to use between trials of spontaneous breathing focus on gradual withdrawal of respiratory support using the techniques described above. Control mode ventilation is usually replaced by either SIMV or A-CMV until the patient has established adequate respiratory effort, following which the number of ventilator breaths can be gradually reduced. Whilst breathing via an artificial airway, some respiratory support is normally required, and this is most commonly provided with PSV, the level of which can again be reduced gradually.

It is important to not place excessive reliance on modern ventilator systems to wean patients from ventilatory support. Close attention must also be paid to nutrition, psychological care such as establishment of normal night:day sleep patterns, and the use of non-invasive ventilation (page 464) following early extubation. Protocols for weaning are now widely used to ensure all these aspects are addressed, but some patients will still remain ventilated for many weeks and specialist units now exist to care for these challenging patients.[34]

POSITIVE END-EXPIRATORY PRESSURE

A great variety of pathological conditions, as well as general anaesthesia, result in a decrease in FRC. The deleterious effect of this on gas exchange has been considered elsewhere (page 342) and it is reasonable to consider increasing the FRC by the application of PEEP, first described by Hill et al in 1965.[35]

Expiratory pressure can be raised during both artificial ventilation and spontaneous breathing, and both forms are best considered together. The terminology is confusing and this chapter adheres to the definitions illustrated in Figure 32.6. Note in particular sPEEP in which a patient inhales spontaneously from ambient pressure but exhales against PEEP. This involves the subject in a considerable amount of additional work of breathing because he must raise his entire minute volume to the level of PEEP that is applied. This is undesirable and CPAP is much to be preferred to sPEEP.

True CPAP is more difficult to achieve than sPEEP. Biased demand valves may be used but usually result in a pronounced dip in inspiratory pressure, increasing the total work of breathing. The simplest approach is a T-piece with a high fresh gas flow venting through a PEEP valve at the expiratory limb throughout the respiratory phase. Electronic ventilators produce CPAP in a similar fashion by circulating high flows of gas around the ventilator circuit at the required positive pressure.

PEEP may be achieved by many techniques. The simplest is to exhale through a preset depth of water but more convenient methods are spring-loaded valves or diaphragms pressed down by gas, a column of water or a spring. It is also possible to use venturis and fans opposing the direction of expiratory gas flow.

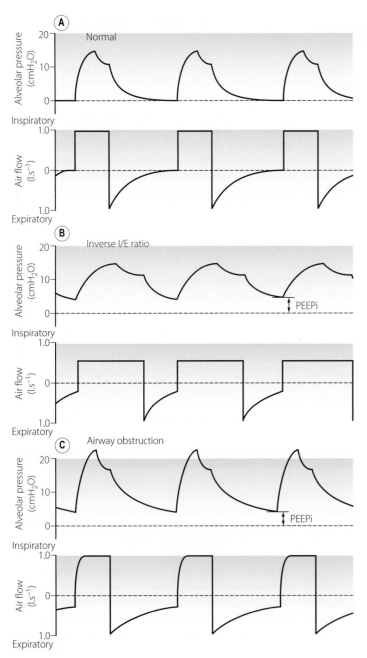

Fig. 32.6 Pressure and flow curves demonstrating generation of intrinsic positive end-expiratory pressure (PEEPi). (A) Normal ventilation with both alveolar pressure and airway flow returning to zero before the next breath. (B) Inverse I:E ratio ventilation. Although the decline in pressure and flow is normal, there is insufficient time for complete expiration to occur. (C) Airway obstruction. Expiratory time is normal, but the decline in pressure and flow is retarded to such an extent that expiration is again incomplete.

INTRINSIC PEEP[18]

If a passive expiration is terminated before the lung volume has returned to FRC, there will be residual end-expiratory raised alveolar pressure variously known as dynamic hyperinflation, auto PEEP or intrinsic PEEP (PEEPi).[36] The elevated alveolar pressure will not be transmitted back to the ventilator pressure sensors, so PEEPi may go undetected,[37] but simple methods to measure it have been described.[36] Artificial ventilation with inverse I:E ratio may result in PEEPi, but it is more commonly a result of increased expiratory flow resistance due to airway disease or retention of mucus, or from the tracheal tube (Figure 32.6). Eventually, alveolar pressure and lung volume increase sufficiently to cause reductions in both lung compliance and airway resistance (pages 32 and 47); expiratory flow rate then increases and so the degree of PEEPi stabilises.

At first sight PEEPi may be perceived as beneficial – for example, leading to increased FRC and alveolar recruitment – and it is likely that improved gas exchange seen with inverse I:E ratio results, at least in part, from this mechanism. However, the first hazard of PEEPi is its variability. Small changes in airway resistance, for example with mucus retention, can lead to rapid increases in the level of PEEPi. The cardiovascular consequences of PEEPi are significant (see below), and have been described as 'applying a tourniquet to the right heart'.[37] Finally, the presence of PEEPi will impede the ability of the patient to trigger ventilators by necessitating a greater fall in alveolar pressure to initiate respiratory support.[18]

Application of external PEEP will, to some extent, attenuate the generation of PEEPi by maintaining airway patency in late expiration and so improving expiratory flow.

PHYSIOLOGICAL EFFECTS OF POSITIVE PRESSURE VENTILATION

A positive pressure in the chest cavity is a significant physiological insult that normally occurs only transiently with coughing, straining, etc., although the pressure achieved in these situations may be very high. Most physiological effects of IPPV are related to the mean pressure throughout the whole respiratory cycle, which is in turn influenced by a large number of ventilatory settings such as mode of ventilation, tidal volume, respiratory rate and I:E ratio. PEEP results in large increases in mean intrathoracic pressure. For example, IPPV in a patient with normal lungs using 10 breaths of $10\,ml.kg^{-1}$ and an I:E ratio of 1:2 will generate mean airway pressures of approximately $5\,cmH_2O$. Addition of a modest $5\,cmH_2O$ of PEEP will therefore double the mean airway pressure, and thus the physiological insult associated with IPPV. For this reason, much research into the physiological effects of artificial ventilation has focused on PEEP.

RESPIRATORY EFFECTS[38]

Artificial ventilation effectively rests the respiratory muscles, and the effect of this on muscle function is described on page 92.

Distribution of ventilation. Intermittent positive pressure ventilation results in a spatial pattern of distribution that is determined by inflation pressure, regional compliance and time constants. Based on external measurements the anatomical pattern of distribution of inspired gas is different from that of spontaneous breathing, there being a relatively greater expansion of the rib cage.[39] However, with spontaneous breathing regional differences in ventilation are small in the supine position (page 120), and in spite of the altered ribcage motion changes in regional ventilation with IPPV in patients with normal lungs are probably minimal.[40] This is not the case in patients with ALI, in whom the spatial distribution of gas becomes very abnormal with areas of collapse and over-inflated lung developing.[39] Application of PEEP increases lung volume and, at high levels, re-expands collapsed alveoli, which changes the compliance of dependent lung regions and so improves ventilation of these areas.

Apparatus dead space. Positive pressure ventilation, whether invasive or non-invasive, requires the provision of an airtight connection to the patient's airway. This inevitably involves the addition of some apparatus dead space. With orotracheal and tracheostomy tubes much of the normal anatomical dead space (page 129) is bypassed, such that overall anatomical dead space may be unchanged or reduced. With non-invasive ventilation using facemasks, apparatus dead space may be substantial. Ventilator tubing used to deliver IPPV is normally corrugated, and expands longitudinally with each inspiration. For an average ventilator circuit, this expansion may amount to 2–3 ml per cmH_2O of positive pressure, and this volume will constitute dead space ventilation.

Physiological dead space. In normal lungs during anaesthesia, IPPV alone seems to have little effect on the V_D/V_T ratio compared with the value obtained with spontaneous breathing.[39] There is a slight widening of the distribution of $\dot{V}/\dot{Q}$ ratios (page 126) mostly as a result of a reduction in pulmonary blood flow from depression of cardiac output (see below). These changes are normally not sufficient to alter gas exchange. The acute application of moderate amounts of PEEP causes only a slight increase in V_D/V_T ratio.[41]

The alveolar component of physiological dead space may be increased by ventilation in patients with lung injury, or when mean intrathoracic pressure is high such as with significant amounts of PEEP. Under the latter conditions, lung volume is

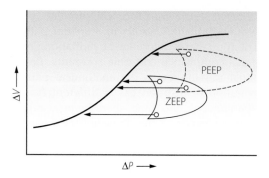

Fig. 32.7 Effect of positive end-expiratory pressure (PEEP) on the relationship between regional pressure and volume in the lung (supine position). Note that compliance is greater in the upper part of the lung with zero end-expiratory pressure (ZEEP) and in the lower part of the lung with PEEP, which thus improves ventilation in the dependent zone of the lung. (Diagram kindly supplied by Professor J. Gareth Jones.)

increased to such an extent that not only does cardiac output fall but pulmonary vascular resistance rises as well (see Figure 7.4).[42] Perfusion to over-expanded alveoli is reduced and areas of lung with high $\dot{V}/\dot{Q}$ ratios develop, which constitute alveolar dead space. In healthy lungs, this effect is not seen until PEEP levels exceed 10–15 cmH$_2$O.[41] However, with IPPV in ALI overdistension occurs in the relatively small number of functional alveoli (page 457), and local perfusion to these lung units is likely to be impeded.

Lung volume. IPPV and ZEEP will have no effect on FRC. However, with PEEP, end-expiratory alveolar pressure will equal the level of applied PEEP and this will reset the FRC in accord with the pressure/volume curve of the respiratory system (see Figure 3.8). For example, PEEP of 10 cmH$_2$O will increase FRC by 500 ml in a patient with a compliance of 0.5 l.kPa^{-1} (50 ml.cmH$_2$O^{-1}). In many patients this may be expected to raise the tidal range above the closing capacity (page 48) and so reduce pulmonary collapse. Prevention of alveolar collapse is probably the greatest single advantage of PEEP. It will also reduce airway resistance according to the inverse relationship between lung volume and airway resistance (see Figure 4.5). It may also change the relative compliance of the upper and lower parts of the lung (Figure 32.7), thereby improving the ventilation of the dependent over-perfused parts of the lung.

Arterial Po$_2$. Neither IPPV nor PEEP improve arterial oxygenation appreciably in patients with healthy lungs. During anaesthesia, it has been repeatedly observed that PEEP does little to improve arterial oxygenation in healthy patients. Pulmonary shunting is decreased, but the accompanying decrease in cardiac output reduces the mixed venous oxygen saturation, which counteracts the effect of a reduction in the shunt, resulting in minimal increase in arterial Po$_2$.[41] There is however no doubt that positive pressure ventilation improves arterial Po$_2$ in a wide range of pathological situations. In most cases, the improvement in Po$_2$ relates to the mean airway pressure achieved, and, as described above, PEEP provides an easy way of elevating airway pressures. Re-expansion of collapsed lung units, improved ventilation of alveoli with low $\dot{V}/\dot{Q}$ ratios, and redistribution of extravascular lung water will all contribute to the observed improvement in oxygenation. The use of PEEP for prevention of atelectasis in anaesthesia is described on page 336, whilst its contribution to the treatment of pulmonary oedema and acute lung injury are described on pages 424 and 457 respectively.

THE VALSALVA EFFECT

It has long been known that an increase in intra-thoracic pressure has complex circulatory effects, characterised as the Valsalva effect, which is the circulatory response to a subject increasing his airway pressure to about 5 kPa (50 cmH$_2$O) against a closed glottis for about 30 seconds. The normal response is in four parts (Figure 32.8A). Initially the raised intrathoracic pressure alters the base line for circulatory pressures and the arterial pressure (measured relative to atmosphere) is consequently increased (phase 1). At the same time, ventricular filling is decreased by the adverse pressure gradient from peripheral veins to the ventricle in diastole, and cardiac output therefore decreases. The consequent decline in arterial pressure in phase 2 is normally mitigated by three factors – tachycardia, increased systemic vascular resistance (afterload) and an increase in peripheral venous pressure, which tends to restore the venous return. As a result of these compensations, the arterial pressure normally settles to a value fairly close to the level before starting the Valsalva manoeuvre. When the intrathoracic pressure is restored to normal, there is an immediate decrease in arterial pressure due to the altered base line. Simultaneously the venous return improves and therefore the cardiac output increases within a few seconds. However, the arteriolar bed remains constricted temporarily, and there is therefore a transient overshoot of arterial pressure.

Figure 32.8B shows the abnormal 'square wave' pattern that occurs with raised end-diastolic pressure

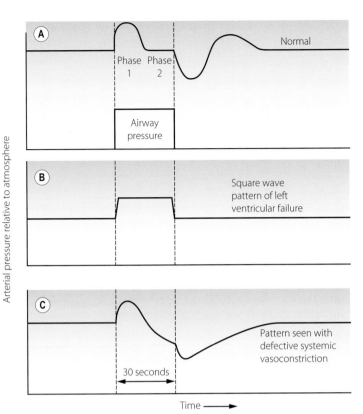

Fig. 32.8 Qualitative changes in mean arterial blood pressure during a Valsalva manoeuvre as seen in the normal subject and for two abnormal responses. See text for explanation of the changes.

or left ventricular failure or both. The initial increase in arterial pressure (phase 1) occurs normally, but the decline in pressure in phase 2 is missing because the output of the congested heart is not usually limited by end-diastolic pressure. Because the cardiac output is unchanged, there is no increase in pulse rate or systemic vascular resistance. Therefore there is no overshoot of pressure when the intra-thoracic pressure is restored to normal.

Figure 32.8C shows a different abnormal pattern, which may be seen with defective systemic vasoconstriction (e.g. autonomic neuropathy or a spinal anaesthetic). Phase 1 is normal, but in phase 2, the decreased cardiac output is not accompanied by an increase in systemic vascular resistance and the arterial pressure therefore continues to decline. The normal overshoot is replaced by a slow recovery of arterial pressure as the cardiac output returns to control values.

CARDIOVASCULAR EFFECTS OF POSITIVE PRESSURE VENTILATION[43,44]

Initially there was great reluctance to use PEEP, partly because of the well-known Valsalva effect, and partly because of the circulatory hazard that had been described in the classic paper of Cournand

and his colleagues in 1948.[45] Not many papers in this field have two Nobel prize winners amongst their authors. The cardiovascular effects of IPPV and PEEP continue to cause problems in clinical practice, and after another half century of investigation, the effects remain incompletely elucidated.

Cardiac output.[43] Bindslev et al[41] reported a progressive decrease in cardiac output with IPPV and PEEP in anaesthetised patients without pulmonary pathology. Compared with when anaesthetised and breathing spontaneously, cardiac output was reduced by 10% with IPPV and ZEEP, 18% with $9\,cmH_2O$ of PEEP, and 36% with $16\,cmH_2O$ of PEEP. Another study, this time in patients with severe acute lung injury, also demonstrated a progressive reduction in cardiac output for PEEP in the range 5–$30\,cmH_2O$, but the effect was partially reversed by blood volume expansion (Figure 32.9).

There is general agreement that the main cause of the reduction in cardiac output is obstruction to filling of the right atrium, caused by the elevated intrathoracic pressure. With spontaneous respiration, the negative intrathoracic pressure during inspiration draws blood into the chest from the major veins, known as the 'thoracic pump'. Positive intrathoracic pressure abolishes this effect and also imposes a further reduction in driving pressure for flow between extra- and intrathoracic vessels. Reduced right ventricle (RV) filling pressures quickly lead to reduced left ventricle (LV) filling, and cardiac output falls.[48] These changes will clearly be more pronounced with hypovolaemia. Paradoxically, this physiological response may be utilised to treat hypovolaemia by imposing an inspiratory resistance to further reduce the negative inspiratory pressure and improve venous return.[49]

A second cause for reduced cardiac output may come into play with high airway pressures, moderate PEEP, or lung hyperinflation such as occurs with PEEPi. As described above, increasing lung volume leads to elevated pulmonary vascular resistance, which will cause an increase in RV volume.[42] There is now good evidence that dilation of the RV has profound effects on LV function, preventing adequate LV filling and reducing LV compliance, both of which lead to a fall in cardiac output.[43] Contractility of the LV is not thought to change with positive intrathoracic pressure. Interactions of some of the factors by which PEEP may influence cardiac output and systemic arterial pressure are shown in Figure 32.10.

Oxygen flux. In many patients with pulmonary disease, PEEP tends to improve the arterial Po_2 while decreasing the cardiac output. As PEEP is increased the oxygen delivery (the product of cardiac output and arterial oxygen content; page 202) tends to rise to a maximum and then falls. Assuming that a normal or high oxygen flux is desirable, use of IPPV or PEEP therefore requires optimisation of cardiac output with fluid replacement (see Figure 32.9) or with positive inotropes, and this is now routine practice in critical care units.

Arterial blood pressure. Figure 32.9 shows the decline in mean arterial pressure closely following the change in cardiac output with increasing PEEP. Although there was some increase in systemic vascular resistance, this was only about half that required for maintenance of the arterial pressure in the face of the declining cardiac output.

Interpretation of vascular pressures. Atrial pressures are normally measured relative to atmospheric pressure. With positive pressure ventilation, atrial pressures tend to be increased relative to atmospheric. However, relative to intrathoracic pressure, they are reduced at higher levels of PEEP (Figure 32.9). It is the transmural pressure gradient and not the level relative to atmosphere that is relevant to cardiac filling.[44]

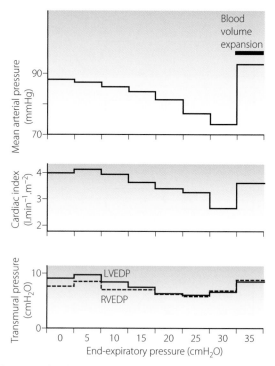

Fig. 32.9 Cardiovascular responses as a function of positive end-expiratory pressure (PEEP) in patients with acute lung injury. Left and right ventricular end-diastolic pressure (LVEDP and RVEDP) were measured relative to intrapleural pressure. (Drawn from data of reference 46 and reproduced from reference 47 by permission of the publishers of International Anesthesiology Clinics.)

Transmission of airway pressure to other intrathoracic structures. The intrapleural pressure is protected from the level of PEEP by the transmural pressure gradient of the lungs. Animal studies have shown that reduced pulmonary compliance is the main factor governing the transmission of airway pressure to other thoracic structures. With reduced compliance the effect of mean intrathoracic pressure on cardiac output is greatly reduced.[48] Patients with diseased lungs tend to have reduced pulmonary compliance, which limits the rise in intrapleural pressure (Figure 32.11). Therefore, their cardiovascular systems are better protected against the adverse effects of IPPV and PEEP.

Haemodynamic response in heart failure. The cardiovascular responses described thus far apply only to patients with normal cardiac function, and, like the Valsalva response, are very different in patients with raised ventricular end-diastolic pressure with or without ventricular failure.[44] Reduction of venous return to an overloaded and failing right

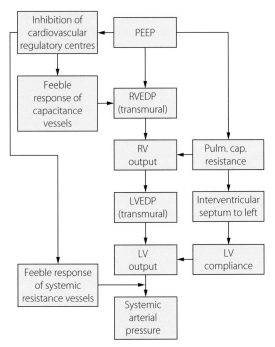

Fig. 32.10 Summary of the possible cardiovascular effects of positive end-expiratory pressure (PEEP). See text for full explanation. RVEDP and LVEDP, right and left ventricular end-diastolic pressure; RV and LV, right and left ventricle.

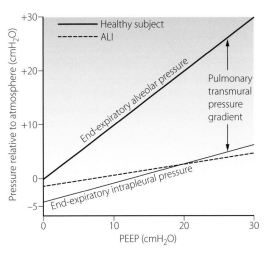

Fig. 32.11 End-expiratory alveolar and intrapleural pressures as a function of positive end-expiratory pressure (PEEP). The lower unbroken line shows intrapleural pressure in the relaxed healthy subject. The broken line shows values of intrapleural pressure in patients with acute lung injury taken from reference 46. Absolute values of pressure probably reflect experimental technique and cannot be compared between studies. (Reproduced from reference 47 by permission of the publishers of International Anesthesiology Clinics.)

heart will return the RV to a more favourable section of its Frank–Starling curve (see Figure 29.3) and so improve its function. Reducing RV end-diastolic volume will overcome some of the adverse ventricular interactions that occur in heart failure and so also improve LV function. These factors almost certainly contribute to the success of CPAP in the treatment of cardiogenic pulmonary oedema (page 424).

OTHER PHYSIOLOGICAL EFFECTS

Renal effects. Patients receiving prolonged IPPV tend to become oedematous. Protein depletion and inappropriate fluid loading may be factors but there is also evidence that PEEP itself reduces glomerular filtration.[50] Arterial pressure tends to be reduced as described above, while central venous pressure is raised. Therefore, the pressure gradient between renal artery and vein is reduced and this has a direct effect on renal blood flow. In addition, PEEP causes elevated levels of antidiuretic hormone, possibly due to activation of left atrial receptors, although this is insufficient to fully explain the changes in urinary flow rate.

Pulmonary neutrophil retention. Neutrophils have a diameter close to that of a pulmonary capillary, and this is important in slowing their transit time through the lung to facilitate margination for pulmonary defence mechanisms (page 435). Any reduction in pulmonary capillary diameter may therefore be expected to increase pulmonary neutrophil retention, which has indeed been demonstrated in humans following a Valsalva manoeuvre[51] or with the application of PEEP.[52] If the neutrophils trapped in this way have already been activated, for example following cardiopulmonary bypass, then lung injury may occur.

VENTILATOR-ASSOCIATED LUNG INJURY[53,54]

The first description of the potential harm that artificial ventilation may cause to the lungs was published in 1745 by John Fothergill.[55,56] Following the successful resuscitation of a patient using expired air respiration rather than bellows, which were fashionable at the time, Fothergill wrote that:

> *the lungs of one man may bear, without injury, as great a force as those of another man can exert; which by the bellows cannot always be determin'd.*

Artificial ventilation may damage *normal* lungs only after prolonged ventilation with high airway pressures or large tidal volumes, and is rarely a problem in clinical practice. However, in abnormal lungs such as during acute lung injury (Chapter 31) VALI may contribute not only to further lung damage, but also to multisystem organ failure affecting other body systems.[57]

BAROTRAUMA

A sustained increase in the transmural pressure gradient can damage the lung. The commonest forms of barotrauma attributable to artificial ventilation with or without PEEP are subcutaneous emphysema, pneumomediastinum and pneumothorax. Pulmonary barotrauma probably starts as disruption of the alveolar membrane, with air entering the interstitial space and tracking along the bronchovascular bundles into the mediastinum, from which it can reach the peritoneum, the pleural cavity or the subcutaneous tissues. Radiological demonstration of pulmonary interstitial gas may provide an early warning of barotrauma.

A second form of barotrauma is bronchiolectasis,[58] which describes gross dilatation of terminal and respiratory bronchioles which used to be commonly seen at autopsy in patients following prolonged artificial ventilation. The development of bronchiolectasis was increased by high PEEP levels, high peak airway pressures, large tidal volumes and the duration of artificial ventilation. The condition of bronchiolectasis appears to be analogous to bronchopulmonary dysplasia described in infants ventilated for respiratory distress syndrome.[59] Hopefully, modern ventilators and ventilatory strategies mean that this condition is now unlikely to develop.

VOLUTRAUMA[55]

Many animal studies have demonstrated pulmonary oedema following artificial ventilation with high inflation pressures. In one of these studies, lung damage with high inflation pressures was attenuated by restricting chest movement to prevent over-distension of the lungs, indicating that alveolar size rather than pressure was responsible for lung injury.[60] Termed volutrauma, this is now believed to contribute significantly to lung damage in patients with acute lung injury, in whom only a small proportion of alveoli may receive the entire tidal volume (page 457).

This form of VALI most commonly manifests itself as interstitial or alveolar pulmonary oedema. There are several possible underlying mechanisms, all of which are closely inter-related.

Alveolar distension causes permeability pulmonary oedema (page 423).[53] With extreme lung distension in animal studies this occurs quickly and probably results from direct trauma to alveolar structures. Recent work on lung cell cultures in vitro has revealed some of the mechanisms of this cellular trauma.[61] Severe stretching of the cells can induce apoptosis, provoke the release of inflammatory cytokines, or damage tight junctions between cells or the plasma membrane. Stretch frequency is also an important determinant of the damage done, supporting the inclination towards slower respiratory rates in injured lungs. In larger animals and humans, the permeability changes occur slowly (several hours) and are likely to result from the alterations in surfactant and inflammatory mediators described below rather than widespread cellular damage.

Airway trauma occurs with repeated closure and reopening of small airways with each breath, and has been termed atelectrauma. Eventually, mucosal oedema will develop and the airways become progressively more difficult to open until collapse occurs. Recruitment of lung units with positive pressure ventilation has beneficial effects on gas exchange, and so encourages the use of higher pressures and volumes to recruit more airways, leading to further VALI.

Surfactant function is affected by artificial ventilation. Animal studies have demonstrated that surfactant *release* is increased by artificial ventilation, but there is also ample evidence that surfactant *function* is reduced.[53] Cyclical closure of airways during expiration causes surfactant to be drawn from the alveoli into the airway,[62] whilst alveolar proteins seen with permeability oedema inactivate surfactant (page 456). The resultant increase in alveolar surface tension will not only affect lung compliance but may also increase local microvascular permeability and encourage alveolar collapse.

Lung inflammation occurs with VALI. Termed biotrauma, this includes a pro-inflammatory response to ventilation that is independent of any infection present, and also includes activation of immunological and coagulation systems, and cellular growth and apoptotic pathways.[54] Pulmonary neutrophils are implicated in biotrauma and their migration into lung tissue has been described above. Once activated – for example, by stretching as described above or by exposure to the alveolar basement membrane – inflammatory mediators will contribute to permeability oedema and further loss of surfactant function.

PREVENTION OF VALI

PEEP. In spite of its contribution to mean airway pressure, animal studies show that modest amounts of PEEP are helpful in reducing VALI.[63] Reduction of interstitial oedema, prevention of cyclical airway closure, and preservation of surfactant function are all possible mechanisms for this effect. Determination of an acceptable level of PEEP in injured lungs is discussed on page 457.

Tidal volume and airway pressure should be minimised as far as possible. Plateau pressure is the ventilator measurement that equates most closely to the degree of alveolar distension. It is currently recommended that in patients with normal chest wall compliance the plateau pressure should not be allowed to exceed $35\,cmH_2O$.[64]

A 'protective' ventilation strategy that combines these requirements is described on page 457, and its use in the clinical setting to reduce VALI is now widely accepted.

ARTIFICIAL VENTILATION FOR RESUSCITATION

Until about 1960, artificial ventilation was usually attempted by application of mechanical forces directly to the trunk. Methods were based on the rescuer manipulating the trunk and arms of the victim to achieve changes in lung volume which, when performed in sequence could produce some degree of pulmonary ventilation. These methods, which undoubtedly saved many lives in the past, are now largely obsolete.

EXPIRED AIR VENTILATION[65]

Recognition of the inadequacy of the manual methods of artificial ventilation led directly to a radical new approach to artificial ventilation in an emergency. Around 1960 there was vigorous re-examination of the concept of the rescuer's expired air being used for inflation of the victim's lungs.

At first sight, it might appear that expired air would not be a suitable inspired air for the victim.

Table 32.4 Alveolar gas concentrations during expired air resuscitation

	NORMAL SPONTANEOUS RESPIRATION	EXPIRED AIR RESUSCITATION WITH DOUBLED VENTILATION	
		DONOR	RECIPIENT
Alveolar CO_2	6%	3%	6%
Alveolar O_2	15%	18%	15%

Doubling the rescuer's ventilation increases his alveolar O_2 concentration to a value midway between the normal alveolar oxygen concentration and that of room air.

However, if the rescuer doubles his ventilation he is able to breathe for two. If neither party had any respiratory dead space, the simple relationship shown in Table 32.4 would apply. In fact, the rescuer's dead space improves the situation. At the start of inflation, the rescuer's dead space is filled with fresh air and this is the first gas to enter the victim's lungs. If the rescuer's dead space is artificially increased by apparatus dead space, this will improve the freshness of the air that the victim receives and will also reduce the likelihood of hypocapnia in the rescuer.

Expired air ventilation has now displaced the manual methods in all except the most unusual circumstances and its success depends on the following factors:

1. It is normally possible to achieve adequate ventilation for long periods of time without fatigue, though symptomatic hypocapnia can occur.[66]
2. The hands of the rescuer are free to control the patency of the victim's airway.
3. The rescuer can monitor the victim's chest expansion visually and can also hear any airway obstruction and sense the tidal exchange from the proprioceptive receptors in his own chest wall.
4. The method is extremely adaptable and has been used, for example, before drowning victims have been removed from the water, and on linesmen electrocuted while working on pylons. No manual method would have any hope of success in such situations.
5. The method seems to come naturally, and many rescuers have achieved success with the minimum of instruction.

In 'out-of-hospital' cardiac arrest situations bystanders are reluctant to attempt cardiopulmonary resuscitation (CPR), usually from an unjustified fear of infection, to such an extent that CPR is attempted in less than a third of victims.[67,68] This has led to several studies of the contribution made by expired-air ventilation in this situation, comparing standard CPR with chest compressions alone. For the first few minutes after a witnessed cardiac arrest, oxygen stores in the blood and lungs may obviate the need for artificial ventilation until trained personnel and equipment arrive. The trials so far have found no difference in outcomes between the groups receiving ventilation or not,[67] and recent recommendations are that for witnessed, out-of-hospital, collapse expired air ventilation is not necessary until help arrives. It is hoped that if avoiding the requirement for ventilation encourages more bystanders to intervene by providing cardiac compressions alone then overall survival may be improved.[68]

EXTRAPULMONARY GAS EXCHANGE

The development of an artificial lung remains only a distant possibility,[69,70] but techniques for short-term replacement of lung function or more prolonged partial respiratory support have existed for many years. Extracorporeal gas exchangers were first developed for cardiac surgery to facilitate cardiopulmonary bypass and so allow surgery on a motionless heart. Subsequently the use of extracorporeal, and more recently intracorporeal, gas exchange was extended into the treatment of respiratory failure.

FACTORS IN DESIGN[71]

The lungs of an adult have an interface between blood and gas of the order of $126 m^2$. It is not possible to achieve this in an artificial substitute, and artificial lungs can be considered to have a very low 'diffusing capacity'. Nevertheless, they function satisfactorily within limits for many reasons.

Factors favouring performance

- The real lung is adapted for maximal exercise, while patients requiring extrapulmonary gas exchange are usually close to basal metabolic rate or less if hypothermia is used, for example during cardiac surgery.
- Under resting conditions at sea level, there is an enormous reserve in the capacity of the lung to achieve equilibrium between pulmonary

capillary blood and alveolar gas (see Figure 9.2). Therefore, a subnormal diffusing capacity does not necessarily result in arterial hypoxaemia.

- It is possible to operate an artificial lung with an 'alveolar' oxygen concentration in excess of 90%, compared with 14% for real alveolar gas under normal circumstances. This greatly increases the oxygen transfer for a given 'diffusing capacity' of the artificial lung.
- The 'capillary transit time' of an artificial lung can be increased beyond the 0.75 second in the real lung. This facilitates the approach of blood Po_2 to 'alveolar' Po_2 (see Figure 9.2).
- It is possible to use countercurrent flow between gas and blood. This does not occur in the lungs of mammals although it is used in the gills of fishes.

Carbon dioxide exchanges much more readily than oxygen because of its greater blood and lipid solubility. Therefore, in general, elimination of carbon dioxide does not present a major problem and the limiting factor of an artificial lung is oxygenation.

Unfavourable factors

Against these favourable design considerations, there are certain advantages of the real lung – apart from its very large surface area – that are difficult to emulate in an artificial lung.

- The pulmonary capillaries have a diameter close to that of a red blood cell (RBC). Therefore, each RBC is brought into very close contact with the alveolar gas (see Figure 2.7). The diffusion distance for artificial lungs is considerably greater and this problem is considered further below.
- The vascular endothelium is specially adapted to prevent undesirable changes in the formed elements of blood, particularly neutrophils and platelets. Most artificial surfaces cause clotting of blood, and artificial lungs therefore require the use of anticoagulants.
- The lung is an extremely efficient filter with an effective pore size of about $10 \mu m$ for flow rates of blood up to about $25 l.min^{-1}$. This is difficult to achieve with any man-made filter.

Bubble oxygenators

By breaking up the gas stream into small bubbles, it is possible to achieve very large surface areas of interface. However, the smaller the bubbles, the greater the tendency for them to remain in suspension when the blood is returned to the patient. This is dangerous during cardiopulmonary bypass because of the direct access of the blood to the systemic circulation. With a mean RBC transit time of 1–2 seconds and an oxygen concentration of more than 90%, bubble oxygenators achieve an acceptable outflow blood Po_2 with blood flow rates up to about $6\,l.min^{-1}$. The Pco_2 of the outflowing blood must be controlled by admixture of carbon dioxide with the inflowing oxygen in the gas phase.

Cellular and protein damage (see below) at the blood–gas interface occurs in bubble oxygenators. This is not considered to have significant clinical effects during short term use, as for example with cardiac surgery, but may become significant when used for prolonged periods in the treatment of respiratory failure.[71]

Membrane oxygenators

Diffusion properties. Unlike their predecessors, currently available membranes offer little resistance to the diffusion of oxygen and carbon dioxide. At $25–50\,\mu m$ thick, artificial membranes are several times thicker than the active side of the alveolar/capillary membrane (Figure 2.8), but they contain small ($<1\,\mu m$) pores, which increase gas transfer substantially. The hydrophobic nature of the membrane material prevents water entering the pores and in normal use membranes can withstand a hydrostatic pressure gradient of the order of normal arterial blood pressure. Over time the pores tend to fill with protein which slowly reduces the membrane efficiency.

Gas diffusion within the blood presents a considerable barrier to efficiency of membrane oxygenators. Slow diffusion of gases through plasma is now thought to limit gas transfer in normal lung, in which the RBC is almost in contact with the capillary wall (page 148). Streamline flow through much wider channels in a membrane oxygenator tends to result in a stream of RBCs remaining at a distance from the interface. It has been estimated that in membrane oxygenators the diffusion path for oxygen is about 25 times further than in lung. Much thought has been devoted to the creation of turbulent flow to counteract this effect by 'mixing' the blood. Unfortunately, this inevitably leads to a greater degree of cell damage (see below) and increased resistance to flow through the oxygenator.

Biocompatibility. Adsorption of proteins, particularly albumin, onto the membrane reduces platelet,

neutrophil and complement activation (see below), and this technique may be used to 'prime' oxygenators before use. Attempts to mimic endothelial cell properties have led to the production of membranes with heparin bonded to the surface, which also reduces activation of most of the processes described below.

DAMAGE TO BLOOD

Damage due to oxygenators is probably far less than that which results from surgical suction in removing blood from the operative site and, during cardiac surgery, this factor outweighs any differences attributable to the type of oxygenator. However, during prolonged extracorporeal oxygenation for respiratory failure, the influence of the type of oxygenator becomes important, and membrane oxygenators are then clearly superior to bubble oxygenators.

Protein denaturation. Contact between blood and either gas bubbles or synthetic surfaces results in protein denaturation, and synthetic surfaces become coated with a layer of protein. With membrane oxygenators this tends to be self-limiting, and the protein products remain bound to the membrane. Bubble oxygenators cause a continuous and progressive loss of protein, including the release of denatured proteins into the circulation where they may have biological effects.

Complement activation. Complement activation occurs when blood comes into contact with any artificial surface and complement C5a is known to be formed after cardiopulmonary bypass surgery.

RBCs. Shear forces, resulting from turbulence or foaming, may cause shortened survival or actual destruction of RBCs. However, without surgical suction, damage to RBCs with membrane oxygenators remains within reasonable limits for many days.

Leukocytes and platelets. Counts of these elements are usually reduced by an amount in excess of the changes attributable to haemodilution. Platelets are lost by adhesion and aggregation, and following cardiac surgery postoperative counts are commonly about half the preoperative value. Neutrophil activation may occur within the extracorporeal circuit leading to pathological effects in distant organs.

Coagulation. No oxygenator can function without causing coagulation of the blood. Anticoagulation is therefore a sine qua non of the technique and heparin is usually employed for this purpose. Heparin-bonded components have significantly reduced the systemic anticoagulant requirement and allowed more prolonged use of circuits, but coagulopathy remains the most common complication of extracorporeal circulation.[72]

SYSTEMS FOR EXTRAPULMONARY GAS EXCHANGE[73]

Cardiopulmonary bypass for cardiac surgery remains the most common situation in which patients are exposed to extrapulmonary gas exchange. The duration of such exposure is normally very short, and causes few physiological disturbances postoperatively. Providing longer term respiratory support is much less common, and also considerably more difficult, but three techniques exist.

Extracorporeal membrane oxygenation (ECMO).[74] A traditional ECMO system requires continuous blood flow from the patient to a reservoir system, from which a pump propels blood through an oxygenator and a heat exchanger back to the patient. Venovenous ECMO is acceptable for treatment of respiratory failure, and may be instituted via percutaneous venous catheters. If circulatory support is also required, then venoarterial ECMO is used, which normally requires surgical access to the vessels. A typical adult ECMO circuit provides $7 m^2$ of membrane for oxygenation using 100% oxygen, with blood flows of approximately $2-4 l.min^{-1}$. The technique is only available in specialised centres, so in recent years ECMO systems have been developed for use whilst transporting the patient to the ECMO facilities.[75]

Technological improvements in the design of ECMO circuits have allowed the development of a simplified system referred to as pumpless extracorporeal lung assist (pECLA). In pECLA arterial and venous cannulae are connected to a small membrane oxygenator and the patient's own blood pressure drives blood flow through the system.[76,77] The surface area of the pECLA device is about $1.3 m^2$, and blood flows of $1.0-2.5 l.min^{-1}$ occur across one side of the membrane and about $10 l.min^{-1}$ of oxygen is passed across the other side. As the name implies, pECLA systems are too small to entirely replace the gas exchange function of the lungs, but it can provide valuable respiratory support in a much less invasive fashion than traditional ECMO. As would be expected, oxygenation with pECLA is less effective than CO_2 removal, with average values for oxygen transfer of $41.7 ml.min^{-1}$ compared with $148.0 ml.min^{-1}$ for CO_2.[78]

Extracorporeal carbon dioxide removal (ECCO₂R). A different approach to artificial gas exchange was attempted by Gattinoni et al.[79] An ECMO system was used only to remove carbon dioxide, and oxygenation maintained by a modification of apnoeic mass movement oxygenation (page 172). The lungs were either kept motionless or were ventilated two to three times per minute.

The technique depended on two important differences between the exchange of carbon dioxide and oxygen. First, membrane oxygenators remove carbon dioxide some 10–20 times more effectively than they take up oxygen. Second, the normal arterial oxygen content ($20 ml.dl^{-1}$) is very close to the maximum oxygen capacity, even with 100% oxygen in the gas phase ($22 ml.dl^{-1}$). Therefore, there is little scope for superoxygenation of a fraction of the cardiac output to compensate for a larger fraction of the cardiac output in which oxygenation does not take place. In contrast, the normal mixed venous carbon dioxide content is $52 ml.dl^{-1}$ compared with an arterial carbon dioxide content of $48 ml.dl^{-1}$. There is therefore ample scope for removing a larger than normal fraction of carbon dioxide from a part of the cardiac output to compensate for the remaining fraction that does not undergo any removal of carbon dioxide. It is therefore possible to maintain carbon dioxide homoeostasis by diversion of only a small fraction of the cardiac output through an extracorporeal membrane oxygenator.[79] Despite this advantage, ECCO₂R was never a widely adopted technique and no improvements in survival were found.

Intravascular oxygenators (IVOX).[80] Siting the gas exchange membrane within the patient's own circulation obviates the need for any extracorporeal circulation. In return, the size of the gas exchange surface is severely limited, and the blood flow around the membrane no longer controlled. However, the development of a heparin-bonded hollow fibre oxygenator suitable for use in humans promoted interest in the technique. The device is inserted via surgical exposure of the femoral vein until it lies throughout the length of both inferior and superior vena cavae, through the right atrium. An IVOX device comes in different sizes between 40–50 cm long with 600–1100 fibres through which oxygen flows, providing a surface area of $0.21-0.52 m^2$ for gas exchange.[81] Blood flow in the vena cavae is thought to be mostly laminar, even with the IVOX in place, and gas exchange is again therefore limited by diffusion within the blood.[80]

The available membrane surface area with IVOX is such that total extrapulmonary gas exchange is currently impossible, and the technique is suitable only for partial respiratory support.

IVOX does allow some improvement in ventilator settings, which should alleviate the risk of lung trauma. Outcome studies are awaited, but it is unlikely that the modest improvement in gas exchange seen with current systems will have significant effects.[82]

CLINICAL APPLICATIONS[83]

Neonates and infants.[73,74] Acute respiratory failure in neonates and infants results from a variety of causes such as meconium aspiration syndrome, congenital diaphragmatic hernia, acute respiratory distress syndrome and a variety of infections. ECMO is indicated for treatment of acute respiratory failure of such severity that predicted survival is less than 20%. Though survival varies with the aetiology, there is general agreement that ECMO improves outcome substantially in infants, with some centres achieving survival figures of almost 80%.[74] Complications of ECMO are, however, numerous. Vascular access in infants is difficult, and venoarterial ECMO using the carotid and jugular vessels is often required, though venovenous ECMO with a double lumen cannula is now widely used. In either case, cerebral blood flow may be affected during ECMO and as result a significant

number of ECMO treated infants develop cerebral damage, which in some infants causes long term disability.[74,84] Improvements in other therapies, including artificial ventilation, for these very sick patients have led to a progressive reduction in the number treated with ECMO.[83]

Adults.[85] Extrapulmonary gas exchange is occasionally used as a therapeutic 'bridge' in patients waiting for lung transplantation, but its main indication is for management of severe acute lung injury (Chapter 30). Ventilator-associated lung injury as a result of artificial ventilation (page 481) contributes to respiratory failure in severe ALI, and the prospect of using extrapulmonary gas exchange to facilitate 'lung rest' is attractive.

Unfortunately, the significant benefits of ECMO use in infants have not been found in adults, and its place in treatment remains controversial.[83,86] The invasive nature of extrapulmonary gas exchange and the serious potential complications mean that ECMO is used only in the most severely ill patients. Even in specialist centres, recruitment of enough patients for randomised trials is difficult, and units have tended to simply publish results of uncontrolled case series, though further clinical trials are in progress.

Current interest in pECLA has led to its use in a variety of circumstances to reduce arterial P_{CO_2} to acceptable levels in artificially ventilated patients.[87] Perhaps the latest technique for partial lung replacement will succeed in the adult clinical environment where its predecessors have mostly failed.

References

1. Hillberg RE, Johnson DC. Noninvasive ventilation. *N Engl J Med.* 1997;337:1746–1752.

2. Mehta S, Hill NS. Noninvasive ventilation. *Am J Respir Crit Care Med.* 2001;163:540–577.

3. Hill NS. Clinical applications of body ventilators. *Chest.* 1986;90:897–905.

4. Drinker P, Shore LA. An apparatus for the prolonged administration of artificial respiration. *J Clin Invest.* 1929;7:229–247.

5. Thomson A. The role of negative pressure ventilation. *Arch Dis Child.* 1997;77:454–458.

6. Grasso F, Engelberts D, Helm E, et al. Negative-pressure

ventilation: Better oxygenation and less lung injury. *Am J Respir Crit Care Med.* 2008;177:412–418.

7. Petros AJ, Fernando SSD, Shenoy VS, Al-Saady NM. The Hayek oscillator. Nomograms for tidal volume and minute ventilation using external high frequency oscillation. *Anaesthesia.* 1995;50:601–606.

8. Dilkes MG, McNeill JM, Hill AC, Monks PS, McKelvie P, Hollamby RG. The Hayek oscillator: a new method of ventilation in microlaryngeal surgery. *Ann Otol Rhinol Laryngol.* 1993;102:455–458.

9. Chiumello D. Is the helmet different than the face mask

in delivering noninvasive ventilation? *Chest.* 2006;129:1402–1403.

10. Claman DM, Pipier A, Sanders MH, Stiller RA, Votteri BA. Nocturnal noninvasive positive pressure ventilatory assistance. *Chest.* 1996;110:1581–1588.

*11. Ambrosino N, Vagheggini G. Noninvasive positive pressure ventilation in the acute care setting: where are we? *Eur Respir J.* 2008;31:874–886.

12. Kolodziej MA, Jensen L, Rowe B, Sin D. Systematic review of noninvasive positive pressure ventilation in severe stable COPD. *Eur Respir J.* 2007;30:293–306.

13. Peter JV, Moran JL, Phillips-Hughes J, Graham P, Bersten AD. Effect of non-invasive positive pressure ventilation (NIPPV) on mortality in patients with acute cardiogenic pulmonary oedema: a meta-analysis. *Lancet*. 2006;367:1155–1163.

14. Antonelli M, Conti G, Esquinas A, et al. A multiple-center survey on the use in clinical practice of noninvasive ventilation as a first-line intervention for acute respiratory distress syndrome. *Crit Care Med*. 2007;35:18–25.

15. L'Her E, Deye N, Lellouche F, et al. Physiologic effects of noninvasive ventilation during acute lung injury. *Am J Respir Crit Care Med*. 2005;172:1112–1118.

16. Burns KEA, Adhikari NKJ, Keenan SP, Meade M. Use of non-invasive ventilation to wean critically ill adults off invasive ventilation: meta-analysis and systematic review. *BMJ*. 2009;338:1305–1308.

17. El Solh AA, Aquilina A, Pineda L, Dhanvantri V, Grant B, Bouquin P. Noninvasive ventilation for prevention of post-extubation respiratory failure in obese patients. *Eur Respir J*. 2006;28:588–595.

18. Rossi A, Appendini L. Wasted efforts and dyssynchrony: is the patient-ventilator battle back? *Intensive Care Med*. 1995;21:867–870.

19. Sassoon CSH, Gruer SE. Characteristics of the ventilator pressure- and flow-trigger variables. *Intensive Care Med*. 1995;21:159–168.

20. Dongelmans DA, Veelo DP, Bindels A, et al. Determinants of tidal volumes with adaptive support ventilation: a multicenter observational study. *Anesth Analg*. 2008;107:932–937.

21. Neumann P, Golisch W, Strohmeyer A, Buscher H, Burchardi H, Sydow M. Influence of different release times on spontaneous breathing pattern during airway pressure release ventilation. *Intensive Care Med*. 2002;28:1742–1749.

22. Dekel B, Segal E, Perel A. Pressure support ventilation. *Arch Intern Med*. 1996;156:369–373.

23. Smith BE. High frequency ventilation: past, present and future? *Br J Anaesth*. 1990;65:130–138.

24. Bouchut J-C, Godard J, Claris O. High-frequency oscillatory ventilation. *Anesthesiology*. 2004;100:1007–1012.

25. Chan KPW, Stewart TE, Mehta S. High-frequency oscillatory ventilation for adult patients with ARDS. *Chest*. 2007;131:1907–1916.

26. Chakrabarti MK, Gordon G, Whitwam JG. Relationship between tidal volume and deadspace during high frequency ventilation. *Br J Anaesth*. 1986;58:11–17.

27. Butler WJ, Bohn DJ, Bryan AC, Froese AB. Ventilation by high-frequency oscillation in humans. *Anesth Analg*. 1980;59:577–584.

28. Nunn JF, Hill DW. Respiratory dead space and arterial to end-tidal CO_2 tension difference in anesthetized man. *J Appl Physiol*. 1960;15:383–389.

29. Hurst JM, Branson RD, Davis K, Barrette RR, Adams KS. Comparison of conventional mechanical ventilation and high-frequency ventilation. A prospective randomized trial in patients with respiratory failure. *Ann Surg*. 1990;211:486–491.

30. MacIntyre N. Discontinuing mechanical ventilator support. *Chest*. 2007;132:1049–1056.

*31. Boles J-M, Bion J, Connors A, et al. Weaning from mechanical ventilation. *Eur Respir J*. 2007;29:1033–1056.

*32. MacIntyre NR, Cook DJ, Ely EW, et al. Evidence-based guidelines for weaning and discontinuing ventilatory support. A collective task force facilitated by the American College of Chest Physicians; the American Association of Respiratory Care; and the American College of Critical Care Medicine. *Chest*. 2001;120:375S–395S.

33. Yang KL, Tobin MJ. A prospective study of indexes predicting the outcome of trials of weaning from mechanical ventilation. *N Engl J Med*. 1991;324:1445–1450.

34. Simonds AK. Streamlining weaning: protocols and weaning units. *Thorax*. 2005;60:175–177.

35. Hill JD, Main FB, Osborn JJ, Gerbode F. Correct use of respirator on cardiac patient after operation. *Arch Surg*. 1965;91:775–778.

36. Gottfried SB, Reissman H, Ranieri M. A simple method for the measurement of intrinsic end-expiratory pressure during controlled and assisted modes of mechanical ventilation. *Crit Care Med*. 1992;20:621–629.

37. Conacher ID. Dynamic hyperinflation – the anaesthetist applying a tourniquet to the right heart. *Br J Anaesth*. 1998;81:116–117.

*38. Soni N, Williams P. Positive pressure ventilation: what is the real cost? *Br J Anaesth*. 2008;101:446–457.

39. Vellody VPS, Nassery M, Balasaraswathi K, Goldberg NB, Sharp JT. Compliances of human rib cage and diaphragm-abdomen pathways in relaxed versus paralyzed states. *Am Rev Respir Dis*. 1978;118:479–491.

40. Hulands GH, Greene R, Iliff LD, Nunn JF. Influence of anaesthesia on the regional distribution of perfusion and ventilation in the lung. *Clin Sci*. 1970;38:451–460.

41. Bindslev LG, Hedenstierna G, Santesson J, Gottlieb I, Carvallhas A. Ventilation-perfusion distribution during inhalational anaesthesia. *Acta Anaesthesiol Scand*. 1981;25:360–371.

42. Biondi JW, Schulman DS, Soufer R, et al. The effect of

incremental positive end-expiratory pressure on right ventricular hemodynamics and ejection fraction. *Anesth Analg.* 1988;67:144–151.

*43. Pinsky MR. The hemodynamic consequences of mechanical ventilation: an evolving story. *Intensive Care Med.* 1997;23:493–503.

44. Tyberg JV, Grant DA, Kingma I, et al. Effects of positive intrathoracic pressure on pulmonary and systemic hemodynamics. *Respir Physiol.* 2000;119:163–171.

45. Cournand A, Motley HL, Werko L, Richards DW. Physiological studies of the effects of intermittent positive pressure breathing on cardiac output in man. *Am J Physiol.* 1948;152:162–174.

46. Jardin F, Farcot J-C, Boisante L, Curien N, Margairaz A, Bourdarias J-P. Influence of positive end-expiratory pressure on left ventricular performance. *N Engl J Med.* 1981;304:387–392.

47. Nunn JF. Positive end-expiratory pressure. *Int Anaesthesiol Clin.* 1984;22:149–164.

48. Mitaka C, Nagura T, Sakanishi N, Tsunoda Y, Amaha K. Two-dimensional echocardiographic evaluation of inferior vena cava, right ventricle, and left ventricle during positive-pressure ventilation with varying levels of positive end-expiratory pressure. *Crit Care Med.* 1989;17:205–210.

49. Ryan KL, Cooke WH, Rickards CA, Lurie KG, Convertino VA. Breathing through an inspiratory threshold device improves stroke volume during central hypovolemia in humans. *J Appl Physiol.* 2008;104:1402–1409.

50. Marquez JM, Douglas ME, Downs JB, et al. Renal function and cardiovascular responses during positive airway pressure. *Anesthesiology.* 1979;50:393–398.

51. Markos J, Hooper RO, Kavanagh-Gray D, Wiggs BR, Hogg JC.

Effect of raised alveolar pressure on leukocyte retention in the human lung. *J Appl Physiol.* 1990;69:214–221.

52. Loick HM, Wendt M, Rötker J, Theissen JL. Ventilation with positive end-expiratory airway pressure causes leukocyte retention in human lung. *J Appl Physiol.* 1993;75:301–306.

53. Dreyfuss D, Saumon G. Ventilator-induced lung injury: lessons from experimental studies. *Am J Respir Crit Care Med.* 1998;157:294–323.

*54. Oeckler RA, Hubmayr RD. Ventilator-associated lung injury: a search for better therapeutic targets. *Eur Respir J.* 2007;30:1216–1226.

55. Slutsky AS. Lung injury caused by mechanical ventilation. *Chest.* 1999;116(supp):9S–15S.

56. Fothergill J. Observations on a case published in the last volume of the medical essays, & c. of recovering a man dead in appearance, by distending the lungs with air. *Philos Trans R Soc Lond.* 1745;43:275–281.

57. Slutsky AS, Tremblay LN. Multiple system organ failure – is mechanical ventilation a contributing factor. *Am J Respir Crit Care Med.* 1998;157: 1721–1725.

58. Slavin G, Nunn JF, Crow J, Doré CJ. Bronchiolectasis – a complication of artificial ventilation. *BMJ.* 1982;285:931–934.

59. Taghizadeh A, Reynolds EOR. Pathogenesis of bronchopulmonary dysplasia following hyaline membrane disease. *Am J Pathol.* 1976;82:241–264.

60. Dreyfuss D, Soler P, Basset G, Saumon G. High inflation pressure pulmonary edema. Respective effects of high airway pressure, high tidal volume and positive end-expiratory pressure. *Am Rev Respir Dis.* 1988;137:1159–1964.

61. Trepat X, Farré R. Alveolar permeability and stretch:

too far, too fast. *Eur Respir J.* 2008;32:826–828.

62. Faridy EE. Effect of ventilation on movement of surfactant in airways. *Respir Physiol.* 1976;27:323–334.

63. Hooper J. Advances in mechanical ventilation. *Can J Anaesth.* 1998;45:R149–R154.

64. Slutsky AS. Consensus conference on mechanical ventilation – January 28–30, 1993 at Northbrook, Illinois, USA. *Intensive Care Med.* 1994; 20: 64–79.

65. Wenzel V, Idris AH, Dörges V, et al. The respiratory system during resuscitation: a review of the history, risk of infection during assisted ventilation, respiratory mechanics, and ventilation strategies for patients with an unprotected airway. *Resuscitation.* 2001;49:123–134.

66. Thierbach AR, Wolcke BB, Krummenauer F, Kunde M, Jänig C, Dick WF. Artificial ventilation for basic life support leads to hyperventilation in first aid providers. *Resuscitation.* 2003;57:269–277.

67. SOS-KANTO study group. Cardiopulmonary resuscitation by bystanders with chest compression only (SOS-KANTO): an observational study. *Lancet.* 2007;369:920–926.

68. Soar J, Nolan JP. Cardiopulmonary resuscitation for out of hospital cardiac arrest. *BMJ.* 2008;336:782–783.

69. Jack D. Artificial lungs on the way – but don't hold your breath. *Lancet.* 1997;349:260.

70. Zwischenberger JB, Alpard SK. Artificial lungs: a new inspiration. *Perfusion.* 2002;17:253–268.

71. Wegner JA. Oxygenator anatomy and function. *J Cardiothorac Vasc Anaesth.* 1997;11:275–281.

72. Briegel J, Hummel T, Lenhart A, Heyduck M, Schelling G, Haller M. Complications during long-term extracorporeal lung assist

(ECLA). *Acta Anaesthesiol Scand Suppl.* 1996;109:121–122.

73. Walker G, Liddell M, Davis C. Extracorporeal life support – state of the art. *Paediatr Respir Rev.* 2003;4:147–152.

74. Cook LN. Update on extracorporeal membrane oxygenation. *Paediatr Respir Rev.* 2004;5(supp A):S329–S337.

75. Rossaint R, Pappert D, Gerlach H, Lewandowski K, Keh D, Falke K. Extracorporeal membrane oxygenation for transport of hypoxaemic patients with severe ARDS. *Br J Anaes.* 1997;78:241–246.

76. Hoeper MM, Welte T. Extracorporeal lung assist: more than kicking a dead horse? *Eur Respir J.* 2008;32:1431–1432.

*77. Bein T, Weber F, Philipp A, et al. A new pumpless extracorporeal interventional lung assist in critical hypoxemia/hypercapnia. *Crit Care Med.* 2006;34:1372–1377.

78. Müller T, Lubnow M, Philipp A, et al. Extracorporeal pumpless interventional lung assist in clinical practice: determinants of efficacy. *Eur Respir J.* 2009;33:551–558.

79. Gattinoni L, Pesenti A, Rossi GP, et al. Treatment of acute respiratory failure with low-frequency positive-pressure ventilation and extracorporeal removal of CO_2. *Lancet.* 1980;2:292–294.

80. Bidani A, Zwischenberger JB, Cardenas V. Intracorporeal gas exchange: current status and future development. *Intensive Care Med.* 1996;22:91–93.

81. Conrad SA, Eggerstedt JM, Grier LR, Morris VF, Romero MD. Intravenacaval membrane oxygenation and carbon dioxide removal in severe acute respiratory failure. *Chest.* 1995;107:1689–1697.

82. Peek GJ, Firmin RK. Extracorporeal membrane oxygenation, a favourable outcome? *Br J Anaesth.* 1997;78:235–236.

83. Schuerer DJE, Kolovos NS, Boyd KV, Coopersmith CM. Extracorporeal membrane oxygenation. Current clinical practice, coding, and reimbursement. *Chest.* 2008;134:179–184.

84. Field D, Davis C, Elbourne D, Grant A, Johnson A, Macrea D UK Collaborative ECMO Trial Group. UK laborative randomised trial of neonatal extracorporeal membrane oxygenation. *Lancet.* 1996;348:75–82.

85. Lewandowski K. Extracorporeal membrane oxygenation for severe acute respiratory failure. *Crit Care.* 2000;4:156–168.

86. Lennartz H. Extracorporeal lung assist in ARDS: history and state of the art. *Acta Anaesthesiol Scand Suppl.* 1996;109:114–116.

87. Hammell C, Forrest M, Barrett P. Clinical experience with a pumpless extracorporeal lung assist device. *Anesthesia.* 2008;63:1241–1244.

Chapter 33

Pulmonary surgery

KEY POINTS

- Surgical resection of lung tissue via a thoracotomy is a routine procedure, used mostly for treating lung cancer, which requires careful assessment of the patient's physiological reserve.
- Less invasive surgical techniques such as video-assisted thoracic surgery are increasing rapidly and associated with less physiological disturbance and complications.
- One-lung ventilation is required for many pulmonary surgery procedures and understanding of the physiology involved is vital for its safe use.
- Lung transplantation is an established technique for treating advanced lung disease, with chronic obstructive pulmonary disease currently being the most common indication.
- Lung transplant results in completely denervated lungs, which leaves the respiratory pattern unaffected but impairs the cough reflex.

In current clinical practice surgery of the lungs, mediastinum and chest wall is routinely performed, and although still high-risk by modern surgical standards the outcome for most patients is favourable. The physiological disturbances caused during and after pulmonary surgery are immense and in this chapter the effects of the more common pulmonary surgical procedures are outlined.

PHYSIOLOGICAL ASPECTS OF COMMON INTERVENTIONS

BRONCHOSCOPY

Bronchoscopy is performed frequently and allows direct visualisation of the airway and if necessary the collection of washings and biopsies of airway and lung tissue. It may also be used therapeutically to, for example, remove inhaled foreign bodies, resect tumours or place stents to overcome airway obstruction. Two types of bronchoscopy are performed:

Flexible bronchoscopy.[1] The flexibility of fibre-optic bronchoscopes allows a view of all the major branches of the tracheobronchial tree with minimal risk of trauma and discomfort for the patient. The procedure can therefore be performed without general anaesthesia, though extensive topical anaesthesia to the airway is required, and most clinicians also provide sedation to relieve the anxiety associated with having a bronchoscopy.[2] Hypoxia during a flexible bronchoscopy is common,[1] occurring in 17% of patients from one study,[2] and supplemental oxygen is therefore normally used. Lung function during bronchoscopy is significantly impaired. Whilst the bronchoscope is in place the functional residual capacity (FRC) is increased by 17%,[3] and forced vital capacity (FVC), forced expiratory volume in one second (FEV_1), and peak expiratory flow are all decreased,[4] indicating airflow obstruction. These observations are not explained simply by the presence of the bronchoscope in the airway, as the observed airway flow limitation begins after the airway local anaesthetic is applied (before insertion of the bronchoscope) and continues for several minutes after the bronchoscope has been removed, suggesting that a bronchoconstrictor action of the topical anaesthesia is responsible.[4] Respiratory depression may also occur during or soon after bronchoscopy, and the causes of this are uncertain but likely to relate either to the sedative drugs or the topical anaesthesia in the airway. The major limitation of flexible bronchoscopy is the size of the

DOI: 10.1016/B978-0-7020-2996-7.00033-7

instruments that may be passed down the broncho-scope, and though very suitable for visualisation of the airway and obtaining biopsies or washings, for removal of foreign bodies or airway surgery a larger portal for access to the tracheobronchial tree is required.

Rigid bronchoscopy. Straight, rigid, bronchoscopes are available with internal diameters up to 8 mm, and these may be passed into the trachea and a variety of instruments used through the bronchoscope. To see around corners in the bronchial tree 30- and 90-degree angled telescopes are used. With rigid bronchoscopy foreign bodies that are wedged in the airway can be removed, tracheal tumours resected, airway haemor-rhage treated, and stents deployed in the trachea or main bronchi to overcome stenosing tumours or air-way leaks. The major disadvantage of the technique is the requirement for general anaesthesia, often in a patient with significant respiratory disease.

Ventilation during a rigid bronchoscopy with general anaesthesia is a challenge and four main techniques may be used:[5]

1. Spontaneous ventilation. A ventilating bronchoscope allows the normal anaesthetic breathing system to be attached to a side port of the bronchoscope, which also must have a glass window to occlude its proximal lumen to prevent escape of the anaesthetic gases. With deep anaesthesia to suppress airway reflexes the patient may breathe during the procedure with anaesthesia maintained by inhalational or intravenous agents. Leaks around the bronchoscope are a problem, particularly if the surgeon wishes to pass instruments down the bronchoscope, so this technique is now only rarely used and usually in children in whom the small size of the cricoid cartilage minimises leakage of inhaled gases from around the bronchoscope.

2. Positive pressure ventilation. This form of ventilation may be achieved via a ventilating bronchoscope as described above, but once again the lack of a seal between the airway and bronchoscope makes the technique problematic. The most common technique used for ventilation is the Sanders injector, which is a high pressure oxygen supply (4 atmospheres) intermittently applied to the proximal end of the rigid bronchoscope through a small diameter 'injector'. As a result of the Venturi effect, the high velocity jet of oxygen entrains room air and increases the pressure along the bronchoscope causing lung inflation.

Anaesthesia must be maintained by intravenous agents, and adequacy of ventilation can only be assessed by observation of the chest rather than the usual capnography (page 174), but this technique does allow the surgeon to operate down the bronchoscope whilst the patient is being ventilated. The Sanders injector system for ventilation is problematic in patients with lung disease, as the inspired oxygen concentration and pulmonary inflation pressure that can be generated are highly variable, being influenced not only by the bronchoscope dimensions and side ports but also by the compliance and airway resistance of the patient's lungs.[6]

3. High frequency jet ventilation (page 473) may be used during bronchoscopy, and the ability of the technique to ventilate the lungs with minimal increase in airway pressure makes it particularly useful in patients with airway leaks such as bronchopleural fistulae.

4. Apnoeic oxygenation may be used during rigid bronchoscopy, but normally only as a last resort and for a short period of time – that is, until hypercapnia develops.

THORACOSCOPY

Insertion of a telescope through the chest wall into the pleural space allows direct inspection of the pleura, lungs, mediastinum and diaphragm to facil-itate diagnosis or therapeutic interventions. Three types of thoracoscopy exist:

1. Medical thoracoscopy.[7] This technique may be used to investigate pleural effusions or pneumothorax when less invasive interventions such as thoracocentesis have failed to reach a diagnosis. One or two ports are inserted into the chest in an awake or sedated patient using local anaesthesia in a similar way to insertion of a chest drain. In most cases the thoracoscope is being inserted into an existing pleural space, i.e. a pleural effusion or pneumothorax, so the physiological insult is less than may be imagined. Minor interventions such as biopsies, breaking down of pleural adhesions or talc pleurodesis (page 496) may be performed if accompanied by suitable analgesia.

2. Thoracoscopy using gas insufflation. This technique is usually performed under general anaesthesia and involves insertion of multiple ports and insufflation of carbon dioxide into the pleural space to create a com-partment in which the operation can be performed. The technique is mostly used by vascular surgeons to perform a sympathectomy of the upper limb.

Increasing the intrapleural pressure above atmospheric in this way effectively causes a tension pneumothorax (page 446) and it is therefore vital that the pressure used is both well-controlled and kept as low as possible (usually less than 10 mmHg).[8] Intermittent positive pressure ventilation of the lung on the operative side may be continued so minimising the effect of the capnothorax on gas exchange, and close monitoring allows any cardiovascular changes to be quickly corrected by releasing carbon dioxide from the chest cavity. Any carbon dioxide left in the pleura at the conclusion of surgery will be quickly reabsorbed (page 448). Despite the significant physiological hazards associated with this technique, mortality is believed to be low, and normally results from damage to lung or vasculature rather than from the insufflation of carbon dioxide.[9]

3. *Video-assisted thoracic surgery* (VATS) is a term used by thoracic surgeons to describe any operation that is facilitated by insertion of a video camera into the chest cavity. Usually a small thoracotomy is made, and the camera and operating instruments all passed through this small opening, though other ports may be inserted elsewhere in the chest wall. This procedure differs from a thoracoscopy as described above in that the chest cavity is open to the atmosphere so a positive intrathoracic pressure cannot occur. One-lung ventilation is therefore needed, and the lung on the operative side collapses under its own elastic recoil or has to be retracted by the surgeon. The small breach of the chest cavity required for VATS has numerous advantages compared with the effects of a thoracotomy (see below) and the technique is widely used for pleural surgery such as pleurodesis (page 496) and for intervention following a pneumothorax. Minor lung surgery such as wedge resections and lung biopsies are also suitable for a VATS approach, and though a lobectomy can be done in this way the operation remains controversial.[10]

THORACOTOMY

A surgical opening in the chest cavity was first used more than 100 years ago, usually for the treatment of empyema (page 448) and tuberculosis. In current surgical practice the indications for thoracotomy have widened to include surgery of the lungs, major vessels, oesophagus and thoracic spine. In most cases, thoracotomy is performed in the lateral position which has significant effects on respiratory physiology (see below) and through a postero-lateral incision. Thoracotomy includes division of the muscles

exterior to the ribcage and entering the pleura, usually through the 5th intercostal space, by separating the intercostal muscles from the rib. The rib adjacent to the thoracotomy is commonly divided or a piece of rib resected to improve access and to minimise rib fractures when the chest wall is retracted.

The effects of thoracotomy on postoperative respiratory function are profound, with significant reductions in chest wall compliance and respiratory muscle activity[11] resulting from chest wall oedema, pain, disruption of muscle anatomy, and later in the recovery phase scarring of chest wall tissues. In the first 24 hours following surgery, FVC and FEV_1 are only 30–50% of the preoperative volumes, with some evidence that the type of thoracotomy incision used may affect these values.[12] Chest wall compliance falls to around 60% of the preoperative value by the third postoperative day before slowly improving.[13] At one week after surgery, FVC and FEV_1 are around 70–80% of preoperative values, and by this stage the different incisions seem to have little effect on recovery.[14,15]

Other measures of respiratory muscle strength such as maximum inspiratory and expiratory mouth pressures are also reduced to about half the preoperative values following thoracotomy, and in one study had not returned to normal 12 weeks after surgery.[16] The same study showed a rapid return to normal of both measures of muscle function following VATS procedures. Older patients, who have poor respiratory muscle strength relative to younger patients, took longer to recover muscle function following surgery, possibly explaining the greater incidence of pulmonary complications with increasing age. Thoracotomy alone therefore impairs respiratory muscle function to such an extent that ventilation may not be able to keep pace with the extra ventilatory requirements associated with having major surgery, and alveolar hypoventilation can occur along with regional pulmonary collapse and impaired oxygenation. Even in patients less severely affected the ability to cough is always weakened with an increased risk of chest complications.[11] For patients who have a lung resection through their thoracotomy, lung compliance is also decreased to about half their preoperative value, compounding the above problems.[13]

Considering the surgical trauma associated with thoracotomy, it is unsurprising that there is commonly severe pain in the postoperative period. Damage to somatic nerves supplying the skin and chest wall structures is exacerbated by trauma to the visceral nerves supplying the pleura and possibly by involvement of the sympathetic chain in the chest cavity. Because all three of these nerve pathways may be involved, treatment of acute postoperative pain is challenging, with multimodal treatment regimes being required. However, of more significance to the patient is the observation that following a thoracotomy almost half of patients develop a chronic pain syndrome, the pathophysiology of which remains unknown, though genetic and psychological factors are believed to be important contributors.[17]

LUNG RESECTION

Assessing patient fitness for lung resection.[18,19] Lung function is assessed using either the FEV_1, or, if the patient has parenchymal lung disease, the diffusing capacity for carbon monoxide (DL_{CO}, page 153). If these are less than 80% of normal predicted values for that patient, an attempt is made to calculate predicted postoperative values based on which anatomical sections of lung need to be removed. Radionucleotide ventilation or perfusion scans or quantitative computerised tomography scans may all be used to measure functional lung units, and are useful techniques as they also show which pathological lung units are already not contributing to overall function. Less invasive is the anatomical method in which the lungs are divided into 19 anatomical segments of equal value, and knowing which segments are to be removed enables estimation of postoperative predicted lung function. For many years a general rule of lung resection was that a predicted postoperative FEV_1 of less than 0.8–1.0 l precluded resection, though evidence for this rule is poor. Using an absolute value for FEV_1 or DL_{CO} is fraught with difficulties as sex, age and height all affect the normal values, and decisions should now always be based on the values as a percentage of the predicted normal for that patient.

Different studies have produced varied results on the association between percentage predicted postoperative FEV_1 or DL_{CO} and outcome, but a value of less than 40% of predicted normal is now generally accepted as being associated with an increased mortality and complication rate. For patients in this situation, measurement of preoperative exercise tolerance has the advantage of also including a cardiovascular component to the assessment and may help to further define risks and outcomes. The most objective way of quantifying exercise activity is by measuring VO_{2max} (page 262). Values of less than 15 ml.min^{-1}.kg^{-1} are again associated with poor outcome. Clinical measures of exercise tolerance have some value, but these

must be performed under supervision as patients' own reported exercise tolerance is normally greatly exaggerated. Tests which have some limited use in predicting outcome after lung resection include the shuttle test (number of times a patient can walk between two markers 10 m apart), 6-minute walk test (distance able to walk within 6 minutes) and stair climbing (the number of stairs or height of stairs the patient is able to climb[20]).

Partial lung resection. The magnitude of lung resection operations varies greatly from removal of a small tumour in the lung periphery to a complete pneumonectomy, with the more minor procedures being performed via VATS and the more major via a thoracotomy. Wherever possible, dissection is made between lobes or in intersegmental planes. Great care is required when operating on pulmonary vessels, particularly pulmonary arteries which have thin walls and are easy to damage, resulting in significant haemorrhage that may be difficult to control. The use of staple systems has made the closure of vessels, bronchi and the resection of lung tissue technically much easier and less hazardous than manual suturing of these structures.

Following lung resection, the remaining lung in the hemithorax quickly expands to fill the available space. Two chest drains are usually placed in the chest cavity and connected to underwater seal systems to allow any air or blood to drain. If the remaining lung does not fully expand, a negative pressure of up to 20 cmH$_2$O may be applied to the drains to encourage the lung to expand.

Pneumonectomy. Resection of an entire lung is usually performed for removal of large, central lung tumours (Figure 33.1A). Following pneumonectomy correct management of the empty hemithorax is crucial. If air is drained from the cavity too quickly mediastinal shift will occur which impairs venous drainage to the heart and can cause cardiovascular collapse. The most common practice is therefore to leave no drain in the chest cavity, and monitor the position of the mediastinum daily with a chest X-ray. Alternatively, a chest drain can be placed (Figure 33.1B), but be clamped for most of the time and only released briefly and intermittently to ensure the pressure in the cavity is approximately atmospheric. A more interventional approach is to measure the pressure in the chest cavity and instill or remove air to maintain a pressure of −2 to −4 cmH$_2$O on inspiration and +2 to +4 cmH$_2$O on expiration. Within a few weeks of pneumonectomy the volume of the hemithorax decreases due to a combination of mediastinal shift, elevation of the diaphragm, and contraction of

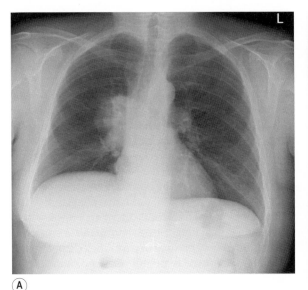

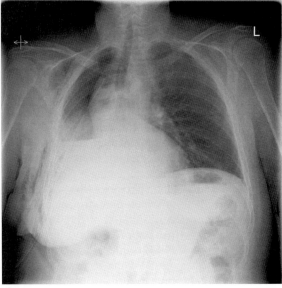

(A)

(B)

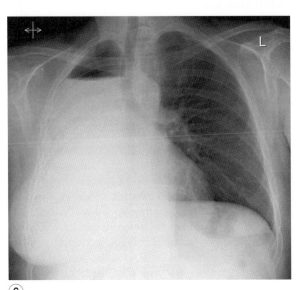

(C)

Fig. 33.1 (A) Chest radiograph showing large lung cancer at the right hilum. (B) The same patient 24 hours after a right pneumonectomy. Note the shifted trachea and mediastinum, contracted right thoracic cage, and early accumulation of fluid in the empty hemithorax. (C) One month later, with the empty hemithorax already almost completely filled with fluid and a hyper-expanded left lung.

the chest wall, and pleural fluid replaces the air in the chest cavity (Figure 33.1C). Over the ensuing months or years, the fluid volume decreases as the mediastinal shift continues, and the other lung herniates anteriorly or posteriorly across the midline to partially fill the vacated hemithorax. Complete replacement of the fluid is however unusual.

Recent studies in animals have demonstrated the intriguing phenomenon of 'neoalveolarisation' following lung resection.[21] Within 20 days of lung resection in mice the number of alveoli in the remaining lung increased by 50%, completely restoring the gas exchanging surface area.[22] Neoalveolarisation probably occurs by new alveoli forming in the walls of existing alveolar ducts and respiratory bronchioles, and is so far only described in young animals, as would be expected from the observation that in mammals formation of alveoli is a post-natal process (page 250). It therefore remains only a distant prospect that adult patients will be able to grow new lung tissue after lung resection.

Lung injury following pneumonectomy.[23,24] Acute lung injury (Chapter 31) is a serious complication that occurs in the postoperative period in between 2.5% and 9% of pneumonectomies, and more rarely follows smaller lung resections such as lobectomy. Mortality is high, with a quarter of patients dying, though this is an improvement compared with only a few years ago. The pathophysiology of post-pneumonectomy acute lung injury is controversial, with perioperative fluid overload being viewed by many clinicians as the main cause, though the pathophysiology is now better elucidated and far more complex than simply administering excessive volumes of intravenous fluid. High-protein pulmonary oedema develops approximately 24 hours postoperatively, and is believed to result from endothelial cell injury in the pulmonary capillaries. How this initial injury occurs is less clear, though the increased capillary blood flow in the remaining lung is likely to cause stretching of endothelial cells or excessive shear forces in the vessels, both of which may disrupt the intercellular junctions. Overdistension of the lung either during surgery with inappropriately large tidal volumes[25] or use of PEEP, or following surgery with sub-optimal management of the contralateral chest cavity may all contribute to further disruption of the alveolar–capillary barrier.[23] Once this initial lung injury has occurred, many other factors will then affect the severity of the clinical picture and its management, including fluid administration, inspired oxygen levels and the ventilation strategy, all of which should follow the same principles as for the management of ALI whatever the cause (Chapter 31).

SURGERY FOR CHRONIC OBSTRUCTIVE PULMONARY DISEASE (COPD)[26]

Surgical treatment is reserved for patients with severe COPD in whom emphysematous changes predominate. When the airspaces created in emphysema become larger than 1 cm in diameter they are referred to as a 'bulla'. Nearby bullae can merge and result in extremely large air spaces, occupying up to one-third of the lung volume. Like emphysema, bullae have little effect on gas exchange as both tidal ventilation and blood flow to the bulla are negligible. However, with giant bullae the airspace acts in a similar fashion to a pneumothorax (page 445) and compresses surrounding lung tissue, causing further worsening of airway collapse and subsequent disturbance of gas exchange. In these cases surgical treatment involves 'bullectomy', and with careful patient selection this can be a useful operation. Improved surgical techniques led to a resurgence of interest in surgery for COPD and extended the indications to include patients who do not have bullae.

Lung volume reduction surgery (LVRS) involves removing 20–30% of lung volume, to include the most emphysematous areas, and can have impressive results. Improved long-term survival compared with best medical therapy has only been proven in patients with poor exercise capacity and upper lobe emphysema,[27,28] and conversely, patients with high exercise capacity and emphysema elsewhere in the lung have a higher mortality following surgery compared with medical treatment. Despite these mixed survival results, in appropriately selected groups of patients LVRS can improve exercise capacity,[27,29] lung volumes, quality of life[30] and arterial Po_2.[31] Understanding of the physiological mechanisms leading to clinical improvements remains incomplete. Potential benefits of LVRS include reduced pulmonary collapse adjacent to emphysematous areas, improved elastic recoil of the remaining lung tissue, and better respiratory muscle function, particularly of the diaphragm,[32] secondary to reduced hyperinflation (see Figure 6.1).

PLEURODESIS[33]

Pleurodesis describes a variety of procedures, all of which aim to induce adhesions between the visceral and parietal pleura. The two most common indications are pneumothorax that has failed to respond to conservative management (page 456) or palliation of malignant pleural effusion. Though the preferred technique varies with the indication, the success of any pleurodesis depends upon inducing inflammation in the pleura whilst simultaneously ensuring the two pleural layers are closely apposed, so allowing the normal inflammation and tissue repair processes to cause scarring in the pleural space. Apposition of the pleura is usually achieved by using a pleural drain, but if required an inflammatory reaction in the pleura can be initiated by various means. A pleurectomy may be performed, with the parietal pleura being simply stripped from the inside of the chest wall, or a less traumatic technique is pleural abrasion in which the pleura is rubbed with a dry gauze or other abrasive surface. Alternatively, sclerosants can be instilled into the pleural cavity, including antibiotics (e.g. doxycycline), antiseptics (e.g. iodopovidone), anticancer drugs or minerals such as talc. Talc pleurodesis is the most common technique, and the talc may either be instilled as a slurry through a small pleural catheter to avoid surgical intervention, or as a dry powder (poudrage) via a surgical approach. Recent work has identified the importance of the particle size of talc in the development of adverse effects from talc pleurodesis.[34] Talc particles have been found to enter the lung parenchyma or systemic circulation following pleurodesis, risking the development of pulmonary fibrosis or systemic inflammation respectively. Use of particle sizes greater than 5μm reduces the complication rate, presumably because the talc particles are unable to pass through the similarly-sized stoma in the pleura (page 445) to gain access to the lymphatics and circulation.

Obliterating the pleura by these techniques may be expected to cause long-term impairment of lung function, but after an initial decline immediately after the procedure, total lung capacity returns to normal approximately 6 months later.[35] This is in keeping with the bizarre observation, first discovered in the 1700s, that elephants have no pleural space with connective tissue binding their lungs tightly to the inside of the chest wall, with no apparent long-term ill effects for the species.[36]

Table 33.1 Indications for one-lung ventilation[37]

ABSOLUTE INDICATIONS	RELATIVE INDICATIONS
Isolation of lung to avoid cross contamination:	*Surgical exposure*:
Lung abscess	Thoracic aortic surgery
Massive haemorrhage	Pneumonectomy
Unilateral ventilation:	Lung resection
Bronchopleural fistula	Thoracoscopy
Giant lung cyst or bulla	Oesophagectomy
Tracheobronchial tree disruption	Thoracic spine surgery
Intensive care:	*Intensive care*:
Life threatening hypoxia from unilateral lung disease	Severe hypoxia from unilateral lung disease

ONE-LUNG VENTILATION

Many of the surgical procedures already described will be facilitated by apnoea of the operative lung during surgery. These, and other indications for one-lung ventilation (OLV), are shown in Table 33.1. Indications are divided into absolute, where without OLV the patient's life is at risk, and relative, when OLV will help manage the patient's condition but is not mandatory.

LUNG ISOLATION TECHNIQUES

Isolation of one lung requires knowledge of some anatomical features of the large airways. First, the angle at which the right and left main bronchi branch from the trachea is highly variable, being on average 25° from the vertical for the right main bronchus and 45° for the left (Figure 33.2). There is however wide individual variation in these angles both in health and disease,[38] but the right main bronchus is almost always at the less acute angle. Second, the distance between the carina and the first segmental bronchus is normally 5 cm in the left main bronchus and only 2.5 cm in the right, making occlusion of the right upper lobe a possibility when a cuffed tube is in the right main bronchus.

There are three options available to isolate one lung:[37]

1. Endobronchial tube. This involves placement of a small diameter cuffed endotracheal tube into the main bronchus of the lung that needs to remain ventilated (Figure 33.2A). Endobronchial intubation,

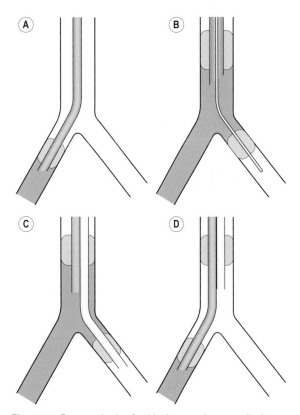

Fig. 33.2 Four methods of achieving one-lung ventilation of the right lung. (A) Single lumen endobronchial tube in the right main bronchus. (B) Bronchial blocker passed through a standard tracheal tube into the left main bronchus. (C) Left sided double-lumen tube with ventilation via the tracheal lumen. (D) Right sided double-lumen tube with ventilation via the bronchial lumen. In each case the blue area shows where ventilation is occurring.

usually of the right main bronchus, is a common accidental occurrence when tracheal tubes are advanced too far into the airway. Deliberate endobronchial intubation is rarely used due to the difficulties of positioning the tube in the correct side (though this may be facilitated by passing the tube over a flexible bronchoscope) and because the technique does not allow ventilation of the other lung without repositioning the tube.

2. Bronchial blockers. A bronchial blocker is a narrow catheter with a balloon at the tip, which may be inserted through a standard tracheal tube into the main bronchus of the lung requiring isolation and the cuff intermittently inflated to block gas flow into that lung (Figure 33.2B). A variety of techniques are available to direct the blocker into the required main bronchus, including blockers with angled tips and guidewires that loop around a bronchoscope allowing the blocker to be guided along the bronchoscope once this is in the correct position. Bronchial blockers have the advantage of being placed through a standard tracheal tube, and the cuff is small compared with a double lumen tube so is less likely to occlude segmental bronchi. Bronchial blockers also have several disadvantages, mostly arising from the small lumen of the device, such as an inability to suction the non-ventilated lung and slow collapse of the non-ventilated lung, though this can be accelerated by use of 100% oxygen immediately before lung isolation (page 502).

3. Double lumen tubes (DLT). This is the most common technique for lung isolation, and the correct position for both left and right DLTs is shown in Figure 33.2C and D respectively. A variety of designs have been developed over the years, all aimed at easing the passage of these quite large tubes through the upper airway and larynx whilst increasing the likelihood of the bronchial tube entering the required side. The advantageous angle of the right main bronchus means right sided DLTs are more likely to enter the correct bronchus, but the close proximity of the right upper lobe bronchus means these tubes usually have modified bronchial cuff shapes to minimise the chances of occlusion of the right upper lobe. Use of a left sided DLT avoids this problem but then the risk of the tube entering the incorrect bronchus is increased. Once correctly sited, irrespective of whether a right or left sided DLT has been used, both lungs can be ventilated or suction catheters passed independently, and the two lungs are isolated from each other to prevent cross contamination with blood or infectious secretions.

PHYSIOLOGY OF ONE–LUNG VENTILATION[39,40]

Despite OLV now being a routine technique in many situations, hypoxia still occurs commonly. A detailed understanding of the physiology of OLV is therefore vital if a logical approach to management is to be adopted. First, the factors that influence lung function during OLV will be considered.

Patient position

Though OLV may be required in a supine patient, the lateral position is most commonly used for thoracic surgery and this position significantly affects ventilation and perfusion of the lungs. The loss of muscle tone in the chest wall and diaphragm associated with general anaesthesia (page 333) causes gravity to affect the volumes of the left and right hemithoraces. The volume of the dependent lung is decreased by the weight of the mediastinum above and by cephalad movement of the diaphragm from the weight of the abdominal contents. Table 8.1 (page 120) shows the distribution of FRC and ventilation in the left and right lungs in both lateral positions when anaesthetised. FRC in the dependent lung is approximately one litre less than the non-dependent lung, and inevitably, under general anaesthesia, atelectasis forms in the dependent lung (Figure 33.3).[41] 'Breaking' the operating table to open the intercostal space on the operative side of the chest will further compress the dependent lung.

These changes in lung volume affect the position of each lung on a regional compliance curve. In a spontaneously breathing awake patient in the lateral position, the lower lung is on a steeper part of the compliance curve than the non-dependent lung and therefore receives more ventilation (Figure 33.4A). Dependent lung ventilation is also enhanced by the cephalad movement of the lower diaphragm increasing its efficiency. When anaesthetised, paralysed and ventilated in the lateral position the effect of the diaphragm position is lost, and the reduction of FRC for both lungs causes the non-dependent lung to reside in the steep middle part of a compliance curve and it is this lung that now receives approximately 60% of ventilation (Figure 33.4B). Due to the larger volume of the right lung, these considerations are affected by which side the patient is on, with a larger differential FRC and ventilation when the left lung is dependent. Perfusion of the dependent lung is always greater

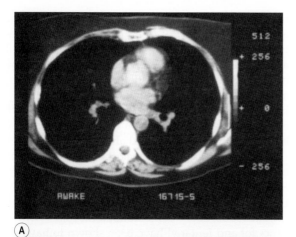

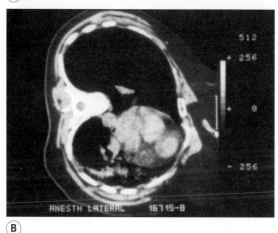

Fig. 33.3 Computerised tomography scans during anaesthesia in the lateral position. (A) Patient awake in the supine position. (B) Patient anaesthetised and turned into the left lateral position. Note the position of the mediastinum and the atelectasis in the left lung. Scans kindly provided by Prof. G. Hedenstierna.

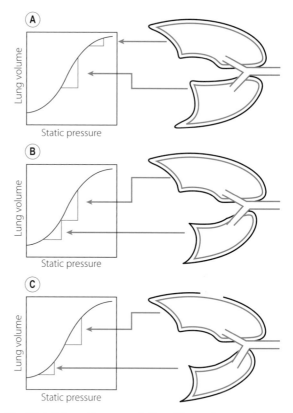

Fig. 33.4 Schematic representation of lung volumes and regional compliance in the right lateral position. (A) Awake patient, spontaneously breathing. The non-dependent (left) lung has a higher FRC than in the supine position so is at a less favourable part of the compliance curve and the dependent (right) lung will receive relatively more ventilation. (B) Anaesthetised and paralysed patient in the same position. The loss of muscle activity in the diaphragm and chest wall reduces FRC in both lungs and the weight of the mediastinum compresses the dependent lung. This changes their position on the compliance curve, and the non-dependent (left) lung is now the better ventilated. (C) Same situation with the chest open. Loss of the negative pleural pressure of the non-dependent lung causes further mediastinal shift, further compromising the function of the dependent lung. In the left lateral position the same physiological changes occur, but the impact is greater when the smaller left lung is the dependent one.

THE OPEN CHEST

Allowing air to enter the pleural space of the non-dependent lung will exacerbate the changes described so far. The negative intrapleural pressure of the upper hemithorax in effect holds up the mediastinum, and when this is lost the full weight of the heart and other mediastinal structures further compresses the

than the non-dependent lung in the lateral position, and this differential is mostly uninfluenced by anaesthesia and paralysis. Thus the ventilation/perfusion ratios of the lung are well matched when in the lateral position and awake, but anaesthesia and artificial ventilation in this position results in significant mismatch with greater ventilation of the non-dependent lung associated with greater perfusion of the dependent lung.

Ceasing ventilation of the non-dependent lung therefore removes the better ventilated lung, leaving the challenge of ventilating the low volume, low-compliance dependent lung, but also removes the larger part of the $\dot{V}/\dot{Q}$ mismatch.

dependent lung (Figure 33.4C). This effect will occur whether the pleura is open to the atmosphere, or if gases have been insufflated into the chest cavity to facilitate surgery, and the effect of a positive intrapleural pressure, as sometimes used in thoracoscopic surgery, will be even more significant. With a thoracotomy, the compliance of the chest wall is in effect removed, and only lung compliance (page 27) will determine ventilation of the non-dependent lung, which will be free to expand to a large volume if ventilation of both lungs continues.

Perfusion of the non–ventilated lung

Once ventilation of the non-dependent lung ceases, matching of ventilation to perfusion becomes almost entirely dependent on the amount of blood flowing through the apnoeic non-dependent lung. Factors affecting pulmonary vascular resistance are described in detail in Chapter 7 and include passive factors such as gravity and lung volume, and active control of pulmonary blood vessel size. During OLV the effect of gravity depends on patient position: in the lateral position perfusion of the upper lung will be reduced, but this will not be the case if OLV is used in the supine position. As a result of this relatively high blood flow in the supine position oxygenation is more often impaired than during OLV in the lateral position.[42] Pulmonary vascular resistance (PVR) is minimal at FRC (see Figure 7.4) so a small reduction in pulmonary blood will occur when the non-ventilated lung collapses towards residual volume. Surgical manipulation of the lung is also likely to reduce its blood flow either by distorting and so occluding pulmonary vasculature or by direct clamping of pulmonary vessels as part of the surgical procedure.

Of the many mechanisms involved in active control of PVR (see Table 7.1) it is hypoxic pulmonary vasoconstriction (HPV, page 108) that is believed to be the most important determinant of pulmonary blood flow in the non-ventilated lung. The 40–50% of cardiac output that would be expected to flow through the non-ventilated lung is believed to be reduced to 20–30% by hypoxic pulmonary vasoconstriction.[39] The passive increase in PVR as a result of reduced lung volume is thought to be small in comparison with the effect of HPV – if during OLV the non-ventilated lung is reinflated and ventilated with nitrogen the blood flow to the lung is unaffected, but performing the same manoeuvre with oxygen increases the blood flow to normal.[43] How much HPV occurs is influenced by both alveolar and mixed venous Po_2 (see Figure 7.8), so changes in cardiac output or oxygen consumption that will affect venous Po_2 may influence blood flow to the non-ventilated lung. A fall in mixed venous Po_2 enhances the HPV response, and an abnormally high mixed venous Po_2 may have the opposite effect as oxygen diffuses from the alveolar capillary blood into the non-ventilated alveoli.[43]

The effect of general anaesthesia on HPV has been controversial for some years (see page 346).[39,44] Results from in-vitro or animal studies have shown that all inhalational anaesthetic agents, including nitrous oxide, cause some inhibition of HPV whilst propofol and fentanyl have been shown to have no effect. Translating these observations into clinical practice is problematic due to the numerous other factors that may affect HPV such as:

- Cardiac output, which is reduced by most general anaesthetic drugs. A fall in cardiac output will reduce blood flow through both shunt and normal regions of lung (page 134) and decrease the mixed venous Po_2, which will affect HPV as described above.

- Individual variation in the HPV response is large and difficult to predict. Evidence for this is seen at high altitude, where varying degrees of HPV between individuals affects their likelihood of developing pulmonary oedema (page 286).

- Non-anaesthetic drugs, particularly vasoactive drugs. Vasodilators such as calcium channel blockers (which are commonly taken by patients having thoracic surgery) are known to attenuate the HPV response. Conversely, routinely used vasoconstrictors such as phenylephrine may preferentially constrict pulmonary vessels in normoxic lung regions.[39]

- Pa_{CO_2} and alkalosis. Hypocapnia or metabolic alkalosis may attenuate HPV whilst hypercapnia and acidosis have the opposite effect. Thus any abnormality of Pa_{CO_2} or acid–base balance may adversely affect relative blood flow between the two lungs during OLV.

- Epidural analgesia is widely used during thoracic surgery and has been described as enhancing the HPV response, but this observation is also likely to be indirectly mediated by changes in the systemic circulation.[45]

- Temperature affects HPV, with animal studies showing an attenuated response during hypothermia and vice versa.[46]

Clinical studies of OLV using various anaesthetic agents have failed to show any consistent differences between anaesthetic techniques. Inhalational anaesthetic agents used at clinically appropriate doses of around 1 MAC produce similar degrees of impaired oxygenation as intravenous anaesthetic techniques,[39] particularly if depth of anaesthesia with the two techniques is equivalent.[47] Thoracic epidural anaesthesia has also been shown to have no effect on oxygenation during OLV irrespective of whether the technique is used with intravenous or inhalational general anaesthesia.[48]

Pharmacological enhancement of HPV can be used to improve oxygenation during OLV. Inhaled nitric oxide (page 111) may be used to improve blood flow to the ventilated lung, though the expected improvement in oxygenation only seems to occur in patients who are already hypoxic or who have existing pulmonary hypertension.[49] Almitrine is a systemically administered peripheral chemoreceptor agonist that can enhance HPV and so improve oxygenation during OLV.[50] Its effects are dose-dependent, and if the dose is too high then generalised pulmonary vasoconstriction occurs, rather than only in hypoxic regions, and pulmonary hypertension and a greater shunt fraction occurs. These two potential therapeutic techniques are therefore not yet in routine clinical use.

MANAGEMENT OF ONE-LUNG VENTILATION

The aim of ventilation during OLV is to maintain arterial Po_2 and Pco_2 as near normal as possible and is achieved by maintaining adequate alveolar ventilation while minimising the amount of shunt through the non-ventilated lung. Understanding of the physiology already described allows a logical approach to management.

Artificial ventilation during OLV

If alveolar minute volume during OLV is maintained at similar values as when ventilating two lungs, then CO_2 elimination is also maintained, though achieving adequate alveolar ventilation, particularly in diseased lungs, may be a significant challenge. The traditional technique is to use smaller tidal volumes than two lung ventilation at a faster respiratory rate, the latter being adjusted to achieve normal end-tidal or arterial Pco_2 values. Reducing tidal volume increases the anatomical dead space (page 130) so significant increases in respiratory rate may be needed to maintain alveolar ventilation. If respiratory rate is too fast, intrinsic PEEP (page 476) may occur and cause overexpansion of the dependent lung, increasing airway pressures and reducing blood flow through the dependent lung leading to a worsening of shunt and oxygenation. This is a particular risk in patients with increased airway resistance of any cause. The optimum size of tidal volume to use for OLV remains controversial.[51,52] Use of a standard two lung ventilation value of 10–15 ml.kg^{-1} will commonly lead to unacceptably high airway pressures, may over-distend alveoli (potentially damaging the lung), cause increased pulmonary vascular resistance (so increasing shunt) and contribute to postoperative lung injury.[25] If small tidal volumes are used such as 5–8 ml.kg^{-1} then alveolar ventilation will be difficult to maintain and atelectasis more likely to occur. Finally, the addition of PEEP to the ventilated lung during OLV seems like a logical response to its reduced lung volume and propensity to develop atelectasis, but PEEP will also increase the pulmonary vascular resistance of the dependent lung and potentially worsen the shunt. Thus numerous studies have reported conflicting results concerning the benefit of dependent lung PEEP on oxygenation during OLV.[39]

So tidal volume, respiratory rate and PEEP each have opposing and undesirable effects at extreme values, risking either inadequate alveolar ventilation with hypoxia or hypercapnia at one extreme, or lung damage that may result in acute lung injury of the ventilated lung at the other. Suggested optimal ventilator settings for OLV have followed the debate regarding ventilation in patients with acute lung injury, who share the challenge of having only a small functional lung (page 457). The suggested 'protective ventilation' strategy requires low tidal volumes of 6–8 ml.kg^{-1} used in conjunction with low levels of PEEP (5 cmH$_2$O), and has been shown to improve oxygenation and reduce the systemic inflammatory response associated with OLV.[53] In addition, this strategy may be more effective with pressure controlled ventilation compared with volume controlled ventilation.[54] Finally, when calculating the required tidal volume an a per kg basis, calculated lean body weight should be used in obese patients rather than total weight. Lung size is more closely related to height rather than weight, and application of a 'per kg' tidal volume in some of today's very obese patients will risk volutrauma to the ventilated lung.

Use of a high inspired oxygen fraction (FI_{O_2}) during OLV is routine to maximise oxygenation of blood in areas of lung with low, but greater than zero, $\dot{V}/\dot{Q}$ ratios. Use of 100% oxygen may risk encouraging atelectasis formation in a lung with an already reduced lung volume (page 336). Conversely, as described above, achievement of a high mixed venous PO_2 may reduce pulmonary vascular resistance in the ventilated lung and so reduce shunt fraction.

As for two-lung ventilation (page 336) a recruitment manoeuvre can be performed during OLV to re-expand atelectasis in the dependent lung, a strategy that has been shown to decrease dead space and improve oxygenation.[55] The recruitment manoeuvre described for OLV involves volume controlled ventilation with a respiratory rate of 12 breaths per minute and inspiratory time of 50%. Every 5 breaths the tidal volume and PEEP are then increased to achieve peak inspiratory pressures and PEEP values (respectively) of 30/10, 35/15 and 40/20, these last settings being maintained for 10 breaths before reducing the settings in the same stepwise manner.

Management of the non–ventilated lung[39]

In some patients no action needs to be taken with the non-ventilated lung which can be allowed to collapse, following which gas exchange will remain acceptable. Sadly this is often not the case. Given that the most likely cause of hypoxia during OLV is shunt through the non-ventilated lung the first approach should be to minimise this blood flow. Ventilation with 100% oxygen before isolating the lung causes it to collapse more quickly, and although in theory this will delay the onset of HPV there were no adverse effects on oxygenation 10 minutes after lung isolation in a clinical study.[56] As described above, encouraging the surgeon to manipulate the lung, or if appropriate to clamp the pulmonary vessels, are direct ways of reducing non-ventilated lung perfusion. Facilitating effective HPV by avoiding the various factors described above that attenuate the response should be routine practice. The second approach is to accept that shunt through the non-ventilated lung is inevitable and to oxygenate this blood by apnoeic oxygenation. Insufflation of a few litres per minute of oxygen at zero end-expiratory pressure (ZEEP) may be effective, but care must be taken to ensure there is a route for gas to flow back out of the non-ventilated lung to avoid lung expansion or even barotrauma.

Using ZEEP, the lung will continue to collapse and the oxygen will therefore not gain access to those areas of lung where the shunt is occurring. A more effective technique is to apply CPAP to the non-ventilated lung which delivers 100% oxygen, limits the maximum pressure that can be attained in the lung, and reduces the amount of lung collapse that occurs. Applying 5–10 cmH$_2$O of CPAP has been shown to not inflate the lung sufficiently to interfere with surgery and to be very effective at improving oxygenation. The timing of the application of CPAP may be important as it will be less effective if lung collapse has already occurred, in which case, provided the surgery permits, the lung may be briefly reinflated and the CPAP applied during the deflation phase.

SUMMARY OF THE CLINICAL MANAGEMENT OF OLV

Prior to commencing OLV initial ventilator settings:
- FI_{O_2} of 0.6 to 0.8
- respiratory rate 15
- pressure controlled ventilation, with inflation pressure adjusted to achieve tidal volume of 6–8 ml.kg^{-1}
- PEEP of 5–10 cmH$_2$O.

If hypoxia occurs:
- establish that the double lumen tube position is still correct and that ventilation of the non-ventilated lung is still occurring with the required gas mixture
- administer 100% oxygen and 5–10 cmH$_2$O of CPAP to the non-ventilated lung, after a single inflation of the lung if surgery permits.

If hypoxia continues:
- perform a recruitment manoeuvre of the dependent lung
- ensure cardiac output is not reduced
- consider whether the blood flow to the non-ventilated lung can be clamped, or the surgery performed with intermittent two-lung ventilation.

LUNG TRANSPLANTATION

Transplantation of a human lung was first performed in 1963,[57] but in the years following this few patients survived for longer than a month.

In the early 1980s improved immunosuppression led to a resurgence of interest and the technique has now become an established form of treatment. The function of a transplanted lung is important for the well-being of the recipient, but also furthers our understanding of certain fundamental issues of pulmonary physiology. The subject has been reviewed recently.[58-63]

CLINICAL ASPECTS[64]

Indications

Patients who are considered for transplant have severe respiratory disease, and are receiving optimal therapy, but still have a life expectancy of less than 2–3 years. Uncontrolled respiratory infection, significant disease of other organs, continued smoking or an age in excess of 55–65 years are normally contraindications. Precise selection criteria for recipients vary between transplant centres and with the respiratory disease, but in general patients referred for transplant have a forced expiratory volume in one second (FEV_1) of less than 30% predicted, resting hypoxia, hypercapnia and commonly pulmonary hypertension. The indications for lung transplant are shown in Table 33.2, where it can be seen that COPD remains the most common.

The number of patients awaiting transplant exceeds the number of donors. In recent years the number of donor organs available has remained static while the number of candidates for lung transplants has risen rapidly.[62] As a result, median waiting time for an organ to become available has increased, and many patients still die while on the waiting list. Cadaveric donor lungs are taken from patients less than 65 years of age with limited smoking history and no evidence of lung disease. Using current selection criteria only about 15% of organ donors are suitable for lung donation. Strategies to improve the number of lung transplants being performed include living-related lobar transplants (see below), extending donor selection criteria using more objective tests of lung function,[66] or using non-heartbeating donors.[67] This last approach potentially offers unique advantages for lung donation, as oxygenation of the donor lung after cessation of circulation can conserve lung function for up to an hour, and in future this may be extended further by ex-vivo ventilation and perfusion of the lung.[62]

Types of transplant

Donor and recipient chest sizes are matched. With current organ preservation solutions, lung transplants must be performed within 6–8 hours of organ removal.

Single lung transplant is the simplest procedure. The recipient's pneumonectomy is undertaken via a thoracotomy using one-lung ventilation (page 497), which presents a significant challenge in these patients.[68] The donor lung is implanted, with anastomoses of the main bronchus, the left or right pulmonary artery and a ring of left atrium containing both pulmonary veins of one side. Cardiopulmonary bypass is required in some cases, particularly those patients with preoperative pulmonary hypertension who are at risk of right-sided heart failure during one-lung ventilation.

Table 33.2 Indications for lung transplantation and the type of operation performed

INDICATION	TOTAL NUMBER	OPERATIONS PERFORMED FOR EACH INDICATION		
		HEART–LUNG (%)	BILATERAL (%)	SINGLE (%)
COPD	7282	1.3	36.2	62.5
α_1-antitrypsin deficiency	1561	3.3	55.4	41.3
Idiopathic pulmonary fibrosis	4041	1.8	36.4	61.8
Cystic fibrosis	3572	9.9	85.4	4.7
Primary pulmonary hypertension	1322	47.9	47.0	5.1
Congenital heart disease	1024	84.9	13.5	1.7

Bilateral lung transplant includes double-lung and bilateral single-lung procedures.
Data are from the Registry of the International Society for Heart and Lung Transplantation,[65] and include transplants performed worldwide between 1995 and June 2007 for the indications shown.

Bilateral lung transplant comes in two forms. Double-lung transplant performed at a single operation is a more complex procedure for which sternotomy and cardiopulmonary bypass are required. The donor lungs are implanted with anastomoses of either the trachea or both bronchi, the main pulmonary artery and the posterior part of the left atrium containing all four pulmonary veins. A simpler alternative is to transplant two lungs sequentially (termed a double single-lung transplant) through bilateral thoracotomies, and this has now almost completely replaced double-lung transplant.

Heart–lung transplant was originally used for patients with primary pulmonary hypertension and Eisenmenger's syndrome, and continues to be the operation of choice for the latter (Table 33.2). Total cardiopulmonary bypass is, of course, essential and the anastomoses involve the right atrium, the aorta and the trachea. The complexity and complication rates of heart–lung transplant are high, and, wherever possible, alternative procedures are now preferred, leading to a decline in the number of heart–lung transplant procedures being performed.[65]

Choice of operation depends on the indication for the transplant, and types of surgery performed are shown in Table 33.2. Single-lung transplantation is favoured, partly because mortality may be lower following this operation, but also because each suitable donor can be used to transplant two recipients. Congenital heart disease commonly requires heart–lung transplant, whilst diseases associated with pulmonary hypertension ideally need either heart–lung transplant or bilateral lung transplant to normalise pulmonary arterial pressure. Lung disease alone is satisfactorily treated with single-lung transplant.

Living-related lung transplants are carried out at several centres in the world.[69,70] Left or right lower lobes of the donor relative are transplanted into the whole hemithorax of the recipient, so the technique is only suitable for children or small adults. The same selection criteria apply as for cadaveric transplantation, so CF patients must have bilateral transplants and therefore two related donors. Survival figures are at least comparable with other forms of lung transplantation, and evidence is emerging of better survival in paediatric lung transplants when living-related, rather than cadaveric, organs are used.[67] The technique is in its infancy, and offers theoretical benefits in the availability of organs and attenuated organ rejection, but the ethical issues for donors are substantial.

Outcome following transplant

The actuarial survival of lung transplant recipients is shown in Figure 33.5. Given the nature of the surgery it is not surprising that there is significant perioperative and early postoperative mortality. Thereafter, mortality rates are low when consideration is given to the two-year predicted survival of recipients prior to transplant.

After lung transplantation FEV_1 is initially poor due to the effects of the surgery, but then shows a gradual improvement, reaching a peak 3–6 months after surgery. From pre-transplant values of 20–30% of predicted normal, recipients of a single-lung transplant achieve values of 50–60% and patients receiving bilateral-lung transplant typically have normal values. These improvements in ventilatory performance contribute to the huge improvement in quality of life following lung transplant.

Exercise performance depends on many factors, which, in addition to pulmonary function, include circulation, condition of the voluntary muscles, motivation and freedom from pain on exertion. Improvement in performance does occur following lung transplantation, but exercise limitation remains common, with maximal oxygen uptake (page 262) of about half normal. There is no evidence that this limitation results from poor pulmonary function, and a muscular origin is more likely,[71] possibly related to myopathy induced by immunosuppressant drugs.

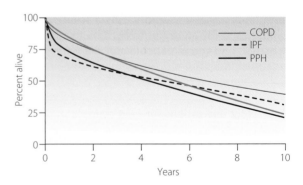

Fig. 33.5 Actuarial survival following lung transplantation for the most common indications. The blue line shows results for all lung transplants; the other lines show results for individual diseases as indicated. Data are from the Registry of the International Society for Heart and Lung Transplantation,[65] and include transplants performed between 1990 and 2006. COPD, chronic obstructive pulmonary disease; IPF, idiopathic pulmonary fibrosis; PPH, primary pulmonary hypertension.

Rejection

Acute rejection occurs following activation of cytotoxic T-lymphocytes by helper T-cells which 'recognise' the foreign tissue. This form of rejection occurs in about 15% of patients and presents as acute lung injury (Chapter 31) within 72 hours of the transplant operation. Treatment involves escalation of immunosuppressive therapy and supportive management as for other forms of lung injury. Recovery of the transplanted lung may occur, but mortality from acute rejection is high.

Chronic rejection in the lung manifests itself as obliterative bronchiolitis syndrome, the origin of which is not clear but which occurs in up to half of patients, normally more than a year after transplantation. Detection of chronic rejection is problematic because in the early stages of acute rejection it is difficult to distinguish rejection from infection on clinical evidence. Both conditions feature arterial hypoxaemia, pyrexia, leukocytosis, dyspnoea and reduced exercise capacity. These changes are followed by a decrease in diffusing capacity and FEV_1, and later by perihilar infiltration or graft opacification on the chest radiograph. Bronchiolitis obliterans, as the name suggests, causes significant air-flow limitation; the FEV_1 is used as a screening test and also to stage the degree of rejection.

Except in the case of identical twins, survival of the transplanted lung depends on immunosuppression.[72] Current therapy involves immunosuppression by three groups of drugs:

1. Steroids to suppress the transcription of numerous pro-inflammatory cytokines.
2. Calcineurin inhibitors, such as cyclosporin-A or tacrolimus, which also reduce cytokine production.
3. Cell-cycle inhibitors, such as azathioprine or mycophenolate mofetil, which suppress cellular production of purines and inhibit lymphocyte subset proliferation.

PHYSIOLOGICAL EFFECTS OF LUNG TRANSPLANT

Transplantation inevitably disrupts the nerve supply, lymphatics and the bronchial circulation. The condition of the recipient is further compromised by immunosuppressive therapy.

The denervated lung. The transplanted lung has no afferent or efferent innervation and there is, as yet, no evidence that re-innervation occurs in patients.[73] However, in dogs, vagal stimulation has been observed to cause bronchoconstriction 3–6 months after lung reimplantation,[74] and sympathetic re-innervation has been demonstrated after 45 months.[75]

In Chapter 5, attention was paid to the weakness of the Hering–Breuer reflex in humans. It was therefore to be expected that denervation of the lung, with block of pulmonary baroreceptor input to the medulla, would have minimal effect on the respiratory rhythm. This is in contrast to the dog and most other laboratory animals, in whom vagal block is known to cause slow deep breathing. Bilateral vagal block in human volunteers was already known to leave the respiratory rhythm virtually unchanged, and it was therefore no great surprise when it was shown that bilateral lung transplant had no significant effect on the respiratory rate and rhythm in patients, after the early postoperative period.[76] Breathing during sleep is also normal.[77]

Bronchial hypersensitivity, i.e. enhanced sensitivity to the bronchoconstrictor effects of inhaled methacholine or histamine can be demonstrated after heart-lung transplantation.[78] This is thought to be due to hypersensitivity of receptors in airway smooth muscle, following denervation of the predominantly constrictor autonomic supply, though not all studies have demonstrated this.[73] In spite of these findings, airway hyper-responsiveness is rarely a problem in transplanted patients.

The cough reflex, in response to afferents arising from below the level of the tracheal or bronchial anastomosis, is permanently lost after lung transplantation.[79] Following single-lung transplant, the remaining diseased lung will continue to stimulate coughing, which will facilitate clearance of secretions from the transplanted lung. Similarly, a bilateral single-lung transplant will be preferable to a double-lung transplant, as the former will maintain intact the potent carinal cough reflex. The abnormality in cough reflex is a major contributor to lung infection following transplant, along with altered mucus clearance as described below.

Ventilation-perfusion ($\dot{V}/\dot{Q}$) relationships. Bilateral lung or heart-lung transplants usually result in normal $\dot{V}/\dot{Q}$ relationships, but following single-lung transplant the situation is more complex. For most indications, including COPD, the single transplanted lung receives the majority of pulmonary ventilation (60–80% of the total) and a similar proportion of pulmonary blood flow, and so $\dot{V}/\dot{Q}$ relationships are acceptable, though not normal.[80,81] However, following single-lung transplant for primary pulmonary hypertension, ventilation to the two lungs remains approximately equal whilst the majority of blood flow (often > 80%) is to the transplanted lung. This $\dot{V}/\dot{Q}$ mismatch fortunately has little effect on arterial oxygenation at rest. During exercise in patients with a single-lung transplant, the already high blood flow to the transplanted lung seems not to increase further, and the normal recruitment of apical pulmonary capillaries (page 103) cannot be demonstrated.[80]

Hypoxic pulmonary vasoconstriction seems to be an entirely local mechanism and, as might be expected, has been shown to persist in the human transplanted lung,[82] though some studies have demonstrated abnormalities, particularly in patients with pulmonary hypertension.[80,81]

Mucociliary clearance. Mucociliary clearance is defective after transplantation.[83] The cause seems to be defective production of mucus, rather than changes in the frequency of cilial beat. This, together with the absent cough reflex below the line of the airway anastomosis, means that the patient is at a disadvantage in clearing secretions. Side effects of immunosuppression compound these changes and lead to enhanced susceptibility to infection of the transplanted lung. Though these factors clearly do not preclude long-term survival of the graft, one-quarter of deaths following lung transplantation result from infection.

References

1. Honeybourne D, Bab J, Bowie P, et al. British Thoracic Society guidelines on diagnostic flexible bronchoscopy. *Thorax.* 2001;56(suppl 1):1–21.

2. Putinati S, Ballerin L, Corbetta L, Trevisani L, Potena A. Patient satisfaction with conscious sedation for bronchoscopy. *Chest.* 1999;115:1437–1440.

3. Matsushima Y, Jones RL, King EG, Moysa G, Alton JD. Alterations in pulmonary mechanics and gas exchange during routine fiberoptic bronchoscopy. *Chest.* 1984;86:184–188.

4. Peacock AJ, Benson-Mitchell R, Godfrey R. Effect of fibreoptic bronchoscopy on pulmonary function. *Thorax.* 1990;45:38–41.

5. Ehrenwerth J, Brull SJ. Anesthesia for thoracic diagnostic procedures. In: Kaplan JA, Slinger PD, eds. *Thoracic Anesthesia.* 3rd ed. Philadelphia: Churchill Livingstone; 2003.

6. Jardine AD, Harrison MJ, Healy TEJ. Automatic flow interruption bronchoscope: A laboratory study. *Br J Anaesth.* 1975;47:385–389.

7. Tassi GF, Davies RJ, Noppen M. Advanced techniques in medical thoracoscopy. *Eur Respir J.* 2006;28:1051–1059.

8. Krasna MJ. Thoracoscopic sympathectomy: a standardized approach to therapy for hyperhidrosis. *Ann Thorac Surg.* 2008;85:S764–S767.

9. Ojimba TA, Cameron AE. Drawbacks of endoscopic thoracic sympathectomy. *Br J Surg.* 2004;91:264–269.

10. Flores RM, Alam N. Video-assisted thoracic surgery (VATS) lobectomy, open thoracotomy, and the robot for lung cancer. *Ann Thorac Surg.* 2008;85:S710–S715.

11. Bolton JWR, Weiman DS. Physiology of lung resection. *Clin Chest Med.* 1993;14:293–303.

12. Lemmer JH, Gomez MN, Symreng T, Ross AF, Rossi NP. Limited lateral thoracotomy. *Arch Surg.* 1990;125:873–877.

13. Peters RM, Wellons HA, Htwe TM, Hill C. Total compliance and work of breathing after thoracotomy. *J Thorac Cardiovasc Surg.* 1969;57:348–355.

14. Hazelrigg SR, Landreneau RJ, Boley TM, et al. The effect of muscle-sparing versus standard posterolateral thoracotomy on pulmonary function, muscle strength, and postoperative pain. *J Thorac Cardiovasc Surg.* 1991;101:394–401.

15. Akçali Y, Demir H, Tezcan B. The effect of standard posterolateral versus muscle-sparing thoracotomy on multiple parameters. *Ann Thorac Surg.* 2003;76:1050–1054.

16. Nomori H, Horio H, Fuyuno G, Kobayashi R, Yashima H. Respiratory muscle strength after lung resection with special reference to age and procedures of thoracotomy. *Eur J Cardiothorac Surg.* 1996;10:352–358.

17. Shaw A, Keefe FJ. Genetic and environmental determinants of post-thoracotomy pain syndrome. *Curr Opin Anaesthesiol.* 2008;21:8–11.

18. Gene L, Colice GL, Shafazand S, Griffin JP, Keenan R, Bolliger CT. Physiologic evaluation of the patient with lung cancer being considered for resectional surgery. ACCP evidenced-based clinical practice guidelines, 2nd ed. *Chest.* 2007;132:161S–177S.

19. van Tilburg PMB, Stam H, Hoogsteden HC, van Klaveren RJ. Pre-operative pulmonary evaluation of lung cancer patients: a review of the literature. *Eur Respir J.* 2009;33:1206–1215.

20. Brunelli A, Al Refai M, Monteverde M, Borri A, Salati M, Fianchini A. Stair climbing test predicts cardiopulmonary complications after lung resection. *Chest*. 2002;121:1106–1110.

*21. Weibel ER. How to make an alveolus. *Eur Respir J*. 2008;31:483–485.

22. Fehrenbach H, Voswinckel R, Michl V, et al. Neoalveolarisation contributes to compensatory lung growth following pneumonectomy in mice. *Eur Respir J*. 2008;31:515–522.

*23. Slinger PD. Postpneumonectomy pulmonary edema. Good news and bad news. *Anesthesiol*. 2006;105:2–5.

24. Slinger PD. Perioperative fluid management for thoracic surgery: the puzzle of postpneumonectomy pulmonary edema. *J Cardiothorac Vasc Anesth*. 1995;9:442–451.

25. Fernández-Pérez ER, Keegan MT, Brown DR, Hubmayr RD, Gajic O. Intraoperative tidal volume as a risk factor for respiratory failure after pneumonectomy. *Anesthesiol*. 2006;105:14–18.

26. Meyers BF, Patterson GA. Chronic obstructive pulmonary disease 10: Bullectomy, lung volume reduction surgery, and transplantation for patients with chronic obstructive pulmonary disease. *Thorax*. 2003;58:634–638.

27. Fishman A, Martinez F, Naunheim K, et al. and the National Emphysema Treatment Trial Research Group. A randomized trial comparing lung-volume-reduction surgery with medical therapy for severe emphysema. *N Engl J Med*. 2003;348:2059–2073.

28. Lenfant C. Will lung volume reduction surgery be widely applied? *Ann Thorac Surg*. 2006;82:385–387.

29. Criner GJ, Belt P, Sternberg AL, et al. Effects of lung volume reduction surgery on gas exchange and breathing pattern during maximum exercise. *Chest*. 2009;135:1268–1279.

30. Miller JD, Malthaner RA, Goldsmith CH, et al. A randomized clinical trial of lung volume reduction surgery versus best medical care for patients with advanced emphysema: a two-year study from Canada. *Ann Thoracic Surg*. 2006;81:314–320.

31. Snyder ML, Goss CH, Neradilek B, et al. and the National Emphysema Treatment Trial Research Group. Changes in arterial oxygenation and self-reported oxygen use after lung volume reduction surgery. *Am J Respir Crit Care Med*. 2008;178:339–345.

32. Gorman RB, McKenzie DK, Butler JE, Tolman JF, Gandevia SC. Diaphragm length and neural drive after lung volume reduction surgery. *Am J Respir Crit Care Med*. 2005;172:1259–1266.

33. Heffner JE, Klein JS. Recent advances in the diagnosis and management of malignant pleural effusions. *Mayo Clin Proc*. 2008;83:235–250.

34. Noppen M. Who's (still) afraid of talc? *Eur Respir J*. 2007;29:619–621.

35. Tschopp JM, Brutsche M, Frey JG. Treatment of complicated spontaneous pneumothorax by simple talc pleurodesis under thoracoscopy and local anaesthesia. *Thorax*. 1997;52:329–332.

36. West JB. Snorkel breathing in the elephant explains the unique anatomy of its pleura. *Respir Physiol*. 2001;126:1–8.

37. Wilson WC, Benumof JL. Anesthesia for thoracic surgery. In: Miller RD, ed. *Miller's Anesthesia*. 6th ed. Philadelphia: Churchill Livingstone; 2005.

38. Karabulut N. CT assessment of tracheal carinal angle and its determinants. *Br J Radiol*. 2005;78:787–790.

39. Triantafillou AN, Benumof JL, Lecamwasam HS. Physiology of the lateral decubitus position, the open chest, and one-lung ventilation. In: Kaplan JA, Slinger PD, eds. *Thoracic anesthesia*. 3rd ed. Philadelphia: Churchill Livingstone; 2003.

40. Szegedi LL. Pathophysiology of one-lung ventilation. *Anesthesiol Clin North America*. 2001;19:435–453.

41. Klingstedt C, Hedenstierna G, Baehrendtz S, et al. Ventilation-perfusion relationships and atelectasis formation in the supine and lateral positions during conventional mechanical and differential ventilation. *Acta Anaesthesiol Scand*. 1990;34:421–429.

42. Watanabe S, Noguchi E, Yamada S, Hamada N, Kano T. Sequential changes of arterial oxygen tension in the supine position during one-lung ventilation. *Anesth Analg*. 2000;90:28–34.

43. Benumof JL. Mechanism of decreased blood flow to atelectatic lung. *J Appl Physiol*. 1979;46:1047–1048.

44. Nagendran J, Stewart K, Hoskinson M, Archer SL. An anesthesiologist's guide to hypoxic pulmonary vasoconstriction: implications for managing single-lung anesthesia and atelectasis. *Curr Opin Anesthesiol*. 2006;19:34–43.

45. Ishibe Y, Shiokawa Y, Umeda T, Uno H, Nakamura M, Izumi T. The effect of thoracic epidural anesthesia on hypoxic pulmonary vasoconstriction in dogs: an analysis of the pressure-flow curve. *Anesth Analg*. 1996;82:1049–1055.

46. Benumof JL, Wahrenbrock EA. Dependency of hypoxic pulmonary vasoconstriction on temperature. *J Appl Physiol*. 1977;42:56–58.

47. Pruszkowski O, Dalibon N, Moutafis M, et al. Effects of propofol vs sevoflurane on arterial oxygenation during one-lung ventilation. *Br J Anaes.* 2007;98:539–544.

48. Özcan PE, Sentürk M, Sungur Ulke Z, et al. Effects of thoracic epidural anaesthesia on pulmonary venous admixture and oxygenation during one-lung ventilation. *Acta Anaesthesiol Scand.* 2007;51:1117–1122.

49. Rocca GD, Passariello M, Coccia C, et al. Inhaled nitric oxide administration during one-lung ventilation in patients undergoing thoracic surgery. *J Cardiothorac Vasc Anesth.* 2001;15:218–223.

50. Dalibon N, Moutafis M, Liu N, Law-Koune J-D, Monsel S, Fischler M. Treatment of hypoxemia during one-lung ventilation using intravenous almitrine. *Anesth Analg.* 2004;98:590–594.

51. Slinger P. Pro: Low tidal volume is indicated during one-lung ventilation. *Anesth Analg.* 2006;103:268–270.

52. Gal T. Con: Low tidal volumes are indicated during one-lung ventilation. *Anesth Analg.* 2006;103:271–273.

53. Michelet P, D'Journo X-B, Roch A, et al. Protective ventilation influences systemic inflammation after esophagectomy. *Anesthesiol.* 2006;105:911–919.

54. Sentürk M, Dilek A, Çamci E, et al. Effects of positive end-expiratory pressure on ventilatory and oxygenation parameters during pressure-controlled one-lung ventilation. *J Cardiothorac Vasc Anesth.* 2005;19:71–75.

55. Tusman G, Böhm SH, Sipmann FS, Maisch S. Lung recruitment improves the efficiency of ventilation and gas exchange during one-lung ventilation anesthesia. *Anesth Analg.* 2004;98:1604–1609.

56. Ko R, McRae K, Darling G, et al. The use of air in the inspired gas mixture during two-lung ventilation delays lung collapse during one-lung ventilation. *Anesth Analg.* 2009;108:1092–1096.

57. Hardy JD, Webb WR, Dalton ML, Walker GR. Lung homotransplantation in man. *JAMA.* 1963;186:1065–1074.

58. Bracken CA, Gurkowski MA, Naples JJ. Lung transplantation: Historical perspectives, current concepts, and anesthetic considerations. *J Cardiothorac Vasc Anesth.* 1997;11:220–241.

59. DeMeo DL, Ginns LC. Lung transplantation at the turn of the century. *Annu Rev Med.* 2001;52:185–201.

60. Snyder LD, Palmer SM. Quality, quantity, or both?: Life after lung transplantation. *Chest.* 2005;128:1086–1087.

61. Pierson RN. Lung transplantation: Current status and challenges. *Transplantation.* 2006;81:1609–1615.

*62. Wilkes DS, Egan TM, Reynolds HY. Lung transplantation: opportunities for research and clinical advancement. *Am J Respir Crit Care Med.* 2005;172:944–955.

63. Corris PA, Christie JD. Update in transplantation 2006. *Am J Respir Crit Care Med.* 2007;175:432–435.

64. Lama VN. Update in lung transplantation 2008. *Am J Respir Crit Care Med.* 2009;179:759–764.

65. Christie JD, Edwards LB, Aurora P, et al. Registry of the International Society for Heart and Lung Transplantation: Twenty-fifth official adult lung and heart/lung transplantation report – 2008. *J Heart Lung Transplant.* 2008;27:957–969.

66. Chang AC, Orens JB. Are there more lungs available than currently meet the eye? *Am J Respir Crit Care Med.* 2006;174:624–625.

67. de Perrot M, Weder W, Patterson GA, Keshavjee S. Strategies to increase limited donor resources. *Eur Respir J.* 2004;23:477–482.

68. Singh H, Bossard RF. Perioperative anaesthetic considerations for patients undergoing lung transplantation. *Can J Anaesth.* 1997;44:284–299.

69. Dark JH. Lung: living related transplantation. *Br Med Bull.* 1997;53:892–903.

70. Starnes VA, Bowdish ME, Woo MS, et al. A decade of living lobar lung transplantation: recipient outcomes. *J Thorac Cardiovasc Surg.* 2004;127:114–122.

*71. Reinsma GD, ten Hacken NHT, Grevink RG, van der Bij W, Koëter GH, van Weert E. Limiting factors of exercise performance 1 year after lung transplantation. *J Heart Lung Transplant.* 2006;25:1310–1316.

72. Knoop C, Haverich A, Fischer S. Immunosuppressive therapy after human lung transplantation. *Eur Respir J.* 2004;23:159–171.

73. Stretton CD, Mak JCW, Belvisi MG, Yacoub MH, Barnes PJ. Cholinergic control of human airways in vitro following extrinsic denervation of the human respiratory tract by heart-lung transplantation. *Am Rev Respir Dis.* 1990;142:1030–1033.

74. Edmunds LH, Graf PD, Nadel JA. Reinnervation of reimplanted canine lung. *J Appl Physiol.* 1971;31:722–727.

75. Lall A, Graf PD, Nadel JA, Edmunds LH. Adrenergic reinnervation of the reimplanted dog lung. *J Appl Physiol.* 1973;35:439–442.

76. Shaw IH, Kirk AJB, Conacher ID. Anaesthesia for patients with transplanted hearts and lungs undergoing non-cardiac surgery. *Br J Anaesth.* 1991;67:772–781.

77. Sanders MH, Costantino JP, Owens GR, et al. Breathing during wakefulness and sleep after human heart-lung transplantation. *Am Rev Respir Dis*. 1989;140:45–51.

78. Glanville AR, Burke CM, Theodore J, et al. Bronchial hyper-responsiveness after human cardiopulmonary transplantation. *Clin Sci*. 1987;73:299–303.

79. Higenbottam T, Jackson M, Woolman P, Lowry R, Wallwork J. The cough response to ultrasonically nebulized distilled water in heart-lung transplantation patients. *Am Rev Respir Dis*. 1989;140:58–61.

80. Ross DJ, Waters PF, Waxman AD, Koerner SK, Mohsenifar Z. Regional distribution of lung perfusion and ventilation at rest and during steady-state exercise after unilateral lung transplantation. *Chest*. 1993;104:130–135.

81. Kuni CC, Ducret RP, Nakhleh RE, Boudreau RJ. Reverse mismatch between perfusion and aerosol ventilation in transplanted lungs. *Clin Nucl Med*. 1993;18:313–317.

82. Robin ED, Theodore J, Burke CM, et al. Hypoxic pulmonary vasoconstriction persists in the human transplanted lung. *Clin Sci*. 1987;72:283–287.

83. Herve P, Silbert D, Cerrina J, Simonneau G, Dartevelle P, and the Paris-Sud Lung Transplant Group. Impairment of bronchial mucociliary clearance in long-term survivors of heart/lung and double-lung transplantation. *Chest*. 1993;103:59–63.

Appendix A

Physical quantities and units of measurement

SI UNITS

A clean transition from the old to the new metric units failed to occur. The old system was based on the centimetre-gram-second (CGS) and was supplemented with many non-coherent derived units such as the millimetre of mercury for pressure and the calorie for work, which could not be related to the basic units by factors which were powers of ten. The new system, the Système Internationale or SI, is based on the metre-kilogram-second (MKS) and comprises base and derived units which are obtained simply by multiplication or division without the introduction of numbers, not even powers of ten.[1]

Base units are metre (length), kilogram (mass), second (time), ampere (electric current), kelvin (thermodynamic temperature), mole (amount of substance) and candela (luminous intensity).

Derived units include newton (force: kilograms metre second^{-2}), pascal (pressure: newton metre^{-2}), joule (work: newton metre) and hertz (periodic frequency: second^{-1}).

Special non-SI units are recognised as having sufficient practical importance to warrant retention for general or specialised use. These include litre, day, hour, minute and the standard atmosphere.

Non-recommended units include the dyne, bar, calorie and gravity-dependent units such as the kilogram-force, centimetre of water and millimetre of mercury, the demise of which has been expected for many years.

The use of SI units in respiratory physiology and clinical practice remains incomplete. The kilopascal has replaced the millimetre of mercury for blood gas partial pressures in Europe but the old units continue to be used in the USA and Australasia. The introduction of the kilopascal for fluid pressures in the medical field has failed to occur for, what appears to be, an entirely specious attachment to the mercury or water manometer. We appear to be condemned to a further period during which we record arterial pressure in mmHg and venous pressure in cmH$_2$O. This absurd situation would be less dangerous if all staff knew the relationship between a millimetre of mercury and a centimetre of water.

As in previous editions of this book, it has proved necessary to make text and figures bilingual, with both SI and CGS units for the benefit of readers who are unfamiliar with one or other of the systems. Some useful conversion factors are listed in Table A.1. There are still some areas of physiology and medicine where non-SI units continue to be extensively used, such as mmHg for most vascular pressures and centimetres of water for airway pressure, so these units are retained throughout this book to aid clarity.

Physical quantities relevant to respiratory physiology are defined below, together with their mass/length/time (MLT) units. These units provide a most useful check of the validity of equations and other expressions which are derived in the course of studies of respiratory function. Only quantities with identical MLT units can be added or subtracted and the units must be the same on both sides of an equation.

VOLUME (DIMENSIONS: L^3)

In this book we are concerned with volumes of blood and gas. Strict SI units would be cubic metres and submultiples. However, the litre (l) and millilitre (ml)

Table A.1 Conversion factors for units of measurement

Force

1 N (newton)	$= 10^5$ dyn

Pressure

1 kPa (kilopascal)	$= 7.50$ mmHg
	$= 10.2$ cmH$_2$O
	$= 0.009\ 87$ standard atmospheres
	$= 10\ 000$ dyn.cm^{-2}
1 standard atmosphere	$= 101.3$ kPa
	$= 760$ mmHg
	$= 1033$ cmH$_2$O
	$= 10$ m of sea water (S.G. 1.033)
1 mmHg	$= 1.36$ cmH$_2$O
	$= 1$ torr (approx)

Compliance

1 l.kPa^{-1}	$= 0.098$ l.cmH$_2$O^{-1}

Flow resistance

1 kPa.l^{-1}.s	$= 10.2$ cmH$_2$O.l^{-1}.sec

Work

1 J (joule)	$= 0.102$ kilopond metres
	$= 0.239$ calories

Power

1 W (watt)	$= 1$ J.s^{-1}
	$= 6.12$ kp.m.min^{-1}

Surface tension

1 N.m^{-1} (Newton/metre or pascal metre)	$= 1000$ dyn.cm^{-1}

In the Figures, Tables and text of this book 1 kPa has been taken to equal 7.5 mmHg or 10 cmH$_2$O.

are recognised as special non-SI units and will remain in use. For practical purposes, we may ignore changes in the volume of liquids which are caused by changes of temperature. However, the changes in volume of gases caused by changes of temperature or pressure are by no means negligible and constitute an important source of error if they are ignored. These are discussed in detail in Appendix C.

FLUID FLOW RATE (DIMENSIONS: L³/T, OR L³.T⁻¹)

In the case of liquids, flow rate is the physical quantity of cardiac output, regional blood flow, etc. The strict SI units would be metre³.second⁻¹, but litres per minute (l.min⁻¹) and millilitres per minute (ml.min⁻¹) are special non-SI units which may be retained. For gases, the dimension is applied to minute volume of respiration, alveolar ventilation, peak expiratory flow rate, oxygen consumption, etc.

The units are the same as those for liquids except that litres per second are used for the high instantaneous flow rates that occur during the course of inspiration and expiration.

In the case of gas flow rates, just as much attention should be paid to the matter of temperature and pressure as when volumes are being measured (Appendix C).

FORCE (DIMENSIONS: MLT⁻²)

Force is defined as mass times acceleration. An understanding of the units of force is essential to an understanding of the units of pressure. Force, when applied to a free body, causes it to change either the magnitude or the direction of its velocity.

The units of force are of two types. The first is the force resulting from the action of gravity on a mass and is synonymous with weight. It includes the kilogram-force and the pound-force (as in the pound per square inch). All such units are non-recommended under the SI and have almost disappeared. The second type of unit of force is absolute and does not depend on the magnitude of the gravitational field. In the CGS system, the absolute unit of force was the dyne and this has been replaced under the MKS system and the SI by the newton (N), which is defined as the force which will give a mass of 1 kilogram an acceleration of 1 metre per second per second.

$$1\text{N} = 1\text{kg.m.s}^{-2}$$

PRESSURE (DIMENSIONS: MLT⁻²/L², OR ML⁻¹T⁻²)

Pressure is defined as force per unit area. The SI unit is the pascal (Pa) which is 1 newton per square metre.

$$1\text{Pa} = 1\text{Nm}^{-2}$$

The pascal is inconveniently small (one hundred-thousandth of an atmosphere) and the kilopascal (kPa) has been adopted for general use in the medical field. Its introduction is simplified by the fact that the kPa is very close to 1% of an atmosphere. Thus a standard atmosphere is 101.3 kPa and the Po_2 of dry air is very close to 21 kPa.

The standard atmosphere may continue to be used under SI. It is defined as $1.013\,25 \times 10^5$ pascals.

The torr came into use only shortly before the move towards SI units. This is unfortunate for the memory of Torricelli, as the torr will disappear from use. The torr is defined as exactly equal to 1/760 of a standard atmosphere and it is therefore very close to the millimetre of mercury, the two units being considered identical for practical purposes. The only distinction is that the torr is absolute, while the millimetre of mercury is gravity based.

The bar is the absolute unit of pressure in the old CGS system and is defined as 10^6 dyn.cm^{-2}. The unit was convenient because the bar is close to 1 atmosphere (1.013 bars) and a millibar is close to 1 centimetre of water (0.9806 millibars).

COMPLIANCE (DIMENSIONS: $M^{-1}L^4T^2$)

The term 'compliance' is used in respiratory physiology to denote the volume change of the lungs in response to a change of pressure. The dimensions are therefore volume divided by pressure, and the commonest units have been litres (or millilitres) per centimetre of water. This continues to slowly change over to litres per kilopascal (l.kPa^{-1}).

RESISTANCE TO FLUID FLOW (DIMENSIONS: $ML^{-4}T^{-1}$)

Under conditions of laminar flow (see Figure 4.2) it is possible to express resistance to gas flow as the ratio of pressure difference to gas flow rate. This is analogous to electrical resistance, which is expressed as the ratio of potential difference to current flow. The dimensions of resistance to gas flow are pressure difference divided by gas flow rate, and typical units in the respiratory field have been cmH$_2$O per litre per second (cmH$_2$O.l^{-1}.s) or dynes. sec.cm^{-5} in absolute units. Appropriate SI units will probably be kPa.l^{-1}.s.

WORK (DIMENSIONS: ML^2T^{-2}, DERIVED FROM $MLT^{-2} \times L$ OR $ML^{-1}T^{-2} \times L^3$)

Work is done when a force moves its point of application or gas is moved in response to a pressure gradient. The dimensions are therefore either force times distance or pressure times volume, in each case simplifying to ML^2T^{-2}. The multiplicity of units of work has caused confusion in the past. Under SI, the erg, calorie and kilopond-metre will disappear in favour of the joule, which is defined as the work done when a force of 1 newton moves its point of application 1 metre. It is also the work done when 1 litre of gas moves in response to a pressure gradient of 1 kilopascal. This represents a welcome simplification.

1 joule = 1 newton metre = 1 litre kilopascal

POWER (DIMENSIONS: ML^2T^{-2}/T OR ML^2T^{-3})

Power is the rate at which work is done and so has the dimensions of work divided by time. The SI unit is the watt, which equals 1 joule per second. Power is the correct dimension for the rate of continuous expenditure of biological energy, although one talks loosely about the 'work of breathing'. This is incorrect and 'power of breathing' is the correct term.

Reference

1. Baron DN. *Units, symbols, and abbreviations. A guide for medical and scientific editors and authors.* 5th edn London: Royal Society of Medicine Press; 1994.

Appendix B

The gas laws

A knowledge of physics is more important to the understanding of the respiratory system than of any other system of the body. Not only gas transfer but also ventilation and perfusion of the lungs occur largely in response to physical forces, with vital processes playing a less conspicuous role than is the case, for example, in brain, heart or kidney.

Certain physical attributes of gases are customarily presented under the general heading of the gas laws. These are of fundamental importance in respiratory physiology.

Boyle's law describes the inverse relationship between the volume and absolute pressure of a perfect gas at constant temperature:

$$PV = K \qquad (1)$$

where P represents pressure and V represents volume. At temperatures near their boiling point, gases deviate from Boyle's law. At room temperature, the deviation is negligible for oxygen and nitrogen and of little practical importance for carbon dioxide or nitrous oxide.

Charles' law describes the direct relationship between the volume and absolute temperature of a perfect gas at constant pressure:

$$V = KT \qquad (2)$$

where T represents the absolute temperature. There are appreciable deviations at temperatures immediately above the boiling point of gases. Equations (1) and (2) may be combined as:

$$PV = RT \qquad (3)$$

where R is the universal gas constant, which is the same for all perfect gases and has the value of 8.1314 joules.degrees kelvin^{-1}.moles^{-1}. From this it may be derived that the mole volume of all perfect gases is 22.4 litres at standard temperature and pressure, dry (STPD). Carbon dioxide and nitrous oxide deviate from the behaviour of perfect gases to the extent of having mole volumes of about 22.2 litres at STPD.

Henry's law describes the solution of gases in liquids with which they do not react. The general principle of Henry's law is simple enough. The number of molecules of gas dissolving in the solvent is directly proportional to the partial pressure of the gas at the surface of the liquid, and the constant of proportionality is an expression of the solubility of the gas in the liquid. This is a constant for a particular gas and a particular liquid at a particular temperature but usually falls with rising temperature.

Unfortunately, confusion often arises from the multiplicity of units that are used. For example, when considering oxygen dissolved in blood, it has been customary to consider the amount of gas dissolved in units of vols% (ml of gas at STPD per 100 ml blood) and the pressure in mmHg. Solubility is then expressed as vols% per mmHg, the value for oxygen in blood at 37°C being about 0.003. However, for carbon dioxide in blood, we tend to use units of mmol.l^{-1} of carbon dioxide per mmHg. The units are then mmol.l^{-1}.mmHg^{-1}, the value for carbon dioxide in blood at 37°C being 0.03. Both vols% and mmol.l^{-1} are valid measurements of the quantity (mass or number of molecules) of the gas in solution and are interchangeable with the appropriate conversion factor.

DOI: 10.1016/B978-0-7020-2996-7.00039-8

Physicists are more inclined to express solubility in terms of the *Bunsen coefficient*. For this, the amount of gas in solution is expressed in terms of volume of gas (STPD) per unit volume of solvent (i.e. one-hundredth of the amount expressed as vols%) and the pressure is expressed in atmospheres.

Biologists, on the other hand, prefer to use the *Ostwald coefficient*. This is the volume of gas dissolved, expressed as its volume under the conditions of temperature and pressure at which solution took place. It might be thought that this would vary with the pressure in the gas phase, but this is not so. If the pressure is doubled, according to Henry's law, twice as many molecules of gas dissolve. However, according to Boyle's law, they would occupy half the volume at double the pressure. Therefore, if Henry's and Boyle's laws are obeyed, the Ostwald coefficient will be independent of changes in pressure at which solution occurs. It will differ from the Bunsen coefficient only because the gas volume is expressed as the volume it would occupy at the temperature of the experiment rather than at 0°C. Conversion is thus in accord with Charles' law and the two coefficients will be identical at 0°C. This should not be confused with the fact that, like the Bunsen coefficient, the Ostwald coefficient falls with rising temperature.

The partition coefficient is the ratio of the number of molecules of gas in one phase to the number of molecules of gas in another phase when equilibrium between the two has been attained. If one phase is gas and the other liquid, the liquid/gas partition coefficient will be identical to the Ostwald coefficient. Partition coefficients are also used to describe partitioning between two media (e.g. oil/water, brain/blood, etc.).

Graham's law of diffusion governs the influence of molecular weight on the diffusion of a gas through a gas mixture. Diffusion rates through orifices or through porous plates are inversely proportional to the square root of the molecular weight. This factor is only of importance in the gaseous part of the pathway between ambient air and the tissues, and is, in general, only of importance when the molecular weight is greater than that of oxygen or carbon dioxide. Graham's law is not relevant to the process of 'diffusion' through the alveolar/capillary membrane (page 147).

Dalton's law of partial pressure states that, in a mixture of gases, each gas exerts the pressure that it would exert if it occupied the volume alone (see Figure 13.8). This pressure is known as the partial pressure (or tension) and the sum of the partial pressures equals the total pressure of the mixture. Thus, in a mixture of 5% carbon dioxide in oxygen at a total pressure of 101 kPa (760 mmHg), the carbon dioxide exerts a partial pressure of $5/100 \times 101 = 5.05$ kPa (38 mmHg). In general terms:

$$P_{CO_2} = F_{CO_2} \times P_B$$

In the alveolar gas at sea level, there is about 6.2% water vapour, which exerts a partial pressure of 6.3 kPa (47 mmHg). The available pressure for other gases is therefore $(P_B - 6.3)$ kPa or $(P_B - 47)$ mmHg. Gas concentrations are usually measured in the dry gas phase and therefore it is necessary to apply this correction for water vapour in the lungs.

Appendix C

Conversion factors for gas volumes

Gas volumes are usually measured at ambient (or environmental) temperature and pressure, either dry (e.g. from a cylinder passing through a rotameter) or saturated with water vapour at ambient temperature (e.g. an expired gas sample). Customary abbreviations are ATPD (ambient temperature and pressure, dry) and ATPS (ambient temperature and pressure, saturated).

CONVERSION OF GAS VOLUME – ATPS TO BTPS

Gas volumes measured by spirometry and other methods usually indicate the volume at ambient temperature and pressure, saturated (ATPS). Tidal volume, minute volume, dead space, lung volumes, and ventilatory gas flow rates, etc. should be converted to the volumes they would occupy in the lungs of the patient at body temperature and pressure, saturated (BTPS).

Conversion from ATPS to BTPS is based on Charles' and Boyle's laws (Appendix B), and conversion factors are listed in Table C.1.

DERIVATION OF CONVERSION FACTORS

$$\text{Volume}_{(BTPS)} = \text{volume}_{(ATPS)} \left(\frac{273 + 37}{273 + t} \right) \left(\frac{P_B - P_{H_2O}}{P_B - 6.3} \right)$$

P_B is barometric pressure (kPa) and Table C.1 has been prepared for a barometric pressure of 100 kPa

Table C.1 Factors for conversion of gas volumes measured under conditions of ambient temperature and pressure, saturated (ATPS) to volumes that would be occupied under conditions of body temperature and pressure, saturated (BTPS)

AMBIENT TEMPERATURE °C	CONVERSION FACTOR	SATURATED WATER VAPOUR PRESSURE	
		kPa	mmHg
15	1.129	1.71	12.8
16	1.124	1.81	13.6
17	1.119	1.93	14.5
18	1.113	2.07	15.5
19	1.108	2.20	16.5
20	1.103	2.33	17.5
21	1.097	2.48	18.6
22	1.092	2.64	19.8
23	1.086	2.80	21.0
24	1.081	2.99	22.4
25	1.075	3.16	23.7
26	1.069	3.66	25.2

(750 mmHg): variations in the range 99–101 kPa (740–760 mmHg) have a negligible effect on the factors.

t is ambient temperature (°C). Table C.1 has been prepared for a body temperature of 37°C: variations in the range 35–39°C are of little importance.

P_{H_2O} is the water vapour pressure of the sample (kPa) at ambient temperature (see Table C.1).

CONVERSION OF GAS VOLUME – ATPS TO STPD

In measurement of absolute amounts of gases such as oxygen uptake, carbon dioxide output and the exchange of 'inert' gases, we need to know the actual quantity (i.e. number of molecules) of gas exchanged and this is most conveniently expressed by stating the gas volume as it would be under standard conditions; i.e. 0°C, 101.3 kPa (760 mmHg) pressure and dry (STPD). Under these conditions, one mole of an ideal gas occupies 22.4 litres.

Conversion from ATPS to STPD is again by application of Charles' and Boyle's laws, as follows:

$$\text{Volume}_{(STPD)} = \text{volume}_{(ATPS)}\left(\frac{273}{273+t}\right)\left(\frac{P_B - P_{H_2O}}{101}\right)$$

P_B is barometric pressure (kPa).

t is ambient temperature (°C).

P_{H_2O} is the saturated water vapour pressure of the sample (kPa) at ambient temperature (see Table C.1).

Appendix D

Symbols and abbreviations

Symbols used in this book are in accord with recommendations for editors of medical and scientific publications in the United Kingdom.[1] There continues to be variation between journals, particularly between Europe and the USA. The use of these symbols is very helpful for an understanding of the quantitative relationships that are so important in respiratory physiology.

Primary symbols (large italic capitals) denoting physical quantities.

F fractional concentration of gas
P pressure, tension or partial pressure of a gas
V volume of a gas
Q volume of blood
C content of a gas in blood
S saturation of haemoglobin with oxygen
R respiratory exchange ratio (RQ)
D diffusing capacity
B binding capacity
  • denotes a time derivative; e.g. $\dot{V}$ ventilation, $\dot{Q}$ blood flow

Secondary symbols denoting location of quantity.

in gas phase (small capitals)	*in blood* (lower case)
ɪ inspired gas	a arterial blood
ᴇ expired gas	v venous blood
ᴀ alveolar gas	c capillary
ᴅ dead space	t total
ᴛ tidal	s shunt
ʙ barometric (usually pressure)	

‾ denotes mixed or mean; e.g. $\bar{v}$ mixed venous blood, $\bar{E}$ mixed expired gas
′ denotes end; e.g. ᴇ′ end-expiratory gas, c′ end-capillary blood

Tertiary symbols indicating particular gases.

O_2 oxygen
CO_2 carbon dioxide
N_2O nitrous oxide
etc
f denotes the respiratory frequency
BTPS, ATPS and STPD – see Appendix C.

Examples of respiratory symbols

$P_{A_{O_2}}$ alveolar oxygen tension
$C\bar{v}_{O_2}$ oxygen content of mixed venous blood
$\dot{V}_{O_2}$ oxygen consumption

Reference

1. Baron DN. *Units, symbols, and abbreviations. A guide for medical and scientific editors and authors.* 5th edn. London: Royal Society of Medicine Press; 1994.

DOI: 10.1016/B978-0-7020-2996-7.00041-6

Appendix E

Mathematical functions relevant to respiratory physiology

This book contains many examples of mathematical statements, which relate respiratory variables under specified conditions. Appendix E is intended to refresh the memory of those readers whose knowledge of mathematics has been attenuated under the relentless pressure of new information acquired in the course of study of the biological sciences.

The most basic study of respiratory physiology requires familiarity with at least four types of mathematical relationship. These are:

a. The linear function.
b. The rectangular hyperbola or inverse function.
c. The parabola or squared function.
d. Exponential functions.

These four types of function will now be considered separately with reference to examples drawn from this book.

THE LINEAR FUNCTION

EXAMPLES

1. Pressure gradient against flow rate with laminar flow (page 40). There is no constant factor and the pressure gradient is zero when flow rate is zero.
2. Respiratory minute volume against P_{CO_2} (page 70). In this case there is a constant factor corresponding to a 'negative' respiratory minute volume when P_{CO_2} is zero.
3. Over a limited range, lung volume is proportional to inflating pressure (page 32). The slope of the line is then the compliance.

Mathematical statement. A linear function describes a change in one variable (dependent or y variable) that is directly proportional to another variable (independent or x variable). There may or may not be a constant factor which is equal to y when x is zero. Thus:

$$y = ax + b$$

where a is the slope of the line and b is the constant factor. In any one particular relationship a and b are assumed to be constant but both may have different values under other circumstances. There are not therefore true constants (like π, for example) and are more precisely termed parameters, whilst y and x are variables.

Graphical representation. Figure E.1 shows a plot of a linear function following the convention that the independent variable (x) is plotted on the abscissa and the dependent variable (y) on the ordinate. Note that the relationship is a straight line and simple regression analysis is based on the assumption that the relationship is of this type. If the slope (a) is positive, the line goes upwards and to the right. If the slope is negative, the line goes upwards and to the left.

THE RECTANGULAR HYPERBOLA OR INVERSE FUNCTION

EXAMPLES

1. The ventilatory response to hypoxia (expressed in terms of P_{O_2}) approximates to a rectangular hyperbola, asymptotic on the horizontal axis

DOI: 10.1016/B978-0-7020-2996-7.00042-8

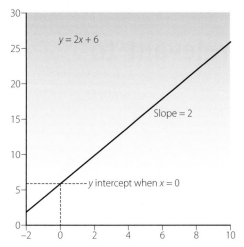

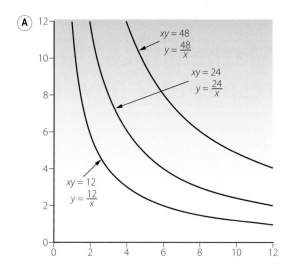

Fig. E.1 A linear function plotted on linear coordinates. Examples include pressure/flow rate relationships with laminar flow (see Figure 4.2) and P_{CO_2}/ventilation response curves (see Figure 5.5).

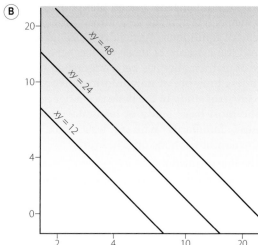

Fig. E.2 Rectangular hyperbolas plotted on (A) linear coordinates and (B) logarithmic coordinates. Examples include the relationships between alveolar gas tensions and alveolar ventilation (see Figures 10.9, 11.2), P_{O_2}/ventilation response curves (see Figure 5.8) and the relationship between airway resistance and lung volume (see Figures 4.5 and 22.13).

to the respiratory minute volume at high P_{O_2} and, on the vertical axis, to the P_{O_2} at which it is assumed ventilation increases towards infinity.

2. The relationships of alveolar gas tensions to alveolar ventilation are conveniently described by rectangular hyperbolas (for carbon dioxide see page 169, and for oxygen see page 181). The curves are concave upwards for gases that are eliminated (e.g. carbon dioxide) and concave downwards for gases that are taken up from the lungs (e.g. oxygen). Curvature is governed by gas output (or uptake) and the asymptotes in each case are zero ventilation and partial pressure of the gas under consideration in the inspired gas. The relationship is extremely helpful for understanding the quantitative relationship between ventilation and alveolar gas tensions.

3. Airway resistance approximates to an inverse function of lung volume (page 48).

Mathematical statement. A rectangular hyperbola describes a relationship when the dependent variable y is inversely proportional to the independent variable x thus:

$$y = a/x + b$$

The asymptote of x is its value when y is infinity and the asymptote of y is its value when x is infinity. If b is zero, then the relationship may be simply represented as follows:

$$xy = a$$

Graphical representation. Figure E.2A shows rectangular hyperbolas with and without constant factors.

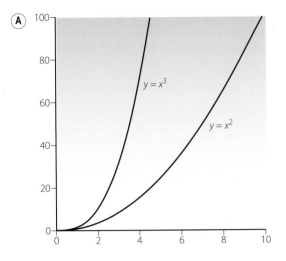

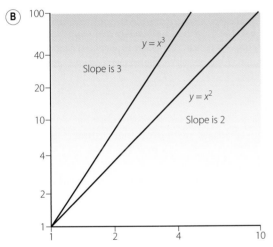

Fig. E.3 Parabolas plotted on (A) linear coordinates and (B) logarithmic coordinates. An example is the pressure/volume relationship with turbulent flow (see Figure 4.3B).

Changes in the value of a alter the curvature but not the asymptotes. Figure E.2B shows the same relationships plotted on logarithmic coordinates. The relationship is now linear but with a negative slope of unity because, if:

$$xy = a$$

then:

$$\log y = -\log x + \log a$$

THE PARABOLA OR SQUARED FUNCTION

EXAMPLE

With fully turbulent gas flow, pressure gradient changes according to the square of gas flow and the plot is a typical parabola (Chapter 4).

Mathematical statement. A parabola is described when the dependent variable (y) changes in proportion to the square of the independent variable (x), thus:

$$y = ax^2$$

Graphical representation. On linear coordinates, a parabola, with positive values of the abscissa, shows a steeply rising curve (Figure E.3A), which may be confused with an exponential function (see below) although it is fundamentally different. On logarithmic coordinates for both abscissa and ordinate, a parabola becomes a straight line with a slope of two (Figure E.3B) because $\log y = \log a + 2 \log x$ (a and $\log a$ are parameters).

EXPONENTIAL FUNCTIONS

GENERAL STATEMENT

An exponential function describes a change in which the rate of change of the dependent variable is proportional to the magnitude of the independent variable at that time. Thus, the rate of change of y with respect to x (i.e. dy/dx)* varies in proportion to the value of y at that instant. That is to say:

$$\frac{dy}{dx} = ky$$

where k is a constant or a parameter.

This general equation appears with minor modifications in three main forms. To the biological worker they may be conveniently described as the tear-away, the wash-out and the wash-in.

---

*dy/dx is the mathematical shorthand for the rate of change of y with respect to x. The 'd' means 'a very small bit of'; therefore dy/dx means a very small bit of y divided by the corresponding very small bit of x. This is equal to the slope of the graph of y against x at that point. In the case of a curve, it is the slope of a tangent drawn to the curve at that point.

THE TEAR-AWAY EXPONENTIAL FUNCTION

This must be described first, as it is the simplest form of the exponential function. It is, however, the least important of the three in relation to respiratory function.

Simple statement. In a tear-away exponential function, the quantity under consideration increases at a rate which is in direct proportion to its actual value – the richer one is, the faster one makes money.

Examples. Classic examples are compound interest, and the mythical water-lily that doubles its diameter every day (Figure E.4). A typical biological example is the free spread of a bacterial colony in which (for example) each bacterium divides every 20 minutes. The doubling time of this example would be 20 minutes.

Mathematical statement. In the case of exponential functions relevant to respiratory function, the independent variable x almost invariably represents time, and so we shall take the liberty of replacing x with t throughout. The tear-away function may thus be represented as follows:

$$\frac{dy}{dt} = ky$$

A little mathematical processing will convert this equation into a more useful form, which will indicate the instantaneous value of y at any time, t.

First multiply both sides by dt/y:

$$\frac{1}{y}dy = kdt$$

Next integrate both sides with respect to t:

$$\log_e y + C_1 = kt + C_2$$

(C_1 and C_2 are constants of integration and may be collected on the right-hand side.)

$$\log_e y = (C_2 - C_1) + kt$$

Finally, take antilogs of each side to the base e:

$$y = e^{(C_2 - C_1)} \times e^{kt}$$

At zero time, $t = 0$ and $e^{kt} = 1$. Therefore the constant $e^{(C_2 - C_1)}$ equals the initial value of y, which we may call y_0. Our final equation is thus:

$$y = y_0 e^{kt}$$

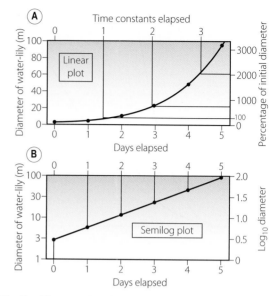

Fig. E.4 The growth of a water-lily that doubles its diameter every day – a typical tear-away exponential function. Initial diameter, 3 metres; size doubled every day (i.e. doubling time = 1 day).

y_0 is the initial value of the variable y at zero time.

e is the base of natural logarithms. This constant (2.71828…) possesses many remarkable mathematical properties.

k is a constant that defines the speed of the particular function. For example, it will differ by a factor of two if our mythical water-lily doubles its size every 12 hours instead of every day. In the case of the wash-out and wash-in, we shall see that k is directly related to certain important physiological quantities, from which we may predict the speed of certain biological changes.

Instead of using e, it is possible to take logs to the more familiar base 10, thus:

$$y = y_0 10^{k_1 t}$$

This is a perfectly valid way of expressing a tear-away exponential function, but you will notice that the constant k has changed to k_1. This new constant does not have the simple relationships of physiological variables mentioned above. It does, however, bear a constant relationship to k, as follows:

$$k_1 = 0.4343k \text{ (approx.)}$$

Graphical representation. On linear graph paper, a tear-away exponential function rapidly disappears

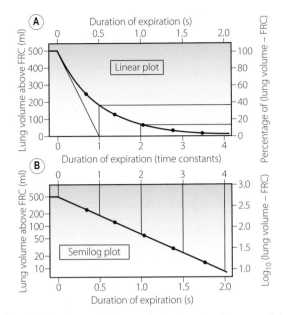

Fig. E.5 Passive expiration – a typical wash-out exponential function. Tidal volume, 500 ml; compliance, 0.5 l.kPa^{-1} (50 ml.cmH$_2$O^{-1}); airway resistance, 1 kPa.l^{-1}.s (10 cmH$_2$O.l^{-1}.s); time constant, 0.5 s; half-life, 0.35 s. The point on the curve indicate the passage of successive half-lives. Note that the logarithmic coordinate has no zero. This accords with the lung volume approaching, but never actually equalling, the FRC.

off the top of the paper (Figure E.4). If plotted on semi-logarithmic paper (time on a linear axis and y on a logarithmic axis), the plot becomes a straight line and this is a most convenient method of presenting such a function. The logarithmic plots in Figures E.4–E.6 are all plotted on semi-log paper.

THE WASH–OUT OR DIE–AWAY EXPONENTIAL FUNCTION

The account of the tear-away exponential function has really been an essential introduction to the wash-out or die-away exponential function, which is of great importance to the biologist in general, and the respiratory physiologist in particular.

Simple statement. In a wash-out exponential function, the quantity under consideration falls at a rate which decreases progressively in proportion to the distance it still has to fall. It approaches but, in theory, never reaches zero.

Examples. Familiar examples are cooling curves, radioactive decay and water running out of the bath. In the last example the rate of flow of bath

water to waste is proportional to the pressure of water, which is proportional to the depth of water in the bath, which in turn is proportional to the quantity of water in the bath (assuming that the sides are vertical). Therefore, the flow rate of water to waste is proportional to the amount of water left in the bath, and decreases as the bath empties. The last molecule of bath water takes an infinitely long time to drain away.

In the field of respiratory physiology, examples include:

1. Passive expiration (Figure E.5).
2. The elimination of inhalational anaesthetics.
3. The fall of arterial $P\text{CO}_2$ to its new level after a step increase in ventilation.
4. The fall of arterial $P\text{O}_2$ to its new level after a step decrease in ventilation.
5. The fall of blood $P\text{CO}_2$ towards the alveolar level as it progresses along the pulmonary capillary.
6. The fall of blood $P\text{O}_2$ towards the tissue level as blood progresses through the tissue capillaries.

Mathematical statement. When a quantity *decreases* with time, the rate of change is *negative*. Therefore, the wash-out exponential function is written thus:

$$\frac{dy}{dt} = -ky$$

from which we may derive the following equations, which give the value of y at any time t:

$$y = y_0 e^{-kt}$$

which is simply another way of saying:

$$y = \frac{y_0}{e^{kt}}$$

y_0 is again the initial value of y at zero time. In Figure E.5, y_0 is the initial value of (lung volume − FRC) at the start of expiration; that is to say, the tidal volume inspired.

e is again the base of natural logarithms (2.718 28…).

k is the constant that defines the rate of decay, and is the reciprocal of a most important quantity known as the *time constant*, represented by the Greek letter tau (τ). Three things should be known about the time constant:

1. Figure E.5 shows a tangent drawn to the first part of the curve. This shows the course events

would take if the initial rate were maintained instead of slowing down in the manner characteristic of the wash-out curve. The time that would then be required for completion would be the time constant (τ) or $1/k$. The wash-out exponential function may thus be written:

$$y = y_0 e^{-t/\tau}$$

2. After 1 time constant, y will have fallen to $1/e$ of its initial value, or approximately 37% of its initial value.
   After 2 time constants, y will have fallen to $1/e^2$ of its initial value, or approximately 13.5% of its initial value.
   After 3 time constants, y will have fallen to $1/e^3$ of its initial value, or approximately 5% of its initial value.
   After 5 time constants, y will have fallen to $1/e^5$ of its initial value, or approximately 1% of its initial value.
3. The time constant is often determined by physiological factors. When air escapes passively from a distended lung, the time constant is governed by two variables, compliance and resistance (see Chapters 3, 4 and 32).

We may now consider the example of passive expiration. Let V represent the lung volume (above FRC), then $-dV/dt$ is the instantaneous expiratory gas flow rate. Assuming Poiseuille's law is obeyed:

$$-\frac{dV}{dt} = \frac{P}{R}$$

when P is the instantaneous alveolar-to-mouth pressure gradient and R is the airway resistance. However, compliance $(C) = V/P$. Therefore:

$$-\frac{dV}{dt} = \frac{1}{CR}V$$

or:

$$\frac{dV}{dt} = -\frac{1}{CR}V$$

Then by integration and taking antilogs as described above:

$$V = V_0 e^{-(t/CR)}$$

By analogy with the general equation of the wash-out exponential function, it is clear that $CR = 1/k = \tau$ (the time constant). Thus the *time constant equals the product of compliance and resistance.*[†] This is analogous to the discharge of an electrical capacitor through a resistance, when the time constant of discharge equals the product of the capacitance and the resistance.

Half-life. It is often convenient to use the half-life instead of the time constant. This is the time required for y to change to half of its previous value. The special attraction of the half-life is its ease of measurement. The half-life of a radioactive element may be determined quite simply. First of all the degree of activity is measured and the time noted. Its activity is then followed and the time noted at which its activity is exactly half the initial value. The difference between the two times is the half-life and is constant at all levels of activity. Half-lives are shown in Figures E.4–E.6 as dots on the curves. For a particular exponential function there is a constant relationship between the time constant and the half-life.

$$\text{Half-life} = 0.69 \times \text{time constant}$$
$$\text{Time constant} = 1.44 \times \text{half-life}$$

Graphical representation. Plotting a wash-out exponential function is similar to the tear-away function (Figure E.5). A semi-log plot is particularly convenient as the curve (being straight) may then be defined by far fewer observations. It is also easy to extrapolate backwards to zero time if the initial value is required but could not be measured directly for some reason. It is, for example, an essential step in the measurement of cardiac output with a dye that is rapidly lost from the circulation (page 115).

THE WASH–IN EXPONENTIAL FUNCTION

The wash-in function is also of special importance to the respiratory physiologist and is the mirror image of the wash-out function.

[†] It is strange at first sight that two quantities as complex as compliance and resistance should have a product as simple as time. In fact, the MLT units (Appendix A) check perfectly well:

$$\text{Compliance} \times \text{resistance} = \text{time}$$
$$M^{-1}L^4T^2 \times ML^{-4}T^{-1} = T$$

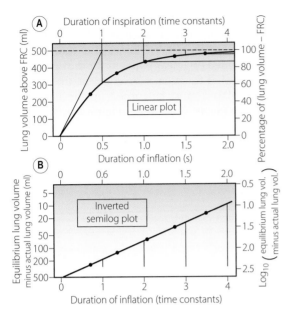

Fig. E.6 Passive inflation of the lungs with a sustained mouth pressure – a typical wash-in exponential function. Final tidal volume, 500 ml; compliance, 0.5 l.kPa^{-1} (50 ml. cmH$_2$O^{-1}); airway resistance, 1 kPa.l^{-1}.s (10 cmH$_2$O.l^{-1}.s); time constant, 0.5 s; half-life, 0.35 s. The points on the curves indicate the passage of successive half-lives. Note that, for the semilog plot, the log scale (ordinate) is from above downwards and indicates the difference between the equilibrium lung volume (inflation pressure maintained indefinitely) and the actual lung volume.

Simple statement. In a wash-in exponential function, the quantity under consideration rises towards a limiting value, at a rate that decreases progressively in proportion to the distance it still has to rise.

Examples. A typical example would be a mountaineer who each day manages to climb half the remaining distance between his overnight camp and the summit of the mountain. His rate of ascent declines exponentially and he will never reach the summit. A graph of his altitude plotted against time would resemble a 'wash-in' curve.

Biological examples include the reverse of those listed for the wash-out function:

1. Inflation of the lungs of a paralysed patient by a sustained increase of mouth pressure (Figure E.6).
2. The uptake of inhalational anaesthetics.
3. The rise of arterial Pco$_2$ to its new level after a step decrease of ventilation.
4. The rise of arterial Po$_2$ to its new level after a step increase of ventilation.

5. The rise of blood Po$_2$ to the alveolar level as it progresses along the pulmonary capillary.
6. The rise of blood Pco$_2$ to the venous level as blood progresses through the tissue capillaries.

Mathematical statement. With a wash-in exponential function, y increases with time and therefore the rate of change is positive. As time advances, the rate of change falls towards zero. The initial value of y is often zero and y approaches a final limiting value that we may designate y_∞ – that is the value of y when time is infinity (∞). A change of this type is indicated thus:

$$\frac{dy}{dt} = k(y_\infty - y)$$

As y approaches y_∞ so the quantity within the parentheses approaches zero, and the rate of change slows down. The corresponding equation that indicates the instantaneous value of y is:

$$y = y_\infty(1 - e^{-kt})$$

y_∞ is the limiting value of y (attained only at infinite time).

e is again the base of natural logarithms.

k is a constant defining the rate of build-up and, as is the case of the wash-out function, it is the reciprocal of the *time constant* the significance of which is described above. It is the time that would be required to reach completion, if the initial rate of change were maintained without slowing down.

After 1 time constant, y will have risen to approximately $100 - 37 = 63\%$ of its final value.

After 2 time constants, y will have risen to approximately $100 - 13.5 = 86.5\%$ of its final value.

After 3 time constants, y will have risen to approximately $100 - 5 = 95\%$ of its final value.

After 5 time constants, y will have risen to approximately $100 - 1 = 99\%$ of its final value.

As in the wash-out function representing passive exhalation, the time constant for the corresponding wash-in exponential function (passive inflation of the lungs) equals the product of compliance and resistance. For the wash-in of a substance into an organ, the time constant equals tissue volume divided by blood flow, or FRC divided by alveolar ventilation as the case may be. As above, the time constant is approximately 1.5 times the half-life.

There are many situations in which the same parameters apply to both wash-in and wash-out functions of the same system. The time constant for each function will then be the same. A classic example is the charging of an electrical capacitor through a resistance, and then allowing it to discharge to earth through the same resistor. The time constant is the same for each process and equals the product of capacitance and resistance. This is approximately true for passive deflation and inflation of the lungs (Figures E.5 and E.6), on the assumption that compliance and airway resistance remain the same.

Graphical representation. The wash-in function may be represented on linear paper as for the other types of exponential function. However, for the semi-log plot, the paper must be turned upside down and the plot made as indicated in Figure E.6. The curve will then be a straight line.

Index